p53 in Breast Cancer

p53 in Breast Cancer: Molecular Mechanisms, Clinical Implications, and Therapeutic Targets comprehensively reviews the role of p53 in breast cancer development, progression, and treatment. It explores the multifaceted functions of p53, from its fundamental connection to breast cancer and pathway mechanisms to its influence on cancer metabolism and the impact of mutational alterations. The initial chapters discuss the complex landscape of p53's involvement in cancer metabolism, the ramifications of its mutations, and its crucial role as a tumor suppressor. The subsequent chapters review the regulatory functions of p53 in cell death, DNA repair, genomic stability, and cell cycle dynamics, highlighting its interactions with transcription factors, DNA repair enzymes, and family members p63 and p73. It further reviews the regulation of mutant p53 via post-translational modifications and delves into the approaches to combat mutated p53, highlighting targeted therapies and efforts to overcome chemoresistance. The chapters also address the role of p53 biomarkers in diagnosis and prognosis, the optimization of treatment responses, and the impact of nutrition on p53 activity. This book is an important resource for oncology and molecular biology researchers.

Key Features

- Provides a thorough examination of the p53 gene and its crucial involvement in breast cancer.
- Explores the critical implications of mutational alterations in p53 on the development and progression of breast cancer.
- Examines the role of p53 in managing apoptosis and contributing to DNA repair and genomic stability.
- Discusses the complex interactions of p53 with transcription factors, DNA repair enzymes, and p63 and p73.
- Highlights the role of p53 as a biomarker in diagnosing and predicting breast cancer prognosis.

p53 in Breast Cancer

Molecular Mechanisms, Clinical Implications, and Therapeutic Targets

Edited by
Manzoor Ahmad Mir

CRC Press
Taylor & Francis Group
Boca Raton London New York

CRC Press is an imprint of the
Taylor & Francis Group, an **informa** business

Designed cover image: Shutterstock

First edition published 2025
by CRC Press
2385 NW Executive Center Drive, Suite 320, Boca Raton FL 33431

and by CRC Press
4 Park Square, Milton Park, Abingdon, Oxon, OX14 4RN

CRC Press is an imprint of Taylor & Francis Group, LLC

ISBN: 9781032859828 (hbk)
ISBN: 9781032859835 pbk)
ISBN: 9781003520771 (ebk)

DOI: 10.1201/ 9781003520771

Typeset in Times
by Deanta Global Publishing Services, Chennai, India

Contents

Introduction

Breast cancer is a major public health concern worldwide, affecting millions of women every year. The field of cancer research has advanced significantly in the last several decades, which has important ramifications for our comprehension and management of different cancers. Given its frequency and impact on millions of lives globally, breast cancer continues to be a major area of emphasis among them. Scientists and physicians are paying close attention to the tumor suppressor protein p53, which has become a key participant in this intricate field of breast cancer research. The goal of this planned book is to thoroughly examine the complex interactions, many functions, and molecular mechanisms that underlie the link between p53 and breast cancer.

Thus, the main aim of the book is to investigate p53's basic roles as a tumor suppressor, which is the first step towards comprehending its role in breast cancer. Twenty carefully chosen chapters make up this extensive book, each providing distinct viewpoints and in-depth studies on different facets of p53 in relation to breast cancer. With chapters covering everything from fundamental science to clinical applications, the book offers researchers, doctors, and students a comprehensive understanding of the subject. The chapters cover important aspects of p53 biology and its significance to the pathophysiology and treatment of breast cancer. They are arranged into discrete topic areas. This book explores the complex relationships between p53 and the advancement of breast cancer, from clarifying the molecular processes underpinning p53's tumor-suppressive capabilities to investigating its interactions with hormone signaling pathways, angiogenesis, and the tumor microenvironment. The book also discusses newly developed p53-targeting therapeutic options, such as gene therapy, immunotherapy, and nutritional therapies, emphasizing the revolutionary potential of these methods to completely alter the breast cancer treatment landscape.

Dr. Manzoor Ahmad Mir

Preface

INTRODUCTION TO THE BOOK

The field of cancer research has made significant strides in the last several decades, greatly enhancing our understanding and management of different cancers. Breast cancer, given its prevalence and impact on millions of lives worldwide, remains a major focus. Scientists and physicians are paying close attention to the tumor suppressor protein p53, which has become a key participant in this intricate field of breast cancer research. The goal of this planned book is to thoroughly examine the complex interactions, many functions, and molecular mechanisms underlying the link between p53 and breast cancer. Our common enthusiasm for expanding knowledge in this important field motivates us as editors and authors, with the ultimate objective of translating bench-to-bedside discoveries to improve patient outcomes. The investigation of p53's basic roles as a tumor suppressor is the first step toward comprehending its role in breast cancer. Often referred to as the "guardian of the genome," p53 is essential for preserving the integrity of cells since it triggers a variety of reactions, including senescence, apoptosis, cell cycle arrest, and DNA repair. Dysregulation of p53 is a major focus of research in cancer biology because it can initiate a series of events that result in unchecked cell proliferation and tumor growth. The importance of p53 in breast cancer is highlighted by the numerous changes including deletions, mutations, and dysregulated expression seen in various disease subtypes. These molecular abnormalities affect the course of the disease, the effectiveness of treatment, and the prognosis of the patient in addition to aiding in the development of tumors. Deciphering the complex biology of p53 in breast cancer thus holds great potential for finding new therapeutic targets and individualized treatment plans.

With chapters spanning fundamental science to clinical applications, the book offers researchers, doctors, and students a comprehensive understanding of the subject. The chapters cover important aspects of p53 biology and its significance to the pathophysiology and treatment of breast cancer. They are arranged into discrete topic areas. This book explores the complex relationships between p53 and the advancement of breast cancer, from clarifying the molecular processes underpinning p53's tumor-suppressive capabilities to investigating its interactions with hormone signaling pathways, angiogenesis, and the tumor microenvironment. The book also explores the clinical ramifications of p53 mutations in breast cancer, including their impact on the prognosis, diagnosis, and treatment outcomes. The chapters provide valuable insights into using p53 for precision medicine approaches in the treatment of breast cancer, from its potential as a predictive biomarker to its role in guiding therapeutic decisions. The book also discusses emerging p53-targeting therapeutic options such as gene therapy, immunotherapy, and nutritional therapies, highlighting the transformative potentials of these strategies to revolutionize the breast cancer treatment landscape.

TARGET AUDIENCE

The book is designed to target broad audiences, including:

- Graduate and postgraduate students of applied medical fields including nursing, oncology, biotechnology, biochemistry, immunology, medical laboratories, biomedical lab technology, and physiotherapy.
- Postgraduate and graduate students pursuing degrees with a focus on cancer biology and medicine.
- Researchers and medical professionals in the field of cancer biology and molecular medicine.

- Health professionals involved in pharmacy, drug design, and oncology.
- Paramedical professionals and students involved in oncology and chemotherapy.
- Pharmaceutical professionals working in oncology and cancer research.

IMPORTANCE OF THE BOOK

- The book is highly significant for its comprehensive coverage of different facets of p53 in relation to breast cancer, each providing distinct viewpoints and in-depth studies. It also explores the clinical implications of p53 mutations in breast cancer, including their impact on prognosis, diagnosis, and therapy outcomes. The chapters offer valuable insights into using p53 for precision medicine approaches in breast cancer treatment, from its potential as a predictive biomarker to its role in guiding therapeutic decisions.
- Additionally, the book discusses emerging p53-targeting therapeutic options, such as gene therapy, immunotherapy, and nutritional therapies, highlighting the transformative potential of these strategies to revolutionize breast cancer treatment.

HIGHLIGHTS OF THE BOOK

1. The book focuses on the complex connection between p53 and breast cancer, offering a focused analysis within the broader field of cancer research.
2. It thoroughly explores p53 biology in breast cancer through 20 well-chosen chapters, covering molecular processes, clinical implications, and treatment strategies.
3. The chapters are organized into discrete sections, allowing for in-depth studies and discussions on a range of topics, including p53 signaling pathways, genetic changes, and therapeutic approaches.
4. The book bridges the gap between fundamental research and clinical practice by highlighting the clinical importance of p53 in breast cancer and discussing its implications for diagnosis, prognosis, and therapeutic decision-making.
5. It highlights the latest developments and potential future directions by delving into cutting-edge research and emerging trends, such as immunotherapy, precision medicine, and innovative treatment methods targeting mutant p53.

FURTHER READING

The following textbooks also give a further understanding of the p53 gene:

- *p53: The Gene that Cracked the Cancer Code* by Sue Armstrong
- *p53 Suppressor Gene* by Tapas Mukhopadhyay, Steven A. Maxwell, and Jack A. Roth
- *Role of p53 in Human Cancers* by Kubra Acikalin Coskun, Merve Tutar, Mervenur Al, Asiye Gok Yurttas, Elif Cansu Abay, Nazlican Yurekli, Bercem Yeman Kiyak, Kezban Ucar Cifci, and Yusuf Tutar
- *The p53 Protein: From Cell Regulation to Cancer* by Guillermina Lozano
- *Mutant p53 and MDM2 in Cancer* by Swati Palit Deb and Sumitra Deb

The following links for video lectures may also be helpful:

https://www.youtube.com/watch?v=2RG9caushI0
https://www.youtube.com/watch?v=Y7KEQQXZxwo
https://www.youtube.com/watch?v=UBDRdPN1OzU
https://www.youtube.com/watch?v=_Isvd01XvSs
https://www.youtube.com/watch?v=-3Di4OgAhmc

For more insight on the topic, we suggest detailed findings from the following links to books by Manzoor Ahmad Mir:

https://doi.org/10.1016/C2021-0-02565-7
https://doi.org/10.1016/C2022-0-00074-X
https://doi.org/10.52305/WXJL6770
https://doi.org/10.1016/C2014-0-02898-5

See also the following links from the cancer.net website:

https://www.cancer.net/cancer-types/breast-cancer/types-treatment
https://discovery.ucl.ac.uk/id/eprint/1472740/
https://www.jmedsciences.com/doi/JMEDS/pdf/10.5005/jp-journals-10045-00138

For diagrammatic illustrations and descriptive tables, see:

http://www.eurekaselect.com/article/49928

Video links on the overall status of cancer, its various types, and current new possible treatment options at:

https://www.sciencedirect.com/science/article/pii/S205970292032278X

Acknowledgments

I would like to take this opportunity to pen down my appreciation for a great number of people whose contributions in numerous ways helped me immensely to move toward my destination. It gives me immense pleasure to express my sense of gratitude and respect to my mentor, Dr. Javed Naim Agrewala, whose constant support, utmost patience, invaluable advice, and guidance rekindled my interest in science from time to time. A special vote of thanks goes to Prof. Neolofar Khan for her efficient guidance to work hard with sincerity, dedication, and devotion both in my professional and personal lives. The staff, scholars (especially Miss Nusrat, Miss Shazia, and Mr. Burhan Ul Haq), and the students in the Department of Bioresources deserve a special mention for all their help rendered in my hour of need. I am also thankful to my soulmate, Miss Sumaira Manzoor, and my parents, Mohammad Abdullah Mir and Zona Begum, and my in-laws, Mohd Ashraf Malik and Posha Begum, for their constant support, love, and care throughout the whole journey. I would like to mention here the affection and love showered by my angels, Ayzel Manzoor and Aariz Manzoor, throughout the writing process of the book. Finally, I would like to thank and acknowledge the Jammu and Kashmir Science Technology and Innovation Council (JKST&IC) for providing financial support vide Project No. JKST&IC/SRE/885-87, dated 27-10-2021, sanctioned to Dr. Manzoor Ahmad Mir (Principal Investigator), and this book is part of the same project titled, "Targeting Drug-Resistant Cancer Stem Cells by Combinational Delivery of Paclitaxel and Quercetin Zerumbone in Breast Cancer."

About the Editor

Manzoor Ahmad Mir is a scientist and head of the Department of Bioresources, University of Kashmir. He holds a master's in zoology with a Gold Medal from HNBG Central University, and a PhD from Jawaharlal Nehru University (New Delhi) and CSIR-Institute of Microbial Technology (Chandigarh) in the field of immunopathology. His research interests are cancer biology with a specialization in drug repurposing, combination therapy of breast cancer and elucidating the molecular mechanism behind it, and the use of natural agents in treating cancer. He is also working on the expression pattern and prognostic significance of chemokines/cytokines of CDKs in breast cancer in addition to virtual screening of drugs for cancer treatment and their mechanistic elucidation. He has published more than 50 high-impact research papers and book chapters, in recognition of which he has received several awards. He has authored more than 16 books with international publishers. He is on the editorial board and a reviewer of prestigious journals and has been an invited speaker at various scientific meetings/conferences within India and abroad. He is a member of many scientific organizations and societies including the American Association of Cancer Research, American Association of Clinical Oncology, and International Immunology Association and a fellow of the Royal British Society. Dr. Mir was awarded the Teachers Associate Research Excellence Fellowship (TARE) by the Department of Science and Technology, Government of India and the Summer Research Fellowship Programme (SRFP-2019) by the Indian Academy of Sciences and National Science Academy. He has developed Massive Open Online Courses (MOOCs) in immunology, human genetics, and endocrinology for undergraduate students sanctioned by the UGC-Consortium for Educational Communication (CEC)–SWAYAM, Ministry of Human Resources Development, Government of India. He has 15 years of research and teaching experience in cancer biology, animal cell and tissue technology, molecular modeling and drug design, and comparative immunology.

Contributors

Inmbisat Altaf
Government College for Women, Srinagar, Jammu and Kashmir, India

Shahnaz Anjum
Department of Botany, School of Bioengineering and Biosciences, Lovely Professional University, Phagwara, Punjab, India

Jahnvi Arora
Biotechnology Engineering, University Institute of Engineering and Technology, Punjab University, Chandigarh, India

Mary Chatterjee
Department of Biotechnology Engineering, University Institute of Engineering & Technology, Punjab University, Chandigarh, India

Adeeba Farooq
Department of Biotechnology, School of Life Sciences, Central University of Kashmir Nunar Campus, Jammu and Kashmir, India

Mehvish Feroz
Department of Bioresources, School of Biological Sciences, University of Kashmir, Srinagar, Jammu and Kashmir, India

Subzar Ah Ganaie
Department of Nanotechnology, University of Kashmir, India

Saima Gul
Department of Bioresources, School of Biological Sciences, University of Kashmir, Srinagar, Jammu and Kashmir, India

Asfer Hamid
Division of Soil Science and Agricultural Chemistry, SKUAST, Jammu, India

Shristi Handa
Biotechnology Branch, University Institute of Engineering and Technology, Punjab University, Chandigarh, India

Kirti Hooda
Centre for Nanoscience and Nanotechnology, Punjab University, Chandigarh, India

Alia Jabar
Department of Bioresources, School of Biological Sciences, University of Kashmir, Srinagar, Jammu and Kashmir, India

Akhil Jamwal
Department of Biotechnology Engineering, UIET, Punjab University, Chandigarh, India

Asma Jan
Department of Bioresources, School of Biological Sciences, University of Kashmir, Srinagar, Jammu and Kashmir, India

Iqra Jan
Department of Bioresources, School of Biological Sciences, University of Kashmir, Srinagar, Jammu and Kashmir, India

Nusrat Jan
Department of Bioresources, School of Biological Sciences, University of Kashmir, Srinagar, Jammu and Kashmir, India

Tabish Javeed
Department of Bioresources, School of Biological Sciences, University of Kashmir, Srinagar, Jammu and Kashmir, India

Arfa Ji
Department of Biotechnology, University of Kashmir, Srinagar, India

Samridhi Kaul
Department of Biotechnology Engineering, University Institute of Engineering & Technology, Punjab University, Chandigarh, India

Gowhar Masoodi
Department of Bioresources, School of Biological Sciences, University of Kashmir, Srinagar, Jammu and Kashmir, India

Manzoor Ahmad Mir
Department of Bioresources, School of Biological Sciences, University of Kashmir, Srinagar, Jammu and Kashmir, India

Ibtisam Mumtaz
Department of Nanotechnology, University of Kashmir, India

Sadaf Qadir
Department of Bioresources, School of Biological Sciences, University of Kashmir, Srinagar, Jammu and Kashmir, India

Aaqib Rashid
Department of Physics, National Institute of Technology, Srinagar, India

Faizan Shakeel
Max Smart Super Specialty Hospital, Saket, New Delhi, India

Shazia Sofi
Department of Bioresources, School of Biological Sciences, University of Kashmir, Srinagar, Jammu and Kashmir, India

Burhan Ul Haq
Department of Bioresources, School of Biological Sciences, University of Kashmir, Srinagar, Jammu and Kashmir, India

Ehtisham-ul Haq
Department of Biotechnology, University of Kashmir, Srinagar, India

Adil Jameel Var
Department of Chemistry, University of Delhi, India

Janifar Yasin
Department of Bioresources, School of Biological Sciences, University of Kashmir, Srinagar, Jammu and Kashmir, India

1 Role of p53 in Cancer Metabolism

Inmbisat Altaf[1], Nusrat Jan[2], Shazia Sofi[2], and Manzoor Ahmad Mir[2]*

[1]Govt. College for Women, Srinagar, J&K
[2]Department of Bioresources, School of Biological Sciences, University of Kashmir, Srinagar, J&K, India
*drmanzoor@kashmiruniversity.ac.in

1.1 INTRODUCTION

p53 is widely regarded as a crucial tumor suppressor due to the prevalence of somatic mutations in TP53 across numerous cancer types and the high risk of early-onset cancers in individuals with germline mutations of TP53, such as those diagnosed with Li–Fraumeni syndrome (LFS). Approximately half of all human tumors exhibit TP53 mutations, while the remaining malignancies with wild-type p53 display functional inactivation of the p53 pathway through alternative mechanisms, including the action of viral oncoproteins or regulators like MDM2 or MDM4. p53 primarily functions as a transcription factor that is activated by various stressors to control the expression of genes involved in proliferation and senescence, DNA repair, and cell death [1, 2]. Research on TP53 has been ongoing since its initial discovery in 1979, and it remains the gene with the strongest correlation to human tumors identified to date. The understanding of p53 has evolved from viewing it as an oncogene to recognizing it as a tumor suppressor gene [3]. TP53, sometimes known as the "guardian of the genome," is essential for reacting to several internal and external stressors, such as hypoxia, food deprivation, oncogene activation, and DNA damage [4–7]. Regretfully, mutations have been found in more than 50% of primary human cancers, indicating that TP53 inactivation is a frequent event in carcinogenesis [8, 9]. The missense type accounts for the majority of these TP53 mutations. These mutant versions contribute to the malignant characteristics of cancer cells by frequently acquiring gain-of-function activity in addition to losing their tumor-suppressive role [10]. With mutations detected in more than 50% of cases, p53, a crucial tumor suppressor, is the gene most commonly altered in human cancers [11]. The emergence and advancement of colorectal cancer have been linked to the accumulation of driver gene alterations. TP53/Trp53 is a significant driver gene implicated in the development of cancer in numerous organs. In humans and mice, it encodes the tumor suppressor p53. Furthermore, it has been demonstrated that certain missense-type mutations in the DNA-binding region of the p53 gene confer carcinogenic properties. Consequently, it is crucial to take into account both the loss of wild-type p53 function and the possible acquisition of oncogenic function by missense mutant p53 when analyzing the significance of p53 mutations in the development of colorectal cancer [12, 13]. The first known tumor suppressor gene was TP53, which was initially reported in 1979 [14–17]. Ten years after its discovery, genetic and functional data revealed that it was a tumor suppressor, contrary to the initial belief that it was an oncogene. Human malignancies frequently exhibit inactivation of TP53 activity or its associated pathway, which is frequently associated with increased malignancy, poor patient survival, and treatment resistance [18–21]. On chromosome 17 (17p13), the TP53 tumor suppressor gene is situated at the short arm. It is composed of 11 exons that span 20 kilobases and codes for a 53 kDa nuclear phosphoprotein. The N-terminus

DOI: 10.1201/9781003520771-1

transactivation domain, the sequence-specific DNA-binding domain, the oligomerization domain, and the C-terminus negative regulatory domain are the four unique functional domains that make up the TP53 protein [22]. Metabolic alterations are a characteristic of tumor cells and have lately been identified as a major contribution to tumor growth [23–25]. Tumor cell proliferation necessitates the use of energy and macromolecule biosynthesis precursors. To meet energy and biosynthetic demands, tumor cells frequently exhibit fundamental metabolic alterations. Interestingly, recent investigations have revealed a novel function of p53 in metabolic control, including glycolysis, the pentose phosphate pathway, mitochondrial oxidative phosphorylation, and lipid metabolism, which contributes to p53's role in tumor suppression

An increasing number of biological processes, such as DNA repair, cell cycle arrest, apoptosis, autophagy, senescence, metabolism, and aging, have been linked to the TP53 gene [19, 26–28]. When the wild-type p53 protein binds to particular DNA response regions, it triggers the production of a large number of genes that ultimately prevent the growth and spread of cancer [29]. Under normal circumstances, the p53 signaling pathway is activated when cells are exposed to various stress signals. This enables the cells to initiate several transcriptional programs, including cell cycle arrest, DNA repair, senescence, and apoptosis, which in turn suppresses the formation of tumors [30]. The majority of human cancers, if not all of them, inactivate the TP53 gene by acquiring loss-of-function mutations or by suppressing the expression of wild-type p53 proteins. Cancer metastasis and progression are aided by the TP53 gene's inactivation, which promotes invasion, proliferation, and cell survival [31]. The actions of p53 in the wild type are lost in more than 75% of TP53 gene mutations. Mutant p53 proteins have the potential to negate the protective role of wild-type p53 [32, 33] or operate as dominant negative over wild-type p53 action [34]. The nuclear p53 phosphoprotein controls normal cell division, and the buildup of mutant p53 that is not functional in tumor cell nuclei is linked to the onset and/or advancement of several neoplastic disorders, including breast cancer [35]. Under extreme oncogenic stress, p53 activation causes senescence and cell cycle arrest, and this is a critical mechanism controlling the suppression of carcinogenesis (Figure 1.1). Key signaling nodes involved in the control of mTOR kinase are frequently the site of convergence of oncogenic stimuli [36, 37].

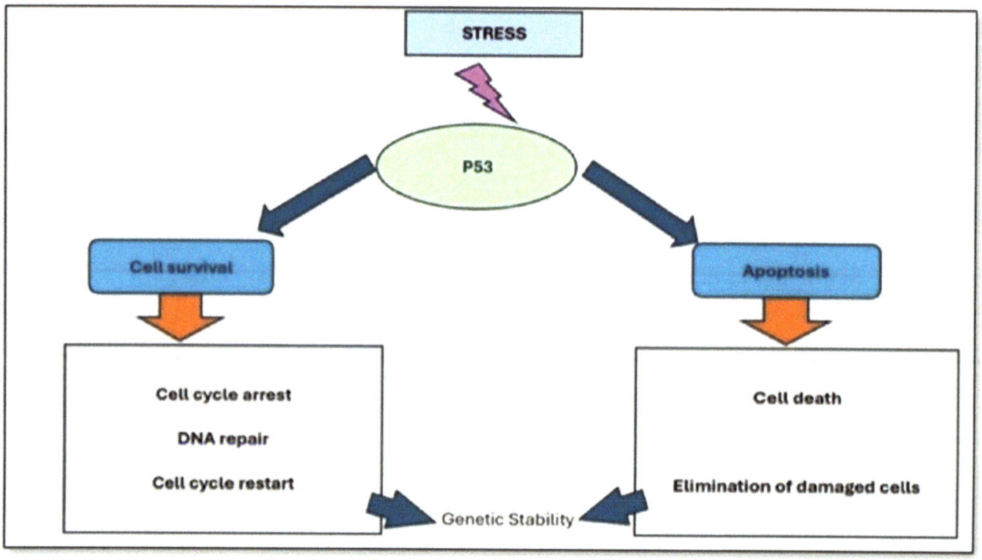

FIGURE 1.1 Stress-induced p53 performs biological activities to preserve genomic integrity.

1.2 p53 AND CELL METABOLISM

It was discovered that cancer cells' metabolism was changed. Cancer cells' metabolic changes affect how they respond to food and oxygen availability, promoting cell proliferation, growth, and survival [38, 39]. Recent research has shown that p53 plays a crucial role in metabolic shifting in malignant cells, implying a new function for p53 in regulating cell metabolism. However, the way p53 regulates metabolism is complex. It is well recognized that glucose availability directly influences cell proliferation, which is mediated by the activation of AMP-activated protein kinase (AMPK) [40, 41]. Metabolic stress activates p53 via AMPK-dependent phosphorylation, which is controlled by mTOR. The mTOR pathway regulates cell proliferation, survival, and energy metabolism.

1.2.1 Role of p53 in Glycolysis

Glycolysis is the metabolic mechanism that transforms glucose into pyruvate and generates ATP and NADH. Glycolysis occurs in practically every species, indicating that it is one of the oldest known metabolic pathways [42]. Recently, it was discovered that p53 regulates glycolysis by controlling the expression of fructose-2,6-bisphosphatase, also known as the TP53-induced glycolysis regulator (TIGAR) [43, 44]. TIGAR inhibits glycolysis by degrading fructose-2,6-bisphosphate (Fru-2,6-P2), a strong allosteric effector of the glycolytic enzyme 6-phosphofructokinase-1 (PFK-1). The expression of TIGAR not only reduces glycolytic activity by dephosphorylating Fru-2,6-P2 to Fru-6-P, but it also switches glucose to an alternate pathway, the pentose phosphate pathway (PPP), while decreasing ROS formation and apoptosis by boosting glutathione production. PPP generates more nicotinamide adenine dinucleotide phosphate (NADPH) [43, 45]. NADPH acts as a reducing agent in anabolic activities including lipid and nucleic acid synthesis. p53 inhibits glycolysis in many ways. GLUT 1–4 facilitates glucose transport across cell plasma membranes, which is the initial rate-limiting step in glucose metabolism. p53 inhibits GLUT1 and GLUT4 expression, reducing glucose absorption in cells [46].

1.2.2 Role of p53 in Pentose Phosphate Pathway

The PPP is an alternative pathway to glycolysis. The PPP has two phases: an oxidative phase that produces NADPH, an important intracellular reductant required for reductive biosynthesis; and a nonoxidative phase that produces ribose-5-phosphate, the precursor for the biosynthesis of nucleotides [47, 48]. Metabolites from glycolysis can be routed into the PPP and utilized to generate NADPH and ribose-5-phosphate [47]. The PPP is frequently activated in malignancies in various ways. Overexpression of PKM2 (pyruvate kinase M2) in many types of tumors has been shown to activate the PPP [49, 50]. PKM2 is the enzyme that converts phosphoenolpyruvate to pyruvate as the final step in glycolysis. PKM2 is active in tetrameric form in differentiated tissues and most normal proliferating cells, but inert in dimeric form in most cancers [49, 50]. Overexpression of the inactive dimeric form of PKM2 in tumor cells slows glycolysis and causes the accumulation of metabolic intermediates, promoting the shuttling of these substrates through the PPP. The G6PD (glucose-6-phosphate dehydrogenase) is the PPP's first and rate-limiting enzyme. It has been observed that p53 binds directly to G6PD and inhibits its function, preventing glycolytic intermediates from being diverted into the PPP [51, 52]. Through negative control of the PPP, p53 can limit the generation of NADPH and ribose-5-phosphate, both of which are required for tumor cell growth and division.

1.2.3 Role of p53 in Fatty Acid Metabolism

Fatty acids are crucial metabolic intermediaries. Fatty acids can be used for lipid synthesis and protein modification, such as palmitoylation, myristoylation, and glycerophosphatidylinositol anchor formation. They can also be destroyed through mitochondrial β-oxidation to provide substrates for oxidative phosphorylation, which generates ATP. p53 regulates fatty acid metabolism via guanidinoacetate methyltransferase (GAMT), which controls the creatine metabolic pathway involved in fatty acid metabolism [40]. GAMT converts guanidinoacetate to creatine, which is connected to energy-generating circuits that regulate ATP homeostasis. Cancer cells have altered energy metabolism, including the fatty acid production route via fatty acid synthase (FAS). FAS, a multifunctional enzyme, converts acetyl-CoA and malonyl-CoA to palmitate through successive processes [42, 53]. Many human malignancies, including breast, prostate, endometrium, and colon carcinomas, exhibit increased FAS expression and aberrant fatty acid synthesis metabolism [43, 44]. GAMT is related to FAS, as creatine therapy increases AMPK and ACC phosphorylation, indicating FAS activation [38]. Metabolic stress activates p53, which promotes β-oxidation of fatty acids [46]. β-oxidation breaks down fatty acids in mitochondria and/or peroxisomes to produce acetyl-CoA, which is the entrance molecule for the Krebs cycle. Research suggests that fatty acid β-oxidation increases in response to glucose restriction, indicating metabolic reprogramming [47, 54]. p53 increases β-oxidation via CPT1 [49]. CPT1, also called carnitine acyltransferase 1, is a mitochondrial enzyme found on the outer membrane. CPT1 initiates fatty acid import by binding to carnitine. Malonyl-CoA can inhibit this enzyme.

1.2.4 Role of p53 in Amino Acid Metabolism

Amino acid metabolism has a significant influence on cancers, and p53 protects cells from metabolic stress and promotes survival. Glutaminolysis converts glutamine to TCA cycle intermediates, allowing cancer cells to proliferate despite glucose shortage [55]. p53 promotes cancer cell proliferation by activating the expression of glutaminase 2 (GLS2), an enzyme responsible for producing energy from glutamine during glucose deprivation. Glutamate reduces both intracellular and extracellular oxidative stress, promoting cell survival [56, 57]. When glucose and glutamine levels are low, aspartate metabolism plays a crucial role in energy production. Under glutamine deficiency, p53 transactivates the aspartate/glutamate transporter solute carrier family 1 member 3 (SLC1A3), according to reports. p53 can increase cellular survival by activating high-affinity amino acid transporters [58]. Serine has a vital role in tumor cell survival and proliferation. p53 stimulates serine synthesis through glutathione (GSH) production, ultimately resulting in cell survival [59, 60]. In summary, p53 increases cellular survival by increasing energy synthesis from amino acids during glucose deprivation.

1.3 REGULATION OF p53

To comprehend molecular coevolution, conservation, adaptation, and the fundamental mechanisms of genetic disorders and cancer, the p53 tumor suppressor and its principal regulator, the MDM2 E3 ubiquitin ligase, offer an invaluable paradigm deprivation [61–65]. The BOX-I motif in the transactivation domain of p53 and its regulator MDM2 have coevolved, according to recent studies, both at the RNA and protein levels. A highly controlled script that has discrete roles in different stress-induced signaling pathways has developed as a result of this coevolution [66]. In response to stress, MDM2 and p53 interact, stabilizing p53, whereas MDM2 functions as a positive regulator [66–68]. There is a complicated connection between autophagy, p53, and cancer. In situations where alternative nutrition sources are scarce, basal autophagy can be stimulated to produce necessary metabolites in addition to acting as an evolutionarily conserved quality control mechanism. Although p53's role in autophagy is mainly understood concerning cancer cells, it also probably plays a role in maintaining normal tissue homeostasis. This involves both transcriptional and non-transcriptional effects. Several genes that encode proteins involved in the autophagy mechanism's core machinery, autophagy regulators, and lysosomal proteins are direct targets of p53 [69–73]. Targeting heat shock protein gp96 may be a tactic to undermine p53's anti-apoptotic properties in hepatoma cells because it can facilitate MDM2's binding to p53 and increase p53's ubiquitination and degradation [74]. Similar in behavior to gp96, the ubiquitin-binding protein SHAPRIN plays a crucial role in encouraging the proliferation of breast cancer cells [75]. One RNA-binding protein that is often altered or deleted in lung cancer is called RNA-binding motif protein 10 (RBM10). RBM10 has been shown

TABLE 1.1
Function, Regulation, and Implications of the p53 Protein

Function/Regulation	Description	Implications
DNA damage response	Activated in response to DNA damage, promotes cell cycle arrest, DNA repair, or apoptosis, to prevent the propagation of damaged DNA and maintain genomic stability. Plays a crucial role in preserving genome integrity and preventing the accumulation of mutations that can lead to cancer development.	Plays a crucial role in preserving genome integrity and preventing the accumulation of mutations that can lead to cancer development.
Tumor suppression	Acts as a tumor suppressor by inhibiting cell proliferation, inducing cell cycle arrest, and promoting apoptosis in response to oncogenic signals or cellular stress.	Loss or mutation of p53 can result in uncontrolled cell growth and increased susceptibility to cancer.
Transcriptional regulation	Binds to specific DNA sequences to activate or repress the expression of target genes involved in cell cycle control, DNA repair, apoptosis, and other cellular processes.	Regulates the expression of genes that are critical for maintaining cellular homeostasis and preventing abnormal cell growth.
Protein stability	Regulated by ubiquitin-mediated proteasomal degradation with Mdm2 playing a crucial role in targeting p53 for degradation.	Dysregulation of p53 degradation can lead to the accumulation of mutant or unstable p53, contributing to cancer development and progression.
Post-translational modifications	Subject to various modifications such as phosphorylation, acetylation, and methylation, which can affect its stability, DNA binding capacity, and transcriptional activity.	Post-translational modifications modulate p53 function and response to cellular signals, influencing its ability to suppress tumor growth and regulate cell fate.

in studies to be able to obstruct MDM2's binding to p53, which in turn inhibits p53 ubiquitination and tumor cell proliferation by inducing apoptosis [76]. p52-ZER6 can increase p53 ubiquitination, improve MDM2 and p53 binding, and accelerate tumor growth [77]. The connection between E3 ligase and p53 can be competitively inhibited by other regulators that can also bind directly to E3 ligase. Mainly found in the liver, heart, and skeletal muscles, β-lactamase-like protein (LACTB) can regulate cell state and lipid metabolism to produce anticancer effects [78]. Intestinal cancer cells' p53 degradation can be inhibited by LACTB's ability to attach directly to the p53 C-terminus, blocking p53's ability to link to MDM2 [79]. Identified to be a negative regulator of SIRT1 and a significant cellular stressor deleted in breast cancer 1 (DBC1), research has demonstrated that DBC1 can directly bind p53 and decrease p53 ubiquitination by competing with MDM2 for p53 binding [80]. Additionally, DBC1 and CREB-binding protein (CBP) can interact to control p53 polyubiquitination that is dependent on CBP, stabilize p53 levels, and encourage p53-dependent tumor cell death [81]. Table 1.1 depicts the function, regulation, and implications of the p53 protein.

1.4 p53 AND CANCER-SPECIFIC METABOLIC ALTERATIONS

Cells are continually subjected to many biological stressors, including DNA damage. Cellular stressors cause genomic aberrations such as mutations, deletions, and translocations, leading to genomic instability (Figure 1.2). Accumulation of genetic abnormalities can lead to cancer [82]. Mutational inactivation is one of the most common molecular pathways behind p53 failure. An

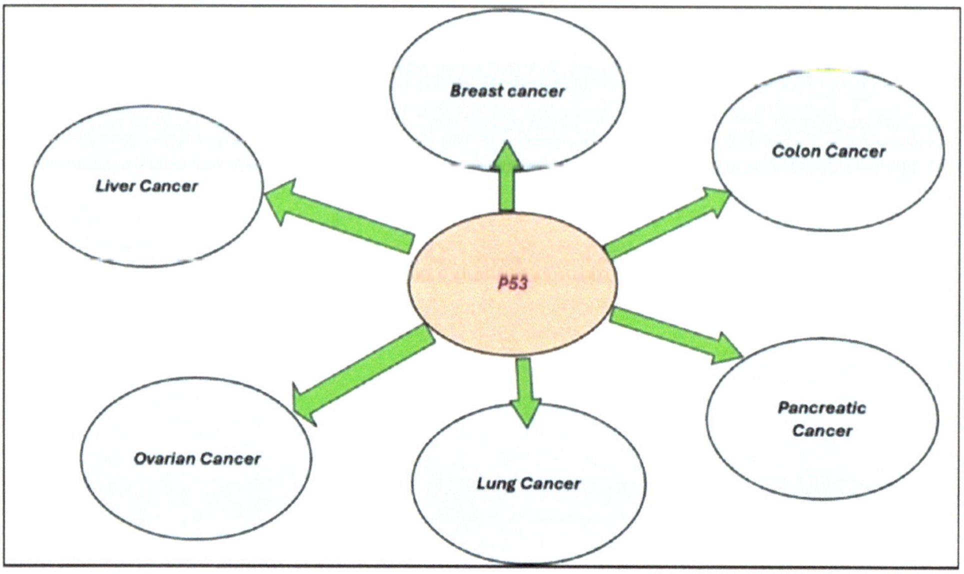

FIGURE 1.2 p53 and different cancer types.

extensive mutation search indicated that p53 loss-of-function mutations are present in more than half of all human malignancies [83]. Among them, 95% of mutations were detectable within the genomic region (exons 5–8) that encodes the DNA-binding domain. A closer look at the mutation profiles indicated that the six most frequently altered amino acid residues in human malignancies are Arg-175, Gly-245, Arg-248, Arg-249, Arg-273, and Arg-282 [84]. These mutations in p53's DNA-binding domain disturb its normal conformation, rendering the mutant p53 deficient in sequence-specific transcriptional activation that is dependent on the wild-type p53-binding consensus element. Furthermore, mutant p53 exhibits dominant-negative behavior toward wild-type p53, forming heterotetramers with wild-type p53, and has carcinogenic potential [85–87].

1.4.1 Mutant p53 in Breast Cancer

The majority of human cancers, including breast cancer, have TP53 mutations, which code for the tumor suppressor protein p53 [88–91]. In general, 30–35% of invasive primary breast tumors have a mutation in the gene. TP53 mutations are found in about 80% of patients with triple-negative (TN) breast cancer, 10% of samples from patients with luminal A disease, 30% of patients with luminal B type, and 70% of patients with the HER2-enriched form of the disease. The frequency of TP53 mutations in breast cancer, however, varies depending on the molecular subtype of the disease [92–97]. The most often altered gene in breast cancer is TP53, as was previously mentioned. Similar to other forms of cancer, missense mutations accounting for 81% of the mutations in breast cancer are located in exons 5–8 [93, 94].

About 10% can be found in exon 4 and 6% in exon 10. Exons 2, 3, 9, and 11 mutations seem to be uncommon (<2% of instances). Only 19% of mutations are modest deletions, and 5% are insertions; 73% of mutations are single-base substitutions [94, 95]. According to the histological and biochemical features of breast cancers, the frequency of mutations varies; it is higher in ductal than lobular, lymph node-positive than lymph node-negative, ER-negative than ER-positive, and HER2-positive than HER2-negative cases. On the other hand, there are several compelling reasons to target mutant p53 in the therapy of breast cancer. First, as was already mentioned, the most often mutated gene in this cancer is p53. Specifically, almost 80% of patients with TN breast cancer have p53 mutations [96]. There is presently no approved targeted therapy for patients with TN breast cancer, in contrast to the circumstances with ER-/PR-positive or HER2-positive patients. Patients with TNBC typically have a bad prognosis because of their inherent aggression and lack of a specific therapy [98]. The fact that over 90% of patients with brain metastases from breast cancer have altered versions of the p53 gene makes it an appealing therapeutic target for the disease [99]. There is presently no effective treatment available for patients who have metastases to this organ. Last, p53 mutations are clonal in at least some breast cancers and should thus be found in every one of the cancer's malignant cells. Breast cancer metabolism is complex and highly dependent on hormone fluctuations [100, 101]. Breast cancer subtypes also have an impact on metabolic rewiring. Mutations in p53 have been linked to abnormal oxidative respiration and glycolysis in breast cancer, which varies depending on the subtype [100, 102]. The majority of hormone-dependent post-menopausal breast tumors (the most common subtype) have wild-type p53. The role of p53 in breast metabolism is complex and influenced by female hormones, as discussed in [103, 104].

1.4.2 Mutant p53 in Colon Cancer

The third most frequent type of cancer and a major global cause of cancer-related mortality is colorectal cancer [105, 106]. For patients with metastases, the five-year survival rate declines dramatically to roughly 14% [107]. To create a unique therapeutic approach, it is crucial to understand the mechanisms underlying the malignant growth process. Benign adenomatous intestinal polyps are the precursor to colorectal cancer, which develops into advanced adenoma with high-grade dysplasia, invasive adenocarcinoma, and spread to other organs. Known as "multistep tumorigenesis," this progressive progression of colorectal cancer is believed to be caused by distinct genetic changes in tumor suppressors or oncogenes at each stage [108–110]. APC, KRAS, SMAD4, and TP53 are among the frequently mutated genes in human colorectal malignancies that have been revealed by recent genome-wide investigations [92, 111]. These mutations are present in roughly 10–80% of non-hypermutated colorectal cancers. The acquisition of stemness, enhanced cell proliferation, suppression of differentiation, and poorer genomic DNA maintenance are believed to result from genetic changes in these genes. These changes may contribute to "hallmarks of cancer" [112] as important elements of the cancer cell signaling pathways [113]. Li–Fraumeni syndrome, a family cancer condition involving a variety of malignancies, is caused by germline mutations in TP53, suggesting that p53 has a tumor suppressor function in a range of tissues [114, 115]. In the Pan-Cancer cohort, TP53 consistently has the highest frequency of mutations (42% of all samples analyzed) [89]. The rate of TP53 mutation in non-hypermutated colorectal cancers is approximately 55–60%, making it the second most common mutation in colorectal cancer (APC mutation is found >80%). In hypermutated colorectal cancers, however, the rate of TP53 mutation is significantly reduced to ~20% [64–66]. Furthermore, a poor prognosis for several cancer types, including colorectal malignancies, has been linked to TP53 mutations [116]. Examining individuals with metastatic advanced colorectal cancer, it was consistently found that 80% of them had TP53 mutations [117]. However, TP53 mutations are uncommon in benign colonic adenomatous polyps [118], and the frequency of their alterations ranges from 15% to 30% [119, 120].

1.4.3 Mutant p53 in Pancreatic Cancer

With a five-year survival rate of only 10%, pancreatic ductal adenocarcinoma (PDAC) is an extremely fatal illness [121]. This bad prognosis is caused by the illness developing to a highly advanced stage without obvious symptoms as well as mostly useless treatments. Gaining further insight into the molecular mechanisms behind PDAC development would help improve the management of this illness. It is essential to comprehend the molecular mechanisms underlying the onset and spread of tumors to create innovative therapeutic approaches and early detection indicators. A model of the pathophysiology of the illness has been developed as a result of the genetic and histological analysis of the development of human PDAC [122, 123]. According to research on human cancer genome sequencing, ~94% of human PDACs have activating mutations in the KRAS oncogene, indicating that PDAC initiation is driven by these mutations [124]. According to early histological studies, pancreatic ductal cells are the source of PDAC. These cells grow into pancreatic intraepithelial neoplasias (PanINs), which are precursor lesions resembling pre-malignant ductal-like lesions. PanINs then progress through progressively more dysplastic stages known as PanIN1A, 1B, 2, and 3, which eventually result in invasive PDACs [125, 126]. Particularly, mutations in SMAD4 and TP53 have been reported in PanIN3 lesions, and mutations in CDKN2A have been found in PanIN2 lesions. These findings suggest that these mutations are critical for the development of higher-grade lesions and eventually PDAC. Notably, loss of heterozygosity (LOH) of TP53 is usually linked to the development from PanIN3 to metastatic PDAC, indicating that p53 acts as a barrier to metastatic disease [127]. This is consistent with research using animal models that demonstrate transformation-related protein 53 (Trp53) inactivation permits malignant progression [128]. Furthermore, TP53 mutations in PanIN3 were mostly deduced using p53 protein immunostaining [129]. However, this method only offers an imprecise evaluation of TP53 status, since positive may indicate the accumulation of mutant p53 or the stability of wild-type p53 in response to a stress signal. Thus, a more thorough examination of these tumor suppressors' functions in PDAC is necessary. Specifically, since p53 is mutated in around 75% of PDACs, comprehending its function will be extremely helpful in understanding the pathogenesis of PDACs. Even though p53 is the most often altered gene in human cancer, the exact processes by which it prevents tumor development are yet unknown. The transcriptional activator p53 is known to inhibit the progression of the cell cycle or trigger apoptosis in response to acute DNA damage. It accomplishes this by transcriptionally activating target genes that contain p53 consensus binding sites, such as those that encode the pro-apoptotic BCL2 family members NOXA and PUMA and the CDK inhibitor p21 [130]. Although this ability was initially thought to explain p53 tumor suppressor activity, research in mouse models has demonstrated that strong p53-mediated activation of these genes is not necessary for tumor suppression and that p53 controls a number of additional cellular responses that may also be involved in tumor suppression [130–136].

1.4.4 Mutant p53 in Lung Cancer

The chance of dying from lung cancer is significantly increased by persistent smoking. The mutagenic effect of tobacco smoke is thought to be the primary cause of lung cancer in humans among all of its other carcinogenic effects [137, 138]. The p53 tumor suppressor gene alterations provided the majority of the evidence in favor of that theory. In physiologically stressed conditions, the "emergency brake" gene p53 exerts its tumor-preventing apoptotic and cell cycle checkpoint functions [26, 139]. Mutations affecting these processes frequently confer a proliferative advantage to p532 mutant cells over p531 wild-type cells. Among the 3,800 possible carcinogens present in tobacco smoke, benzo[a]pyrene diol epoxide (BPDE), a metabolite of benzo[a]pyrene, a polycyclic aromatic hydrocarbon present in cigarette smoke, is the most likely to play a causal mediatory role between smoking, p53 mutations, and lung cancer. At the N2 position of guanines, BPDE attaches itself to DNA and creates large adducts [140]. The mutational characteristic of BPDE is the preponderance of G3T transversions (70%) caused by DNA polymerase misreading the adducts during replication if they are not corrected. G3T transversions are widespread (35%) in human lung cancer but uncommon (10%) in the majority of other malignancies, suggesting a potential association between BPDE and lung cancer [137, 141, 142]. The TP53 gene is located on chromosome 17p13; abnormalities in this gene have been linked to increased cellular resistance to therapy and a poorer prognosis for survival in lung cancers [142–144]. LOH has been frequently detected in lung cancer cell lines and tumor samples, suggesting that this gene is likely involved in the pathogenesis of lung cancer. The specimens with small cell lung cancers have the highest prevalence of TP53 mutations. Conversely, among non-small cell lung cancer tumor samples, TP53 mutation frequency is highest in squamous cell carcinomas and lowest in adenocarcinomas [145, 146]. Somatic mutations and elevated TP53 expression are present in about 23% and 65% of non-small cell lung cancers, respectively. Tumors with and without gene loss at 17p13 are known to harbor TP53 mutations, which are primarily identified in the protein's DNA-binding domain [147]. The acquired TP53 mutations are maintained during tumor growth and metastatic dissemination because coding mutations of TP53 occur relatively early in the development of lung cancer and may be necessary for maintaining the malignant phenotype [148, 149].

1.4.5 Mutant p53 in Ovarian Cancer

Ovarian cancer is the fifth most common female malignancy and the top cause of mortality for gynecologic cancer patients [150]. Unfortunately, there are no effective preventive treatments for this swiftly lethal condition. The five-year survival rate for ovarian cancer is 95% when discovered and treated early. However, 70% of patients are diagnosed late and have a poor prognosis [151]. Patients with advanced disease (stages III and IV) receive excellent surgical debulking followed by chemotherapy. The conventional chemotherapeutic therapy for ovarian cancer patients is taxane and platinum-based regimens. Although the regimen is highly effective, 50% of women will die from the condition [152]. Traditional clinicopathologic criteria do not effectively predict patient prognosis. CA 125 is the only validated marker for ovarian cancer and can be seen in the serum of almost 80% of women with the disease [151]. CA 125 is reliable for monitoring therapy response and illness recurrence, but not as a diagnostic or prognostic marker. Identifying molecular prognostic markers can help guide therapy decisions. Cell cycle regulators are often changed in human cancer, making them of particular relevance. p53, a tumor suppressor gene on 17 p13, encodes a nuclear phosphoprotein that negatively regulates the cell cycle [152]. p53, a tumor suppressor gene, is mutated in 50% of advanced ovarian cancer cases [153]. p53 expression is elevated by oncogene activation, hypoxia, and DNA damage, leading to apoptosis or cell cycle arrest. Normally, p53 is tightly regulated by its interaction with MDM2, a negative regulator. Viral proteins such as HPV E6, simian virus 40 big T antigen, adenovirus E1a, and hepatitis B x antigen can all inhibit p53 action.

1.4.6 Mutant p53 in Liver Cancer

Liver cancer is the sixth most prevalent cancer in males and the ninth most common cancer in women, with the third highest fatality rate among all malignancies worldwide [154, 155]. Approximately 80% of cases occur in Eastern Asia, South-Eastern Asia, Mid-Africa, and West Africa as a result of viral hepatitis [155–157]. Hepatocellular carcinoma (HCC) is primarily caused by viral hepatitis, as well as exposure to extrinsic factors like aflatoxin B1, polyvinyl chloride (PVC), a poor diet, non-alcoholic fatty liver disease (NAFLD), and excess iron exposure. Genetic etiologies for HCC include hereditary hemochromatosis and α1-antitrypsin deficiency [158, 159]. Countries continue to face challenges in avoiding liver cancer, despite efforts such as immunizations for hepatitis B virus (HBV), novel treatments for hepatitis C virus (HCV), controls on PVC manufacture, and restrictions on AFB1 contamination [159, 160]. The molecular processes underlying liver carcinogenesis remain unknown. Mutations in the tumor suppressor p53, which regulates cell cycle progression, apoptosis, DNA repair, senescence, and metabolism, are prevalent in HCC [24, 161]. p53 is the most often altered human gene, accounting for about 50% of all malignancies [10]. In HCC, high amounts of gankyrin, a 26S proteasome regulatory protein, and murine double minute 2 (MDM2), a p53-specific ubiquitin ligase, can reduce p53 protein levels [162, 163]. MicroRNAs (miRNAs) can suppress p53 activity. In HCC, dysregulated miRNA-24 promotes invasion and metastasis by reducing p53 levels [164]. Multiple mechanisms in HCC reduce p53 activity, which contributes to its origin. Table 1.2 depicts the impact of mutant p53 in different types of cancers.

1.5 p53 AND MITOCHONDRIAL FUNCTION

Maintaining metabolic homeostasis requires both the action of tumor suppressor proteins like p53 and mitochondrial control. Controlling mitochondrial size, number, and shape involves fusion, fission, and intracellular transit [144, 165]. Mitochondrial dynamics optimize bioenergetic performance to meet the cell's energy demands [166, 167]. p53 has been shown to alter mitochondrial dynamics [168–170]. The shape of mitochondria is closely related to their functional condition.

TABLE 1.2
Impact of Mutant p53 in Different Cancer Types

Cancer Type	Presence of Mutant p53	Impact of Mutant p53
Breast cancer	Frequently detected	Tumor growth, invasion, and resistance to therapy
Colon cancer	Common occurrence	Increased invasiveness, metastasis, and therapy resistance
Pancreatic cancer	Significant proportion	Tumor initiation, progression, and therapy resistance
Lung cancer	Frequent occurrence	Aggressive tumor behavior, chemotherapy resistance, poor prognosis
Ovarian cancer	Common occurrence	Tumor progression, chemotherapy resistance, poor survival outcomes
Liver cancer (hepatocellular carcinoma)	Frequently observed	Increased proliferation, invasion, metastasis, and therapy resistance

Mitochondrial fission and fusion play a crucial role in maintaining mitochondrial function under various metabolic and environmental stressors. This includes preserving mitochondrial biomass, number, biogenesis, and degradation. Unopposed fission leads to mitochondrial fragmentation, resulting in excess glucose, stress, cell death, and defective oxidative phosphorylation (OXPHOS). Fission plays a crucial role in producing new mitochondria (mitochondrial biogenesis) and removing damaged mitochondria to ensure appropriate mitochondrial activity [166, 167].

Unopposed mitochondrial fusion reduces stress during food withdrawal and improves OXPHOS rates. Defective mitochondria are removed by fusing them with healthy mitochondria in a complementation process. There is evidence that p53 regulates mitochondrial fission and fusion. Mitofusin 2 (mfn2), a membrane-bound component of fusion, is a direct downstream target of p53, which inhibits cellular proliferation and increases cell death [166, 168]. In muscle physiology research, p53 regulates fission and fusion proteins. p53 knockout (KO) mice show abrupt changes in mitochondrial architecture and impaired respiratory capacity [171]. A previous study found that p53 KO mice lose mitochondrial function and biomass, but wild-type p53 mice maintain mitochondrial biogenesis [170] and researchers are now investigating the impact of p53 on mitochondrial dynamics in breast cancer metabolism, as well as its involvement in balancing glycolysis and OXPHOS. Mitochondrial dynamics play a crucial role in shifting metabolic demands and the bioenergetic efficiency of cells.

1.6 p53-BASED CANCER THERAPY

After 30 years of study, the structure and function of p53 have been thoroughly understood. Based on the nearly universal loss of p53 activity in tumors, a great deal of work has been done to create novel cancer treatments. Complex animal models have demonstrated that even in advanced cancers, stimulation of the p53 response can be therapeutic [172]. Gene therapy targeting p53, known as Gendicine, has received approval in China, while Advexin, the US equivalent, has demonstrated efficacy in several clinical trials. Tumor immunologists are presently evaluating several p53-based vaccines in cancer patients due to the tumor-specific modification in p53 processing, which raises the p53 protein level in many tumors due to an increase in the protein's half-life [173]. It was demonstrated in the late 1980s and early 1990s that transfection of the wild-type p53 gene may cause apoptosis and growth suppression in a range of human tumor cells. A curative response is shown in murine model systems when the p53 function is precisely revived within the tumor. This demonstrated that p53 might still limit tumor growth even in more advanced stages. It's interesting to note that p53 activity that produced anticancer activity in lymphoma models was observed to be apoptotic [174], while p53 activity produced a senescent phenotype in a liver tumor model. This was demonstrated in a spectacular trial to subsequently trigger a strong macrophage response that eradicated the tumor [175]. A few of them have undergone testing in cells, and there are varying degrees of evidence indicating that their actions are due to p53 activation. It is believed that three of these drugs (CP-31398, PRIMA-1, and PhiKan083) reactivate mutant p53, whereas RITA may decrease p53's interaction with mdm2. Using the wild-type-specific antibody PAb1620, CP-31398 was chosen from a biochemical screen for compounds supporting the stability of p53's DNA-binding domain (DBD) [176, 177]. Because PRIMA-1 can kill tumor cells that express mutant p53 more efficiently than tumor cells that lack p53, it was chosen from the NCI Diversity Set of chemicals [178]. When PRIMA-1 is injected intravenously or intraperitoneally, it inhibits the growth of human tumor xenografts that are generated from osteosarcoma, lung, and breast cancer [178]. Restoring the wild-type features of p53 mutants, which are frequently overexpressed in cancer, is a feasible therapeutic approach because wild-type p53 is an effective activator of apoptosis and senescence [179] in tumor cells. It is possible that restoring normal p53 expression and function could serve as the basis for a gene therapy approach to treat cancer, as multiple studies have demonstrated that transfection of cancer cells with plasmids expressing wild-type p53 can cause apoptosis and/or growth arrest. Thus far, a number of clinical research studies have been carried out utilizing viral and non-viral vectors that transport p53 genes, either independently or in conjunction with other therapeutic agents [180]. It is possible to reverse some tumor-derived mutations that result in loss of function in wild-type p53 by introducing other point mutations that support p53 protein stability [84]. This suggests that the structural alteration is reversible.

1.7 p53 AND WARBURG EFFECT

Otto Heinrich Warburg proposed the Warburg effect, which links malignant tumor growth to altered energy metabolism. Malignant tumors mostly rely on non-oxidative glycolysis for energy, whereas normal cells primarily rely on the oxidative breakdown of pyruvate, a byproduct of glycolysis, within the mitochondria [184]. The Warburg effect distinguishes between normal and cancerous cells based on their glycolysis to respiration ratio. Recent research suggests that p53 loss in cancer cells increases glycolysis while decreasing OXPHOS. These findings establish a relationship between the p53 protein and energy metabolism, revealing a new mechanism for the Warburg effect and p53's role in tumor suppression through metabolic regulation. Given the significance of p53 in tumor suppression and its high mutation rate (>50%) in human tumors, mutations in the p53 gene and loss of function of the p53 protein may contribute to the Warburg effect (Figure 1.3).

The Warburg effect explains why positron emission tomography imaging was created to detect tumors because tumors absorb more fluorodeoxyglucose, a glucose analog [134], than normal cells. Recent research suggests that the Warburg effect plays a significant role in carcinogenesis and may be the target of tumor therapy [24, 181, 182]. Nevertheless, nothing is known about the mechanism underlying the Warburg effect. The Warburg effect is typified by significantly elevated lactate generation and glucose absorption in tumor cells [24, 183]. The first rate-limiting step in glucose metabolism is the transport of glucose across the PM of cells, which is mediated by glucose transporters (GLUTs), such as GLUT1-4. The primary glucose transporter expressed in muscle and fat tissues that respond to insulin is GLUT4. Insulin significantly increases GLUT4's translocation to the PM, which facilitates muscle and fat cells' absorption of glucose.

A few types of normal cells include pyruvate kinase isoform M2 (PKM2), but cancer cells have significant levels of this isoform. The rate-limiting stage of glycolysis is catalyzed by PKM2, which regulates the production of ATP by converting phosphoenolpyruvate (PEP) to pyruvate. PKM2 counteracts the Warburg effect by preventing glycolysis and ATP synthesis in tumors, despite this seeming contradiction. The contrary is true, even though this effect could initially appear to be harmful to the formation of tumors. PKM2 facilitates the transfer of metabolites via the PPP and other alternative pathways by delaying their passage through glycolysis. This process results in the

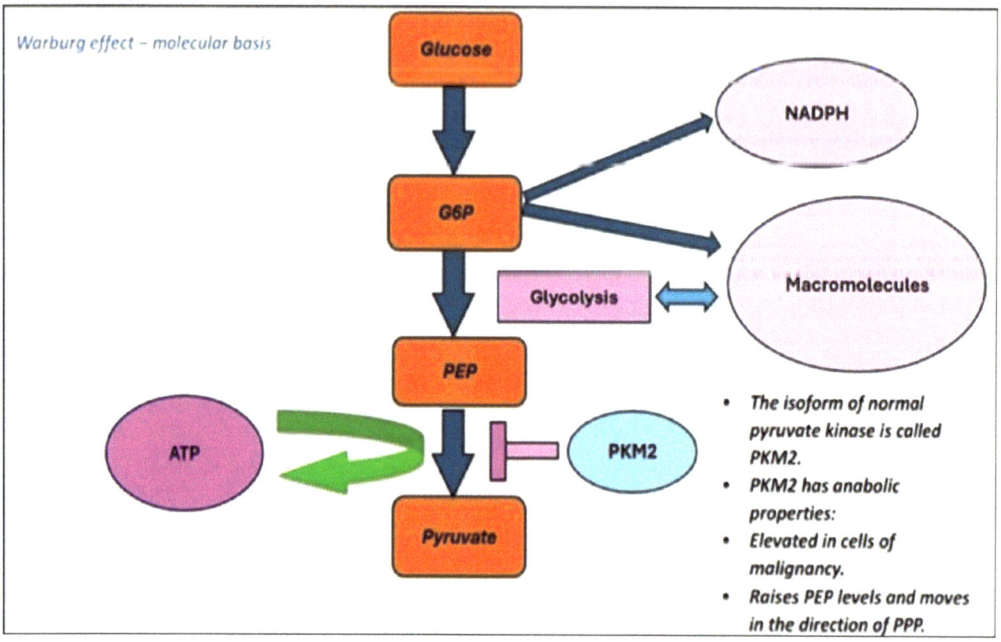

FIGURE 1.3 PKM2 and its impact on the pentose phosphate pathway and glycolysis.

production of significant amounts of reduced NADPH and other macromolecules. These molecules are necessary for the production of macromolecules and for maintaining the redox balance, which is necessary to sustain the fast cell division that takes place inside a tumor.

The basal absorption of glucose by cells and organs is controlled by GLUT1–3 [184]. Of these, GLUT1 is the most broadly expressed in practically all cell types and tissues, and it is in charge of their basal absorption of glucose; in contrast, basal uptake of glucose is controlled by GLUT2 and 3 in certain particular tissues [184]. Tumor cell metabolism has recently attracted renewed attention, notwithstanding Otto Warburg's 1927 discovery that tumors prefer to use glycolysis over oxidative phosphorylation [185]. The Warburg effect [183] refers to the utilization of glycolysis even in the presence of oxygen, which gives the tumor cell less ATP efficiency than oxidative phosphorylation. Nevertheless, the tumor cell also gains from the breakdown of glucose by glycolysis, which supplies substrates for anabolic activities such as the lipid metabolism route, the pentose phosphate pathway, and the citric acid cycle-mediated synthesis of amino acids and nucleotides [186]. Additionally, it may provide a growth advantage in hypoxic environments, enabling tumor cells to endure oxygen-free environments [187]. According to Warburg's concept, the first stage of cancer is this malfunction in cellular respiration and the consequent switch to glycolysis [183]. However, it is still unclear if altered metabolism causes cancer formation or if these changes occur after cancer development, except for a small fraction of malignancies in which mutation of one of the genes encoding the tricarboxylic acid (TCA) cycle enzymes results in tumorigenesis [188].

1.8 CONCLUSION

p53 is a critical regulator of numerous biological functions that is overexpressed in many illnesses. The significance of p53 in carcinogenesis and development has been extensively researched, and an increasing number of studies have discovered that p53 also plays a significant role in infection, metabolism, neurodevelopment, and, most notably, cancer. As a result, biomedical researchers have conducted extensive studies into p53-targeted treatment techniques. Mutations in oncogenes and tumor suppressor genes disrupt various intracellular signaling pathways, affecting tumor cell metabolism and reengineering it to improve survival and growth. Indeed, metabolic changes are likely essential for tumor cells to respond to proliferative signals supplied by oncogenic signaling pathways. The involvement of p53 in cancer metabolism is a fascinating and important topic of oncology study, spanning a wide range of cancers including lung cancer, colon cancer, breast cancer, pancreatic cancer, and liver cancer. The discovery of the complicated link between p53 and the Warburg effect sheds light on the metabolic reprogramming that happens in cancer cells. As the "guardian of the genome," p53 regulates metabolic processes in cancer cells. p53 functions as a tumor suppressor by managing a complex network of metabolic pathways such as glycolysis, oxidative phosphorylation, and fatty acid metabolism, ensuring a careful balance between anabolic and catabolic activities. Dysregulation of the p53 signaling pathway can cause the Warburg effect, which is characterized by increased glycolysis and decreased oxidative phosphorylation, allowing cancer cells to adapt to harsh conditions and accelerate tumor growth.

REFERENCES

1. Kruiswijk, F., C.F. Labuschagne, and K.H. Vousden, p53 in survival, death and metabolic health: a lifeguard with a licence to kill. *Nature Reviews Molecular Cell Biology*, 2015. **16**(7): p. 393–405.
2. Jan, N., et al., Exploring the role of trifarotene against RAR-α: an investigation of expression pattern and clinicopathological significance of RAR-α in breast cancer. *Frontiers in Pharmacology*, 2024. **15**. https://doi.org/10.3389/fphar.2024.1361679
3. Levine, A.J. and M. Oren, The first 30 years of p53: growing ever more complex. *Nature Reviews Cancer*, 2009. **9**(10): p. 749–758.
4. Boutelle, A.M. and L.D. Attardi, p53 and tumor suppression: it takes a network. *Trends in Cell Biology*, 2021. **31**(4): p. 298–310.
5. Wang, Z., A. Strasser, and G.L. Kelly, Should mutant TP53 be targeted for cancer therapy? *Cell Death & Differentiation*, 2022. **29**(5): p. 911–920.
6. Hafner, A., et al., The multiple mechanisms that regulate p53 activity and cell fate. *Nature Reviews Molecular Cell Biology*, 2019. **20**(4): p. 199–210.
7. Jan, N., et al., Targeting breast cancer stem cells through retinoids: a new hope for treatment. *Critical Reviews in Oncology/Hematology*, 2023: p. 104156.
8. Vaddavalli, P.L. and B. Schumacher, The p53 network: cellular and systemic DNA damage responses in cancer and aging. *Trends in Genetics*, 2022. **38**(6): p. 598–612.
9. Jan, N., et al., Metronomic chemotherapy and drug repurposing: a paradigm shift in oncology. *Heliyon*, 2024.
10. Parrales, A. and T. Iwakuma, Targeting oncogenic mutant p53 for cancer therapy. *Frontiers in Oncology*, 2015. **5**: p. 288.
11. Basu, S. and M.E. Murphy, Genetic modifiers of the p53 pathway. *Cold Spring Harbor Perspectives in Medicine*, 2016. **6**(4): p. a026302.
12. Nakayama, M. and M. Oshima, Mutant p53 in colon cancer. *Journal of molecular cell biology*, 2019. **11**(4): p. 267–276.
13. Sofi, S., et al., Elucidation of interleukin-19 as a therapeutic target for breast cancer by computational analysis and experimental validation. *Saudi Journal of Biological Sciences*, 2023. **30**(9): p. 103774–103774.
14. Lane, D.P. and L.V. Crawford, T antigen is bound to a host protein in SY40-transformed cells. *Nature*, 1979. **278**(5701): p. 261–263.
15. Linzer, D.I. and A.J. Levine, Characterization of a 54K dalton cellular SV40 tumor antigen present in SV40-transformed cells and uninfected embryonal carcinoma cells. *Cell*, 1979. **17**(1): p. 43–52.
16. Kress, M., et al., Simian virus 40-transformed cells express new species of proteins precipitable by anti-simian virus 40 tumor serum. *Journal of Virology*, 1979. **31**(2): p. 472–483.
17. Melero, J., et al., Identification of new polypeptide species (48–55K) immunoprecipitable by antiserum to purified large T antigen and present in SV40-infected and-transformed cells. *Virology*, 1979. **93**(2): p. 466–480.
18. Munro, A., S. Lain, and D. Lane, P53 abnormalities and outcomes in colorectal cancer: a systematic review. *British Journal of Cancer*, 2005. **92**(3): p. 434–444.

19. Vogelstein, B., D. Lane, and A.J. Levine, Surfing the p53 network. *Nature*, 2000. **408**(6810): p. 307–310.
20. Vousden, K.H. and X. Lu, Live or let die: the cell's response to p53. *Nature Reviews Cancer*, 2002. **2**(8): p. 594–604.
21. Sofi, S., et al., Clinicopathological and prognostic significance of Bcl2 in breast cancer: a comprehensive in silico and in vitro study. *Saudi Journal of Biological Sciences*, 2023. https://doi.org/10.1016/j.sjbs.2023.103916
22. McKinney, K. and C. Prives, Regulation of p53 DNA binding. *25 Years of p53 Research,* 2005: p. 27–51. https://doi.org/10.1007/1-4020-2922-5_2
23. Cairns, R.A., I.S. Harris, and T.W. Mak, Regulation of cancer cell metabolism. *Nature Reviews Cancer*, 2011. **11**(2): p. 85–95.
24. Vousden, K.H. and K.M. Ryan, p53 and metabolism. *Nature Reviews Cancer*, 2009. **9**(10): p. 691–700.
25. Vander Heiden, M.G., L.C. Cantley, and C.B. Thompson, Understanding the Warburg effect: the metabolic requirements of cell proliferation. *Science*, 2009. **324**(5930): p. 1029–1033.
26. Levine, A.J., p53, the cellular gatekeeper for growth and division. *Cell*, 1997. **88**(3): p. 323–331.
27. Jin, S. and A.J. Levine, The p53 functional circuit. *Journal of Cell Science*, 2001. **114**(23): p. 4139–4140.
28. Riley, T., et al., Transcriptional control of human p53-regulated genes. *Nature Reviews Molecular Cell Biology*, 2008. **9**(5): p. 402–412.
29. Levine, A.J., The many faces of p53: something for everyone. *Journal of Molecular Cell Biology*, 2019. **11**(7): p. 524–530.
30. Vousden, K.H. and C. Prives, Blinded by the light: the growing complexity of p53. *Cell*, 2009. **137**(3): p. 413–431.
31. Muller, P.A. and K.H. Vousden, p53 mutations in cancer. *Nature Cell Biology*, 2013. **15**(1): p. 2–8.
32. Brosh, R. and V. Rotter, When mutants gain new powers: news from the mutant p53 field. *Nature Reviews Cancer*, 2009. **9**(10): p. 701–713.
33. Oren, M. and V. Rotter, Mutant p53 gain-of-function in cancer. *Cold Spring Harbor Perspectives in Biology*, 2010. **2**(2): p. a001107.
34. Petitjean, A., et al., Impact of mutant p53 functional properties on TP53 mutation patterns and tumor phenotype: lessons from recent developments in the IARC TP53 database. *Human Mutation*, 2007. **28**(6): p. 622–629.
35. Allred, D.C., et al., Association of p53 protein expression with tumor cell proliferation rate and clinical outcome in node-negative breast cancer. *JNCI: Journal of the National Cancer Institute*, 1993. **85**(3): p. 200–206.
36. Loayza-Puch, F., et al., p53 induces transcriptional and translational programs to suppress cell proliferation and growth. *Genome Biology*, 2013. **14**: p. 1–12.
37. Sofi, S., et al., A comprehensive analysis of notch signaling genes in breast cancer: expression pattern and prognostic significance. *Advances in Cancer Biology-Metastasis*, 2023. **7**: p. 100104.
38. Gottlieb, E. and K.H. Vousden, p53 regulation of metabolic pathways. *Cold Spring Harbor Perspectives in Biology*, 2010. **2**(4): p. a001040.
39. Mir, M.A., N. Jan, and H. Qayoom, Conventional Chemotherapy vs. Metronomic Chemotherapy, in *Novel Approaches in Metronomic Chemotherapy for Breast Cancer Treatment.* 2024, CRC Press. p. 27–42.
40. Hardie, D.G., The AMP-activated protein kinase pathway–new players upstream and downstream. *Journal of Cell Science*, 2004. **117**(23): p. 5479–5487.
41. Mir, M.A., N. Jan, and S. Sofi, Introduction to Metronomic Chemotherapy, in *Novel Approaches in Metronomic Chemotherapy for Breast Cancer Treatment.* 2024, CRC Press. p. 1–14.
42. Romano, A. and T. Conway, Evolution of carbohydrate metabolic pathways. *Research in Microbiology*, 1996. **147**(6–7): p. 448–455.
43. Bensaad, K., et al., TIGAR, a p53-inducible regulator of glycolysis and apoptosis. *Cell*, 2006. **126**(1): p. 107–120.
44. Matoba, S., et al., p53 regulates mitochondrial respiration. *Science*, 2006. **312**(5780): p. 1650–1653.
45. Mir, M.A., N. Jan, and I. Noor, Therapeutic Implications of Cytokines and Chemokines Network in Cancer, in *Cytokine and Chemokine Networks in Cancer.* 2023, Springer. p. 385–414.
46. Schwartzenberg-Bar-Yoseph, F., M. Armoni, and E. Karnieli, The tumor suppressor p53 down-regulates glucose transporters GLUT1 and GLUT4 gene expression. *Cancer Research*, 2004. **64**(7): p. 2627–2633.
47. Wamelink, M., E. Struys, and C. Jakobs, The biochemistry, metabolism and inherited defects of the pentose phosphate pathway: a review. *Journal of Inherited Metabolic Disease: Official Journal of the Society for the Study of Inborn Errors of Metabolism*, 2008. **31**(6): p. 703–717.

48. Mir, M.A., et al., Metronomics: toward personalized chemotherapy. *Novel Approaches in Metronomic Chemotherapy for Breast Cancer Treatment*, 2024. p. 99–119. https://doi.org/10.1201/9781032632674-8
49. Harris, I., S. McCracken, and T.W. Mak, PKM2: a gatekeeper between growth and survival. *Cell Research*, 2012. **22**(3): p. 447–449.
50. Luo, W. and G.L. Semenza, Emerging roles of PKM2 in cell metabolism and cancer progression. *Trends in Endocrinology & Metabolism*, 2012. **23**(11): p. 560–566.
51. Jiang, P., et al., p53 regulates biosynthesis through direct inactivation of glucose-6-phosphate dehydrogenase. *Nature Cell Biology*, 2011. **13**(3): p. 310–316.
52. Mir, M.A., M. Bashir, and N. Jan, The Role of Interleukin (IL)-6/IL-6 Receptor Axis in Cancer, in *Cytokine and Chemokine Networks in Cancer.* 2023, Springer. p. 137–164.
53. Mir, M.A., A. Shabir, and N. Jan, Metronomic Chemotherapy in Breast Cancer, in *Novel Approaches in Metronomic Chemotherapy for Breast Cancer Treatment.* CRC Press. p. 72–86.
54. Mir, M.A., et al., Imaging Techniques, Biomarkers, and Methods for Metronomic Chemotherapy, in *Novel Approaches in Metronomic Chemotherapy for Breast Cancer Treatment.* CRC Press. p. 58–71.
55. Pavlova, N.N. and C.B. Thompson, The emerging hallmarks of cancer metabolism. *Cell Metabolism*, 2016. **23**(1): p. 27–47.
56. Suzuki, S., et al., Phosphate-activated glutaminase (GLS2), a p53-inducible regulator of glutamine metabolism and reactive oxygen species. *Proceedings of the National Academy of Sciences*, 2010. **107**(16): p. 7461–7466.
57. Mir, M.A., et al., Proteomics: A Groundbreaking Development in Cancer Biology, in *Proteomics.* 2023, Elsevier. p. 31–53.
58. Tajan, M., et al., A role for p53 in the adaptation to glutamine starvation through the expression of SLC1A3. *Cell Metabolism*, 2018. **28**(5): p. 721–736.e6.
59. Maddocks, O.D., et al., Serine starvation induces stress and p53-dependent metabolic remodelling in cancer cells. *Nature*, 2013. **493**(7433): p. 542–546.
60. Mir, M.A., et al., Proteomics: Application of Next-Generation Proteomics in Cancer Research, in *Proteomics.* 2023, Elsevier. p. 55–76.
61. Lane, D.P., et al., Mdm2 and p53 are highly conserved from placozoans to man. *Cell Cycle*, 2010. **9**(3): p. 540–547.
62. Abegglen, L.M., et al., Potential mechanisms for cancer resistance in elephants and comparative cellular response to DNA damage in humans. *Jama*, 2015. **314**(17): p. 1850–1860.
63. Coffill, C.R., et al., The p53–Mdm2 interaction and the E3 ligase activity of Mdm2/Mdm4 are conserved from lampreys to humans. *Genes & Development*, 2016. **30**(3): p. 281–292.
64. Karakostis, K., et al., p53 mRNA and p53 protein structures have evolved independently to interact with MDM2. *Molecular Biology and Evolution*, 2016. **33**(5): p. 1280–1292.
65. Åberg, E., et al., Evolution of the p53-MDM2 pathway. *BMC Evolutionary Biology*, 2017. **17**: p. 1–12.
66. Gajjar, M., et al., The p53 mRNA-Mdm2 interaction controls Mdm2 nuclear trafficking and is required for p53 activation following DNA damage. *Cancer Cell*, 2012. **21**(1): p. 25–35.
67. Candeias, M.M., et al., P53 mRNA controls p53 activity by managing Mdm2 functions. *Nature Cell Biology*, 2008. **10**(9): p. 1098–1105.
68. Medina-Medina, I., et al., Allosteric interactions by p53 mRNA govern HDM2 E3 ubiquitin ligase specificity under different conditions. *Molecular and Cellular Biology*, 2016. **36**(16): p. 2195–2205.
69. Broz, D.K., et al., Global genomic profiling reveals an extensive p53-regulated autophagy program contributing to key p53 responses. *Genes & Development*, 2013. **27**(9): p. 1016–1031.
70. Eby, K.G., et al., ISG20L1 is a p53 family target gene that modulates genotoxic stress-induced autophagy. *Molecular Cancer*, 2010. **9**: p. 1–14.
71. Gao, W., et al., Upregulation of human autophagy-initiation kinase ULK1 by tumor suppressor p53 contributes to DNA-damage-induced cell death. *Cell Death & Differentiation*, 2011. **18**(10): p. 1598–1607.
72. Crighton, D., et al., DRAM, a p53-induced modulator of autophagy, is critical for apoptosis. *Cell*, 2006. **126**(1): p. 121–134.
73. Martoriati, A., et al., dapk1, encoding an activator of a p19ARF-p53-mediated apoptotic checkpoint, is a transcription target of p53. *Oncogene*, 2005. **24**(8): p. 1461–1466.
74. Wu, B., et al., Heat shock protein gp96 decreases p53 stability by regulating Mdm2 E3 ligase activity in liver cancer. *Cancer Letters*, 2015. **359**(2): p. 325–334.
75. Yang, H., et al., SHARPIN facilitates p53 degradation in breast cancer cells. *Neoplasia*, 2017. **19**(2): p. 84–92.
76. Jung, J.H., et al., RNA-binding motif protein 10 induces apoptosis and suppresses proliferation by activating p53. *Oncogene*, 2020. **39**(5): p. 1031–1040.

77. Huang, C., et al., Zinc-finger protein p52-ZER6 accelerates colorectal cancer cell proliferation and tumour progression through promoting p53 ubiquitination. *EBioMedicine*, 2019. **48**: p. 248–263.
78. Keckesova, Z., et al., LACTB is a tumour suppressor that modulates lipid metabolism and cell state. *Nature*, 2017. **543**(7647): p. 681–686.
79. Zeng, K., et al., LACTB, a novel epigenetic silenced tumor suppressor, inhibits colorectal cancer progression by attenuating MDM2-mediated p53 ubiquitination and degradation. *Oncogene*, 2018. **37**(41): p. 5534–5551.
80. Qin, B., et al., DBC1 functions as a tumor suppressor by regulating p53 stability. *Cell Reports*, 2015. **10**(8): p. 1324–1334.
81. Akande, O.E., et al., DBC1 regulates p53 stability via inhibition of CBP-dependent p53 polyubiquitination. *Cell Reports*, 2019. **26**(12): p. 3323–3335. e4.
82. Elledge, S.J., Cell cycle checkpoints: preventing an identity crisis. *Science*, 1996. **274**(5293): p. 1664–1672.
83. Hollstein, M., et al., p53 mutations in human cancers. *Science*, 1991. **253**(5015): p. 49–53.
84. Joerger, A. and A.R. Fersht, Structure–function–rescue: the diverse nature of common p53 cancer mutants. *Oncogene*, 2007. **26**(15): p. 2226–2242.
85. Herskowitz, I., Functional inactivation of genes by dominant negative mutations. *Nature*, 1987. **329**(6136): p. 219–222.
86. Herskowitz, I., A regulatory hierarchy for cell specialization in yeast. *Nature*, 1989. **342**(6251): p. 749–757.
87. Chen, P.-L., et al., Genetic mechanisms of tumor suppression by the human p53 gene. *Science*, 1990. **250**(4987): p. 1576–1580.
88. Lawrence, M.S., et al., Discovery and saturation analysis of cancer genes across 21 tumour types. *Nature*, 2014. **505**(7484): p. 495–501.
89. Kandoth, C., et al., Mutational landscape and significance across 12 major cancer types. *Nature*, 2013. **502**(7471): p. 333–339.
90. Hoadley, K.A., et al., Multiplatform analysis of 12 cancer types reveals molecular classification within and across tissues of origin. *Cell*, 2014. **158**(4): p. 929–944.
91. Yaeger, R., et al., Clinical sequencing defines the genomic landscape of metastatic colorectal cancer. *Cancer Cell*, 2018. **33**(1): p. 125–136. e3.
92. Brigham, et al., Comprehensive molecular portraits of human breast tumours. *Nature*, 2012. **490**(7418): p. 61–70.
93. Shah, S.P., et al., The clonal and mutational evolution spectrum of primary triple-negative breast cancers. *Nature*, 2012. **486**(7403): p. 395–399.
94. Silwal-Pandit, L., et al., TP53 mutation spectrum in breast cancer is subtype specific and has distinct prognostic relevance. *Clinical Cancer Research*, 2014. **20**(13): p. 3569–3580.
95. Nik-Zainal, S., et al., Landscape of somatic mutations in 560 breast cancer whole-genome sequences. *Nature*, 2016. **534**(7605): p. 47–54.
96. Kriegsmann, M., et al., Mutational profiles in triple-negative breast cancer defined by ultradeep multigene sequencing show high rates of PI3K pathway alterations and clinically relevant entity subgroup specific differences. *Oncotarget*, 2014. **5**(20): p. 9952.
97. Haq, B.U., et al., Targeting p53 misfolding conundrum by stabilizing agents and their analogs in breast cancer therapy: a comprehensive computational analysis. *Frontiers in Pharmacology*, 2024. **14**: p. 1333447.
98. Duffy, M.J., P.M. McGowan, and J. Crown, Targeted therapy for triple-negative breast cancer: where are we? *International journal of cancer*, 2012. **131**(11): p. 2471–2477.
99. Lo Nigro, C., et al., High frequency of complex TP53 mutations in CNS metastases from breast cancer. *British Journal of Cancer*, 2012. **106**(2): p. 397–404.
100. Harrelson, J.P. and M.W. Lee, Expanding the view of breast cancer metabolism: promising molecular targets and therapeutic opportunities. *Pharmacology & Therapeutics*, 2016. **167**: p. 60–73.
101. Mir, M.A., Sumaya, N. Jan, Implications of Chemokine Heterogenicity in Cancer Metastasis, in *Cytokine and Chemokine Networks in Cancer*. 2023, Springer. p. 115–136.
102. Ogrodzinski, M.P., J.J. Bernard, and S.Y. Lunt, Deciphering metabolic rewiring in breast cancer subtypes. *Translational Research*, 2017. **189**: p. 105–122.
103. McGowan, E.M., Y. Lin, and D. Hatoum, Good guy or bad guy? The duality of wild-type p53 in hormone-dependent breast cancer origin, treatment, and recurrence. *Cancers*, 2018. **10**(6): p. 172.
104. Mir, M.A., A. Manzoor, and N. Jan, CCL5/CCR5 Axis in Cancer, in *Cytokine and Chemokine Networks in Cancer*. 2023, Springer. p. 219–240.

105. Ferlay, J., et al., Cancer incidence and mortality patterns in Europe: estimates for 40 countries in 2012. *European Journal of Cancer*, 2013. **49**(6): p. 1374–1403.
106. Siegel, R.L., K.D. Miller, and A. Jemal, Cancer statistics, 2018. *CA: A Cancer Journal for Clinicians*, 2018. **68**(1): p. 7–30.
107. Howlader, N., et al., Cancer-specific mortality, cure fraction, and noncancer causes of death among diffuse large B-cell lymphoma patients in the immunochemotherapy era. *Cancer*, 2017. **123**(17): p. 3326–3334.
108. Fearon, E.R. and B. Vogelstein, A genetic model for colorectal tumorigenesis. *Cell*, 1990. **61**(5): p. 759–767.
109. Markowitz, S.D. and M.M. Bertagnolli, Molecular origins of cancer: Molecular basis of colorectal cancer. *The New England Journal of Medicine*, 2009. **361**(25): p. 2449–60.
110. Fearon, K., et al., Definition and classification of cancer cachexia: an international consensus. *The Lancet Oncology*, 2011. **12**(5): p. 489–495.
111. Giannakis, M., et al., Genomic correlates of immune-cell infiltrates in colorectal carcinoma. *Cell Reports*, 2016. **15**(4): p. 857–865.
112. Hanahan, D. and R.A. Weinberg, Hallmarks of cancer: the next generation. *Cell*, 2011. **144**(5): p. 646–674.
113. Vogelstein, B., et al., Cancer genome landscapes. *Science*, 2013. **339**(6127): p. 1546–1558.
114. Malkin, D., et al., Germ line p53 mutations in a familial syndrome of breast cancer, sarcomas, and other neoplasms. *Science*, 1990. **250**(4985): p. 1233–1238.
115. Srivastava, S., et al., Germ-line transmission of a mutated p53 gene in a cancer-prone family with Li–Fraumeni syndrome. *Nature*, 1990. **348**(6303): p. 747–749.
116. Olivier, M., M. Hollstein, and P. Hainaut, TP53 mutations in human cancers: origins, consequences, and clinical use. *Cold Spring Harbor Perspectives in Biology*, 2010. **2**(1): p. a001008.
117. Brannon, A.R., et al., Comparative sequencing analysis reveals high genomic concordance between matched primary and metastatic colorectal cancer lesions. *Genome Biology*, 2014. **15**: p. 1–10.
118. Borras, J.M., et al., How many new cancer patients in Europe will require radiotherapy by 2025? An ESTRO-HERO analysis. *Radiotherapy and Oncology*, 2016. **119**(1): p. 5–11.
119. Baker, A.J. and P.L. Walker, Ecophysiology of metal uptake by tolerant plants. *Heavy Metal Tolerance in Plants: Evolutionary Aspects*, 1990. **2**: p. 155–165.
120. Hao, X., et al., Chemical retardation of phosphate diffusion in an acid soil as affected by liming. *Nutrient Cycling in Agroecosystems*, 2002. **64**: p. 213–224.
121. Park, W., A. Chawla, and E.M. O'Reilly, Pancreatic cancer: a review. *Jama*, 2021. **326**(9): p. 851–862.
122. Hezel, A.F., et al., Genetics and biology of pancreatic ductal adenocarcinoma. *Genes & Development*, 2006. **20**(10): p. 1218–1249.
123. Ying, H., et al., Genetics and biology of pancreatic ductal adenocarcinoma. *Genes & Development*, 2016. **30**(4): p. 355–385.
124. Waters, A.M. and C.J. Der, KRAS: the critical driver and therapeutic target for pancreatic cancer. *Cold Spring Harbor Perspectives in Medicine*, 2018. **8**(9): p. a031435.
125. Bardeesy, N. and R.A. DePinho, Pancreatic cancer biology and genetics. *Nature Reviews Cancer*, 2002. **2**(12): p. 897–909.
126. Hingorani, S.R., et al., Preinvasive and invasive ductal pancreatic cancer and its early detection in the mouse. *Cancer Cell*, 2003. **4**(6): p. 437–450.
127. Lüttges, J., et al., Allelic loss is often the first hit in the biallelic inactivation of the p53 and DPC4 genes during pancreatic carcinogenesis. *The American Journal of Pathology*, 2001. **158**(5): p. 1677–1683.
128. Hingorani, S.R., et al., Trp53R172H and KrasG12D cooperate to promote chromosomal instability and widely metastatic pancreatic ductal adenocarcinoma in mice. *Cancer cell*, 2005. **7**(5): p. 469–483.
129. Maitra, A., et al., Multicomponent analysis of the pancreatic adenocarcinoma progression model using a pancreatic intraepithelial neoplasia tissue microarray. *Modern Pathology*, 2003. **16**(9): p. 902–912.
130. Bieging, K.T., S.S. Mello, and L.D. Attardi, Unravelling mechanisms of p53-mediated tumour suppression. *Nature Reviews Cancer*, 2014. **14**(5): p. 359–370.
131. Brady, C.A., et al., Distinct p53 transcriptional programs dictate acute DNA-damage responses and tumor suppression. *Cell*, 2011. **145**(4): p. 571–583.
132. Mello, S.S., et al., A p53 super-tumor suppressor reveals a tumor suppressive p53-Ptpn14-Yap axis in pancreatic cancer. *Cancer Cell*, 2017. **32**(4): p. 460–473. e6.
133. Valente, L.J., et al., p53 efficiently suppresses tumor development in the complete absence of its cell-cycle inhibitory and proapoptotic effectors p21, Puma, and Noxa. *Cell Reports*, 2013. **3**(5): p. 1339–1345.

134. Li, T., et al., Tumor suppression in the absence of p53-mediated cell-cycle arrest, apoptosis, and senescence. *Cell*, 2012. **149**(6): p. 1269–1283.
135. Valente, L.J., et al., p53 deficiency triggers dysregulation of diverse cellular processes in physiological oxygen. *Journal of Cell Biology*, 2020. **219**(11): p. e201908212.
136. Mir, M.A., M. Rashid, and N. Jan, Cytokines and Chemokines in Tumor Growth and Progression, in *Cytokine and Chemokine Networks in Cancer*. 2023, Springer. p. 33–77.
137. Greenblatt, M.S., A.P. Grollman, and C.C. Harris, Deletions and insertions in the p53 tumor suppressor gene in human cancers: confirmation of the DNA polymerase slippage/misalignment model. *Cancer Research*, 1996. **56**(9): p. 2130–2136.
138. Hernandez-Boussard, T.M. and P. Hainaut, A specific spectrum of p53 mutations in lung cancer from smokers: review of mutations compiled in the IARC p53 database. *Environmental Health Perspectives*, 1998. **106**(7): p. 385–391.
139. Kinzler, K.W. and B. Vogelstein, Life (and death) in a malignant tumour. *Nature*, 1996. **379**(6560): p. 19–20.
140. Friedberg, E.C., et al., DNA repair and mutagenesis. 2005: American Society for Microbiology Press.
141. Ruggeri, B., et al., Benzo[a]pyrene-induced murine skin tumors exhibit frequent and characteristic G to T mutations in the p53 gene. *Proceedings of the National Academy of Sciences*, 1993. **90**(3): p. 1013–1017.
142. Viktorsson, K., L. De Petris, and R. Lewensohn, The role of p53 in treatment responses of lung cancer. *Biochemical and Biophysical Research Communications*, 2005. **331**(3): p. 868–880.
143. Baumann, M., D. Zips, and S. Appold, Radiotherapy of lung cancer: technology meets biology meets multidisciplinarity. *Radiotherapy and Oncology*, 2009. **91**(3): p. 279–281.
144. Steels, E., et al., Role of p53 as a prognostic factor for survival in lung cancer: a systematic review of the literature with a meta-analysis. *European Respiratory Journal*, 2001. **18**(4): p. 705–719.
145. Kishimoto, Y., et al., Aberrations of the p53 tumor suppressor gene in human non-small cell carcinomas of the lung. *Cancer Research*, 1992. **52**(17): p. 4799–4804.
146. Tammemagi, M.C., J.R. McLaughlin, and S.B. Bull, Meta-analyses of p53 tumor suppressor gene alterations and clinicopathological features in resected lung cancers. *Cancer Epidemiology Biomarkers & Prevention*, 1999. **8**(7): p. 625–634.
147. Chiba, I., et al., Mutations in the p53 gene are frequent in primary, resected non-small cell lung cancer. Lung Cancer Study Group. *Oncogene*, 1990. **5**(10): p. 1603–1610.
148. Sozzi, G., et al., Genetic evidence for an independent origin of multiple preneoplastic and neoplastic lung lesions. *Cancer Research*, 1995. **55**(1): p. 135–140.
149. Harris, C.C., COMMENTARY: p 53 Tumor suppressor gene: from the basic research laboratory to the clinic—an abridged historical perspective. *Carcinogenesis*, 1996. https://doi.org/10.1093/carcin/17.6.1187
150. Ahmedin Jemal, D., et al., Cancer statistics. *CA: A Cancer Journal for Clinicians*, 2004. **54**(1): p. 8–29.
151. Niloff, J.M., et al., CA125 antigen levels in obstetric and gynecologic patients. *Obstetrics & Gynecology*, 1984. **64**(5): p. 703–707.
152. Milner, B.J., et al., p53 mutation is a common genetic event in ovarian carcinoma. *Cancer Research*, 1993. **53**(9): p. 2128–2132.
153. Lamb, P. and L. Crawford, Characterization of the human p53 gene. *Molecular and Cellular Biology*, 1986.
154. Bray, F., et al., Global estimates of cancer prevalence for 27 sites in the adult population in 2008. *International Journal of Cancer*, 2013. **132**(5): p. 1133–1145.
155. Ferlay, J., et al., Cancer incidence and mortality worldwide: sources, methods and major patterns in GLOBOCAN 2012. *International Journal of Cancer*, 2015. **136**(5): p. E359–E386.
156. Jemal, A., et al., Global cancer statistics. *CA: A Cancer Journal for Clinicians*, 2011. **61**(2): p. 69–90.
157. Dhanasckaran, R., A. Limaye, and R. Cabrera, Hepatocellular carcinoma: current trends in worldwide epidemiology, risk factors, diagnosis, and therapeutics. *Hepatic Medicine: Evidence and Research*, 2012. **4**: p. 19–37.
158. Chuang, S.-C., C. La Vecchia, and P. Boffetta, Liver cancer: descriptive epidemiology and risk factors other than HBV and HCV infection. *Cancer Letters*, 2009. **286**(1): p. 9–14.
159. Magnussen, A. and M.A. Parsi, Aflatoxins, hepatocellular carcinoma and public health. *World Journal of Gastroenterology: WJG*, 2013. **19**(10): p. 1508.
160. Guyton, K.Z. and T.W. Kensler, Prevention of liver cancer. *Current Oncology Reports*, 2002. **4**: p. 464–470.

161. Lane, D. and A. Levine, p53 Research: the past thirty years and the next thirty years. *Cold Spring Harbor Perspectives in Biology*, 2010. **2**(12): p. a000893.
162. Iakova, P., L. Timchenko, and N.A. Timchenko. Intracellular signaling and hepatocellular carcinoma. in Seminars in cancer biology. 2011. Elsevier.
163. Ranjan, A., K. Bera, and T. Iwakuma, Murine double minute 2, a potential p53-independent regulator of liver cancer metastasis. *Hepatoma Research*, 2016. **2**: p. 114.
164. Chen, L., et al., MicroRNA-24 increases hepatocellular carcinoma cell metastasis and invasion by targeting p53: miR-24 targeted p53. *Biomedicine & Pharmacotherapy*, 2016. **84**: p. 1113–1118.
165. Westermann, B., Bioenergetic role of mitochondrial fusion and fission. *Biochimica et Biophysica Acta (BBA)-Bioenergetics*, 2012. **1817**(10): p. 1833–1838.
166. Wai, T. and T. Langer, Mitochondrial dynamics and metabolic regulation. *Trends in Endocrinology & Metabolism*, 2016. **27**(2): p. 105–117.
167. Youle, R.J. and A.M. Van Der Bliek, Mitochondrial fission, fusion, and stress. *Science*, 2012. **337**(6098): p. 1062–1065.
168. Wang, W., et al., Mitofusin-2 is a novel direct target of p53. *Biochemical and Biophysical Research Communications*, 2010. **400**(4): p. 587–592.
169. McGowan, E.M., et al., Evaluation of cell cycle arrest in estrogen responsive MCF-7 breast cancer cells: pitfalls of the MTS assay. *PLoS One*, 2011. **6**(6): p. e20623.
170. Saleem, A., P.J. Adhihetty, and D.A. Hood, Role of p53 in mitochondrial biogenesis and apoptosis in skeletal muscle. *Physiological Genomics*, 2009. **37**(1): p. 58–66.
171. Saleem, A., et al., Effect of p53 on mitochondrial morphology, import, and assembly in skeletal muscle. *American Journal of Physiology-Cell Physiology*, 2015. **308**(4): p. C319-C329.
172. Kastan, M.B., Wild-type p53: tumors can't stand it. *Cell*, 2007. **128**(5): p. 837–840.
173. Speetjens, F.M., et al., Induction of p53-specific immunity by a p53 synthetic long peptide vaccine in patients treated for metastatic colorectal cancer. *Clinical Cancer Research*, 2009. **15**(3): p. 1086–1095.
174. Ventura, A., et al., Restoration of p53 function leads to tumour regression in vivo. *Nature*, 2007. **445**(7128): p. 661–665.
175. Xue, W., et al., Senescence and tumour clearance is triggered by p53 restoration in murine liver carcinomas. *Nature*, 2007. **445**(7128): p. 656–660.
176. Foster, B.A., et al., Pharmacological rescue of mutant p53 conformation and function. *Science*, 1999. **286**(5449): p. 2507–2510.
177. Mayer, T.U., et al., Small molecule inhibitor of mitotic spindle bipolarity identified in a phenotype-based screen. *Science*, 1999. **286**(5441): p. 971–974.
178. Bykov, V.J., et al., Restoration of the tumor suppressor function to mutant p53 by a low-molecular-weight compound. *Nature Medicine*, 2002. **8**(3): p. 282–288.
179. Alessio, N., et al., Misidentified human gene functions with mouse models: the case of the retinoblastoma gene family in senescence. *Neoplasia*, 2017. **19**(10): p. 781–790.
180. Valente, J.F., J.A. Queiroz, and F. Sousa, p53 as the focus of gene therapy: past, present and future. *Current Drug Targets*, 2018. **19**(15): p. 1801–1817.
181. Fantin, V.R., J. St-Pierre, and P. Leder, Attenuation of LDH-A expression uncovers a link between glycolysis, mitochondrial physiology, and tumor maintenance. *Cancer Cell*, 2006. **9**(6): p. 425–434.
182. Christofk, H.R., et al., The M2 splice isoform of pyruvate kinase is important for cancer metabolism and tumour growth. *Nature*, 2008. **452**(7184): p. 230–233.
183. Warburg, O., On the origin of cancer cells. *Science*, 1956. **123**(3191): p. 309–314.
184. Bogan, J.S., Regulation of glucose transporter translocation in health and diabetes. *Annual Review of Biochemistry*, 2012. **81**: p. 507–532.
185. Warburg, O., F. Wind, and E. Negelein, The metabolism of tumors in the body. *The Journal of General Physiology*, 1927. **8**(6): p. 519.
186. Kroemer, G. and J. Pouyssegur, Tumor cell metabolism: cancer's Achilles' heel. *Cancer Cell*, 2008. **13**(6): p. 472–482.
187. Pouysségur, J., F. Dayan, and N.M. Mazure, Hypoxia signalling in cancer and approaches to enforce tumour regression. *Nature*, 2006. **441**(7092): p. 437–443.
188. Frezza, C. and E. Gottlieb. Mitochondria in Cancer: Not Just Innocent Bystanders. *Seminars in Cancer Biology*. 2009. Elsevier.

2 Exploring the Intricacies of p53 and Its Connection to Breast Cancer

*Sadaf Qadir, Nusrat Jan, Saima Gul, and Manzoor Ahmad Mir**

Department of Bioresources, School of Biological Sciences, University of Kashmir, Srinagar, J&K, India
*drmanzoor@kashmiruniversity.ac.in

2.1 INTRODUCTION

The tumor suppressor protein, which is formed by the TP53 gene, present on chromosome 17, inhibits the development of cancer. To mediate the suppression of tumors, tumor suppressor protein binds itself to specific genetic material response regions and influences the production of genes implicated in different subsequential activities: cell cycle arrest, ferroptosis, aging, cell death, repairing of DNA, cell eating, or catabolism. Its moniker, "guardian of the genome," is thus fitting. MDM2, an E3 ligase, strictly controls the amount of p53 under normal physiological settings. It does this by inducing p53 degradation via the ubiquitin proteasome-dependent route. Through connecting to MDM2's promoter, p53 can also cause the gene to express. As a result, a negative feedback loop is created that encourages p53 degradation and keeps cellular p53 levels low [1]. Modifications after translation in tumor suppressor protein in response to any cell stress comprise (1) sequence-specific DNA binding, which stabilizes p53, (2) phosphorylation, which disrupts p53's interaction with MDM2, and (3) transactivation. To induce senescence and apoptosis, repair DNA, and control the cell cycle, p53 has to either activate or suppress particular genes. Figure 2.1 illustrates this protein's critical function, which is involved in many biological activities, including ferroptosis, senescence, DNA repair, cell death, autophagy, metabolism of cells, and general regulation of gene expression. These processes may all potentially and in different ways contribute to p53's tumor suppressor function. Worldwide, cancer present in the breast has more frequency in the women population. An estimated occurrence of novel cases is about 2.3 million or about 11.7% of all cases of cancer. It has already overtaken cancer of the lungs as the primary cause of incidence of cancer globally [2–4]. According to epidemiological research, by 2030, the number of individuals affected by breast cancer globally is estimated to be 2.7 million [5, 6]. The incidence in India rose dramatically between 1965 and 1985—nearly 50% [7]. In 2016, it was estimated that there were 118,000 new cases of breast cancer in India, with a 95% uncertainty range of 107,000 to 130,000, and 526,000 (ranging from 474,000 to 574,000) were the most commonly diagnosed cases. Of these cases, 98.1% were in females. The standardized age incidence rate of breast cancer in women increased by 39.1% (95% confidence interval, 5.1 to 85.5) from 1990 to 2016, with this rise observed across all 50 states over the last 26 years [8]. As per the GLOBOCAN data for 2020, breast cancer carried a cumulative risk of 2.81 and accounted for 13.5% (178,361) of total cancer incidences and 10.6% (90,408) of overall cancer-related deaths in India [9, 10]. A notable portion of individuals with Li–Fraumeni syndrome, which predisposes them to a higher risk of breast cancer, carry inherited mutations in the p53 gene

 DOI: 10.1201/9781003520771-2

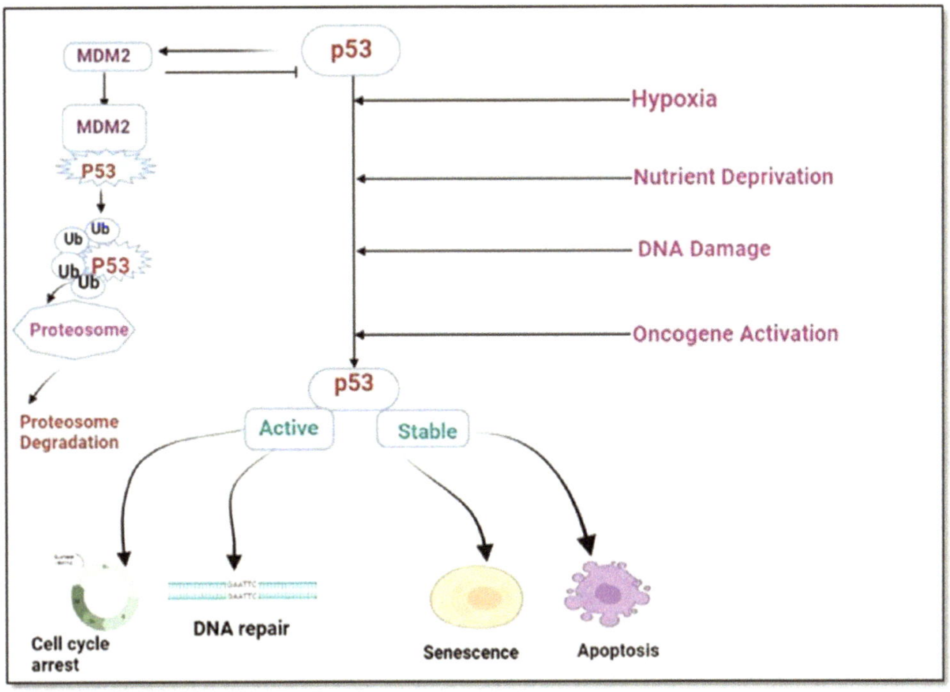

FIGURE 2.1 Normal circumstances result in MDM2 controlling the p53 protein. To control cell division, apoptosis, repairing of DNA and aging, hypoxia, oncogene regulation, DNA damage, and starvation all cause p53 to become activated.

[11–13]. The structure and expression of p53 have been thoroughly investigated in breast cancer, indicating that p53 inactivation is crucial in the development of breast cancer. Initial studies on breast cancer cell lines revealed the presence of mutated p53 [14]. It was shown that the p53 gene often exhibits loss of heterozygosity (LOH) in primary breast cancers [15]. In some cases, this is followed by a mutation in the remaining allele. The majority of p53 alleles left behind from colon cancers are mutant, whereas in breast cancer (BC), a minimum of 60% of reports with loss of hair still have a wild-type p53 allele [15]. However, p53 coding mutations have been found in various research related to BC. A thorough analysis showed that about 20% of patients show altered tumor suppressor protein [16]. Finding the level of tumorigenesis in the breast to which alterations of tumor suppressor protein take place has been the subject of numerous investigations. A thorough examination of micro-dissected tumor material reveals that mutations are more prevalent in high-grade ductal carcinoma in situ in comparison to low-grade ductal carcinoma in situ that is free from mutations [17]. About 20% of cases of breast cancer have p53 mutations overall [16]. There are increased frequencies linked to specific illness categories. For example, multiple studies have discovered that carriers of germ-line mutations in breast cancer 1 (BRCA1) early onset, and breast cancer 2 (BRCA2) early onset have an increased incidence of tumor suppressor protein mutations in malignancies [18, 19]. Additionally, a particular range of tumor suppressor protein alterations is present in these tumors [20]. Surprisingly, 100% of typical medullary breast cancer cases have a p53 mutation [21]. This is especially noteworthy because it is now widely acknowledged that medullary breast tumors and instances linked to BRCA1 have similar clinicopathologies. That's right—methylation-dependent BRCA1 expression suppression is frequently seen in medullary breast tumors [4, 22, 23]. In this chapter, we strive to synthesize the vast body of literature surrounding p53 and its connection to breast cancer, providing insights into the underlying mechanisms, clinical implications, and therapeutic opportunities. Through a multidisciplinary approach that integrates molecular biology, genetics, oncology, and transitional research, we aim to unravel the complexities of p53 biology concerning BC paving the way for improved evaluation, prognostic, and therapeutic strategies in the fight against this formidable disease.

2.2 MOLECULAR FUNCTIONS OF p53

p53 regulates a large number of signaling networks. The questions of precisely how, when, and on what p53 acts are not easily answered. However, p53 responds to environmental disturbances in a very flexible and diverse manner, deciding whether to maintain cellular homeostasis or cause cell death. By acting as a connecting element for several cellular signaling pathways, p53 regulates a vast number of cellular activities tastefully and harmoniously through gene transcriptional control and the interaction of proteins [24]. p53, which is commonly called a tumor suppressor gene, is important for repairing DNA, cell death, and cell cycle arrest due to cellular stress [24–27]. Approximately 50% of tumors found in humans have been shown to have tumor suppressor protein alterations, underscoring the protein's critical function in cancer suppression.

The complete p53 protein consists of the N-terminal transactivation domain (TAD), proline-rich region, DNA-binding domain (DBD), tetramerization domain, and C-terminal regulatory domain. In humans, p53 operates as a homotetramer. Upon binding to DNA, the p53 DBD not only forms a tetramer via the tetramerization domain but also establishes a homotetramer structure composed of two dimers upon DNA binding [28]. The ability of p53 to limit tumor growth depends on the generation of apoptosis [29]. p53 is a nuclear regulator protein that controls a vast number of genes related to cell death. Notably, it has been discovered that p53 migrates to the mitochondria and mediates the intrinsic mechanism, which is also known as the mitochondrial apoptosis pathway, mainly by direct protein–protein interactions with proteins in the B-cell lymphoma-2 family [30]. The B-cell lymphoma family of proteins regulates the activation of the caspase cascade via controlling MOMP, which involves pro- and anti-apoptotic members [31, 32]. B-cell lymphoma 2 (BCL-2) and B-cell lymphoma xL (BCL-xL), both belonging to the B-cell lymphoma-2 group, possess anti-apoptotic properties. They prevent apoptosis by either sequestering pro-apoptotic BH3-only members or directly interacting with the effector proteins BAK and BAX [33]. BCL-2 and BCL-xL dysregulation are frequently linked to chemotherapy resistance and carcinogenesis. According to reports, p53 directly interacts with and irritates BCL-2 and BCL-xL, which activates effectors and eventually causes apoptosis. The p53 DNA-binding domain facilitates its interactions on a surface separate from the hydrophobic groove for Bcl-2 homology 3 peptide binding with BCL-2 and BCL-xL. The binding to B-cell lymphoma-xL17 is enhanced by p53 tetramerization. Using the HADDOCK docking approach, a structural representation of the p53/BCL-xL complex was introduced [34, 35]. Patients with p53 gene alterations for breast cancer frequently show impaired repairing of genetic material. In breast cancer masses with tumor suppressor protein alterations, inhibiting poly(adenosine diphosphate-ribose) and poly(ADP-ribose) polymerase appears to be a viable way to improve therapy responses [36]. In preclinical models, nucleotide analogs in combination with PARP inhibitors exhibit increased efficacy, suggesting that this aggregate helps evaluate strategy for p53 mutant BC. Moreover, the complex role of p53 in disease progression is underscored by its relationship with clinical features of BC, including tumor dimensions, generation, grade, lymphatic spread, nodal involvement, estrogen receptor expression, and estrogen receptor (ER) profile. Being the master of transcription regulation, p53 specifically binds to genetic material and regulates various genomic pathways [37]. It is present in the nucleus as well as in extranuclear material [38]. The complex functioning of tumor suppressor protein holds a vast genomic network in the case of breast cancer [39].

p53 modulates several components of genomic activity to affect the course of the disease by orchestrating a broad and adaptable network (Figure 2.2) [40]. This extensive regulatory influence underscores the intricate and crucial role of tumor suppressor protein in shaping the genomic landscape associated with breast cancer [45]. Understanding the varied effects of tumor suppressor protein functioning provides valuable insights into potential therapeutic strategies for targeting this gene in breast cancer treatment [41]. For many years, tumor suppressor protein's role as a cancer

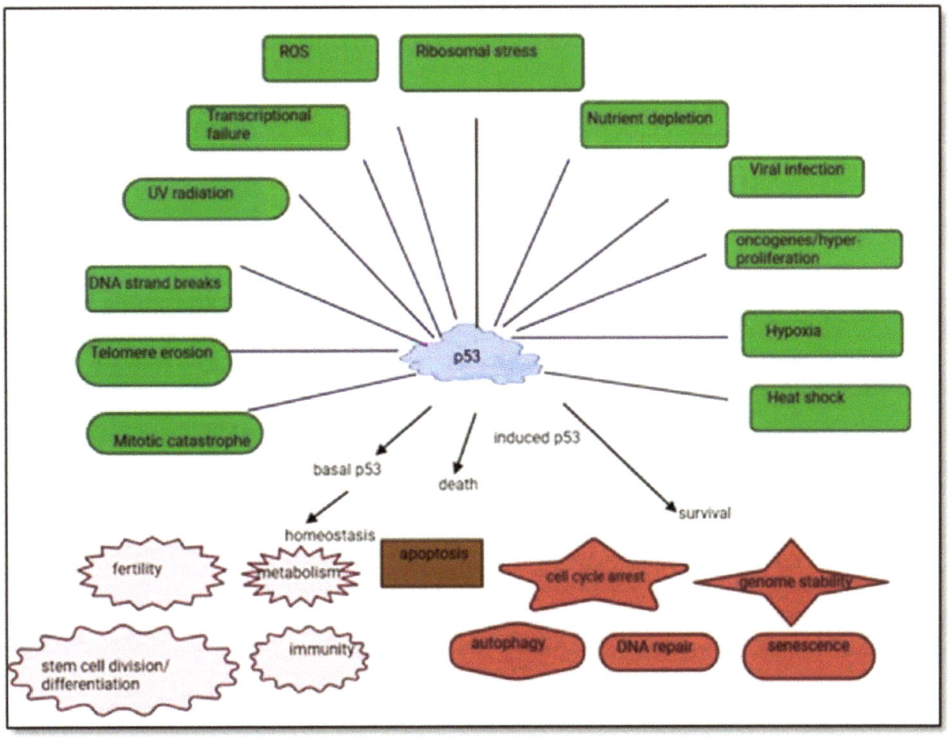

FIGURE 2.2 A wide range of cellular stresses activate p53, which sets off coordinated changes in gene expression and several biological reactions. The type of cell as well as the kind, degree, and length of the initial stress all affect the results. The stress events that trigger the stimulation of p53 via genomic repair response pathways are highlighted in a lilac hue on the left. Baseline or low levels of p53 can influence the homeostatic regulation of some biological processes. ROS stands for reactive oxygen species.

suppressor has been the main focus of attention and is regarded as the "guardian of the genome." By supervising multiple cellular processes at once in a particular setting, p53 controls a wide range of cellular functions [42]. It regulates several biological processes, including DNA repair, metabolism, angiogenesis prevention, and the start of cell senescence [43]. Additionally, p53 influences intracellular redox homeostasis and metabolism via transcription-dependent and transcription-independent mechanisms. Furthermore, researchers came to know that p53 regulates the differentiation and proliferation of progenitor cells. In addition to its potential to accelerate aging and reduce lifespans, p53 plays a critical protective role in maintaining skin color [44]. The relationship that exists between p53 and the mitochondrial antioxidant enzyme determines the destiny of the cell and synchronizes the body's reaction to stress [45, 46]. A wide range of cellular stresses activate p53, which sets off coordinated changes in gene expression and several biological reactions. The type of cell as well as the kind, degree, and length of the initial stress all affect the results. The stress events activate p53 through genetic material damage response pathways. Baseline or low levels of p53 can influence the homeostatic regulation of some biological processes.

2.3 ABNORMALITIES IN TUMOR SUPPRESSOR GENE

Examining the variety of TP53 mutational events in relation to breast cancer reveals a complicated terrain that greatly adds to the disease's heterogeneity. A key component in preserving genomic stability, the TP53 gene undergoes a variety of mutational events, each of which has unique consequences for the development of disease. These mutations frequently cause the p53 protein to become dysfunctional because they might appear as missense mutations, which result in amino acid changes. Furthermore, a reading frame shift brought on by frameshift mutations may result in a shortened and non-functional protein. Splice-site mutations, deletions, and insertions add to the complex array of TP53 changes, each offering a different set of difficulties and chances for therapeutic intervention [47].

Additionally, the spectrum of TP53 mutations encompasses both structural alterations to the gene and different kinds of alterations including gain-of-function mutations that bestow new cancer-promoting properties on p53 proteins [48]. This variation highlights the necessity of tailored strategies for treating breast cancer, taking into account the various functional effects linked to various TP53 mutations. Comprehending this variability is crucial to formulating focused therapeutic approaches customized to the distinct mutational terrain of individual cases of breast cancer [49]. A key area of research is the intricate connection between the diverse TP53 gene mutations and medical results in BC patients, opening the door to more sophisticated and successful strategies in the realm of personalized medicine for BC therapy [50].

2.4 THE LANDSCAPE OF BREAST CANCER

Breast cancer, with approximately 2.3 million new cases globally, stands as one of the prevailing malignancies diagnosed and ranks as the fifth-highest contributor to cancer-related fatalities [2]. When contrasting countries in transition (Melanesia, Western Africa, Micronesia/Polynesia, and the Caribbean) with transitioned nations (Australia/New Zealand, Western Europe, Northern America, and Northern Europe), the mortality rate from breast cancer is roughly 88% higher in the transitioning countries [2].

The BC mortality-to-incidence ratio serves as a reliable indicator of five-year survival rates [9] and was 0.30 worldwide in 2020 [5]. When looking at the seriousness of BC clinically, in areas with advanced healthcare systems like Hong Kong, Singapore, and Turkey, the five-year survival rates for localized and regional cancer were 75.4% and 89.6%, respectively. In contrast, in less developed countries such as India, the Philippines, and Thailand, the survival rates for localized and regional BC were 76.3% and 47.4%, respectively.

In the last 30 years, there has been a notable rise in both the occurrence and death rates related to breast cancer. Between 1990 and 2016, in over half of the countries examined, including Afghanistan, the Philippines, Brazil, and Argentina, the number of new cases of breast cancer increased by more than fourfold. Likewise, the number of deaths due to breast cancer doubled in nearly half of the countries studied, such as Yemen, Paraguay, Libya, and Saudi Arabia [11]. According to current forecasts, it is expected that each year by 2030, approximately 2.7 million new instances of BC will be detected globally, resulting in 870,000 fatalities [12]. Improved cancer registration and detection methods, combined with the adoption of Westernized lifestyles (including later pregnancies, decreased breastfeeding, early onset of menstruation, sedentary behavior, and unhealthy eating habits), are predicted to lead to an increase in breast cancer occurrences in low- and middle-income nations [51].

2.5 DETERMINANTS OF BREAST CANCER

Numerous factors contribute to the risk of developing breast cancer, including factors that can be changed and those that cannot. Table 2.1 gives a brief account of these factors.

2.5.1 Modifiable Determinants

2.5.1.1 Active Lifestyle

The protective impact of physical exercise on the occurrence of BC is accounted for by several theories. These include the possibility that engaging in physical activity helps prevent cancer by reducing the body's exposure to internal sex hormones, modifying immune system reactions, or elevating insulin-like growth factor-1 levels [52–54].

TABLE 2.1
Modifiable and Non-Modifiable Factors in Breast Cancer

Modifiable Factors	Non-Modifiable Factors
Physical activity	Hereditary lineage (associated with breast or ovarian cancer)
Adiposity	DNA alterations
Alcohol intake	Ethnic background
Smoking	Maternity and nursing
Intake of processed food	Thickness of mammary tissue
Prolonged exposure to artificial illumination	Past occurrence of breast cancer
Exposure to chemicals	Benign breast conditions

2.5.1.2 Overweight/Obesity

Based on epidemiological data, obesity is linked to an increased peril of BC. While most overweight postmenopausal women face an increased risk of developing estrogen receptor-positive breast cancer due to this association, obese women experience poorer clinical outcomes irrespective of menopausal status [55].

2.5.1.3 Liquor Intake

For instance, it has been found that drinking alcohol raises the incidence of estrogen-positive BC [56]. When ingested before the initial pregnancy, it significantly contributes to the development of structural alterations in tissue present in the breast, which puts it at risk for additional carcinogenic events [57].

2.5.1.4 Smoking

Carcinogenic substances from nicotine products are carried to mammary tissue, raising the likelihood of alterations in cancer-causing genes and tumor suppressor genes, particularly in the tumor suppressor protein p53 encoded by the Tp53 gene. Consequently, smoking and passive smoking elevates the risk of cancer development [58].

2.5.1.5 Intake of Processed Food

The abundance of fat, sugar, and sodium in highly processed foods contributes to obesity, which poses another risk factor for BC. A 10% increase in the consumption of ready-made foods is associated with an 11% higher risk of BC. Conversely, a diet abundant in fruits, vegetables, whole grains, legumes, and lean protein is linked to a reduced risk of breast cancer [59].

2.5.1.6 Prolonged Exposure to Artificial Illumination

The vulnerability of BC has recently been associated with artificial light at night (ALAN). Disruption of the melatonin cycle and subsequent epigenetic alterations may be the probable cause. Studies to date indicate that compared to individuals with lower ALAN exposure, those with higher exposure are connected to a noticeably higher vulnerability to BC [60].

2.5.1.7 Exposure to Chemicals

Numerous chemicals have been associated with the onset of BC, but the most extensively researched thus far are PCB and DDT. Initial contact with these substances has been found to hinder the proper development of mammary glands [61].

2.5.2 Non-Modifiable Factors

2.5.2.1 Family History

A heightened likelihood of developing BC can also result from a familial background of ovarian cancer, especially when there are BRCA1 and BRCA2 mutations present [62].

2.5.2.2 Genetic Mutations

An elevated likelihood of BC has been associated with several genetic abnormalities. Located on chromosomes 13 and 17, respectively, BRCA1 and BRCA2 are two prominent genes with a high penetrance. The primary association between them and breast carcinogenesis is higher. Inherited mostly in an autosomal dominant manner, the mutations present in the aforementioned genes can also occur sporadically, as is frequently documented. Genes such as tumor protein p53 cadherin 1 (also known as E-cadherin), phosphatase and tensin homolog, and serine/threonine kinase 11 (also known as LKB1) are also highly permeant for BC [63].

2.5.2.3 Race/Ethnicity

Typically, White non-Hispanic women consistently show the highest occurrence of BC. In contrast, Black women have the highest mortality rate from this disease and exhibit the minimum longevity chances [64].

2.5.2.4 Pregnancy and Breastfeeding

Numerous research has solidified the link between the likelihood of female breast cancer and exposure to natural hormones like progesterone and estrogen. Therefore, factors including gestation, lactation, the beginning of menstruation, and menopause, as well as their period and accompanying hormone-mediated imbalances, play a crucial role in potentially triggering cancer-inducing occurrences in the breast. Early full-term pregnancy, especially in one's early 20s, and future increases in the incidence of BC are associated with a lower vulnerability with an increased number of deliveries [65]. Besides the risk factors, through gene expression profiling, researchers have categorized BC based on differences in the frequency of occurrence, treatment efficacy, disease advancement, and survival outcomes. Imaging properties are evident across the luminal A, luminal B, HER2-enriched, and basal-like subtypes. The most prevalent tumors, accounting for 60% to 70% of cases, are those that express the ER. Out of all the subtypes, luminal A cancers have the greatest prognosis. Individuals diagnosed with luminal B tumors typically experience notably reduced overall survival and shorter disease-free survival when compared to other subtypes. It is critical to distinguish between these cancers, as luminal B tumors require additional care. On mammograms, both typically present as irregular masses without associated calcifications; however, after diagnosis, luminal B tumors are more likely to involve the axillary lymph nodes. Overexpression is a characteristic of HER2-enriched malignancies.

2.6 HETEROGENEITY OF BREAST CANCER

It is suggested that the diversity observed in BC stems from differences in cancer cells' genetic, epigenomic, transcriptomic, and proteomic features. These variables impact tumor characteristics including proliferation, apoptosis, and responsiveness to therapy. In individuals with tumor tissues, both intratumor heterogeneity and intertumoral heterogeneity (metastasis) are found [23]. Additionally, the heterogeneity is spatiotemporal. The dynamic term "temporal heterogeneity" describes changes in the molecular composition of tumor cells as the cancer grows. The intricate organization and interplay among different cell groups within tumor formations are defined by spatial heterogeneity. Numerous researchers argue that breast cancer stands as the most diverse cancer affecting women on a global scale. The heterogeneity of breast cancer makes early diagnosis more challenging [66]. The three biggest issues with treating breast cancer are metastasis, recurrence, and therapeutic resistance [69]. It is impossible to fully isolate these issues from one another. Chemotherapy can eradicate cancer cells that are receptive to it, but the resistant cells that remain can lead to metastasis and potentially a recurrence of cancer [67]. Important processes like cell cycle, metabolism, tumor microenvironment (TME), epithelial–mesenchymal transition (EMT), circulating tumor cells (CTCs); and genetic, transcriptomic, epigenetic, proteomic, and clinical and histological information should all be taken into account when developing precise treatments for breast cancer, given the heterogeneity of the disease. Based on breast cancer heterogeneity, numerous standard treatment plans have been extensively used in clinical practice. Treatments for all kinds of breast cancer often involve surgery, radiation, and chemotherapy [68, 69]. Conventional breast surgery involves either a lumpectomy, which leaves the breast intact, or a mastectomy, which removes the entire breast and is typically followed by reconstruction. Axillary excision involves removing the axillary lymph nodes to identify the spread of cancer cells and eradicate them. High-energy radiation is referred to as radiotherapy when it is delivered to the chest wall following a mastectomy, the breast, or just a portion of it, as well as the local lymph nodes [70]. Patients who have metastatic breast cancer in lymph nodes or patients with a high frequency of recurrence are treated with adjuvant chemotherapy. As a result of adjuvant chemotherapy, patients with ER-negative breast cancer have lower chances of recurrence and mortality rates in contrast to ER-positive patients. This is similar to the findings with neoadjuvant chemotherapy [71]. The standard treatment for hormone receptor-positive and HER2-negative breast cancer involves endocrine therapy, which encompasses selective estrogen receptor modulators (SERMs), selective estrogen receptor degraders (SERDs), and aromatase inhibitors (AIs). SERMs include raloxifene, which binds to the ER competitively and thus inactivates the estrogen. The combination of endocrine therapy and CDK4/6 has to be a compulsory method for treating metastatic or advanced hormone receptor-positive breast cancer. For example, ribociclib, a cyclin-dependent kinase 4/6 (CDK4/6) inhibitor, plus AIs, such as tamoxifen, work better together than endocrine therapy alone [4, 72]. The traditional approach to treating triple-negative breast cancer (TNBC), which is well-known for its difficulties in treating intratumor heterogeneity, combines chemotherapy, radiation therapy, and surgery. Even with the introduction of novel biological and targeted therapies, cytotoxic chemotherapy is still the mainstay of care for TNBC patients. Chemotherapies including paclitaxel and cyclophosphamide have been suggested for treating early TNBC before undergoing surgery [73, 74].

2.7 p53 MUTATIONS IN BREAST CANCER

Gain-of-function (GOF) processes can confer carcinogenic characteristics to p53 gene mutations. Accordingly, the mutated p53 protein may interact with various cofactors or transcription factors, changing the transcription and expression of genes to encourage the growth of cancer [13]. Furthermore, these mutations show dominant-negative activity, which prevents the wild-type p53 protein from performing its activities.

2.7.1 Genome Instability

All forms of human cancer are characterized by innate genome instability. It has been shown that the GOF activity of mutant tumor suppressor protein promotes genomic instability. In BC specimens, aberrant copy number 25 is associated with mutations in the tumor suppressor gene. Specifically, the p53 R172H mutation (corresponding to the R175H mutation in mice) disrupts the activity of cyclin E-cyclin-dependent kinase 2 (cdk2) at the centrosome, leading to an increase in centrosome numbers. Studies have shown that mutant p53 can bind to chromatin-regulated genes, such as the methyltransferases [75].

2.7.2 Avoiding Apoptosis

Mutant p53 avoids apoptosis by working with p63 and p73, members of the p53 gene cluster, to inhibit their tumor-suppressive functions. Several p53 mutations, such as the R273H and R175H, were reported to inhibit apoptosis by suppressing the expression of BCL2-modifying factor via enhanced AKT signaling and reducing p73 transcriptional activity on Bax promoter respectively. Thus, cell death is inhibited [76].

2.7.3 Proliferation

In contrast to the original form, mutant tumor suppressor proteins can trigger the transcription of multiple genes, including CCNE2, MAP2K3, c-MYC, and CXCL1, that are involved in cell growth and division. Additionally, it has been demonstrated that mutant tumor suppressor proteins interact with various proteins and transcription factors that support BC development, such as nuclear transcription factor Y (NF-Y), poly(ADP-ribose) polymerase (PARP), and SREBPs, which activate the isoprenoid pathway or HMG-CoA reductase pathway [77].

2.7.4 Metastasis

It has also been observed that mutant p53 increases tumor aggressiveness and potential for metastasis through several pathways, for example, increased cell invasion and metastasis in cancer cells. The stability of the mutant p53 protein could potentially arise due to alterations in its degradation, resilience, or persistence, which is made possible by the Rab coupling protein-regulated release of Hsp90. Additionally, mutant p53 interacts with G-protein coupled receptors, Pin1, and the adenosine A2b receptor (ADORA2B). These interactions correlate with unfavorable clinical outcomes in BC and promote invasion and metastasis through various mechanisms [78].

2.8 p53 MUTATIONS INFLUENCE THE PROGRESSION AND PROGNOSIS OF BREAST CANCER

BC is a varied illness with numerous molecular kinds, each possessing different characteristics and treatment responses. It is estimated that TP53 mutations are involved in about 30% of BC cases. This gene is frequently altered in this type of cancer, making it the most prevalent mutation observed. Missense point mutations, which hinder p53's ability to transcribe, are the main reason behind the maximum number of tumor suppressor protein alterations that usually happen within the DNA-binding domain. These mutations are strongly correlated with tumor subtypes 17 and are associated with an unfavorable forecast for patients with breast cancer [79]. Based on patterns of gene expression, breast tumors are primarily classified into four types: normal, luminal, basal, and HER-2 positive. p53 mutations are rare in the luminal-like kind of BC (26%), with luminal A exhibiting a lower mutation rate (17%) than luminal B (41%). In addition to this, p53 mutations are identified in 53% of HER2-amplified tumors and are most common in malignancies that resemble basal tissues (88%). In comparison to other subtypes, tumor suppressor protein alterations and human epidermal growth factor receptor 2 overabundance are linked to a noticeably inferior prognosis [80]. Additionally, research has demonstrated that inflammatory breast cancer exhibits a higher frequency of p53 mutations (50%) compared to non-inflammatory BC (20–30%). Recent research suggests that the occurrence of p53 mutations across all metastatic BC subtypes is connected to diminished overall survival rates. Additionally, high-grade and advanced-stage malignancies tend to harbor more p53 mutations. These changes are also associated with aggressive forms of breast cancer, such as human epidermal growth factor receptor 2 amplified breast cancer and TNBC [81].

2.9 INTERPLAY BETWEEN p53 AND OTHER MOLECULAR PATHWAYS

A cell signaling system called PI3K/Akt/mTOR is involved in immune response control, motility, growth, proliferation, survival, and metabolism. Furthermore, this pathway has been associated with numerous diseases and conditions, such as vascular disorders, Parkinson's disease, and tuberous sclerosis [82, 83]. Cancer research has also been a focus of PI3K/Akt/mTOR studies. Tumors present in humans like BC have changes to this system; in fact, up to 60% of tumors have various variants that exaggerate this pathway [84]. Deregulation of this system has been linked to multiple hallmarks of cancer, such as unregulated cell proliferation, genetic instability of the genome, and metabolic reprogramming of tumor cells [85]. Furthermore, one of the primary factors contributing to cancer cells' resistance to antitumor medicines is the activation of the phosphoinositide 3-kinase, protein kinase B, and mammalian target of the rapamycin pathway [86]. Because of this, research on the phosphoinositide 3-kinase, protein kinase B, and mammalian target of the rapamycin pathway is essential to comprehending the onset and course of the disease, its function as a putative target for therapy, and its diagnostic and prognostic significance concerning breast cancer patients [87, 88]. PKB also known as Akt is a serine-threonine kinase with three distinct variants that are formed by three separate genes: protein kinase B alpha, protein kinase B beta, and protein kinase B gamma. However, the protein most closely linked to cancer is Akt1 [89]. Through pleckstrin homology (PH) domains, Akt1 interacts with PIP3 [90]. Through this connection, Akt is localized to the cell membrane, thereafter PDK1 and PDK2 phosphorylate the Thr308 and Ser473 residues. PIP3 activates PDK1, although PDK2 is a component of the mTORC2 complex [91].

2.10 CROSSTALK BETWEEN p53 AND OTHER HORMONE RECEPTOR GENES

Two different genes encode different isoforms of the ER protein: ERα, which participates in the survival and growth or multiplication of breast cancer cells, and ERβ, whose role in breast cancer is yet unknown. Empirical data suggests that ERβ could counteract ERα's capacity to promote cell division in response to estrogen (E2) [92, 93]. The ERs main job is to trigger nuclear transcription factors in response to hormones. Following the conventional ER nuclear genomic pathway, it binds to certain DNA sequences known as estrogen response elements (EREs) that are situated in the enhancer/regulatory regions of target genes that control cell division and survival [92]. Interestingly, many coregulators (coactivators and corepressors) can control this conventional ER transcriptional activity. ER can also stimulate the expression of genes by binding to additional transcription factors like NFκB, SP-1, and AP-1 among others [94, 95]. Under the name non-classical ER nuclear genomic route, this alternative genomic signaling target genes to be modified by the indirect action of ER and do not contain the estrogen-response elements (EREs) in their promoters' regions [96, 97].

2.11 THERAPEUTIC IMPLICATIONS AND FUTURE DIRECTIONS

Given the high genetic and epigenetic heterogeneity of cancer genomes, it is likely that the genes that are synthetically deadly to p53 depend on the kind of tissue and cell. The majority of synthetic lethal screens were conducted in one or two cell lines because of throughput limitations. Consequently, it is yet unknown if the hits from the screens are unique to a certain cell type. Future screenings utilizing a wider range of cell lines are therefore required to find more widespread synthetic lethal genes to p53. One type of cancer immunotherapy that has great clinical promise for advanced malignancies, including metastatic melanomas, is adoptive cell transfer, or ACT [98]. Fifty percent of people with metastatic melanomas respond to treatment, and some have very long-lasting remissions. ACTs come in a variety of forms. Tumor-infiltrating lymphocytes (TILs) are a particular kind of T-cells that are present in cancer patients grown in huge amounts outside of the body and then reinfused into the patients to combat the cancer. TCR-T cell transfer is another form of ACT. TCRs used in

T-cell receptors and ACT cloning from T-cells can identify tumor antigens, a little peptide found on tumor cells. Cloned TCRs are encapsulated within lentiviruses and retroviruses, using the baculovirus system Sleeping Beauty, which is then employed to transduce T-cells. After being reinfused into the patient, these modified T-cells (TCR-T) may now selectively target the cancer cells and mediate cancer regression. The CAR-T cell is the third class of ACT. The T-cell receptor in CAR-T cells is designed to have both antigen binding and T-cell stimulation modules (chimeric), which sets them apart from TCR-T cells. The Food and Drug Administration (FDA) has approved three chimeric antigen receptor T-cell treatments for acute lymphoblastic leukemia derived from B-cells, large B-cell lymphoma that has relapsed or is resistant to treatment, and mantle cell lymphoma (MCL) that has relapsed or is resistant to treatment.

2.12 DRUGS TARGETING p53 MUTATIONS

Various approaches have been employed to target p53 mutations. The initial strategy focuses on targeting missense mutp53 to stabilize the wtp53 conformation or restore wtp53 activity. Reactivators are substances or drugs that provide this action. Presently involved in numerous phase II or III clinical trials, APR-246 (eprenetapopt/PRIMA-1MET) stands out as the most prominent medication within this category. APR-246 has been demonstrated to have effective tumor-suppressive effects on mutp53-carrying tumors in mice models; however, the FDA has not yet approved it [99]. Using the fact that cancer cells are addicted to mutp53, the second tactic is to cause missense mutp53 to degrade or become less abundant. This might potentially activate some tumor suppressors that mutp53 has been suppressing, such as p63 and p73. This technique makes use of medications or substances such as statins or HSP90 inhibitors, which are known to cause mutp53 degradation and thereby reduce tumors [100, 101]. The third tactic, known as p53 synthetic lethality, involves selectively causing cancer cells with p53 mutations or deletions to die [102]. Instead of directly targeting mutp53, this approach often focuses on exploiting vulnerabilities caused by tumor suppressor protein deficiency. This strategy employs drugs like Weel inhibitors and inhibitors of DNA damage response signaling, such as ataxia telangiectasia and Rad3-related protein (ATR) inhibitors or checkpoint kinase 1/2 (Chk1/2) inhibitors [103–105]. Other tactics include inhibiting the retrotransposon that is activated with p53 deficit, using wtp53 to rescue non-sense mutations in p53 [106, 107], and suppressing the mutp53-activated YAP/TAZ function [108, 109].

The main suppressor of p53 is MDM2/MDMX [110]. The N-terminal section of mouse double minute 2 (MDM2) interacts with the transactivation domain of p53 (p53-TAD), inhibiting the transcriptional activity of p53. In contrast, wild-type p53 stimulates the transcription of MDM2 [111]. This is the MDM2–p53 negative feedback regulatory loop. Furthermore, E3 ubiquitin ligase, an enzyme present in the C-terminus of MDM2, facilitates nuclear export and p53 degradation [112, 113]. Mouse double minute X, also known as MDM4, is a homolog of MDM2 that shares structural similarities with MDM2 but does not have ubiquitination or ubiquitin conjugation activity. Instead, it can increase ubiquitination or ubiquitin conjugation activity by creating a dimer with MDM 2 [114, 115]. Many human malignancies include overexpression or activation of MDM2/MDM4, which results in p53 inactivation. The MDM2/MDMX–p53 interactions are the focus of many anticancer medications that have been recently discovered [110, 116, 117].

2.13 WTP53 RESTORATION OR STABILIZATION CONFIRMATION FROM MUTP53 THAT IS A MISSENSE

Wtp53 acts as a transcriptional regulator and tumor suppressor and is lost in the majority of mutp53. Conversely, increasing research indicates that specific conditions, such as temperature changes, exposure to synthetic peptides derived from 53BP2 like "CDB3," and the p53 C-terminal domain "Peptide 46," as well as the introduction of second-site mutations or an N-terminal deletion, can restore tumor-suppressive activity [118–120]. Numerous researchers have pursued small molecule drugs that can restore transcriptional activity, tumor-suppressive function, and wtp53 conformation [121]. For instance, CP-31398 is among the oldest compounds identified to reactivate mutated p53, possibly stabilizing the active form of p53 and enhancing its role in cancer suppression mediated by p53 [122, 123]. Moreover, JC744 has recently been discovered as a new compound that can bind to and stabilize the p53Y220C mutant in laboratory conditions through a small surface pocket formed by the p53Y220C mutant, effective at nanomolar concentrations. Still, there aren't many molecules undergoing clinical studies. These include arsenic trioxide (ATO/Trisenox), phenethyl isothiocyanate (PEITC), and APR-246 (eprenetapopt/PRIMA-1MET).

2.14 THERAPEUTIC STRATEGIES TARGETING p53

The increased prevalence of BC worldwide prompted the study of tumor molecular markers to spot potential targets for targeted-evaluating approaches, such as focusing on a specific molecular marker component to restore cellular function without inducing drug toxicity that would otherwise lead to additional cell death.

The body of research on TP53 mutations and its interacting partners, which include activators and repressors, as well as molecular changes in TP53, offers fresh perspectives for the creation of tailored treatments for breast cancers with TP53 mutations. However, most of these specific therapies are still in the preclinical phase. Presently, only two compounds—APR-246 and COTI-2—have progressed to clinical trials [124]. Negative regulators of TP53 as well as wild-type TP53 are targets of treatment methods for breast cancers with TP53 mutations. Targeting TP53 mutations is another of the primary tactics presently in use.

2.15 TP53 NEGATIVE REGULATORS TO BE TARGETED

Several malignancies, particularly breast cancer, have been linked to p53's decreased activity due to increased negative regulators like MDM2 expression. The original type of tumor suppressor protein resumes its original work when MDM2 is inhibited [125–127]. The human MDM2 gene generates a 491 amino acid protein, equivalent to 90 kDa, which exhibits estrogen receptor 3 ubiquitin ligase activity. This activity can either facilitate or impede the degradation of p53. The protein comprises a p53-binding N-terminal domain and a RING domain located at the C-terminus [128, 129]. By utilizing MDM2 inhibitors to disrupt the MDM2–p53 complex, wtp53 will be reactivated, causing necrosis or apoptosis in DNA-damaged cells and halting the growth of tumors. For an MDM2 inhibitor to be therapeutically valuable, it needs to demonstrate strong binding affinity and specificity toward MDM2. Furthermore, in cancer cells expressing wtp53, these negative regulators ought to demonstrate enhanced cellular activity and a highly desired pharmacokinetic profile. Nutlins, benzodiazepine compounds, and MI-series analogs are among the substances that are employed to suppress the p53-negative regulators in breast cancer [130, 131].

2.16 NUTLINS

By screening a variety of chemical libraries, nutlins, which are cis-imidazoline analogs, were discovered as inhibitors of the p53–MDM2 complex, displaying an increased affinity for MDM2. In laboratory and animal studies, nutlin-3, a member of the series, demonstrates a synergistic effect on cancer cells that contain wild-type p53 when used alongside other anticancer drugs such as TNF-related apoptosis-inducing ligand (TRAIL) or bortezomib. In ten arbitrarily chosen cancer cell lines from seven different cancer types—colon, breast, lung, prostate, melanoma, osteosarcoma, and renal—it causes arresting of the cell cycle in the G1/S or G2/M phase and triggers apoptosis [132]. A nutlin derivative called RG7112 (2g) is said to be the first therapeutic small molecule MDM2 inhibitor created to prevent MDM2 from attaching to the p53 site in cancer cells that express the original type of p53 [102]. Apoptosis, inhibition, and cell cycle arrest are all facilitated by stabilizing and reactivating the p53 pathways. In breast tumors where there is a greater presence of wild-type p53 upon diagnosis, nutlins can serve as a substitute for existing cytotoxic therapies, thus preventing excessive cell death associated with drug toxicity [133].

Investigating new strategies to target the p53 gene in breast cancer, the Y220C mutation offers a distinctive way to assess potential low molecular weight inhibitors specific to mutant p53. Notably, the compound PC14586 has proven effective in reactivating and stabilizing the p53 Y220C mutant protein in cells harboring this mutation. This intervention activates the transcription of essential genes associated with wild-type p53 and triggers cell cycle arrest [114]. A phase I/II clinical trial is presently in progress to assess the pharmacodynamics, safety, pharmacokinetics, and potential efficacy of PC14586 as a monotherapy in patients with advanced solid tumors harboring the p53 Y220C mutation. Initial positive results shared at the American Society of Clinical Oncology (ASCO) meeting suggest that PC14586 is generally well-tolerated.

2.17 PROSPECTS FOR THE FUTURE AND DIFFICULTIES IN CREATING THERAPEUTIC APPROACHES AGAINST p53

It is difficult to create inhibitors against p53 as a target protein. The reason for this is that it is a transcription factor that cannot be accessed by an enzyme active site or receptor-ligand pairing. However, the knowledge of the structure of p53 and the molecules that interact with it has made it easier to find and create a variety of substances that may help p53's tumor-suppressive properties to emerge again.

Pre-clinical development is still underway for the majority of small molecule medications intended to target p53-bearing tumors, whether they are mutant or wild type [134, 135]. Despite encouraging pre-clinical results, only a limited number of promising drugs have been investigated in early-stage clinical trials for BC. The results have been mixed, with high-grade toxicity and few signs of efficacy. Although the precise causes of the differences in patient reactions to small molecule inhibitors are still unknown, it is important to take into account the unanticipated consequences of focusing on a particular p53-related pathway. For instance, in tumors with functioning p53, blocking or eliminating MDM2 may activate additional carcinogenic pathways [136]. Furthermore, focusing on p53's negative regulators may cause extensive p53 activation, which could impact both healthy and malignant cells. The efficacy of small molecule drugs for p53 reactivation is constrained by the range of p53 mutations, each showing unique structural changes and molecular behaviors. None of the compounds discussed in this study can address all p53 mutations. Moreover, some of the tactics may exacerbate unfavorable outcomes since they inhibit mutant p53. Intratumoral heterogeneity is an additional topic of concern. The primary issue that has to be addressed, given the heterogeneous character of breast cancers, is whether long-term use of these drugs can restrict their clinical benefits by creating de novo mutations or by exerting selection pressure on already resistant cells. It makes sense to combine the majority of the assessed substances with other therapeutic agents because their clinical efficacy has been demonstrated to be limited. Additionally, research involving patients with breast cancer has examined fulvestrant as well as different Hsp90 and HDAC inhibitors, illuminating the fundamental mechanisms of their anti-cancer action. Although they show secondary effects against p53 models that are mutant or wild type, it is unknown how they relate to patients' p53 mutational status. Further clinical trials that take into account the tumor suppressor protein's mutational update of the tumor may be necessary to ascertain whether these medications have different effects on tumors with original type versus mutant tumor suppressor protein.

2.18 CONCLUSION

In the relentless pursuit of understanding the molecular underpinnings of BC, the multifaceted role of the tumor suppressor gene p53 stands out as a central protagonist. Through decades of meticulous research, the intricate dance between p53 and breast cancer has gradually unfolded, revealing a complex narrative where genetic alterations, signaling pathways, and microenvironmental cues converge to dictate tumor fate. At the heart of this saga lies the enigmatic tumor suppressor protein, rightly called the "guardian of the genome" for its pivotal contribution to safeguarding cellular infrastructure. Emerging from the crucible of DNA damage and cellular stress, p53 orchestrates a collection of responses, ranging from cell cycle arrest, repairing of genetic material, and aging. However, this guardian can be both a shield and a sword, as dysregulation of p53 unleashes a series of events that result in malignant transformation. In the context of breast cancer, the intricate interplay between p53 and its network of interactors exerts a profound influence on tumor initiation, progression, and therapeutic response. Mutational inactivation of p53, a hallmark feature of many cancers including breast cancer, dismantles its tumor-suppressive functions, unleashing the malignant potential of affected cells. Additionally, the complex spectrum of p53 mutations in BC mirrors the heterogeneous nature of the disease. With distinct mutational spectra associated with different molecular subtypes and clinical outcomes. Beyond its canonical functions in DNA damage response, p53 intersects with an array of signaling pathways implicated in breast cancer pathogenesis. From the intricate web of hormone signaling cascades to the dynamic crosstalk between tumor and stromal compartments, p53 exerts nuanced regulatory effects that shape the tumor microenvironment and influence therapeutic outcomes. Moreover, recent advances in single-cell sequencing and spatial profiling techniques offer unprecedented insights into the spatial and temporal dynamics of p53 signaling within the tumor ecosystem, illuminating new opportunities in therapeutic intervention.

In the era of precision medicine, unraveling the intricacies of p53 biology holds profound significance for the clinical handling of breast cancer. Stratification of patients based on p53 mutational status offers a potential avenue for personalized therapy, guiding treatment decisions toward tailored regimens that maximize efficacy while minimizing toxicity. Moreover, leveraging emerging technologies such as CRISPR-based genome editing and small molecule modulators of p53 activity holds promise for targeted manipulation of p53 signaling pathways, offering new hope for patients with refractory disease.

However, the journey toward harnessing the full treatment possibilities of p53 in BC is fraught with challenges and uncertainties. The formidable heterogeneity of p53 mutations within and across tumors presents a formidable obstacle to targeted therapy, necessitating innovative strategies to overcome tumor evolution and therapeutic resistance. Moreover, the intricate interplay between p53 and the tumor microenvironment introduces a layer of complexity that demands comprehensive interrogation and integration into therapeutic paradigms. As we stand at the crossroads of discovery, the nexus of p53 and breast cancer beckons us to venture further into the uncharted territories of cancer biology. By unraveling the intricacies of p53 signaling and its dynamic interplay with the tumor ecosystem, we may unlock novel therapeutic avenues that hold the promise of transforming breast cancer from a formidable foe into a manageable chronic condition. Yet, this journey requires not only scientific acumen but also unwavering dedication and collaboration across disciplines, transcending the boundaries of academia and industry to usher in a new era of precision oncology. The saga of p53 and breast cancer epitomizes the intricate tapestry of cancer biology, where molecular intricacies intertwine with clinical realities to shape the destiny of millions. As we embark on the next chapter of this odyssey, let us heed the lessons learned from the past and embrace the challenges of the future with courage and conviction. For in the crucible of adversity lies the seeds of innovation, and in the nexus of p53 and BC lies the promise of a brighter tomorrow for generations to come.

REFERENCES

1. Haupt, Y., et al., Mdm2 promotes the rapid degradation of p53. *Nature*, 1997. **387**(6630): p. 296–299.
2. Sung, H., et al., Global cancer statistics 2020: GLOBOCAN estimates of incidence and mortality worldwide for 36 cancers in 185 countries. *CA: A Cancer Journal for Clinicians*, 2021. **71**(3): p. 209–249.

3. Sofi, S., et al., A comprehensive analysis of notch signaling genes in breast cancer: expression pattern and prognostic significance. *Advances in Cancer Biology-Metastasis*, 2023. **7**: p. 100104.
4. Jan, N., et al., Targeting breast cancer stem cells through retinoids: a new hope for treatment. *Critical Reviews in Oncology/Hematology*, 2023: p. 104156.
5. Siegel, R., P. Bandi, and A. Jemal, Breast cancer statistics, 2011. *CA: A Cancer Journal for Clinicians*, 2011. **61**: p. 409–418.
6. Jan, N., et al., Metronomic chemotherapy and drug repurposing: a paradigm shift in oncology. *Heliyon*, 2024.
7. Saxena, S., et al., BRCA1 and BRCA2 in Indian breast cancer patients. *Human Mutation*, 2002. **20**(6): p. 473–474.
8. Dhillon, P.K., et al., The burden of cancers and their variations across the states of India: the Global Burden of Disease Study 1990–2016. *The Lancet Oncology*, 2018. **19**(10): p. 1289–1306.
9. International Agency for Research on Cancer, India Source: Globocan 2020. [cited 11 June 2021].
10. Jan, N., et al., Exploring the role of trifarotene against RAR-α: an investigation of expression pattern and clinicopathological significance of RAR-α in breast cancer. *Frontiers in Pharmacology*, 2024. **15**: p. 1361679.
11. Malkin, D., et al., Germ line p53 mutations in a familial syndrome of breast cancer, sarcomas, and other neoplasms. *Science*, 1990. **250**(4985): p. 1233–1238.
12. Haq, B.U., et al., Targeting p53 misfolding conundrum by stabilizing agents and their analogs in breast cancer therapy: a comprehensive computational analysis. *Frontiers in Pharmacology*, 2024. **14**: p. 1333447.
13. Mir, M.A., M. Bashir, and N. Jan, The Role of Interleukin (IL)-6/IL-6 Receptor Axis in Cancer, in *Cytokine and Chemokine Networks in Cancer*. 2023, Springer. p. 137–164.
14. Bartek, J., et al., Genetic and immunochemical analysis of mutant p53 in human breast cancer cell lines. *Oncogene*, 1990. **5**(6): p. 893–899.
15. Davidoff, A.M., et al., Genetic basis for p53 overexpression in human breast cancer. *Proceedings of the National Academy of Sciences*, 1991. **88**(11): p. 5006–5010.
16. Pharoah, P., N. Day, and C. Caldas, Somatic mutations in the p53 gene and prognosis in breast cancer: a meta-analysis. *British Journal of Cancer*, 1999. **80**(12): p. 1968–1973.
17. Done, S.J., et al., p53 missense mutations in microdissected high-grade ductal carcinoma in situ of the breast. *Journal of the National Cancer Institute*, 2001. **93**(9): p. 700–704.
18. Smith, P.D., et al., Novel p53 mutants selected in BRCA-associated tumours which dissociate transformation suppression from other wild-type p53 functions. *Oncogene*, 1999. **18**(15): p. 2451–2459.
19. Phillips, K.-A., et al., Frequency of p53 mutations in breast carcinomas from Ashkenazi Jewish carriers of BRCA1 mutations. *Journal of the National Cancer Institute*, 1999. **91**(5): p. 469–473.
20. Greenblatt, M.S., et al., TP53 mutations in breast cancer associated with BRCA1 or BRCA2 germline mutations: distinctive spectrum and structural distribution. *Cancer Research*, 2001. **61**(10): p. 4092–4097.
21. de Cremoux, P., et al., p53 mutation as a genetic trait of typical medullary breast carcinoma. *Journal of the National Cancer Institute*, 1999. **91**(7): p. 641–643.
22. Esteller, M., et al., Promoter hypermethylation and BRCA1 inactivation in sporadic breast and ovarian tumors. *JNCI: Journal of the National Cancer Institute*, 2000. **92**(7): p. 564–569.
23. Mir, M.A., Sumaya, N. Jan, Implications of Chemokine Heterogenicity in Cancer Metastasis, in *Cytokine and Chemokine Networks in Cancer*. 2023, Springer. p. 115–136.
24. Joerger, A.C. and A.R. Fersht, The p53 pathway: origins, inactivation in cancer, and emerging therapeutic approaches. *Annual Review of Biochemistry*, 2016. **85**: p. 375–404.
25. Kastenhuber, E.R. and S.W. Lowe, Putting p53 in context. *Cell*, 2017. **170**(6): p. 1062–1078.
26. Mir, M.A., N. Jan, and S. Sofi, Introduction to Metronomic Chemotherapy, in *Novel Approaches in Metronomic Chemotherapy for Breast Cancer Treatment*. 2024, CRC Press. p. 1–14.
27. Mir, M.A., M. Rashid, and N. Jan, Cytokines and Chemokines in Tumor Growth and Progression, in *Cytokine and Chemokine Networks in Cancer*. 2023, Springer. p. 33–77.
28. Chen, Y., R. Dey, and L. Chen, Crystal structure of the p53 core domain bound to a full consensus site as a self-assembled tetramer. *Structure*, 2010. **18**(2): p. 246–256.
29. Green, D.R. and G. Kroemer, Cytoplasmic functions of the tumour suppressor p53. *Nature*, 2009. **458**(7242): p. 1127–1130.
30. Chipuk, J.E., et al., Direct activation of Bax by p53 mediates mitochondrial membrane permeabilization and apoptosis. *Science*, 2004. **303**(5660): p. 1010–1014.

31. Singh, R., A. Letai, and K. Sarosiek, Regulation of apoptosis in health and disease: the balancing act of BCL-2 family proteins. *Nature Reviews Molecular Cell Biology*, 2019. **20**(3): p. 175–193.
32. Mir, M.A., et al., Proteomics: Application of Next-Generation Proteomics in Cancer Research, in *Proteomics*. 2023, Elsevier. p. 55–76.
33. Li, M., et al., Bcl-XL: A multifunctional anti-apoptotic protein. *Pharmacological Research*, 2020. **151**: p. 104547.
34. Dominguez, C., R. Boelens, and A.M. Bonvin, HADDOCK: a protein–protein docking approach based on biochemical or biophysical information. *Journal of the American Chemical Society*, 2003. **125**(7): p. 1731–1737.
35. Sofi, S., et al., Clinicopathological and prognostic significance of Bcl2 in breast cancer: a comprehensive in silico and in vitro study. *Saudi Journal of Biological Sciences*, 2023. **31**(2): p. 103916.
36. Valente, J.F., J.A. Queiroz, and F. Sousa, p53 as the focus of gene therapy: past, present and future. *Current Drug Targets*, 2018. **19**(15): p. 1801–1817.
37. Hafner, A., et al., The multiple mechanisms that regulate p53 activity and cell fate. *Nature Reviews Molecular Cell Biology*, 2019. **20**(4): p. 199–210.
38. Wei, C.L., et al., A global map of p53 transcription-factor binding sites in the human genome. *Cell*, 2006. **124**: p. 207–219.
39. Bieging, K.T., S.S. Mello, and L.D. Attardi, Unravelling mechanisms of p53-mediated tumour suppression. *Nature Reviews Cancer*, 2014. **14**(5): p. 359–370.
40. Gu, B. and W.-G. Zhu, Surf the post-translational modification network of p53 regulation. *International Journal of Biological Sciences*, 2012. **8**(5): p. 672.
41. Huo, R., et al., Kinetic analysis of p53 gene network with time delays and PIDD. *International Journal of Biomathematics*, 2024. **17**(03): p. 2350024.
42. Valente, L.J. and L.D. Attardi, P53 orchestrates a complex symphony of cellular processes during oncosuppression. *Molecular & Cellular Oncology*, 2021. **8**(1): p. 1852066.
43. Valente, L.J., et al., p53 deficiency triggers dysregulation of diverse cellular processes in physiological oxygen. *Journal of Cell Biology*, 2020. **219**(11): p. e201908212.
44. Meek, D.W., Regulation of the p53 response and its relationship to cancer. *Biochemical Journal*, 2015. **469**(3): p. 325–346.
45. Sun, Y., A.K. Holley, and D.K. St Clair, p53 regulation of energy metabolism and mitochondria regulation of p53 in cancer cells: an insight into the role of manganese superoxide dismutase. *Current Pharmaceutical Biotechnology*, 2013. **14**(3): p. 261–273.
46. Mir, M.A., et al., Metronomics: toward personalized chemotherapy. *Novel Approaches in Metronomic Chemotherapy for Breast Cancer Treatment*, 2024. p. 99–119. https://doi.org/10.1201/9781032632674-8
47. Monti, P., et al., Heterogeneity of TP53 mutations and P53 protein residual function in cancer: does it matter? *Frontiers in Oncology*, 2020. **10**: p. 593383.
48. Dutta, S., et al., Functional classification of TP53 mutations in acute myeloid leukemia. *Cancers*, 2020. **12**(3): p. 637.
49. Levine, A.J., Spontaneous and inherited TP53 genetic alterations. *Oncogene*, 2021. **40**(41): p. 5975–5983.
50. Levine, A.J., p53: 800 million years of evolution and 40 years of discovery. *Nature Reviews Cancer*, 2020. **20**(8): p. 471–480.
51. Porter, P., “Westernizing” women’s risks? Breast cancer in lower-income countries. *New England Journal of Medicine*, 2008. **358**(3): p. 213.
52. Bernstein, L. and R.K. Ross, Endogenous hormones and breast cancer risk. *Epidemiologic Reviews*, 1993. **15**(1): p. 48–65.
53. Hoffman-Goetz, L., Influence of physical activity and exercise on innate immunity. *Nutrition Reviews*, 1998. **56**(1): p. S126.
54. Hoffman-Goetz, L., et al., Possible mechanisms mediating an association between physical activity and breast cancer. *Cancer: Interdisciplinary International Journal of the American Cancer Society*, 1998. **83**(S3): p. 621–628.
55. Kolb, R. and W. Zhang, Obesity and breast cancer: a case of inflamed adipose tissue. *Cancers*, 2020. **12**(6): p. 1686.
56. Zeinomar, N., et al., Alcohol consumption, cigarette smoking, and familial breast cancer risk: findings from the Prospective Family Study Cohort (ProF-SC). *Breast Cancer Research*, 2019. **21**: p. 1–14.
57. Liu, Y., N. Nguyen, and G.A. Colditz, Links between alcohol consumption and breast cancer: a look at the evidence. *Women’s Health*, 2015. **11**(1): p. 65–77.
58. Terry, P.D. and T.E. Rohan, Cigarette smoking and the risk of breast cancer in women: a review of the literature. *Cancer Epidemiology Biomarkers & Prevention*, 2002. **11**(10): p. 953–971.

59. Castelló, A., et al., Spanish Mediterranean diet and other dietary patterns and breast cancer risk: case–control EpiGEICAM study. *British Journal of Cancer*, 2014. **111**(7): p. 1454–1462.
60. Johns, L.E., et al., Domestic light at night and breast cancer risk: a prospective analysis of 105 000 UK women in the Generations Study. *British Journal of Cancer*, 2018. **118**(4): p. 600–606.
61. Rodgers, K.M., et al., Environmental chemicals and breast cancer: an updated review of epidemiological literature informed by biological mechanisms. *Environmental Research*, 2018. **160**: p. 152–182.
62. Çelik, A., et al., Relationship of breast cancer with ovarian cancer. *A Concise Review of Molecular Pathology of Breast Cancer*, 2015: p. 87–202. https://doi.org/10.5772/59682
63. Shahbandi, A., H.D. Nguyen, and J.G. Jackson, TP53 mutations and outcomes in breast cancer: reading beyond the headlines. *Trends in Cancer*, 2020. **6**(2): p. 98–110.
64. Society, A.C., *Breast Cancer Facts & Figures*. 2007: American Cancer Society.
65. Bernstein, L., Epidemiology of endocrine-related risk factors for breast cancer. *Journal of Mammary Gland Biology and Neoplasia*, 2002. **7**: p. 3–15.
66. Saleem, M.Z., et al., Inhibition of JNK-mediated autophagy promotes proscillaridin A-induced apoptosis via ROS generation, intracellular Ca+ 2 oscillation and inhibiting STAT3 signaling in breast cancer cells. *Frontiers in Pharmacology*, 2020. **11**: p. 01055.
67. Mansoori, B., et al., The different mechanisms of cancer drug resistance: a brief review. *Advanced Pharmaceutical Bulletin*, 2017. **7**(3): p. 339.
68. Loibl, S., et al., Epidemiology and risk factors. *The Lancet Breast Cancer*, 2021. **397**: p. 1750–1769.
69. Mir, M.A., A. Shabir, and N. Jan, Metronomic Chemotherapy in Breast Cancer, in *Novel Approaches in Metronomic Chemotherapy for Breast Cancer Treatment*. CRC Press. p. 72–86.
70. Boyages, J., Radiation therapy and early breast cancer: current controversies. *The Medical Journal of Australia*, 2017. **207**(5): p. 216–222.
71. Berry, D.A., et al., Estrogen-receptor status and outcomes of modern chemotherapy for patients with node-positive breast cancer. *Jama*, 2006. **295**(14): p. 1658–1667.
72. Im, S.-A., et al., Overall survival with ribociclib plus endocrine therapy in breast cancer. *New England Journal of Medicine*, 2019. **381**(4): p. 307–316.
73. Loibl, S., P. Poortmans, and M. Morrow, Breast cancer (vol 397, pg 1750, 2021). *Lancet*, 2021. **397**(10286): p. 1710–1710.
74. Mir, M.A., et al., Imaging Techniques, Biomarkers, and Methods for Metronomic Chemotherapy, in *Novel Approaches in Metronomic Chemotherapy for Breast Cancer Treatment*. CRC Press. p. 58–71.
75. Zhu, J., et al., Gain-of-function p53 mutants co-opt chromatin pathways to drive cancer growth. *Nature*, 2015. **525**(7568): p. 206–211.
76. Di Como, C.J., C. Gaiddon, and C. Prives, p73 function is inhibited by tumor-derived p53 mutants in mammalian cells. *Molecular and Cellular Biology*, 1999. **19**(2): p. 1438–1449.
77. Valentino, E., et al., Mutant p53 potentiates the oncogenic effects of insulin by inhibiting the tumor suppressor DAB2IP. *Proceedings of the National Academy of Sciences*, 2017. **114**(29): p. 7623–7628.
78. Girardini, J.E., et al., A Pin1/mutant p53 axis promotes aggressiveness in breast cancer. *Cancer Cell*, 2011. **20**(1): p. 79–91.
79. Lai, H., et al., Spectrum of p53 tumor suppressor gene mutations and breast cancer survival. *Breast Cancer Research and Treatment*, 2004. **83**: p. 57–66.
80. Dumay, A., et al., Distinct tumor protein p53 mutants in breast cancer subgroups. *International Journal of Cancer*, 2013. **132**(5): p. 1227–1231.
81. Curtis, C., et al., The genomic and transcriptomic architecture of 2,000 breast tumours reveals novel subgroups. *Nature*, 2012. **486**(7403): p. 346–352.
82. Switon, K., et al., Tuberous sclerosis complex: from molecular biology to novel therapeutic approaches. *IUBMB Life*, 2016. **68**(12): p. 955–962.
83. Ortega, M.A., et al., Implication of the PI3K/Akt/mTOR pathway in the process of incompetent valves in patients with chronic venous insufficiency and the relationship with aging. *Oxidative Medicine and Cellular Longevity*, 2018. **2018**. https://doi.org/10.1155/2018/1495170
84. Engelman, J.A., Targeting PI3K signalling in cancer: opportunities, challenges and limitations. *Nature Reviews Cancer*, 2009. **9**(8): p. 550–562.
85. Hanahan, D. and R.A. Weinberg, Hallmarks of cancer: the next generation. *Cell*, 2011. **144**(5): p. 646–674.
86. Martini, M., et al., PI3K/AKT signaling pathway and cancer: an updated review. *Annals of Medicine*, 2014. **46**(6): p. 372–383.
87. Fruman, D.A. and C. Rommel, PI3K and cancer: lessons, challenges and opportunities. *Nature Reviews Drug Discovery*, 2014. **13**(2): p. 140–156.

88. Davis, N.M., et al., Deregulation of the EGFR/PI3K/PTEN/Akt/mTORC1 pathway in breast cancer: possibilities for therapeutic intervention. *Oncotarget*, 2014. **5**(13): p. 4603.
89. Vara, J.Á.F., et al., PI3K/Akt signalling pathway and cancer. *Cancer Treatment Reviews*, 2004. **30**(2): p. 193–204.
90. Toker, A. and L.C. Cantley, Signalling through the lipid products of phosphoinositide-3-OH kinase. *Nature*, 1997. **387**(6634): p. 673–676.
91. Sarbassov, D.D., et al., Phosphorylation and regulation of Akt/PKB by the rictor-mTOR complex. *Science*, 2005. **307**(5712): p. 1098–1101.
92. Osborne, C.K., et al., Estrogen receptor: current understanding of its activation and modulation. *Clinical Cancer Research*, 2001. **7**(12): p. 4338s–4342s.
93. Mir, M.A., et al., Proteomics: A Groundbreaking Development in Cancer Biology, in *Proteomics*. 2023, Elsevier. p. 31–53.
94. McKenna, N.J., R.B. Lanz, and B.W. O'Malley, Nuclear receptor coregulators: cellular and molecular biology. *Endocrine Reviews*, 1999. **20**(3): p. 321–344.
95. Mir, M.A., N. Jan, and H. Qayoom, Conventional Chemotherapy vs. Metronomic Chemotherapy, in *Novel Approaches in Metronomic Chemotherapy for Breast Cancer Treatment*. CRC Press. p. 27–42.
96. Kushner, P.J., et al., Estrogen receptor pathways to AP-1. *The Journal of Steroid Biochemistry and Molecular Biology*, 2000. **74**(5): p. 311–317.
97. Mir, M.A., A. Manzoor, and N. Jan, CCL5/CCR5 Axis in Cancer, in *Cytokine and Chemokine Networks in Cancer*. 2023, Springer. p. 219–240.
98. Rosenberg, S.A., et al., Durable complete responses in heavily pretreated patients with metastatic melanoma using T-cell transfer immunotherapy. *Clinical Cancer Research*, 2011. **17**(13): p. 4550–4557.
99. Bykov, V.J., et al., Restoration of the tumor suppressor function to mutant p53 by a low-molecular-weight compound. *Nature Medicine*, 2002. **8**(3): p. 282–288.
100. Alexandrova, E.M., et al., Improving survival by exploiting tumour dependence on stabilized mutant p53 for treatment. *Nature*, 2015. **523**(7560): p. 352–356.
101. Parrales, A., et al., DNAJA1 controls the fate of misfolded mutant p53 through the mevalonate pathway. *Nature Cell Biology*, 2016. **18**(11): p. 1233–1243.
102. Harada, N., et al., Identification of a checkpoint modulator with synthetic lethality to p53 mutants. *Anti-Cancer Drugs*, 2011. **22**(10): p. 986–994.
103. Hirai, H., et al., Small-molecule inhibition of Wee1 kinase by MK-1775 selectively sensitizes p53-deficient tumor cells to DNA-damaging agents. *Molecular Cancer Therapeutics*, 2009. **8**(11): p. 2992–3000.
104. Reaper, P.M., et al., Selective killing of ATM-or p53-deficient cancer cells through inhibition of ATR. *Nature Chemical Biology*, 2011. **7**(7): p. 428–430.
105. Origanti, S., et al., Synthetic lethality of Chk1 inhibition combined with p53 and/or p21 loss during a DNA damage response in normal and tumor cells. *Oncogene*, 2013. **32**(5): p. 577–588.
106. Floquet, C., et al., Rescue of non-sense mutated p53 tumor suppressor gene by aminoglycosides. *Nucleic Acids Research*, 2011. **39**(8): p. 3350–3362.
107. Zhang, M., et al., Synergistic rescue of nonsense mutant tumor suppressor p53 by combination treatment with aminoglycosides and Mdm2 inhibitors. *Frontiers in Oncology*, 2018. **7**: p. 323.
108. Parrales, A., E. Thoenen, and T. Iwakuma, The interplay between mutant p53 and the mevalonate pathway. *Cell Death & Differentiation*, 2018. **25**(3): p. 460–470.
109. Zhou, Z., et al., *A Hippo's View: From Molecular Basis to Translational Medicine*. 2021, Frontiers Media SA. p. 729155.
110. Manfredi, J.J., Mdm2 and MdmX: partners in p53 destruction. *Cancer Research*, 2021. **81**(7): p. 1633–1634.
111. Kussie, P.H., et al., Structure of the MDM2 oncoprotein bound to the p53 tumor suppressor transactivation domain. *Science*, 1996. **274**(5289): p. 948–953.
112. Freedman, D., L. Wu, and A. Levine, Functions of the MDM2 oncoprotein. *Cellular and Molecular Life Sciences CMLS*, 1999. **55**: p. 96–107.
113. Deng, L., et al., The role of ubiquitination in tumorigenesis and targeted drug discovery. *Signal Transduction and Targeted Therapy*, 2020. **5**(1): p. 11.
114. Linke, K., et al., Structure of the MDM2/MDMX RING domain heterodimer reveals dimerization is required for their ubiquitylation in trans. *Cell Death & Differentiation*, 2008. **15**(5): p. 841–848.
115. Iyappan, S., et al., Turning the RING domain protein MdmX into an active ubiquitin-protein ligase. *Journal of Biological Chemistry*, 2010. **285**(43): p. 33065–33072.
116. Wade, M., Y.V. Wang, and G.M. Wahl, The p53 orchestra: Mdm2 and Mdmx set the tone. *Trends in Cell Biology*, 2010. **20**(5): p. 299–309.

117. Bhattacharya, S., et al., Emerging insights into HAUSP (USP7) in physiology, cancer and other diseases. *Signal Transduction and Targeted Therapy*, 2018. **3**(1): p. 17.
118. Bykov, V.J., et al., Reactivation of mutant p53 and induction of apoptosis in human tumor cells by maleimide analogs. *Journal of Biological Chemistry*, 2005. **280**(34): p. 30384–30391.
119. Nikolova, P.V., et al., Mechanism of rescue of common p53 cancer mutations by second-site suppressor mutations. *The EMBO Journal*, 2000. https://doi.org/10.1093/emboj/19.3.370
120. Liu, W.-L., et al., Biological significance of a small highly conserved region in the N terminus of the p53 tumour suppressor protein. *Journal of Molecular Biology*, 2001. **313**(4): p. 711–731.
121. Parrales, A. and T. Iwakuma, Targeting oncogenic mutant p53 for cancer therapy. *Frontiers in Oncology*, 2015. **5**: p. 288.
122. Foster, B.A., et al., Pharmacological rescue of mutant p53 conformation and function. *Science*, 1999. **286**(5449): p. 2507–2510.
123. El-Deiry, W.S., Targeting mutant p53 shows promise for sunscreens and skin cancer. *The Journal of Clinical Investigation*, 2007. **117**(12): p. 3658–3660.
124. Akkiprik, M., et al., Analysis of p53 gene polymorphisms and protein over-expression in patients with breast cancer. *Pathology & Oncology Research*, 2009. **15**: p. 359–368.
125. Chiurillo, M.A., et al., Distribution of GSTM1, GSTT1, GSTP1 and TP53 disease-associated gene variants in native and urban Venezuelan populations. *Gene*, 2013. **531**(1): p. 106–111.
126. Faghani, M., et al., TP53 PIN3 polymorphism associated with breast cancer risk in Iranian women. *Indian Journal of Cancer*, 2011. **48**(3): p. 298–302.
127. Duffy, M.J., et al., p53 as a target for the treatment of cancer. *Cancer Treatment Reviews*, 2014. **40**(10): p. 1153–1160.
128. Levine, A.J., p53, the cellular gatekeeper for growth and division. *Cell*, 1997. **88**(3): p. 323–331.
129. Burgess, A., et al., Clinical overview of MDM2/X-targeted therapies. *Frontiers in Oncology*, 2016. **6**: p. 7.
130. Jiang, M., et al., p21/waf1/cip1 and mdm-2 expression in breast carcinoma patients as related to prognosis. *International Journal of Cancer*, 1997. **74**(5): p. 529–534.
131. Turbin, D.A., et al., MDM2 protein expression is a negative prognostic marker in breast carcinoma. *Modern Pathology*, 2006. **19**(1): p. 69–74.
132. Wang, Z. and Y. Sun, Targeting p53 for novel anticancer therapy. *Translational Oncology*, 2010. **3**(1): p. 1–12.
133. Shangary, S., et al., Temporal activation of p53 by a specific MDM2 inhibitor is selectively toxic to tumors and leads to complete tumor growth inhibition. *Proceedings of the National Academy of Sciences*, 2008. **105**(10): p. 3933–3938.
134. Chen, X., et al., Mutant p53 in cancer: from molecular mechanism to therapeutic modulation. *Cell Death & Disease*, 2022. **13**(11): p. 974.
135. Mir, M.A., N. Jan, and I. Noor, Therapeutic Implications of Cytokines and Chemokines Network in Cancer, in *Cytokine and Chemokine Networks in Cancer*. 2023, Springer. p. 385–414.
136. Shostak, K., et al., MDM2 restrains estrogen-mediated AKT activation by promoting TBK1-dependent HPIP degradation. *Cell Death & Differentiation*, 2014. **21**(5): p. 811–824.

3 p53 Pathways in the Progression of Breast Cancer

Ibtisam Mumtaz[1], Arfa Ji[2], Subzar Ah Ganaie[1], Faizan Shakeel[3], Adil Jameel Var[4], and Manzoor Ahmad Mir[5]*

[1]Department of Nanotechnology, University of Kashmir
[2]Department of Biotechnology, University of Kashmir Srinagar
[3]Max Smart Super Specialty Hospital, Saket, New Delhi,
[4]Department of Chemistry, University of Delhi,
[5]Department of Bioresources, School of Biological Sciences, University of Kashmir, Srinagar, J&K, India
*drmanzoor@kashmiruniversity.ac.in

3.1 INTRODUCTION

Various biochemical pathways contribute to the intricate progression of breast cancer, but one pivotal controller stands out: the TP53 gene pathway [1, 2]. Sometimes called the "guardian of the genome," the TP53 gene is an essential tumor suppressor that is essential for preserving the integrity of the genome and preventing aberrant cell division. Genetic mutations in the setting of breast cancer, especially those that occur within the TP53 gene, are crucial in causing the malignant transformation of breast tissue [3, 4]. Since TP53 mutations are the most common genetic abnormalities found in many types of cancers, including breast cancer, occurring in up to 50% of cases, their significance in breast cancer is undeniable [5]. These mutations disrupt vital cellular functions that are necessary for preserving tissue homeostasis by impairing TP53's normal function. Significantly, it has been suggested that the pathophysiology of breast cancer is significantly influenced by the decrease of wild-type TP53 function [6]. The protein product that the TP53 gene codes for consists of multiple unique domains, each of which has a distinct function at the molecular level. These consist of the C-terminal negative regulatory domain [7], the tetramerization domain, the central DNA binding domain, and the N-terminal transactivation domain. Notably, mutations in the DNA binding domain are more prevalent in human malignancies, impacting TP53's capacity to interact in a sequence-specific way with genomic DNA. The transcription factor function of TP53, which controls the expression of target genes involved in cell cycle regulation and tumor suppression, depends critically on this interaction [8, 9]. Mdm-2 and p21 are two important target genes among the many that TP53 regulates [10–12]. As a crucial negative regulator of TP53, Mdm-2, which is encoded by the mdm-2 gene, limits its biological activity and directs it toward destruction [13, 14]. On the other hand, p21, sometimes referred to as CDKN1A, functions as a mediator of TP53-dependent growth arrest by preventing cyclin-dependent kinase (CDK) complex activity, which stops cell cycle progression at the G1 phase [15]. Moreover, changes in protein structure brought about by TP53 gene mutations can enhance protein stability and accumulation in tumor cells [16, 17]. The extended existence of the mutant TP53 protein is in contrast to the short half-life of the wild-type TP53, which makes it detectable and potentially useful as a biomarker for the diagnosis and prognosis of cancer [18, 19]. Deciphering the complex functions of the TP53 pathway in the advancement of

DOI: 10.1201/9781003520771-3

breast cancer is essential to figuring out the fundamental causes of carcinogenesis and finding new treatment targets for the efficient treatment of this diverse illness.

3.2 FUNCTIONAL EFFECTS OF p53

3.2.1 DNA Repair

As a tumor suppressor, p53 is essential for preserving the stability of the genome because it gives DNA repair systems enough time to remove damaged lesions before permitting cell division to start again [20]. It controls several DNA repair mechanisms, such as those that repair nucleotides, bases, and mismatches, as well as those that repair double-strand breaks in DNA by homologous recombination and non-homologous end joining [21, 22].

3.2.2 Cell Cycle Regulation

Cell cycle checkpoints are necessary to ensure that cells do not advance to the subsequent phase until the previous phase has been precisely finished. p53 is activated to regulate the G1-S and G2-M phase restriction points when DNA damage occurs. When p53 is activated, it synchronizes the transcriptional control of multiple important proteins, including p21, 14-3-3σ, Cdc25c, and GADD45, to cause cell cycle arrest [23]. It primarily causes G1 arrest by activating p21, which prevents retinoblastoma (Rb) from being hyperphosphorylated and stops E2F-mediated transcription of cell cycle genes that are essential for the G1 to S phase transition. Furthermore, p53 prevents the advancement of G2/M by upregulating the expression of 14-3-3σ, which impairs the activity of cyclin B1/cdc2 in response to DNA damage [24].

3.2.3 Apoptosis

Several research works have shown how important p53 is in starting apoptosis. p53 controls both the internal and extrinsic apoptotic mechanisms, which spread apoptosis. When cell death receptors such as Fas, Death Receptor 5, and TRAIL death-domain containing receptor are expressed in the extrinsic route, it is p53 that causes the development of the Death-inducing signaling complex and the subsequent activation of caspases, such as caspase-8 and caspase-3 [25]. Concurrently, the intrinsic pathway involves the activation of proapoptotic Bcl2 family genes by p53, including BAX, Noxa, PUMA, and BID. This process facilitates the release of cytochrome c and the activation of caspase 9 via BAX multimerization [26–30].

3.2.4 Senescence

Senescence can be brought on by a variety of cellular stressors and is characterized by an irreversible cell cycle stop. When senescence is triggered, the Rb pathway is initiated through p53's activation by ATM/ATR or Chk1/2 proteins, which then activate p21 [31]. Crucially, nevertheless, it should be remembered that stressor doses, timing, and intensity thresholds can dictate whether a cell experiences apoptosis or senescence [32, 33] (Figure 3.1).

3.3 p53 AND CANCER PROGRESSION

Approximately 50% of human malignancies including breast, colon, lung, liver, prostate, bladder, and skin are known to have TP53 gene mutations. The wild-type p53 prevents the spread of defective DNA and the start of malignant features by acting to stop cell replication when DNA damage occurs and waiting for the damage to be repaired. On the other hand, TP53 mutations cause the cell

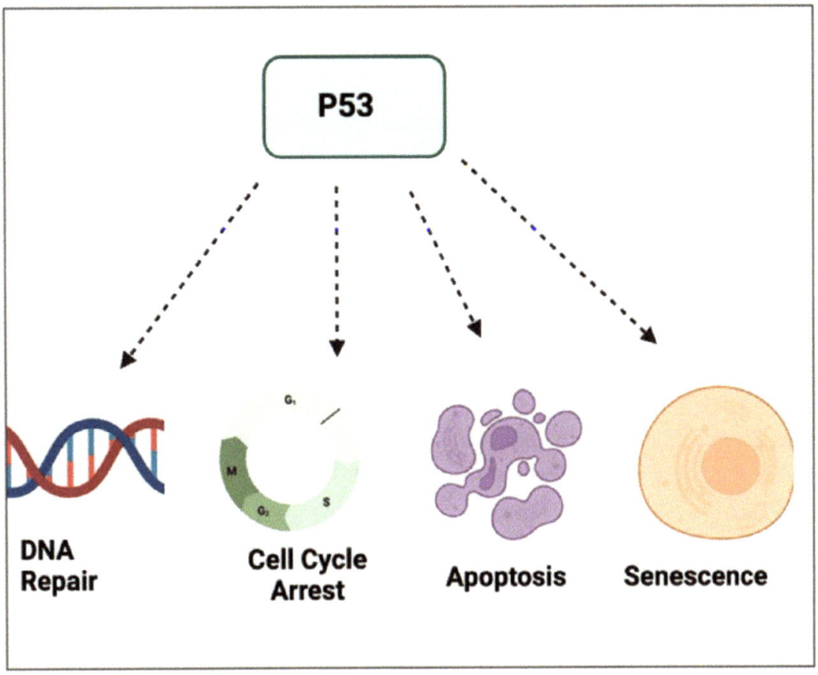

FIGURE 3.1 Functional effects of p53.

cycle to be disrupted, which results in a loss of control over the proliferation of cells and permits damaged DNA to be passed down to the next cell generations, which in turn causes cancer. The p53 proteins that are produced by a healthy TP53 gene are transcription factors that are essential for coordinating several cellular responses, such as DNA repair, cell cycle arrest, senescence, death, differentiation, and metabolism. Together, these actions prevent the spread of cancer, preserving genomic integrity and gaining p53 the title "guardian of the genome." While the accumulation of non-functionally altered p53 in tumor cell nuclei is associated with the start and/or progression of several malignant illnesses, including breast cancer, nuclear p53 phosphoprotein regulates normal cell proliferation [34–37].

Under extreme oncogenic stress, p53 activation initiates cellular senescence and cell cycle arrest, which is an essential strategy to prevent carcinogenesis. Key signaling nodes involved in the control of mTOR kinase are often the site of convergence of oncogenic signals. Disabling the p53/p21 CDK-interacting protein 1 (Cipl) complex through Ras-dependent and Ras-independent activation of the Raf/MEK/ERK cascade promotes cell growth. These results highlight the importance of p53 inactivation and Ras oncogenic activity in human cancer [38–40]. Furthermore, the G2/M phase, apoptosis, and cell proliferation are among the biological processes that are influenced by the p53/p21/p27 and p53/Bcl-2/Bax pathways. The recruitment or control of additional tumor suppressor proteins, such as the inter-alpha-trypsin inhibitor heavy chain 5 protein produced by the ITIH5 gene, may also be a mechanism by which p53 carries out its tumor-suppressive activity. The promoter of ITIH5 in melanoma cells is directly bound by p53, which stimulates ITIH5 transcription and, as a result, inhibits melanoma cell migration and proliferation. This is probably achieved by modifying KLF4 transcriptional activity [41, 42]. Moreover, ZEB1 and ZEB2 transcription factors stimulate the epithelial–mesenchymal transition (EMT), whereas p53 suppresses the expression of ZEB1 and ZEB2 to prevent EMT. These complex interactions highlight the varied functions of the p53 pathway in regulating different cellular processes linked to the advancement of cancer [43, 44].

3.4 MUTANT p53 CONTRIBUTES TO THE PROGRESSION OF CANCER

3.4.1 Promotion of Genetic Instability

Wild-type p53, which is frequently referred to as the "guardian of the genome," is essential for preserving genetic stability in breast cancer because it stops mutations from spreading to daughter cells [45, 46]. The ability of p53-deficient cells to repair DNA damage is still there, but the cells' increased levels of genomic instability—such as chromosomal translocations and aneuploidy—contribute to the advancement of breast cancer [47–49]. The way that typical p53 mutations work is that they interfere with the recruitment of the Mre11/Rad50/NBS1 complex, which in turn causes the ATM sensor to become inactive and the G2/M checkpoint to be impaired [50]. This process interferes with the first response to DNA double-strand breaks and promotes the development of breast cancer. Furthermore, by disrupting the processes involved in DNA replication, mutant p53 can cause genomic anomalies. The replication of aberrant genomic DNA is promoted, and breast cancer progression is exacerbated when, for example, certain mutant p53 proteins activate cyclin A to aid in the creation of DNA replication origins and CHK1 to stabilize replication forks [51].

3.4.2 Accelerating Proliferation

An increasing amount of data points to the role of mutant p53 in facilitating two essential aspects of cancer development: the unbridled capacity for replication and the insensitivity to signals that impede growth [52, 53]. Mutant p53 physically interacts with nuclear transcription factor Y (NF-Y), a fundamental regulator of the cell cycle, and recruits YAP, a crucial component of the Hippo pathway, or acetyltransferase p300 to activate NF-Y target genes, including cyclin A, cyclin B, cdk1, and cdc25C [54, 55]. A transcriptional complex that includes mutant p53, YAP, and TEAD also promotes the expression of circular RNA circPVT1, which in turn activates genes linked to proliferation including mki67 and AURKA [56]. Additionally, microRNA miR-27a, which maintains the activation of ERK1/2 in response to EGF and encourages cellular proliferation and carcinogenesis, is expressed under the control of mutated p53 [57]. Additionally, significant chromatin regulators including MLL1, MLL2, and MOZ are targeted by p53 mutants, which results in a broad increase in active histone modifications that promote proliferation [58]. Furthermore, the TP53 R249S mutation, which is frequently detected in HBV-positive hepatocellular carcinoma, plays a special function in controlling the growth and viability of cancer cells by encouraging c-Myc-dependent rDNA transcription, which is essential for ribosomal biogenesis [59].

3.4.3 Influencing Metabolism

Cell viability depends on the metabolism of glucose, lipids, and nucleotides, which are all altered significantly during cancer growth. Recent research has shown that certain facets of these processes are mediated by mutant p53 proteins [60, 61]. The Warburg effect describes how tumor cells, which proliferate quickly, mainly depend on aerobic glycolysis to meet their high energy and biosynthetic requirements [62]. It has been demonstrated that mutant p53 activates RhoA and its downstream effector ROCK, facilitating GLUT1 translocation to the cell membrane and boosting the rate at which glucose is absorbed and glycolyzed [63]. Mutant p53 preferentially binds to the AMPK alpha subunit when energy is scarce, blocking AMPK signaling's metabolic processes and causing increased aerobic glycolysis and lipid synthesis [64]. Interestingly, the mevalonate pathway—which is in charge of cholesterol synthesis and the generation of significant derivatives of nonsterol isoprenoid—is involved in the promotion of lipid metabolism by mutant p53. Through its association with the master transcription factor SREBP1/SREBP2, mutant p53 is attracted to the promoters of many genes involved in the mevalonate pathway, thereby stimulating their expression [28, 65, 66]. Additionally, the STAT3-mevalonate pathway axis and the mevalonate pathway-DNAJA1 axis block CHIP ubiquitin ligase's ability to degrade mutant p53, creating a positive feedback loop that guarantees quick lipid synthesis [67, 68]. Additionally, through their interaction with ETS2, mutant p53 proteins activate a large number of genes involved in the de novo and salvage pathways necessary for nucleotide synthesis. As a result, GTPase activity is raised and nucleotide pools are expanded. These results collectively highlight the part that mutant p53 plays in the metabolic reprogramming of cancer cells [69, 70].

3.4.4 Metastasis

Most cancer-related deaths are caused by metastasis, a critical component of cancer growth [71, 72]. The first stage of metastasis is called EMT, which allows cells to change morphologically and become more migratory and invasive. Important EMT-related transcription factors including ZEB1, SLUG, and TWIST1 have been demonstrated to be upregulated in expression by mutant p53 via a variety of processes that may vary depending on the type of cell [73–75]. For example, mutant p53 lowers miR-130b, which negatively controls ZEB1, in endometrial cancer [76]; in non-small-cell lung malignancies (NSCLCs), it inhibits MDM2-mediated SLUG degradation, leading to increased SLUG and decreased E-cadherin expression [77]. Furthermore, mutant p53 lessens H3K27me3 repression on the TWIST1 promoter in prostate cells [78]. Moreover, data point to p63's function as an effector of mutant p53-mediated metastasis. In the presence of TGF-b signaling, mutant p53 phosphorylates Smad2 and forms a complex with p63, which inhibits the activation of p63 downstream metastasis suppressor genes [79]. ζ5ζ1-integrin and EGFR are more likely to be trafficked to the cell membrane by mutant p53, which also prevents p63-mediated inactivation of Rab-coupling protein (RCP). This constitutive activation of EGFR/integrin and pro-metastatic Akt signaling results from this [80, 81]. Furthermore, HSP90a production is increased by mutant p53 activation of RCP, which promotes cell motility through ECM interaction [82]. The metastasis caused by mutant p53 is also linked to metabolism reprogramming. Research employing a model of p53R172H/+ mice revealed that the interaction between mutant p53 and ETS2 results in the production of Pla2g16, which facilitates migration and metastasis by catalyzing the conversion of phosphatidic acid into lysophosphatidic acid and free fatty acid [83–85]. Furthermore, the Pro72Arg polymorphism in mutant p53 regulates PGC-1a target genes involved in mitochondrial biogenesis and oxidative phosphorylation, which increases tumor migration and metastasis [86, 87].

3.4.5 Fostering a Cancer-Promoting Microenvironment

It is now understood that the extracellular matrix (ECM), stromal cells, immune cells, and blood vessels, as well as the tumor microenvironment, have an impact on both the course of the tumor and its reaction to therapy. By encouraging angiogenesis and triggering the release of pro-inflammatory cytokines, mutant p53 can change the tumor microenvironment [59, 88, 89]. By downregulating TIMP3 transcription, some mutant p53 variants, including p53R248W and D281G, increase the activity of matrix metalloproteinases (MMPs) and cause enhanced ECM breakdown and metastasis [90, 91]. Additionally, it has been demonstrated that mutant p53 forms complexes with HIF1, which causes the overexpression of ECM elements including collagen and laminin, and accelerates the growth of tumors [92]. Moreover, the NF-kB pathway, a master regulator of inflammation, and mutant p53 exhibit substantial interaction that affects tumor formation and migration by upregulating genes linked to inflammation, cancer, and extracellular matrix remodeling. Furthermore, mutant p53 promotes tumor neo-angiogenesis, another characteristic of cancer, by upregulating the production of pro-angiogenic proteins, such as IL-8, GRO-a, and VEGF [93, 94] (Figure 3.2).

3.5 UNDERSTANDING THE MULTIFACETED MECHANISMS OF p53 INACTIVATION IN HUMAN CANCERS

Around 50% of all cases of human malignancies include p53 common gene mutations. These mutations—especially missense mutations—often result in the protein losing its capacity to bind to particular DNA sequences and activate genes, two essential activities of the p53 protein in its wild-type

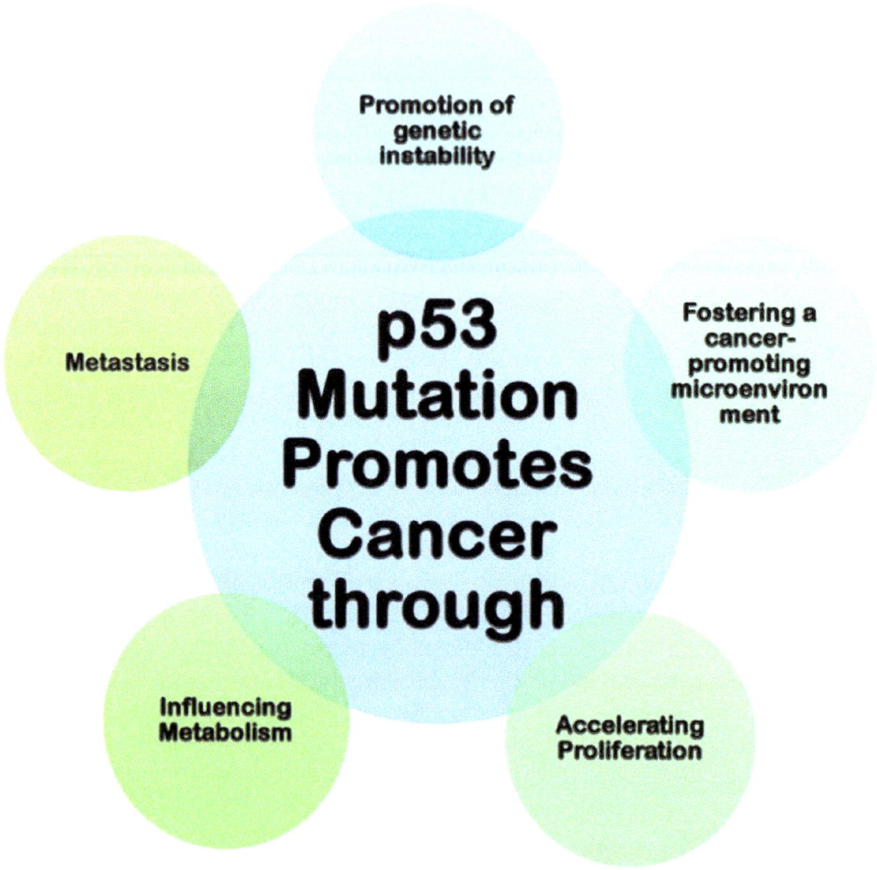

FIGURE 3.2 Different mechanisms by which mutant p53 contributes to cancer progression.

form [95]. When compared to other tumor suppressor genes, p53 has an interestingly greater prevalence of missense mutations, indicating that the production of mutant p53 may have benefits beyond merely losing its wild-type function [96].

The function of p53 can be affected by various methods in many cases of malignancies that do not include p53 mutations. For example, in malignancies linked to viruses, interactions with viral proteins may result in the sequestration or enhanced degradation of p53. Furthermore, p53 is actively degraded by the protein MDM2, whereas p14ARF stabilizes p53 by blocking its interaction with MDM2. p53 may be incorrectly degraded if p14ARF is lost, either by deletion or epigenetic silencing or by overexpressing MDM2. The sequestration of p53 in the cytoplasm, which stops it from localizing to the nucleus and thus reduces its activity, is another method [97, 98].

3.6 UNDERSTANDING p53 INACTIVATION MECHANISMS IN BREAST CANCER

Hereditary mutations in the p53 gene are prevalent among individuals diagnosed with the Li–Fraumeni cancer susceptibility syndrome, heightening the vulnerability to breast cancer [99]. This emphasizes the crucial role of p53 inactivation in breast cancer onset. Substantial research has delved into understanding the structure and activity of p53 in breast cancer, uncovering the presence of mutated p53 in breast cancer cell lines [100]. Loss of heterozygosity (LOH) in the p53 gene frequently occurs in primary breast carcinomas, often alongside mutation of the remaining allele. Unlike colon carcinomas, where the remaining p53 allele tends to be mutant, breast cancer cases with LOH retain a wild-type p53 allele in at least 60% of instances [101]. While p53 coding mutations are detected in breast cancer cases, they are not universally found, with comprehensive meta-analyses indicating that only about 20% of cases exhibit mutant p53 [102]. Efforts have been made to pinpoint the stage of breast tumor development where p53 mutation emerges, revealing that low-grade ductal carcinoma in situ (DCIS) typically lacks mutations, while high-grade DCIS exhibits higher mutation rates [103].

Although the overall prevalence of p53 mutation in breast cancer hovers around 20% [102], certain subtypes demonstrate elevated mutation rates. For example, breast cancers occurring in carriers of germ-line BRCA1 and BRCA2 mutations display heightened rates of p53 mutations, characterized by a distinct spectrum of mutations [104, 105]. Notably, medullary breast carcinomas consistently exhibit p53 mutation in all cases, aligning with the clinicopathological similarities shared with BRCA1-associated cases [106]. Methylation-driven suppression of BRCA1 expression is frequently observed in medullary breast cancers, further accentuating the intricate interplay between p53 and BRCA1 in breast cancer development [98, 107].

3.7 UPSTREAM REGULATOR MODIFICATIONS OF p53 IN BREAST CANCER

Besides BRCA1 and BRCA2, mutations in genes with lower penetrance may significantly contribute to hereditary breast cancer cases. ATM, associated with ataxia-telangiectasia (A-T), has been linked to p53 regulation, as defective p53 activation has been observed in A-T cells following irradiation [108]. Research indicates that ATM phosphorylates both p53 and BRCA1 in response to γ-irradiation. A-T patients, predisposed to various cancers including breast carcinomas, often carry heterozygous truncating mutations in ATM. Additionally, some breast cancer patients exhibit decreased or absent ATM expression, sometimes in conjunction with p53 mutations, suggesting simultaneous inactivation of these genes [109, 110]. Chk2, another protein implicated in transmitting DNA damage signals to p53, is activated by ATM and subsequently phosphorylates p53 [111]. Germ-line mutations in Chk2 have been detected in certain Li–Fraumeni families lacking p53 mutations, suggesting its potential as a tumor suppressor gene [112, 113]. While rare in families with hereditary breast cancer, diminished or lacking Chk2 expression is evident in a notable portion of sporadic breast cancer cases, irrespective of p53 status [114, 115]. In many breast cancers, the mRNA level of p53 is lower compared to normal breast epithelium. Aberrant methylation of the HoxA5 promoter reduces HoxA5 expression, which typically activates p53 transcription. This epigenetic silencing of HoxA5 limits basal p53 mRNA expression, representing a novel mechanism attenuating p53 signaling in breast cancer. Further investigation is needed to understand if other pathway components are similarly regulated [116, 117].

3.8 CHANGES IN p53 COFACTORS IN BREAST CANCER

Other than the phosphorylation-dependent modulation of p53 stability and activity by proteins like ATM, ATR, and Chk2, a new class of proteins is becoming apparent that enhances p53's inherent functions. Among them, breast cancer may be influenced by the apoptosis-stimulating protein of the p53 (ASPP) family, which includes ASPP1 and ASPP2m [118].

By intensifying the activation of apoptotic effectors such as PIG3 and Bax, ASPP1 and ASPP2 augment the pro-apoptotic activity of wild-type p53. The expression of ASPP1 and ASPP2 is frequently decreased in primary breast malignancies with functional p53, which may attenuate p53-driven apoptosis and give breast carcinomas a growth advantage [119]. BRCA1 is known to be a transcriptional coactivator of p53 and is significant in ovarian and breast cancer susceptibility. After DNA damage, BRCA1, which is phosphorylated by ATR, ATM, and Chk2, interacts with wild-type p53 to increase transcription from promoters that respond to p53 [120]. Despite the rarity of somatic mutations in BRCA1 in sporadic breast cancer, its expression is typically downregulated, which may hinder p53 action through methylation-dependent silencing mechanisms [121]. Histone acetyltransferase p300 catalyzes the acetylation of lysine residues in the C-terminus of p53, increasing its ability to activate transcription. In primary breast cancer samples and breast cancer cell lines, truncating mutations in p300 have been found occasionally in conjunction with p53 alterations. This implies that the selection pressure for p53 mutation is not always lessened by p300 mutation [122, 123].

3.9 ASSESSING p53 MUTATIONS AS DIAGNOSTIC MARKERS IN BREAST CANCER

Mutated p53 has become a useful diagnostic marker in the field of breast cancer, particularly in cases that are familial and associated with Li–Fraumeni syndrome [124, 125]. This condition manifests as a variety of malignancies, including brain, breast, adrenocortical, bone/soft tissue sarcomas, leukemia, and others [126, 127]. It is characterized by an autosomal dominant familial pattern. DNA collected from peripheral blood samples of family members can be analyzed, with a focus on specific "codons" or "hot spots," to identify p53 mutations linked to these tumors. Penetrance of the disease is predicted to be 50% by age 30 and 90% by age 60 [28, 128]. A significant fraction of these families exhibit p53 germ-line mutations [129] and new research suggests that the rate may be as high as 70% [130]. Despite the rarity of Li–Fraumeni families, p53 mutation identification is a useful diagnostic tool in clinical settings. Missense mutations, on the other hand, account for the majority of occurrences of sporadic breast cancer and result in altered p53 protein activity [48]. In contrast to many common epithelial cancers, only 15–35% of instances of breast cancer have unique p53 mutations; instead, abnormalities in the function of the p53 protein are more common [131, 132]. Table 3.1 and Table 3.2 depict the compounds and genes targeting mutant p53 tumors that have been tested in breast cancer models or patients.

TABLE 3.1

Compounds and Genes Targeting Mutant p53 Tumors That Have Been Tested in Breast Cancer Models or Patients

Compound/Gene	Mechanism of Action	Stage of Development	Reference
Synthetic Lethal Inhibitors			
THZ-P1-2	Disrupts cell energy metabolism required for mutant p53	Pre-clinical	[133]
Deoxyuridine analogues + PARP inhibitors	Arrest cells at G2 with induction of DNA damage	Pre-clinical	[134]
Roscovitine → Doxorubicin	Arrest cells at G2 with induction of DNA damage	Pre-clinical	[135]
MK-1775	Suppresses G2 arrest via Wee1 inhibition, leading to mitotic catastrophe	Up to Phase II clinical trial in breast cancer but not specifically developed against with mutant p53 tumors	[136]
Onvansertib	Loss of G2/M checkpoint control by PLK1 inhibition	Pre-clinical in breast cancer, up to Phase II clinical trial in other cancers but not specifically developed against mutant p53 tumors	[137]
Chk1 inhibitor (UCN-01, AZD7762)	Suppresses G2 arrest via Chk1 inhibition, leading to mitotic catastrophe	Up to Phase II clinical trial in breast cancer but not specifically developed against mutant p53 tumors	[138]

TABLE 3.2
Compounds and Genes Targeting Mutant p53 Tumors That Have Been Tested in Breast Cancer Models or Patients

Compound/Gene	Mechanism of Action	Stage of Development	Reference
Mutant p53 Reactivators			
PRIMA-1, APR-246	Michael addition: target cysteine residue to restore the DNA binding ability of p53 and prevent aggregation of mutant p53	Pre-clinical in breast cancer, up to Phase III clinical trial (APR-246 in combination with azacitidine) in myelodysplastic syndrome (NCT03745716)	[139]
PC14586	Binds to crevices of Y220C mutant, leading to increased thermal stability of DNA binding domain of p53 Y220	Phase I/II in advanced solid tumors, including breast cancer, with TP53 Y220C mutation (NCT04585750)	[140]
HBAP	Binds to DNA binding domain of p53 through hydroxyl group; restores transcriptional activity of wild-type p53	Pre-clinical	[141]
Spautin-1	Inhibits deubiquitinating proteins; promotes chaperone-mediated autophagy leading to lysosomal degradation of mutant p53	Pre-clinical	[142]
YK-3-237	Activates SIRT1 to reduce mutant p53 acetylation and its stability	Pre-clinical	[143]
THZ1	Inhibits CDK7, which is critical for mutant p53 expression	Pre-clinical	[144]
Disulfiram	Induces glutathionylation of p53, targeting it for proteasomal degradation	Phase II clinical trial with copper in breast cancer but not specifically developed against mutant p53 tumors	[145]
ZIF-8 (and Z1-RGD)	Zn^{2+} chelator; increased mutant p53 glutathionylation	Pre-clinical	[138]

3.10 THERAPEUTIC APPROACHES OF RESTORING p53 FUNCTION

3.10.1 Through Gene Therapy

The potential of gene therapy to restore p53 activity is becoming more and more obvious as our understanding of gene editing and viral vectors advances. This pathway may lead to the introduction of novel treatments for several cancers, including breast cancer, such as viral recombinant p53 gene transfer [146, 147]. Viral vectors such as adenovirus have been used to deliver a minigene encoding wild-type p53, which has been shown in vitro [148, 149] studies and in vivo [150, 151] animal models to be capable of inducing apoptosis and inhibiting tumor growth in breast cancer. More recently, studies have looked into augmenting therapeutic efficacy against a variety of cancer types, including breast cancer, by combining gene therapy with conventional systemic chemotherapy [152].

3.10.2 Releasing Active p53

The creation of drugs that target p53 reactivation via methods other than gene therapy is gaining popularity. Targeting tumors with functioning (wild-type) but inactive p53 is one area of concentration.

This strategy is based on the idea that p53 is coupled to other proteins in these tumors, like MDM-2 [10] or the molecular chaperone HSP90, both of which are important for the development and behavior of breast tumors. Efforts to break up the complex that these "p53 inactivating proteins" form have provided important information about how to treat this particular subtype of cancer [153].

3.10.3 Restoring p53 Function

Additional approaches to regaining p53 function center on enhancing its transcriptional and tumor-suppressive capacities, which depend on the p53 DNA binding domain's capacity to attach to particular DNA sequences. According to research, p53's DNA binding and tumor suppressor capabilities may be interfered with by post-translational changes of the p53 C-terminus [7, 154]. This has led to efforts being made to eliminate a negative regulatory domain located at the C-terminus of p53. Synthetic short peptides produced from the p53 C-terminus or antibodies targeting the C-terminus have been used to do this; both have been shown to induce a p53-dependent response in specific cell lines expressing mutant p53 [155]. As an alternative, it has been discovered that certain substances improve the stability of wild-type p53 and allow mutant p53 to maintain an active state by maintaining and stabilizing the DNA binding domain in an active conformation [156].

3.11 CONCLUSION

The TP53 gene pathway holds significant importance in the advancement of breast cancer, acting as a pivotal controller of genomic stability and cellular growth. Alterations in the TP53 gene impede its typical operation, resulting in the disturbance of critical cellular functions and fostering tumor development. Grasping the diverse functions of p53 in breast cancer, encompassing DNA repair, cell cycle management, apoptosis, and senescence, is essential for unraveling the underlying mechanisms of tumorigenesis and pinpointing prospective targets for therapy. Moreover, the intricate interplay between p53 and various cofactors, regulators, and upstream modifiers further highlights the complexity of p53 signaling in breast cancer development. From ASPP proteins to BRCA1 and p300, alterations in these molecules influence p53 function and contribute to tumor progression. Additionally, the diagnostic significance of p53 mutations, particularly in familial breast cancer cases, underscores the clinical relevance of understanding p53 biology. Therapeutically, restoring p53 function emerges as a promising strategy for combating breast cancer. Gene therapy approaches, along with novel drug development targeting p53 activation and inhibition of p53-inactivating proteins, offer potential avenues for restoring the tumor-suppressive functions of p53. Moreover, elucidating the mechanisms of p53 inactivation in breast cancer provides insights into personalized treatment strategies and the development of targeted therapies. Overall, a comprehensive understanding of the multifaceted mechanisms underlying p53 inactivation in breast cancer is essential for advancing our knowledge of tumor biology, improving diagnostic techniques, and developing effective therapeutic interventions to combat this heterogeneous disease.

REFERENCES

1. Bishop, J.M. and R.A. Weinberg, Scientific American molecular oncology. *(No Title)*, 1996.
2. Haq, B.U., et al., Targeting p53 misfolding conundrum by stabilizing agents and their analogs in breast cancer therapy: a comprehensive computational analysis. *Frontiers in Pharmacology*, 2024. **14**: p. 1333447.
3. Lane, D.P., p53, guardian of the genome. *Nature*, 1992. **358**(6381): p. 15–16.
4. Janus, F., et al., The dual role model for p53 in maintaining genomic integrity. *Cellular and Molecular Life Sciences CMLS*, 1999. **55**: p. 12–27.
5. Hollstein, M., et al., Database of p53 gene somatic mutations in human tumors and cell lines. *Nucleic Acids Research*, 1994. **22**(17): p. 3551.

6. Ball, H.M., et al., Differential p53 protein expression in breast cancer fine needle aspirates: the potential for in vivo monitoring. *British Journal of Cancer*, 2001. **85**(8): p. 1102–1105.
7. Hupp, T., Regulation of p53 protein function through alterations in protein-folding pathways. *Cellular and Molecular Life Sciences CMLS*, 1999. **55**: p. 88–95.
8. El-Deiry, W.S., et al., Definition of a consensus binding site for p53. *Nature Genetics*, 1992. **1**(1): p. 45–49.
9. Bourdon, J.-C., et al., Further characterisation of the p53 responsive element–identification of new candidate genes for trans-activation by p53. *Oncogene*, 1997. **14**(1): p. 85–94.
10. Bueso-Ramos, C.E., et al., Abnormal expression of MDM-2 in breast carcinomas. *Breast Cancer Research and Treatment*, 1996. **37**: p. 179–188.
11. Jiang, M., et al., p21/waf1/cip1 and mdm-2 expression in breast carcinoma patients as related to prognosis. *International Journal of Cancer*, 1997. **74**(5): p. 529–534.
12. Kato, Y., et al., Augmentation of lipopolysaccharide-induced thymocyte apoptosis by interferon-γ. *Cellular Immunology*, 1997. **177**(2): p. 103–108.
13. Barak, Y., et al., mdm2 expression is induced by wild type p53 activity. *The EMBO Journal*, 1993. **12**(2): p. 461–468.
14. Haupt, Y., et al., Mdm2 promotes the rapid degradation of p53. *Nature*, 1997. **387**(6630): p. 296–299.
15. Harper, J.W., et al., The p21 Cdk-interacting protein Cip1 is a potent inhibitor of G1 cyclin-dependent kinases. *Cell*, 1993. **75**(4): p. 805–816.
16. Siegel, J., et al., Enhanced p53 activity and accumulation in response to DNA damage upon DNA transfection. *Oncogene*, 1995. **11**(7): p. 1363–1370.
17. Lane, D., Exploiting the p53 pathway for cancer diagnosis and therapy. *British Journal of Cancer*, 1999. **80**.
18. Finlay, C., et al., Activating mutations for transformation by p53 produce a gene product that forms an hsc70-p53 complex with an altered half-life. *Molecular and Cellular Biology*, 1988. https://doi.org/10.1128/mcb.8.2.531-539.1988
19. Lane, D., On the expression of the p53 protein in human cancer. *Molecular Biology Reports*, 1994. **19**: p. 23–29.
20. Georgakilas, A.G., O.A. Martin, and W.M. Bonner, p21: a two-faced genome guardian. *Trends in Molecular Medicine*, 2017. **23**(4): p. 310–319.
21. Williams, A.B. and B. Schumacher, p53 in the DNA-damage-repair process. *Cold Spring Harbor Perspectives in Medicine*, 2016. **6**(5): p. a026070.
22. Mir, M.A., et al., Proteomics: A Groundbreaking Development in Cancer Biology, in *Proteomics*. 2023, Elsevier. p. 31–53.
23. Giono, L.E. and J.J. Manfredi, The p53 tumor suppressor participates in multiple cell cycle checkpoints. *Journal of Cellular Physiology*, 2006. **209**(1): p. 13–20.
24. Helton, E.S. and X. Chen, p53 modulation of the DNA damage response. *Journal of Cellular Biochemistry*, 2007. **100**(4): p. 883–896.
25. Clarke, A., et al., Thymocyte apoptosis induced by p53-dependent and independent pathways. *Nature*, 1993. **362**(6423): p. 849–852.
26. Lowe, C. and A. Masters, The long-time behaviour of the velocity autocorrelation function in a Lorentz gas. *Physica A: Statistical Mechanics and its Applications*, 1993. **195**(1–2): p. 149–162.
27. Mir, M.A., et al., Proteomics: Application of Next-Generation Proteomics in Cancer Research, in *Proteomics*. 2023, Elsevier. p. 55–76.
28. Jan, N., et al., Targeting breast cancer stem cells through retinoids: a new hope for treatment. *Critical Reviews in Oncology/Hematology*, 2023: p. 104156.
29. Mir, M.A., A. Shabir, and N. Jan, Metronomic Chemotherapy in Breast Cancer, in *Novel Approaches in Metronomic Chemotherapy for Breast Cancer Treatment*. 2024, CRC Press. p. 72–86.
30. Sofi, S., et al., Elucidation of interleukin-19 as a therapeutic target for breast cancer by computational analysis and experimental validation. *Saudi Journal of Biological Sciences*, 2023. **30**(9): p. 103774–103774.
31. Dolan, D.W., et al., Integrated stochastic model of DNA damage repair by non-homologous end joining and p53/p21-mediated early senescence signalling. *PLoS Computational Biology*, 2015. **11**(5): p. e1004246.
32. Riley, T., et al., Transcriptional control of human p53-regulated genes. *Nature Reviews Molecular Cell Biology*, 2008. **9**(5): p. 402–412.
33. Mir, M.A., N. Jan, and I. Noor, Therapeutic Implications of Cytokines and Chemokines Network in Cancer, in *Cytokine and Chemokine Networks in Cancer*. 2023, Springer. p. 385–414.

34. George, P., p53 how crucial is its role in cancer. *International Journal of Current Pharmaceutical Research*, 2011. **3**(2): p. 19–25.
35. Suh, Y. A., et al., Multiple stress signals activate mutant p53 in vivo. *Cancer Research*, 2011. **71**(23): p. 7168–7175.
36. Sofi, S., et al., A comprehensive analysis of notch signaling genes in breast cancer: expression pattern and prognostic significance. *Advances in Cancer Biology-Metastasis*, 2023. **7**: p. 100104.
37. Mir, M.A., N. Jan, and H. Qayoom, Conventional Chemotherapy vs. Metronomic Chemotherapy, in *Novel Approaches in Metronomic Chemotherapy for Breast Cancer Treatment*. 2024, CRC Press. p. 27–42.
38. Allred, D.C., et al., Association of p53 protein expression with tumor cell proliferation rate and clinical outcome in node-negative breast cancer. *JNCI: Journal of the National Cancer Institute*, 1993. **85**(3): p. 200–206.
39. Loayza-Puch, F., et al., p53 induces transcriptional and translational programs to suppress cell proliferation and growth. *Genome Biology*, 2013. **14**: p. 1–12.
40. Drosten, M., et al., Loss of p53 induces cell proliferation via Ras-independent activation of the Raf/Mek/Erk signaling pathway. *Proceedings of the National Academy of Sciences*, 2014. **111**(42): p. 15155–15160.
41. Qiu, L., et al., FKBP11 promotes cell proliferation and tumorigenesis via p53-related pathways in oral squamous cell carcinoma. *Biochemical and Biophysical Research Communications*, 2021. **559**: p. 183–190.
42. Liu, J., et al., ITIH5, a p53-responsive gene, inhibits the growth and metastasis of melanoma cells by downregulating the transcriptional activity of KLF4. *Cell Death & Disease*, 2021. **12**(5): p. 438.
43. Kim, T., et al., p53 regulates epithelial–mesenchymal transition through microRNAs targeting ZEB1 and ZEB2. *Journal of Experimental Medicine*, 2011. **208**(5): p. 875–883.
44. Mir, M.A., A. Manzoor, and N. Jan, CCL5/CCR5 Axis in Cancer, in *Cytokine and Chemokine Networks in Cancer*. 2023, Springer. p. 219–240.
45. Lane, D.P., p53, guardian of the genome. *Nature*, 1992. **358**(6381): p. 15–16.
46. Mir, M.A., M. Rashid, and N. Jan, Cytokines and Chemokines in Tumor Growth and Progression, in *Cytokine and Chemokine Networks in Cancer*. 2023, Springer. p. 33–77.
47. Levine, A.J., p53: 800 million years of evolution and 40 years of discovery. *Nature Reviews Cancer*, 2020. **20**(8): p. 471–480.
48. Hollstein, M., et al., p53 mutations in human cancers. *Science*, 1991. **253**(5015): p. 49–53.
49. Kandoth, C., et al., Mutational landscape and significance across 12 major cancer types. *Nature*, 2013. **502**(7471): p. 333–339.
50. Brosh, R. and V. Rotter, When mutants gain new powers: news from the mutant p53 field. *Nature Reviews Cancer*, 2009. **9**(10): p. 701–713.
51. Raj, N. and L.D. Attardi, The transactivation domains of the p53 protein. *Cold Spring Harbor Perspectives in Medicine*, 2017. **7**(1): p. a026047.
52. Levine, A.J., N.A. Jenkins, and N.G. Copeland, The roles of initiating truncal mutations in human cancers: the order of mutations and tumor cell type matters. *Cancer Cell*, 2019. **35**(1): p. 10–15.
53. Song, H., M. Hollstein, and Y. Xu, p53 gain-of-function cancer mutants induce genetic instability by inactivating ATM. *Nature Cell Biology*, 2007. **9**(5): p. 573–580.
54. Amelio, I. and G. Melino, Context is everything: extrinsic signalling and gain-of-function p53 mutants. *Cell Death Discovery*, 2020. **6**(1): p. 16.
55. D'Orazi, G. and M. Cirone, Mutant p53 and cellular stress pathways: A criminal alliance that promotes cancer progression. *Cancers*, 2019. **11**(5): p. 614.
56. Liu, D., H. Song, and Y. Xu, A common gain of function of p53 cancer mutants in inducing genetic instability. *Oncogene*, 2010. **29**(7): p. 949–956.
57. Hanel, W. and U.M. Moll, Links between mutant p53 and genomic instability. *Journal of Cellular Biochemistry*, 2012. **113**(2): p. 433–439.
58. Singh, S., et al., Mutant p53 establishes targetable tumor dependency by promoting unscheduled replication. *The Journal of Clinical Investigation*, 2017. **127**(5): p. 1839–1855.
59. Hanahan, D. and R.A. Weinberg, The hallmarks of cancer. *Cell*, 2000. **100**(1): p. 57–70.
60. Hanahan, D. and R.A. Weinberg, Hallmarks of cancer: the next generation. *Cell*, 2011. **144**(5): p. 646–674.
61. Di Agostino, S., et al., Gain of function of mutant p53: the mutant p53/NF-Y protein complex reveals an aberrant transcriptional mechanism of cell cycle regulation. *Cancer Cell*, 2006. **10**(3): p. 191–202.

62. Di Agostino, S., et al., YAP enhances the pro-proliferative transcriptional activity of mutant p53 proteins. *EMBO Reports*, 2016. **17**(2): p. 188–201.
63. Verduci, L., et al., The oncogenic role of circPVT1 in head and neck squamous cell carcinoma is mediated through the mutant p53/YAP/TEAD transcription-competent complex. *Genome Biology*, 2017. **18**: p. 1–24.
64. Wang, W., et al., Mutant p53-R273H gains new function in sustained activation of EGFR signaling via suppressing miR-27a expression. *Cell Death & Disease*, 2013. **4**(4): p. e574–e574.
65. Zhu, J., et al., Gain-of-function p53 mutants co-opt chromatin pathways to drive cancer growth. *Nature*, 2015. **525**(7568): p. 206–211.
66. Jan, N., et al., Exploring the role of trifarotene against RAR-α: an investigation of expression pattern and clinicopathological significance of RAR-α in breast cancer. *Frontiers in Pharmacology*, 2024. **15**: p. 1361679.
67. Liao, P., et al., Mutant p53 gains its function via c-Myc activation upon CDK4 phosphorylation at serine 249 and consequent PIN1 binding. *Molecular Cell*, 2017. **68**(6): p. 1134–1146.e6.
68. Eriksson, M., et al., Effect of mutant p53 proteins on glycolysis and mitochondrial metabolism. *Molecular and Cellular Biology*, 2017. **37**: p. e00328.
69. Liu, J., et al., Tumor suppressor p53 and metabolism. *Journal of Molecular Cell Biology*, 2019. **11**(4): p. 284–292.
70. Vana, A.C., et al., Arachidonyl trifluoromethyl ketone ameliorates experimental autoimmune encephalomyelitis via blocking peroxynitrite formation in mouse spinal cord white matter. *Experimental Neurology*, 2011. **231**(1): p. 45–55.
71. Zhang, C., et al., Tumour-associated mutant p53 drives the Warburg effect. *Nature Communications*, 2013. **4**(1): p. 2935.
72. Zhou, G., et al., Gain-of-function mutant p53 promotes cell growth and cancer cell metabolism via inhibition of AMPK activation. *Molecular Cell*, 2014. **54**(6): p. 960–974.
73. Freed-Pastor, W.A., et al., Mutant p53 disrupts mammary tissue architecture via the mevalonate pathway. *Cell*, 2012. **148**(1): p. 244–258.
74. Parrales, A., et al., DNAJA1 controls the fate of misfolded mutant p53 through the mevalonate pathway. *Nature Cell Biology*, 2016. **18**(11): p. 1233–1243.
75. Romeo, M.A., et al., STAT3 and mutp53 engage a positive feedback loop involving HSP90 and the mevalonate pathway. *Frontiers in Oncology*, 2020. **10**: p. 1102.
76. Kollareddy, M., et al., Regulation of nucleotide metabolism by mutant p53 contributes to its gain-of-function activities. *Nature Communications*, 2015. **6**(1): p. 7389.
77. Schneider, G., et al., Tissue-specific tumorigenesis: context matters. *Nature Reviews Cancer*, 2017. **17**(4): p. 239–253.
78. Gupta, G.P. and J. Massagué, Cancer metastasis: building a framework. *Cell*, 2006. **127**(4): p. 679–695.
79. Dong, P., et al., Mutant p53 gain-of-function induces epithelial–mesenchymal transition through modulation of the miR-130b–ZEB1 axis. *Oncogene*, 2013. **32**(27): p. 3286–3295.
80. Wang, S.-P., et al., p53 controls cancer cell invasion by inducing the MDM2-mediated degradation of Slug. *Nature Cell Biology*, 2009. **11**(6): p. 694–704.
81. Kogan-Sakin, I., et al., Mutant p53R175H upregulates Twist1 expression and promotes epithelial–mesenchymal transition in immortalized prostate cells. *Cell Death & Differentiation*, 2011. **18**(2): p. 271–281.
82. Adorno, M., et al., A mutant-p53/Smad complex opposes p63 to empower TGFβ-induced metastasis. *Cell*, 2009. **137**(1): p. 87–98.
83. Selivanova, G. and J. Ivaska, Integrins and mutant p53 on the road to metastasis. *Cell*, 2009. **139**(7): p. 1220–1222.
84. Muller, P.A., et al., Mutant p53 drives invasion by promoting integrin recycling. *Cell*, 2009. **139**(7): p. 1327–1341.
85. Zhang, S., et al., Mutant p53 drives cancer metastasis via RCP-mediated Hsp90α secretion. *Cell Reports*, 2020. **32**(1): p. 107879.
86. Xiong, S., et al., Pla2g16 phospholipase mediates gain-of-function activities of mutant p53. *Proceedings of the National Academy of Sciences*, 2014. **111**(30): p. 11145–11150.
87. Mills, G.B. and W.H. Moolenaar, The emerging role of lysophosphatidic acid in cancer. *Nature Reviews Cancer*, 2003. **3**(8): p. 582–591.
88. Stein, Y., R. Aloni-Grinstein, and V. Rotter, Mutant p53—a potential player in shaping the tumor–stroma crosstalk. *Journal of Molecular Cell Biology*, 2019. **11**(7): p. 600–604.

89. Cordani, M., et al., Mutant p53 proteins alter cancer cell secretome and tumour microenvironment: Involvement in cancer invasion and metastasis. *Cancer Letters*, 2016. **376**(2): p. 303–309.
90. Loging, W.T. and D. Reisman, Inhibition of the putative tumor suppressor gene TIMP-3 by tumor-derived p53 mutants and wild type p53. *Oncogene*, 1999. **18**(52): p. 7608–7615
91. Jan, N., et al., Metronomic chemotherapy and drug repurposing: a paradigm shift in oncology. *Heliyon*, 2024..
92. Rahnamoun, H., et al., Mutant p53 shapes the enhancer landscape of cancer cells in response to chronic immune signaling. *Nature Communications*, 2017. **8**(1): p. 754.
93. Kieser, A., et al., Mutant p53 potentiates protein kinase C induction of vascular endothelial growth factor expression. *Oncogene*, 1994. **9**(3): p. 963–970
94. Mir, M.A., M. Bashir, and N. Jan, The Role of Interleukin (IL)-6/IL-6 Receptor Axis in Cancer, in *Cytokine and Chemokine Networks in Cancer*. 2023, Springer. p. 137–164.
95. Vogelstein, B., D. Lane, and A.J. Levine, Surfing the p53 network. *Nature*, 2000. **408**(6810): p. 307–310.
96. Sigal, A. and V. Rotter, Oncogenic mutations of the p53 tumor suppressor: the demons of the guardian of the genome. *Cancer Research*, 2000. **60**(24): p. 6788–6793.
97. Hussain, S.P. and C.C. Harris, Molecular epidemiology and carcinogenesis: endogenous and exogenous carcinogens. *Mutation Research/Reviews in Mutation Research*, 2000. **462**(2–3): p. 311–322.
98. Mir, M.A., et al., Metronomics: toward personalized chemotherapy. *Novel Approaches in Metronomic Chemotherapy for Breast Cancer Treatment*, 2024. p. 99–119. https://doi.org/10.1201/9781032632674-8
99. Malkin, D., et al., Germ line p53 mutations in a familial syndrome of breast cancer, sarcomas, and other neoplasms. *Science*, 1990. **250**(4985): p. 1233–1238.
100. Bartek, J., et al., Genetic and immunochemical analysis of mutant p53 in human breast cancer cell lines. *Oncogene*, 1990. **5**(6): p. 893–899.
101. Davidoff, A.M., et al., Genetic basis for p53 overexpression in human breast cancer. *Proceedings of the National Academy of Sciences*, 1991. **88**(11): p. 5006–5010.
102. Pharoah, P., N. Day, and C. Caldas, Somatic mutations in the p53 gene and prognosis in breast cancer: a meta-analysis. *British Journal of Cancer*, 1999. **80**(12): p. 1968–1973.
103. Done, S.J., et al., p53 missense mutations in microdissected high-grade ductal carcinoma in situ of the breast. *Journal of the National Cancer Institute*, 2001. **93**(9): p. 700–704.
104. Smith, P.D., et al., Novel p53 mutants selected in BRCA-associated tumours which dissociate transformation suppression from other wild-type p53 functions. *Oncogene*, 1999. **18**(15): p. 2451–2459.
105. Phillips, K.-A., et al., Frequency of p53 mutations in breast carcinomas from Ashkenazi Jewish carriers of BRCA1 mutations. *Journal of the National Cancer Institute*, 1999. **91**(5): p. 469–473.
106. de Cremoux, P., et al., p53 mutation as a genetic trait of typical medullary breast carcinoma. *Journal of the National Cancer Institute*, 1999. **91**(7): p. 641–643.
107. Esteller, M., et al., Promoter hypermethylation and BRCA1 inactivation in sporadic breast and ovarian tumors. *JNCI: Journal of the National Cancer Institute*, 2000. **92**(7): p. 564–569.
108. Stankovic, T., et al., ATM mutations and phenotypes in ataxia-telangiectasia families in the British Isles: expression of mutant ATM and the risk of leukemia, lymphoma, and breast cancer. *The American Journal of Human Genetics*, 1998. **62**(2): p. 334–345.
109. Dörk, T., et al., Spectrum of ATM gene mutations in a hospital-based series of unselected breast cancer patients. *Cancer Research*, 2001. **61**(20): p. 7608–7615.
110. Angele, S., et al., Abnormal expression of the ATM and TP53 genes in sporadic breast carcinomas. *Clinical Cancer Research*, 2000. **6**(9): p. 3536–3544.
111. Bell, D.W., et al., Heterozygous germ line hCHK2 mutations in Li-Fraumeni syndrome. *Science*, 1999. **286**(5449): p. 2528–2531.
112. Allinen, M., et al., Mutation analysis of the CHK2gene in families with hereditary breast cancer. *British Journal of Cancer*, 2001. **85**(2): p. 209–212.
113. Vahteristo, L., et al., Functionality of endogenous folates from rye and orange juice using human in vivo model. *European Journal of Nutrition*, 2002. **41**: p. 271–278.
114. Sullivan, A., et al., Concomitant inactivation of p53 and Chk2 in breast cancer. *Oncogene*, 2002. **21**(9): p. 1316–1324.
115. Mir, M.A., N. Jan, and S. Sofi, Introduction to Metronomic Chemotherapy, in *Novel Approaches in Metronomic Chemotherapy for Breast Cancer Treatment*. 2024, CRC Press. p. 1–14.
116. Raman, V., et al., Compromised HOXA5 function can limit p53 expression in human breast tumours. *Nature*, 2000. **405**(6789): p. 974–978.

117. Mir, M.A., et al., Imaging Techniques, Biomarkers, and Methods for Metronomic Chemotherapy, in *Novel Approaches in Metronomic Chemotherapy for Breast Cancer Treatment.* 2024, CRC Press. p. 58–71.
118. Samuels-Lev, Y., et al., ASPP proteins specifically stimulate the apoptotic function of p53. *Molecular Cell*, 2001. **8**(4): p. 781–794.
119. Sgroi, D.C., et al., In vivo gene expression profile analysis of human breast cancer progression. *Cancer Research*, 1999. **59**(22): p. 5656–5661.
120. Zhang, H., et al., BRCA1 physically associates with p53 and stimulates its transcriptional activity. *Oncogene*, 1998. **16**(13): p. 1713–1721.
121. Catteau, A., et al., Methylation of the BRCA1 promoter region in sporadic breast and ovarian cancer: correlation with disease characteristics. *Oncogene*, 1999. **18**(11): p. 1957–1965.
122. Gayther, S.A., et al., Mutations truncating the EP300 acetylase in human cancers. *Nature Genetics*, 2000. **24**(3): p. 300–303.
123. Sofi, S., et al., Clinicopathological and prognostic significance of Bcl2 in breast cancer: a comprehensive in silico and in vitro study. *Saudi Journal of Biological Sciences*, 2023. **31**(2): p. 103916.
124. Li, F.P. and J.F. Fraumeni Jr, Rhabdomyosarcoma in children: epidemiologic study and identification of a familial cancer syndrome. *Journal of the National Cancer Institute*, 1969. **43**(6): p. 1365–1373.
125. Li, F.P. and J.F. Fraumeni Jr, Soft-tissue sarcomas, breast cancer, and other neoplasms: a familial syndrome? *Annals of Internal Medicine*, 1969. **71**(4): p. 747–752.
126. Kleihues, P., et al., Tumors associated with p53 germline mutations: a synopsis of 91 families. *The American Journal of Pathology*, 1997. **150**(1): p. 1.
127. Mir, M.A., Sumaya, N. Jan, Implications of Chemokine Heterogenicity in Cancer Metastasis, in *Cytokine and Chemokine Networks in Cancer.* 2023, Springer. p. 115–136.
128. Williams, W. and L. Strong, *Familial Cancer.* Muller HR, Weber W, eds. 1985: Karger.
129. Malkin, D., p53 and the Li-Fraumeni syndrome. *Cancer Genetics and Cytogenetics*, 1993. **66**(2): p. 83–92.
130. Varley, J.M., et al., Germ-line mutations of TP53 in Li-Fraumeni families: an extended study of 39 families. *Cancer Research*, 1997. **57**(15): p. 3245–3252.
131. Thompson, A.M., p53 and breast cancer. *The Breast*, 1993. **2**(1): p. 8–10.
132. Andersen, T.I. and A.-L. Børresen, Alterations of the TP53 gene as a potential prognostic marker in breast carcinomas: advantages of using constant denaturant gel electrophoresis in mutation detection. *Diagnostic Molecular Pathology*, 1995. **4**(3): p. 203–211.
133. Emerling, B.M., et al., Depletion of a putatively druggable class of phosphatidylinositol kinases inhibits growth of p53-null tumors. *Cell*, 2013. **155**(4): p. 844–857.
134. Zonneville, J., et al., Selective therapeutic strategy for p53-deficient cancer by targeting dysregulation in DNA repair. *Communications Biology*, 2021. **4**(1): p. 862.
135. Jabbour-Leung, N.A., et al., Sequential combination therapy of CDK inhibition and doxorubicin is synthetically lethal in p53-mutant triple-negative breast cancer. *Molecular Cancer Therapeutics*, 2016. **15**(4): p. 593–607.
136. Ha, D.-H., et al., Antitumor effect of a WEE1 inhibitor and potentiation of olaparib sensitivity by DNA damage response modulation in triple-negative breast cancer. *Scientific Reports*, 2020. **10**(1): p. 9930.
137. Giordano, A., et al., Polo-like kinase 1 inhibitor onvansertib synergizes with paclitaxel in breast cancer carrying p53 mutation. *Annals of Oncology*, 2019. **30**: p. v125–v126.
138. Zhang, Y., et al., Glutathionylation-dependent proteasomal degradation of wide-spectrum mutant p53 proteins by engineered zeolitic imidazolate framework-8. *Biomaterials*, 2021. **271**: p. 120720.
139. Rangel, L.P., et al., p53 reactivation with induction of massive apoptosis-1 (PRIMA-1) inhibits amyloid aggregation of mutant p53 in cancer cells. *Journal of Biological Chemistry*, 2019. **294**(10): p. 3670–3682.
140. Dumbrava, E.E., et al., First-in-human study of PC14586, a small molecule structural corrector of Y220C mutant p53, in patients with advanced solid tumors harboring a TP53 Y220C mutation. *Journal of Clinical Oncology*, 2022. **40**(16): p. 3003.
141. Xu, C., J. Zhuang, and X. Zhang, 2-[(4-Hydroxybenzyl) Amino] Phenol (HBAP) Restores the Mutated p53 to the Level Similar to That of Wild-Type p53 Protein and Inhibits Breast Cancer Growth in vivo to by Inducing Tumor Cells Apoptosis. *Frontiers in Cell and Developmental Biology*, 2020. **8**: p. 574799.
142. Vakifahmetoglu-Norberg, H., et al., Chaperone-mediated autophagy degrades mutant p53. *Genes & Development*, 2013. **27**(15): p. 1718–1730.
143. Yi, Y.W., et al., Targeting mutant p53 by a SIRT1 activator YK-3-237 inhibits the proliferation of triple-negative breast cancer cells. *Oncotarget*, 2013. **4**(7): p. 984.

144. Peng, J., et al., Targeting mutated p53 dependency in triple-negative breast cancer cells through CDK7 inhibition. *Frontiers in Oncology*, 2021. **11**: p. 664848.
145. Paranjpe, A. and K.S. Srivenugopal, Degradation of NF-κB, p53 and other regulatory redox-sensitive proteins by thiol-conjugating and-nitrosylating drugs in human tumor cells. *Carcinogenesis*, 2013. **34**(5): p. 990–1000.
146. Beaudry, G.A., A.H. Bertelsen, and M.I. Sherman, Therapeutic targeting of the p53 tumor suppressor gene. *Current Opinion in Biotechnology*, 1996. **7**(6): p. 592–600.
147. Su, N., et al., Breast cancer gene therapy: transgenic immunotherapy. *Breast Cancer Research and Treatment*, 1994. **31**: p. 349–356.
148. Wills, K.N., et al., Development and characterization of recombinant adenoviruses encoding human p53 for gene therapy of cancer. *Human Gene Therapy*, 1994. **5**(9): p. 1079–1088.
149. Li, P., et al., Therapeutic potential of recombinant p53 overexpression in breast cancer cells expressing endogenous wild-type p53. *Breast Cancer Research and Treatment*, 1998. **48**: p. 273–286.
150. Casey, G., et al., Growth suppression of human breast cancer cells by the introduction of a wild-type p53 gene. *Oncogene*, 1991. **6**(10): p. 1791–1797.
151. Chen, Q.-R. and A.J. Mixson, Systemic gene therapy with p53 inhibits breast cancer: recent advances and therapeutic implications. *Frontiers in Bioscience*, 1998. **3**: p. D997–D1004.
152. Gurnani, M., et al., Adenovirus-mediated p53 gene therapy has greater efficacy when combined with chemotherapy against human head and neck, ovarian, prostate, and breast cancer. *Cancer Chemotherapy and Pharmacology*, 1999. **44**: p. 143–151.
153. Whitesell, L., et al., The physical association of multiple molecular chaperone proteins with mutant p53 is altered by geldanamycin, an hsp90-binding agent. *Molecular and Cellular Biology*, 1998. **18**(3): p. 1517–1524.
154. Hupp, T.R., A. Sparks, and D.P. Lane, Small peptides activate the latent sequence-specific DNA binding function of p53. *Cell*, 1995. **83**(2): p. 237–245.
155. Selivanova, G., et al. Reactivation of Mutant p53: A New Strategy for Cancer Therapy, in *Seminars in Cancer Biology*. 1998. Elsevier.
156. Foster, B.A., et al., Pharmacological rescue of mutant p53 conformation and function. *Science*, 1999. **286**(5449): p. 2507–2510.

4 Mutational Alterations in p53

Their Impact on the Development of Breast Cancer

*Burhan Ul Haq, Asma Jan, and Manzoor Ahmad Mir**

Department of Bioresources, School of Biological Sciences, University of Kashmir, Srinagar, J&K, India

*drmanzoor@kashmiruniversity.ac.in

4.1 INTRODUCTION

Since its initial announcement in 1979, TP53 has been highly researched. Currently, TP53 is the gene most strongly correlated with human cancers; its previous classification as an oncogene has been replaced with that of a tumor suppressor gene [1]. Because of its function in responding to a variety of internal and external stimuli, including nutrition scarcity, hypoxia, activation of oncogenes, and DNA damage, TP53 is regarded as the "guardian of the genome" [2–4]. The mutations in over 50% of human initial tumors result in TP53 inactivation, which is a frequent occurrence in carcinogenesis [5]. Missense mutations account for the majority of TP53 mutations. These mutations frequently exhibit gain-of-function activity in addition to loss of tumor-suppressive function, which adds to the malignant characteristics of cancer cells (Figure 4.1) [6]. Dittmer et al., for example, transformed p53-deficient fibroblasts into p53 V143A, R175H, R248W, R273H, and D281G mutants, which increased the tumorigenic potential in nude mice [7]. p53 K117R mutant knock-in mice were created by Li et al., and they eliminated p53-mediated apoptosis [8]. The cancers containing mutp53 are more aggressive and metastatic than p53-deficient or p53 wild-type cancers [9–11]. Li–Fraumeni syndrome, which predisposes to a range of early-onset cancers including adrenal cortical carcinomas, brain tumors, sarcomas, and breast carcinomas, is caused by germline TP53 mutations [12–14]. Sporadic malignancies such as head and neck cancer, lung cancer, colorectal cancer, ovarian cancer, and breast cancer are influenced by somatic TP53 mutations [9, 10, 15]. More significantly, TP53 mutations are linked to a poor prognosis in cancers of the bladder, breast, and hematopoietic system [16–18]. Moreover, the spectrum of TP53 mutations varies in different cancers [19, 20]. This chapter provides an overview of our knowledge of the mutp53 spectrum and kinds of cancer. A synopsis of the mutant p53 accumulation and gain-of-function pathways is also provided. We also highlight the factors that contribute to mutp53's gain-of-function in malignancies, including genomic instability, ferroptosis, the microenvironment, and stemness. Finally, we describe the new approaches being developed to target mutp53 in cancer treatment. As a result, this chapter will aid in improving comprehension of the significance of mutant p53 as a target for treatment approaches.

DOI: 10.1201/9781003520771-4

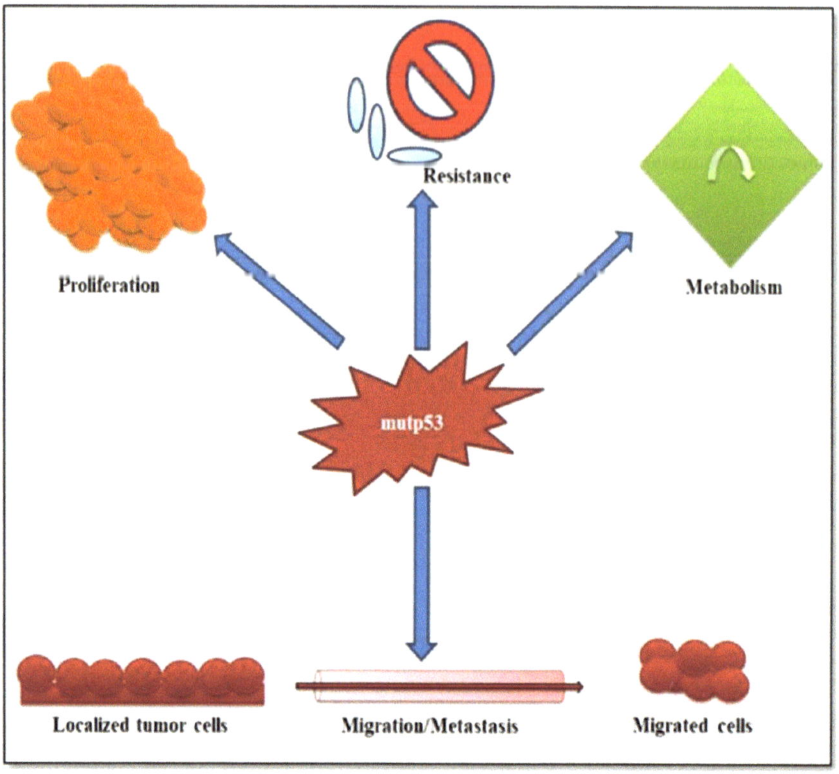

FIGURE 4.1 The mutp53 gets engaged in resistance, proliferation, metabolism, and metastasis.

4.2 GAIN-OF-FUNCTION OF MUTP53 IN CANCER

4.2.1 Genetic Instability

It is known that genomic instability is a characteristic of human malignancies [21]. As the protector of the genome, wtp53 is crucial in preserving genome stability, whereas mutp53 may encourage genomic instability. It was discovered that mutp53 encourages chromosomal instability and amplification [21–24]. For example, in osteosarcoma, mutp53 interacts with topoisomerase I to induce gene amplification [21]. Mutp53 causes interchromosomal translocation in pre-tumor thymocytes [23]. Mutp53 promotes the development of DNA replication origins and stabilizes replication forks in lung cancer, resulting in the formation of micronuclei and the growth of cells with aberrant genomes [25, 26]. Additionally, mutp53 prevents the MRE11-RAD50-NSB1 complex from attaching to DNA damage sites, which inactivates ATM and causes genetic instability [23]. Mutp53 inhibits BRCA1 and RAD17 expression in lung and breast cancer, which results in genomic instability and hinders DNA damage repair [25, 27]. Notably, a significant number of solid tumors have been observed to have cell-in-cell structures. While mutp53 aids in the development of cell-in cell formations in lung adenocarcinomas by engulfing living cells and causing abnormal mitosis, wtp53 promotes the demise of the cells that form these structures [28, 29]. Therefore, mutp53 and genomic instability interact in a way that is crucial to the genesis of cancer.

4.2.2 Tumor Microenvironment and Mutp53

Mutp53 may be able to control the tumor microenvironment, according to mounting data (Table 4.1). Solid tumors are associated with TAMs, or tumor-associated macrophages. By encouraging an anti-tumor milieu and modifying the M1 polarization pattern in nearby macrophages, wtp53

TABLE 4.1
Role of Mutp53 and the Underlying Modulatory Mechanisms

Role	Target	Mechanism	Reference
Genetic instability	E2F4	Inhibits DNA damage repair	[30]
Microenvironment	NF-κB	Leads to an enhanced inflammatory reaction	[31]
Stemness	MiR-200c	Promotes cancer stemness	[32]

inhibits the growth of tumors [33, 34]. Moreover, mutp53 may encourage the neo-angiogenesis of tumors. The ID4 protein stimulates the production of pro-angiogenic proteins IL8 and GRO-α in non-small cell lung carcinoma (NSCLC). On the other hand, mutp53 activates ID4, while mutp53 depletion reduces ID4 expression [35]. Mutp53 can encourage the synthesis of VEGF in leukemia, creating a milieu that is conducive to cell proliferation [36, 37]. Furthermore, malignancies also exhibit persistent inflammation. Mutp53 influences TNF-induced NF-κB activation in breast cancer (BC), exacerbating the inflammatory response [31]. By inhibiting the expression of sIL-1Ra in colon adenocarcinoma, mutp53 can create a pro-inflammatory tumor microenvironment that can result in tumor malignancy [38, 39].

4.2.3 Cancer Stemness

It was discovered that mutp53 has a role in the phenotypic acquisition of cancer stem cells (CSCs). The capacity of CSCs to generate diverse tumor cells, which are essential to the development and spread of cancer, is one of their defining characteristics [40]. Wtp53 often prevents the development of CSCs and suppresses the expression of CSC markers [41]. On the other hand, mutp53 increases the expression of CSC markers such as ALDH, Lgr5, and CD44, and boosts the growth of CSC subpopulations to encourage the development of colorectal cancer [42, 43]. Overexpression of mutp53 in BC and glioblastoma not only raises the expression of markers for CSCs but also encourages their proliferation [44]. Furthermore, the expression of long noncoding RNAs (lncRNAs) such as lnc273-31 and lnc273-34 in colorectal cancer can be regulated by the p53 R273H mutant, which encourages CSC self-renewal and tumor growth [45]. Mutp53 regulates miRNA, which further enhances cancer stemness. For example, in basal-like BC, mutp53 increases cancer stemness by modifying the miR-200c-PCK2 axis [32]. Mutp53 promotes cancer stemness in lung adenocarcinomas by controlling the miR-324-5p-CUEDC2-NF-κB pathway [46].

4.3 STRATEGIES OF TUMOR TREATMENT

4.3.1 Restoration of Wild-Type Activity

Reactivating mutp53's wild-type activity is a useful tactic for halting the growth of tumors. Numerous investigations have revealed that peptide medications and small molecule substances, including CP-31398, can cause modifications to the spatial conformation and folding pattern of mutp53 [47], RITA [48], PEITC [49], NSC319726 [50], chetomin [51], ReACp53 [52], and pCAPs [52]. Notably, clinical trials are presently being conducted for APR-246, COT1-2, PC14586, and arsenic trioxide (ATO). Methylene quinuclidinone is APR-246's active form in vivo; it is sometimes referred to as PRIMA-1MET. It binds mutp53's DNA binding domain covalently to restore anti-tumor transcriptional activity and wild-type conformation [53, 54]. In triple-negative breast cancer, acute myeloid leukemia, and esophageal adenocarcinoma, APR-246 exhibits strong anti-tumor action [55–57]. Increasing the dosage of APR-246 in addition to other anti-cancer medications can improve treatment outcomes. APR-246 can strengthen the inhibitory effect on esophageal cancer when paired with cisplatin and 5-fluorouracil, according to research by Liu et al. [55]. Additionally, research has revealed that APR-246 exhibits mutp53-independent actions that lead to increased ROS via glutathione depletion and, eventually, lipid peroxidation cell death. Moreover, COTI-2 can restore DNA binding properties and reactivate mutp53, which prevents cell division and induces apoptosis [58]. Transcriptional activity can be restored by ATO by targeting structural mutp53. Additionally, mouse xenograft models show that ATO reactivates mutp53 to inhibit tumor growth [59]. Accordingly, our data indicate that mutp53's restoration to its wild-type conformation represents a viable anti-cancer tactic. A direct tactic to restore p53 activity in cancer cells is the delivery of wtp53 via adenovirus. Gendicine is the first gene therapy medication authorized to treat several cancer types, such as head and neck, lung, breast, cervical, ovarian, liver, and pancreatic cancers [60, 61]. Compared to standard therapy alone, the combination of chemotherapy and radiation with gendicine typically results in much greater response rates [60]. More critically, patients treated with gendicine do not see a substantial change in the outcome or long-term survival based on their p53 mutational status [60, 61]. Adenovirus ONYX-015, which has had its E1B section removed, is capable of replicating and causing cytolysis in cancer cells lacking wtp53. Treatment with ONYX-015 dramatically increases the survival rate of mice harboring mutp53 in comparison to those carrying wtp53 [62].

4.4 ROLE OF p53 IN BREAST CANCER

4.4.1 Mutant p53's Role in the Onset and Spread of Cancer

In addition to displaying a dominant-negative activity that prevents the functioning of wild-type p53, gain-of-function (GOF) processes, in which the mutant protein combines with other transcription factors or cofactors to control gene transcription and expression, might provide carcinogenic activity to p53 mutations and promote the growth of cancer [63, 64] (Figure 4.2).

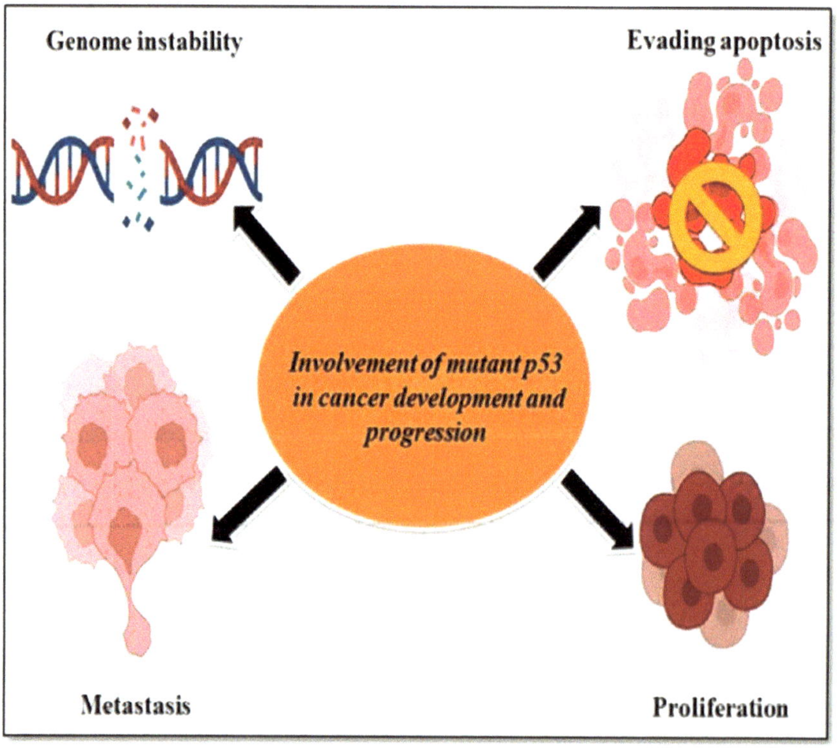

FIGURE 4.2 The role of mutant p53 in the development of cancer.

4.4.1.1 Genome Instability

All forms of human cancer are characterized by innate genome instability. It has been demonstrated that mutant p53's GOF activity encourages genomic instability. Mutant p53 is linked to aberrant copy numbers in breast cancer samples [65]. Centrosome amplification results from the p53 R172H mutant's (R175H equivalent in mice) modulation of cyclinE-cdk2 activity at the centrosome, which causes centrosome abnormalities [66–68]. According to separate research, methyltransferases MLL1 and MLL2, which increase histone methylation and acetylation and are connected to the onset of cancer and genomic instability, are examples of chromatin-regulated genes that mutant p53 can bind to and stimulate the expression [69, 70].

4.4.1.2 Avoiding Apoptosis

Mutant p53 avoids apoptosis by working with p63 and p73, members of the p53 family, to inhibit their tumor-suppressive functions [71]. It has been shown that several p53 mutations, including R273H and R175H, prevent apoptosis by inhibiting BCL2-modifying factor production through increased AKT signaling [72] and decreasing, respectively, the transcriptional activity of p73 on the Bax promoter [73].

4.4.1.3 Proliferation

Different from their wild-type counterparts, mutant p53 proteins can trigger the transcription of many genes linked to cell proliferation [74]. A few of them are CXCL1, MAP2K3, c-MYC, and CCNE2. Furthermore, it has been documented that mutant p53 interacts with several transcription factors or proteins that promote the growth of breast cancer, including the sterol regulatory element-binding protein (SREBP) through the activation of the mevalonate pathway, DAB2IP, NF-Y, and PARP [75–79].

4.4.1.4 Metastasis

It has also been observed that mutant p53 increases tumor aggressiveness and potential for metastasis through several pathways. One such mechanism is the enhancement of cell invasion and metastasis in cancer cells through the stability of mutant p53 protein by Rab coupling protein-mediated release of Hsp90 [80]. Additionally, mutant p53 interacts with the adenosine A2b receptor (ADORA2B), a G-protein coupled receptor [81], and Pin1 [82, 83]. Both interactions are linked to poor clinical outcomes in BC and enhance invasion and metastasis.

4.5 p53 AS A THERAPEUTIC TARGET: A TWO-SIDED APPROACH

The majority of BC instances belong to the luminal-like subtype, with almost two-thirds being of the wild-type, despite TP53 being the most frequently altered gene in breast cancer [84, 85]. The overexpression of MDM2 or MDMX in these malignancies mostly suppresses the p53 activity. The majority of the mutations that inactivate p53 function in the remaining one-third of breast cancer patients are found in HER2-positive and basal-like subtypes [86]. Therefore, to reactivate p53's tumor-suppressive properties, several mutation status-differentiated treatment approaches have been investigated. These strategies focus on these two primary p53 inactivation pathways.

4.6 TREATMENTS FOR BREAST CANCER WITH WILD-TYPE p53 EXPRESSION

In normal cells, an imbalance between MDM2 and p53 can result in cancerous alterations. Every human tumor has MDM2 gene amplification in about 7% of cases [87]. MDM2 now possesses an oncogene-like characteristic. About 38% of patients with breast cancer have elevated MDM2 protein expression [43, 88]. Moreover, MDM2 expression and the presence of estrogen receptors (ER) are linked; ER-positive (ER+) cell lines have increased MDM2 expression [89]. This makes MDM2 a desirable target for therapeutics, particularly in p53-wild-type malignancies. Most medicines targeting MDM2 try to either (1) disrupt the MDM2–p53 connection, (2) downregulate the expression of MDM2, or (3) inhibit its E3 ligase function and its association with the proteasome to minimize degradation of p53 and p53-dependent tumor suppressor pathways activation.

4.7 INHIBITING THE MDM2-p53 INTERACTION

A hydrophobic surface pocket was discovered in the high-resolution crystal structure of the MDM2-p53 interaction (Phe19, Trp23, Leu26) [85, 90]. This makes it possible to create tiny compounds that inhibit the MDM2-p53 connection and cause p53 to become active in cancerous cells. More than 20 distinct chemical classes assert their ability to prevent this kind of interaction [91]. The majority of research, however, focuses on four groups of substances: benzodiaze, pinediones, spirooxindoles, and nutlins (Figure 4.3). We will also concentrate on nutlin-based and spirooxindole class chemicals in this chapter because they are the most frequently used MDM2-p53 interaction inhibitor classes in BC research and because they have the characteristics of drugs.

4.7.1 Nutlins

Nutlins work by sterically blocking MDM2 at its p53 binding pocket. In turn, this causes MDM2-overexpressing cancer cells to undergo apoptosis and p53-associated cell cycle arrest [92]. The nutlin family's initial examples of these chemicals are nutlin-1, -2, and -3. The nutlin molecule has undergone several revisions over time, including RG7112 and idasanutlin (RG7388), which have better binding, potency, and pharmacological characteristics [93]. In cells containing wild-type p53, these substances demonstrated dose-dependent stabilization of p53 and sensitivity; however, they were unable to produce any p53-regulated tumor-suppressive effects in cells containing mutant or non-functional p53 [94]. Since nutlins only bind to the p53 binding pocket of MDM2, their action is restricted by the overexpression of MDMX, another p53 negative regulator [95, 96]. Combining doxorubicin, an anthracycline-based DNA damaging agent that causes direct MDM2 ubiquitination and the subsequent destruction of MDMX, with nutlins is one method of overcoming p53 inactivation caused by MDMX [97]. Another method of circumventing MDMX inactivation involves the use of small molecule MDMX inhibitors, like XI-011, XI-006, and SJ-172550. When combined

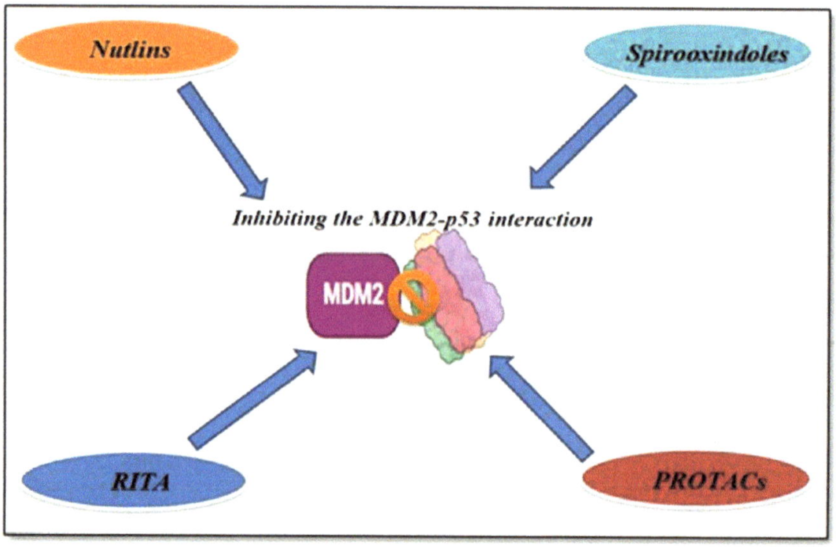

FIGURE 4.3 Inhibiting the association of MDM2 with p53.

with nutlin-3a, these inhibitors produce cumulative effects and cause apoptosis in the ER+ MCF-7 cell line that expresses wild-type p53 [98–100].

4.7.2 Spirooxindoles

Also known as the MI-series, spirooxindoles are structurally related to nutlins. These resemble the hydrophobic pocket residues that are crucial for binding in MDM2-p53. Like nutlins, these medicines show particular potency in p53 wild-type cells and only slight effects on p53 mutant cells. Many of these small molecule compounds are being studied in breast cancer models; however, they are all still in the pre-clinical phases [101–108]. Only in wild-type p53-bearing breast cancer cell lines or xenografts did any of these drugs exhibit anti-proliferative effects by triggering p53 downstream genes linked to cell cycle arrest and death.

4.8 OTHER SMALL MOLECULE MDM2–p53 INHIBITORS

Several other small molecule MDM2–p53 inhibitors have been studied in BC models in addition to nutlins and spirooxindoles. RITA is one such example; it binds to the N-terminus of p53 and causes a conformational change that breaks the MDM2-p53 connection and causes the accumulation of p53. The reactivation of p53 and the promotion of apoptosis in tumor cells is known as RITA [109]. Additionally, it has been documented that RITA causes MDMX deterioration via ATM [26, 110]. Other substances that influence the MDM2–p53 interaction include NVP CGM097, tricetin, and prenylchalcone 2e. Particularly in cells that contain wild-type p53, these substances cause an increase in the expression of p53 in proteins and the downstream effectors, resulting in cell cycle arrest and apoptosis [111–113].

4.8.1 PROTACs

MDM2–p53 binding inhibition is a concept that goes beyond tiny drugs. Using these chemicals, for instance, can be used to create MDM2-based proteolysis targeting chimeras (PROTACs), which exploit MDM2's E3 ligase activity to break down a target protein. Currently, three PROTACs use a derivative based on nutlin to attract MDM2 and cause BRD4, androgen receptor, and PARP1 degradation, respectively [114]. These substances not only degrade pro-oncogenic proteins but also play a secondary function in sequestering MDM2, which in turn stabilizes wild-type p53. Additionally, MDM2 can be the target of a PROTAC aimed to degrade it. The IMiD-based PROTAC MD-224 binds to the E3 ligase cereblon and MDM2 with lenalidomide and MI-1061, respectively, causing MDM2 protein degradation that lowers MDM2's capacity to degrade p53 [115].

4.9 DOWNREGULATING MDM2 EXPRESSION

MDM2 inhibition or downregulation is an additional therapeutic approach for malignancies expressing wild-type p53. Although the technique results in enhanced p53 activity, it suppresses MDM2 directly, which is different from how suppression of MDM2-p53 interaction works [91]. JapA is one of several substances that can directly bind to MDM2 and cause its downregulation or degradation [116], inulanolide A, and lineariifolianoid A. These substances not only cause the MDM2 protein to degrade and suppress its transcription, but the latter two also prevent the expression of the MDM2 transactivator NFAT1, which is often highly expressed in BC [117, 118]. Another illustration is SP-141, which exhibits direct binding to MDM2 and inhibits its expression by encouraging its degradation and autoubiquitination [119]. Regardless of the presence of p53 mutations, these substances cause G2/M arrest, apoptosis, and cytotoxicity in addition to suppressing tumor growth in xenograft models. According to reports, MDM2 can also be inhibited by CPI-7c, which binds to the RING and N-terminal domains of the protein to cause ubiquitin proteasome-mediated destruction. This not only keeps p53 stable but also encourages it to attach to the death receptor promoters, DR4 and

DR5, to trigger TRAIL-induced apoptosis [120]. Apart from new compounds that target MDM2, several clinically approved medications also have secondary activities against MDM2. Albendazole and fenbendazole, for example, significantly reduce MDMX and MDM2 expression in cell lines of BC and melanoma, thereby upregulating p53 and its downstream effector, p21 [121]. It has also been shown that fulvestrant, a commonly used selective estrogen receptor degrader, increases the rate of MDM2 protein turnover and decreases estrogen-dependent MDM2 upregulation without changing MDM2 gene expression or p53 activity. Fulvestrant reduces MDM2 regardless of the presence or absence of p53 mutations [122]. This supports its continued use as a successful treatment in advanced ER+ breast tumors, which frequently overexpress MDM2. Natural substances also show anti-MDM2 properties. Natural goods like genistein, melatonin, makaluvamine analogs (FBATPQ, BA-TPQ, DPA-TPQ, MPA-TPQ, PEA-TPQ), platycodin D, ginsenosides (25-OCH3-PPD), hispolon, gossypol, oroxylin A, gambogic acid and curcumin [123–130] have all been demonstrated to downregulate expression of MDM2; however, only pre-clinical studies have been conducted to assess their relationship with MDM2. Though it is still in the pre-clinical stages, direct targeting of MDM2 is a potential therapeutic option against cancers with wild-type p53. It is important to note that, according to the findings cited in this chapter, MDM2 inhibition affects both wild-type and mutant p53-carrying cells. One theory for the mechanism of action is independent p53-independent p21 overexpression. Therefore, in mutant p53 tumors, the use of direct MDM2 inhibitors may be advantageous over inhibitors of the MDM2–p53 relationship.

4.10 INHIBITING MDM2'S E3 LIGASE ACTIVITY AND ITS BINDING TO PROTEASOME

Minimizing the degradation of wild-type p53 can also be achieved by inhibiting MDM2's E3 ligase activity or its interaction with the 26S proteasome. By attaching to the RING finger domain of MDM2, which is in charge of its E3 ligase function, the family of 7-nitro-5-deazaflavin compounds (HLI98s, HLI373, and HLI393) supports p53 stabilization without reducing its expression. As a result, degradation of p53 mediated by MDM2 is inhibited, restoring p53 activity to specifically destroy cancer cells that harbor p53 that is wild-type [131, 132]. Similarly, sempervirine, a naturally occurring substance, prevents MDM2 E3 ligase activity, which causes cancer cells to undergo apoptosis [133]. The MEL compounds MEL23 and MEL24 are another type of MDM2 E3 ligase inhibitors; they work by reducing the ubiquitination of the RING domains of the MDM2–MDMX heterocomplex, hence inhibiting MDM2–MDMX E3 ligase activity. These chemicals demonstrated p53-independent/MDM2-dependent activity in p53-null cells, indicating that their potential applications extend beyond malignancies expressing wild-type p53. They also promoted cell death in cells expressing wild-type p53 in a p53-dependent manner [134]. A phase I trial involving seven patients with advanced BC has successfully moved this drug forward (NCT00676910). Tumor samples revealed a 102% increase in p53 levels, and one patient had a partial response to JNJ26854165 [135]. It was also found that JNJ26854165 had anti-tumoral actions beyond MDM2/p53, as it caused cells with p53 mutation(s) to undergo S-phase arrest and E2F1-mediated apoptosis [136].

4.11 THERAPIES AGAINST MUTANT p53-BEARING BREAST CANCER

Tumor growth, progression, and metastasis are mediated by mutant p53, which is commonly seen in HER2-enriched and triple-negative breast cancer (TNBC) subtypes [137]. This makes it a desirable target for BC therapy. In TNBC, p53 mutation is also most commonly clonal [138], offering a unique homogeneity characteristic in a heterogenic malignancy such as breast cancer. Targeting mutant p53 is therapeutically valuable, as evidenced by the intrinsic aggressiveness of TNB and the relative dearth of targeted treatments available. For tumors with p53 mutations, the main objectives of targeted therapies are to (1) bring mutant p53 back to normal, (2) promote degradation, (3) induce synthetic lethality, (4) obstruct interactors or pathways that lead to its gain-of-function, (5) utilize immunotherapies, and (6) use gene therapies via vectors to transfer the wild-type p53 gene into tumor cells.

4.12 RESTORING MUTANT p53 TO WILD-TYPE-LIKE CONFORMATIONS OR FUNCTIONS

The majority of TP53 mutations are missense, meaning that the p53 protein has one amino acid changed, which prevents the protein from binding DNA [139]. Many substances, including pyrazoles, quinuclidines, thiosemicarbazones, and 2-sulfonylpyrimidines have been created to help mutant p53 regain functions similar to those of wild-type p53.

MQ, or 2-methylene-3-quinuclidinone, is the active metabolite and is produced during in vivo metabolism of quinuclidine-based prodrugs, such as PRIMA-1 and its methylated counterpart, APR-246 (also known as PRIMA-1MET). By focusing on exposed cysteine residues in the core domain of the mutant p53 protein, MQ, a nucleophile acceptor, corrects the folding of the protein and restores its ability to bind DNA. It does this by changing thiol groups through the Michael addition reaction. Cys-124 and Cys-277 are recognized targets of MQ and are essential residues in stabilizing mutant p53 R175H [54]. PRIMA-1 not only reverses the dominant-negative effect of mutant p53 by reactivating it but also prevents it from aggregating [140]. Additionally, in several cancers, particularly BC, it activates caspase-2, -3, and -9 to enhance apoptosis and upregulate p53's downstream genes, such as p21, PUMA, BAX, and NOXA [141]. It has been observed that mice xenografts and PRIMA-1 and APR-246 selectively suppress mutant p53 over wild-type p53 breast cancer cell lines [140]. It's interesting to note that in a variety of breast cancer cell lines, there is a link between high endogenous p53 expression and higher sensitivity to APR-246 [142]. Future studies will mostly focus on PRIMA-1 and its analog. It is yet unknown how some of the targeted cysteine residues in the core domain reactivate mutant p53 because not all of them have been found.

4.13 SYNTHETIC LETHALITY

An inactivation of the G2/M checkpoint will result in an unintentional entry into mitosis and a mitotic catastrophe, even with substantial DNA damage. This could be a promising therapeutic target for p53-mutant cancers.

4.13.1 G2 Checkpoint Targeting

Weel kinase mediates cell cycle arrest by suppressing CDK1 activity, which is a crucial part of G2/M checkpoint regulation. Breast cancer is among the tumors where Weel is overexpressed [143]. MK-1775, also known as AZD1775 or adavosertib, is a Weel inhibitor that encourages cancer cells to evade the G2/M checkpoint, which results in a mitotic catastrophe. In several cancer models, this drug demonstrated greater anti-tumor action in cells containing mutant p53 compared to wild-type p53; however, this difference is not as noticeable in ER-positive cell lines [144, 145].

Another substance that takes advantage of the G2/M dependence of mutant p53 is UCN-01, a Chk1 (upstream of Weel). Although this drug exhibited a preferential cytotoxic impact over wild-type p53 in mutant p53-overexpressing cells, its phase I clinical trial outcomes were not up to par [146]. Reviving Chk1 as a therapeutic target against mutant p53, AZD7762, a more selective inhibitor of Chk1, showed enhanced responsiveness and higher survival in TNBC animal models including p53 mutation [147]. Additionally, in the mutant p53 T47D breast model, AZD7762 promotes radiation-induced apoptosis and mitotic catastrophe by reversing radiation-induced G2/M arrest and DNA double-strand repair, which limits tumor xenograft growth [148].

Numerous combination therapy plans for breast cancer are also based on the G2 checkpoint susceptibility of mutant p53. For instance, it has been demonstrated that doxorubicin and pan-CDK inhibitor roscovitine were administered in order to cause synthetic lethality in mutant p53 TNBC cells only. When combined with doxorubicin, roscovitine stops these cells in the G2/M phase, increases DNA double-strand breaks, and prevents DNA repair by reducing proteins linked to homologous recombination. In comparison to single-agent or concurrent treatment, the sequential administration of roscovitine and doxorubicin results in a greater reduction in tumor volume and enhanced overall survival in mutant p53 TNBC xenografts [149].

DNA damage is also increased by a different combination therapy that uses PARP inhibitors and deoxyuridine analogs. Mutant p53 cells cannot, however, initiate the p53–p21 signaling pathway to halt at G1 for DNA repair, in contrast to wild-type p53 cells. Consequently, these cells accumulate damage to their DNA and are stopped at G2. It should come as no surprise that this combination works well only in p53 mutant breast cancer, as it dramatically slows the growth of the xenografts and increases their overall survival rate [150].

4.13.2 Other Targets of Synthetic Lethality

G2 dependency is not the only way that mutant p53 is thought to exhibit synthetic lethality. Using mutant p53, computational gene expression profiling identified several potential gene targets implicated in synthetic lethality. PLK1, PLK4, and AURKA are a few of these potential genes for which inhibitors are now accessible [151].

When compared to wild-type p53-prevalent luminal cell lines, the therapy with PLK1 inhibitor onvansertib in mutant p53-prevalent TNBC showed a more substantial effect. In xenografts and mutant p53 breast cancer cell lines, onvansertib and paclitaxel exhibit selective synergy [152]. PI5P4K, or phosphatidylinositol 5-phosphate 4-kinase, is another dangerous synthetic target. It has been documented that PI5P4K is increased in a subgroup of breast tumors and is linked to p53 deletions or mutations. When this kinase was depleted in p53-deficient breast cancer cells, in vitro growth was inhibited and the lifetime of p53-knockout mice was extended [153]. The only PI5P4K inhibitor currently on the market is THZ-P1-2, however, it hasn't been investigated in breast cancer. In addition to the aforementioned targets, there may be still unidentified synthetic lethal targets connected to mutant p53. These findings might open up other treatment options for cancers containing p53 mutations.

4.14 GENETIC APPROACHES

Tumor cells can be targeted for senescence or cell death by introducing viral or plasmid vectors containing the wtp53 gene [154]. A noteworthy construct is gentacine, also known as Ad-p53, which is a combination of the human wtp53 gene and an adenovirus serotype-5 vector. In vitro, gentacine and gefitinib, an EGFR inhibitor, demonstrated synergistic growth inhibition and a reduction in tumor burden in MDA–MB-468 xenografts [155]. In a clinical trial, gentacine was tested as a treatment for TNBC. Half of the patients received gentacine in addition to capecitabine, and the other half received capecitabine alone. Compared to capecitabine alone (71.8%), gentacine plus capecitabine had greater response rates (84.4%), indicating that gentacine may have therapeutic promise as a therapy for mutant p53-prevalent TNBC [60]. A couple of other viral-based constructs that are comparable are ONYX015 and Advexin (also known as Ad5CMV-p53), both of which have undergone clinical trial evaluation. A phase II trial that combined intratumoral injection of Ad5CMV-p53 with doxorubicin and docetaxel was terminated early due to the lack of pathologic full response in any patient with locally advanced breast cancer. On the other hand, all 12 patients exhibited objective clinical responses with broad tumor-infiltrating leukocytes in scattered tumor cells [156]. Although utilizing wild-type p53-containing vectors for genetic methods yields encouraging outcomes, its applicability is restricted to malignancies deficient in p53 and lacking either GOF or dominant-negative actions of mutant p53 [157]. This offers an alternate plan of action to counteract the p53 mutant's predominant detrimental effect. Additional methods for reversing p53 mutations in cancer cells include CRISPR-Cas9 and synthetic small interfering RNA (siRNA). According to a study, applying certain siRNA to distinct p53 hotspot mutations reduced cancer cell viability while not affecting p53 mRNA that is wild type [158]. Additionally, p53 mutations in HCC1954 breast cancer cell lines were successfully repaired by base editing using CRISPR-Cas9 at a rate of 3.3–7.6% [159]. Targeting tumors with mutant p53 may eventually lead to the development of these systems as viable treatment options, even though further optimization is necessary to increase the delivery and editing efficiency of these systems before clinical application.

4.15 CONCLUSION AND SUMMARY

It can be difficult to create inhibitors against the protein p53 as a target. This is explained by the fact that it is a transcription factor without an accessible receptor-ligand interaction or active site of an enzyme. However, knowledge of the structure of p53 and its interaction partners has made it easier to find and manufacture a variety of substances that may help p53's tumor-suppressive properties to be restored. Many different small molecule compounds of varying degrees of complexity have been developed to target both wild-type and mutant p53-bearing tumors, albeit the majority are still in the pre-clinical phases of development [160]. Only a few prospective drugs have been investigated in early phase clinical studies including cases of breast cancer, despite their promising pre-clinical outcomes. There have been conflicting findings, including high-grade toxicity and minimal effectiveness signs.

The unexpected effects of blocking a specific target linked to p53 should be taken into account, even though the precise causes of the variations in patient response to the small molecule inhibitors are still unknown. For instance, MDM2 inhibition or deletion might cause the activation of additional carcinogenic pathways in tumors with functional p53 [161]. Furthermore, p53 negative regulators may be targeted to cause widespread p53 activation, which could impact both healthy and unhealthy cells. Since most of the compounds under investigation have shown poor clinical efficacy when used alone, it is imperative to combine these substances with additional therapeutic agents. Furthermore, fulvestrant and several Hsp90 and HDAC inhibitors are notable compounds that have been studied in breast cancer patients and have additional primary mechanisms of action against cancer. They exhibit secondary effects against p53 models that are mutant and wild type, but it is unclear how they relate to a patient's p53 mutational status. Such medications may have therapeutic value if additional clinical studies are conducted taking into account the tumor's p53 mutational status to examine whether they have differential activities. The tumor suppressor p53 is one crucial regulator of cellular responses. Both wild-type and mutant p53 proteins are attractive therapeutic targets because breast tumors have distinct subtype-based predominances of the p53 protein. This chapter compiles the different therapy strategies that are being researched to target p53-bearing cells in breast cancer models that are both wild type and mutant. All of these strategies seek to minimize the quantity of wild-type p53 being degraded and/or increase the amount of mutant p53 produced by chemical or genetic means. In summary, additional clinical research is needed on p53, especially for patients with high p53 mutational burden who also have TNBC and HER2-positive subtypes. p53 is a highly relevant therapeutic target for breast cancer. An important future path will be the optimization of p53-associated therapeutic techniques, including logical combinations.

REFERENCES

1. Levine, A.J. and M. Oren, The first 30 years of p53: growing ever more complex. *Nature Reviews Cancer*, 2009. **9**(10): p. 749–758.
2. Boutelle, A.M. and L.D. Attardi, p53 and tumor suppression: it takes a network. *Trends in Cell Biology*, 2021. **31**(4): p. 298–310.
3. Wang, Z., A. Strasser, and G.L. Kelly, Should mutant TP53 be targeted for cancer therapy? *Cell Death & Differentiation*, 2022. **29**(5): p. 911–920.
4. Hafner, A., et al., The multiple mechanisms that regulate p53 activity and cell fate. *Nature Reviews Molecular Cell Biology*, 2019. **20**(4): p. 199–210.
5. Vaddavalli, P.L. and B. Schumacher, The p53 network: cellular and systemic DNA damage responses in cancer and aging. *Trends in Genetics*, 2022. **38**(6): p. 598–612.

6. Parrales, A. and T. Iwakuma, Targeting oncogenic mutant p53 for cancer therapy. *Frontiers in Oncology*, 2015. **5**: p. 288.
7. Dittmer, D., et al., Gain of function mutations in p53. *Nature Genetics*, 1993. **4**(1). p. 42–46.
8. Li, T., et al., Tumor suppression in the absence of p53-mediated cell-cycle arrest, apoptosis, and senescence. *Cell*, 2012. **149**(6): p. 1269–1283.
9. Muller, P.A.J. and K.H. Vousden, Mutant p53 in cancer: new functions and therapeutic opportunities. *Cancer Cell*, 2014. **25**(3): p. 304–317.
10. Zhang, Y., et al., Somatic Trp53 mutations differentially drive breast cancer and evolution of metastases. *Nature Communications*, 2018. **9**(1): p. 3953.
11. Hanel, W., et al., Two hot spot mutant p53 mouse models display differential gain of function in tumorigenesis. *Cell Death & Differentiation*, 2013. **20**(7): p. 898–909.
12. Malkin, D., et al., Germ line p53 mutations in a familial syndrome of breast cancer, sarcomas, and other neoplasms. *Science*, 1990. **250**(4985): p. 1233–1238.
13. Olivier, M., M. Hollstein, and P. Hainaut, TP53 mutations in human cancers: origins, consequences, and clinical use. *Cold Spring Harbor Perspectives in Biology*, 2010. **2**(1): p. a001008.
14. Olivier, M., et al., Li-Fraumeni and related syndromes: correlation between tumor type, family structure, and TP53 genotype. *Cancer Research*, 2003. **63**(20): p. 6643–6650.
15. Olivier, M., et al., The clinical value of somatic TP53 gene mutations in 1,794 patients with breast cancer. *Clinical Cancer Research: An Official Journal of the American Association for Cancer Research*, 2006. **12**(4): p. 1157–1167.
16. Brosh, R. and V. Rotter, When mutants gain new powers: news from the mutant p53 field. *Nature Reviews Cancer*, 2009. **9**(10): p. 701–713.
17. Silwal-Pandit, L., et al., TP53 mutation spectrum in breast cancer is subtype specific and has distinct prognostic relevance. *Clinical Cancer Research*, 2014. **20**(13): p. 3569–3580.
18. Petitjean, A., et al., TP53 mutations in human cancers: functional selection and impact on cancer prognosis and outcomes. *Oncogene*, 2007. **26**(15): p. 2157–2165.
19. Pfeifer, G.P. and A. Besaratinia, Mutational spectra of human cancer. *Human Genetics*, 2009. **125**: p. 493–506.
20. Giacomelli, A.O., et al., Mutational processes shape the landscape of TP53 mutations in human cancer. *Nature Genetics*, 2018. **50**(10): p. 1381–1387.
21. El-Hizawi, S., et al., Induction of gene amplification as a gain-of-function phenotype of mutant p53 proteins. *Cancer Research*, 2002. **62**(11): p. 3264–3270.
22. Blandino, G. and S. Di Agostino, New therapeutic strategies to treat human cancers expressing mutant p53 proteins. *Journal of Experimental & Clinical Cancer Research*, 2018. **37**: p. 1–13.
23. Song, H., M. Hollstein, and Y. Xu, p53 gain-of-function cancer mutants induce genetic instability by inactivating ATM. *Nature Cell Biology*, 2007. **9**(5): p. 573–580.
24. Jan, N., et al., Exploring the role of trifarotene against RAR-α: an investigation of expression pattern and clinicopathological significance of RAR-α in breast cancer. *Frontiers in Pharmacology*, 2024. **15**: p. 1361679.
25. Singh, S., et al., Mutant p53 establishes targetable tumor dependency by promoting unscheduled replication. *The Journal of Clinical Investigation*, 2017. **127**(5): p. 1839–1855.
26. Mir, M.A., A. Ishrat, and N. Jan, *Prognostic and Diagnostic Significance of Chemokines and Cytokines in Cancer, in Cytokine and Chemokine Networks in Cancer.* 2023, Springer. p. 353–384.
27. Jan, N., et al., Metronomic chemotherapy and drug repurposing: a paradigm shift in oncology. *Heliyon*, 2024. https://doi.org/10.1016/j.heliyon.2024.e24670
28. Mackay, H.L., et al., Genomic instability in mutant p53 cancer cells upon entotic engulfment. *Nature Communications*, 2018. **9**(1): p. 3070.
29. Sofi, S., et al., Elucidation of interleukin-19 as a therapeutic target for breast cancer by computational analysis and experimental validation. *Saudi Journal of Biological Sciences*, 2023. **30**(9): p. 103774–103774.
30. Valenti, F., et al., Gain of function mutant p53 proteins cooperate with E2F4 to transcriptionally downregulate RAD17 and BRCA1 gene expression. *Oncotarget*, 2015. **6**(8): p. 5547.
31. Di Minin, G., et al., Mutant p53 reprograms TNF signaling in cancer cells through interaction with the tumor suppressor DAB2IP. *Molecular Cell*, 2014. **56**(5): p. 617–629.
32. Chao, C.-H., et al., Mutant p53 attenuates oxidative phosphorylation and facilitates cancer stemness through downregulating miR-200c–PCK2 axis in basal-like breast cancer. *Molecular Cancer Research*, 2021. **19**(11): p. 1900–1916.
33. Lujambio, A., et al., Non-cell-autonomous tumor suppression by p53. *Cell*, 2013. **153**(2): p. 449–460.

34. Sofi, S., et al., Clinicopathological and prognostic significance of Bcl2 in breast cancer: a comprehensive in silico and in vitro study. *Saudi Journal of Biological Sciences*, 2023. **31**(2): p. 103916.
35. Fontemaggi, G., et al., The execution of the transcriptional axis mutant p53, E2F1 and ID4 promotes tumor neo-angiogenesis. *Nature Structural & Molecular Biology*, 2009. **16**(10): p. 1086–1093.
36. Narendran, A., et al., Mutant p53 in bone marrow stromal cells increases VEGF expression and supports leukemia cell growth. *Experimental hematology*, 2003. **31**(8): p. 693–701.
37. Sofi, S., et al., A comprehensive analysis of notch signaling genes in breast cancer: expression pattern and prognostic significance. *Advances in Cancer Biology-Metastasis*, 2023. **7**: p. 100104.
38. Ubertini, V., et al., Mutant p53 gains new function in promoting inflammatory signals by repression of the secreted interleukin-1 receptor antagonist. *Oncogene*, 2015. **34**(19): p. 2493–2504.
39. Haq, B.U., et al., Targeting p53 misfolding conundrum by stabilizing agents and their analogs in breast cancer therapy: a comprehensive computational analysis. *Frontiers in Pharmacology*, 2024. **14**: p. 1333447.
40. Wang, J., et al., Autophagy augments the self-renewal of lung cancer stem cells by the degradation of ubiquitinated p53. *Cell Death & Disease*, 2021. **12**(1): p. 98.
41. Park, E.K., et al., Transcriptional repression of cancer stem cell marker CD133 by tumor suppressor p53. *Cell Death & Disease*, 2015. **6**(11): p. e1964–e1964.
42. Solomon, H., et al., Mutant p53 gain of function underlies high expression levels of colorectal cancer stem cells markers. *Oncogene*, 2018. **37**(12): p. 1669–1684.
43. Mir, M.A., M. Rashid, and N. Jan, Cytokines and Chemokines in Tumor Growth and Progression, in *Cytokine and Chemokine Networks in Cancer*. 2023, Springer. p. 33–77.
44. Escoll, M., et al., Mutant p53 oncogenic functions in cancer stem cells are regulated by WIP through YAP/TAZ. *Oncogene*, 2017. **36**(25): p. 3515–3527.
45. Zhao, Y., et al., P53-R273H mutation enhances colorectal cancer stemness through regulating specific lncRNAs. *Journal of Experimental & Clinical Cancer Research*, 2019. **38**: p. 1–16.
46. Ghatak, D., et al., MicroRNA-324-5p–CUEDC2 Axis mediates gain-of-function mutant p53-driven cancer stemness. *Molecular Cancer Research*, 2021. **19**(10): p. 1635–1650.
47. Chollat-Namy, M., et al., The pharmalogical reactivation of p53 function improves breast tumor cell lysis by granzyme B and NK cells through induction of autophagy. *Cell Death & Disease*, 2019. **10**(10): p. 695.
48. Shin, D., et al., RITA plus 3-MA overcomes chemoresistance of head and neck cancer cells via dual inhibition of autophagy and antioxidant systems. *Redox Biology*, 2017. **13**: p. 219–227.
49. Aggarwal, M., et al., Reactivation of mutant p53 by a dietary-related compound phenethyl isothiocyanate inhibits tumor growth. *Cell Death & Differentiation*, 2016. **23**(10): p. 1615–1627.
50. Yu, X., et al., Allele-specific p53 mutant reactivation. *Cancer Cell*, 2012. **21**(5): p. 614–625.
51. Hiraki, M., et al., Small-molecule reactivation of mutant p53 to wild-type-like p53 through the p53-Hsp40 regulatory axis. *Chemistry & Biology*, 2015. **22**(9): p. 1206–1216.
52. Tal, P., et al., Cancer therapeutic approach based on conformational stabilization of mutant p53 protein by small peptides. *Oncotarget*, 2016. **7**(11): p. 11817.
53. Sallman, D.A., et al., Eprenetapopt (APR-246) and azacitidine in TP53-mutant myelodysplastic syndromes. *Journal of Clinical Oncology*, 2021. **39**(14): p. 1584.
54. Zhang, Q., et al., APR-246 reactivates mutant p53 by targeting cysteines 124 and 277. *Cell Death & Disease*, 2018. **9**(5): p. 439.
55. Liu, D.S.H., et al., APR-246 potently inhibits tumour growth and overcomes chemoresistance in preclinical models of oesophageal adenocarcinoma. *Gut*, 2015. **64**(10): p. 1506–1516.
56. Birsen, R., et al., APR-246 induces early cell death by ferroptosis in acute myeloid leukemia. *Haematologica*, 2022. **107**(2): p. 403.
57. Walerych, D., et al., Proteasome machinery is instrumental in a common gain-of-function program of the p53 missense mutants in cancer. *Nature Cell Biology*, 2016. **18**(8): p. 897–909.
58. Salim, K.Y., et al., COTI-2, a new anticancer drug currently under clinical investigation, targets mutant p53 and negatively modulates the PI3K/AKT/mTOR pathway. *European Journal of Cancer*, 2016. **1**(69): p. S19.
59. Chen, S., et al., Arsenic trioxide rescues structural p53 mutations through a cryptic allosteric site. *Cancer Cell*, 2021. **39**(2): p. 225–239.
60. Zhang, W.-W., et al., The first approved gene therapy product for cancer Ad-p53 (Gendicine): 12 years in the clinic. *Human Gene Therapy*, 2018. **29**(2): p. 160–179.

61. Su, X., et al., Effect and safety of recombinant adenovirus-p53 transfer combined with radiotherapy on long-term survival of locally advanced cervical cancer. *Human Gene Therapy*, 2016. **27**(12): p. 1008–1014.
62. Heise, C., et al., ONYX-015, an E1B gene-attenuated adenovirus, causes tumor-specific cytolysis and antitumoral efficacy that can be augmented by standard chemotherapeutic agents. *Nature Medicine*, 1997. **3**(6): p. 639–645.
63. Bargonetti, J. and C. Prives, Gain-of-function mutant p53: history and speculation. *Journal of Molecular Cell Biology*, 2019. **11**(7): p. 605–609.
64. Mir, M.A., et al., Proteomics: A Groundbreaking Development in Cancer Biology, in *Proteomics*. 2023, Elsevier. p. 31–53.
65. Jain, A.N., et al., Quantitative analysis of chromosomal CGH in human breast tumors associates copy number abnormalities with p53 status and patient survival. *Proceedings of the National Academy of Sciences*, 2001. **98**(14): p. 7952–7957.
66. Murphy, K.L., A.P. Dennis, and J.M. Rosen, A gain of function p53 mutant promotes both genomic instability and cell survival in a novel p53-null mammary epithelial cell mode. *The FASEB Journal*, 2000. **14**(14): p. 2291–2302.
67. Mir, M.A., et al., Proteomics: Application of Next-Generation Proteomics in Cancer Research, in *Proteomics*. 2023, Elsevier. p. 55–76.
68. Mir, M.A., N. Jan, and H. Qayoom, Conventional Chemotherapy vs. Metronomic Chemotherapy, in *Novel Approaches in Metronomic Chemotherapy for Breast Cancer Treatment*. CRC Press. p. 27–42.
69. Zhu, J., et al., Gain-of-function p53 mutants co-opt chromatin pathways to drive cancer growth. *Nature*, 2015. **525**(7568): p. 206–211.
70. Mir, M.A., N. Jan, and S. Sofi, Introduction to Metronomic Chemotherapy, in *Novel Approaches in Metronomic Chemotherapy for Breast Cancer Treatment*. 2024, CRC Press. p. 1–14.
71. Lim, L.Y., et al., Mutant p53 mediates survival of breast cancer cells. *British Journal of Cancer*, 2009. **101**(9): p. 1606–1612.
72. Tan, B.S., et al., Mutant p53-R273H mediates cancer cell survival and anoikis resistance through AKT-dependent suppression of BCL2-modifying factor (BMF). *Cell death & disease*, 2015. **6**(7): p. e1826–e1826.
73. Di Como, C.J., C. Gaiddon, and C. Prives, p73 function is inhibited by tumor-derived p53 mutants in mammalian cells. *Molecular and Cellular Biology*, 1999. **19**(2): p. 1438–1449.
74. Kim, E. and W. Deppert, Transcriptional activities of mutant p53: when mutations are more than a loss. *Journal of Cellular Biochemistry*, 2004. **93**(5): p. 878–886.
75. Freed-Pastor, W.A., et al., Mutant p53 disrupts mammary tissue architecture via the mevalonate pathway. *Cell*, 2012. **148**(1): p. 244–258.
76. Xiao, G., et al., Gain-of-function mutant p53 R273H interacts with replicating DNA and PARP1 in breast cancer. *Cancer Research*, 2020. **80**(3): p. 394–405.
77. Di Agostino, S., et al., Gain of function of mutant p53: the mutant p53/NF-Y protein complex reveals an aberrant transcriptional mechanism of cell cycle regulation. *Cancer Cell*, 2006. **10**(3): p. 191–202.
78. Valentino, E., et al., Mutant p53 potentiates the oncogenic effects of insulin by inhibiting the tumor suppressor DAB2IP. *Proceedings of the National Academy of Sciences*, 2017. **114**(29): p. 7623–7628.
79. Mir, M.A., N. Jan, and I. Noor, Therapeutic Implications of Cytokines and Chemokines Network in Cancer, in *Cytokine and Chemokine Networks in Cancer*. 2023, Springer. p. 385–414.
80. Zhang, S., et al., Mutant p53 drives cancer metastasis via RCP-mediated Hsp90α secretion. *Cell Reports*, 2020. **32**(1): p. 107879.
81. Horigome, E., et al., Mutant TP53 modulates metastasis of triple negative breast cancer through adenosine A2b receptor signaling. *Oncotarget*, 2018. **9**(77): p. 34554.
82. Girardini, J.E., et al., A Pin1/mutant p53 axis promotes aggressiveness in breast cancer. *Cancer Cell*, 2011. **20**(1): p. 79–91.
83. Mir, M.A., et al., Metronomics: toward personalized chemotherapy. *Novel Approaches in Metronomic Chemotherapy for Breast Cancer Treatment*, 2024. p. 99–119. https://doi.org/10.1201/9781032632674-8
84. Ungerleider, N.A., et al., Breast cancer survival predicted by TP53 mutation status differs markedly depending on treatment. *Breast Cancer Research*, 2018. **20**: p. 1–8.
85. Mir, M.A., M. Rashid, and N. Jan, *The Interleukin-8 Pathway in Cancer, in Cytokine and Chemokine Networks in Cancer*. 2023, Springer. p. 165–190.
86. Mir, M.A., A. Manzoor, and N. Jan, *CCL5/CCR5 Axis in Cancer, in Cytokine and Chemokine Networks in Cancer*. 2023, Springer. p. 219–240.

87. Forslund, A., et al., MDM2 gene amplification is correlated to tumor progression but not to the presence of SNP309 or TP53 mutational status in primary colorectal cancers. *Molecular Cancer Research*, 2008. **6**(2): p. 205–211.
88. Yu, Q., et al., Amplification of Mdmx and overexpression of MDM2 contribute to mammary carcinogenesis by substituting for p53 mutations. *Diagnostic Pathology*, 2014. **9**: p. 1–8.
89. Kundu, N., et al., Estrogen-activated MDM2 disrupts mammary tissue architecture through a p53-independent pathway. *Oncotarget*, 2017. **8**(29): p. 47916.
90. Baek, S., et al., Structure of the stapled p53 peptide bound to Mdm2. *Journal of the American Chemical Society*, 2012. **134**(1): p. 103–106.
91. Nag, S., et al., Targeting MDM2-p53 interaction for cancer therapy: are we there yet? *Current Medicinal Chemistry*, 2014. **21**(5): p. 553–574.
92. Vassilev, L.T., et al., In vivo activation of the p53 pathway by small-molecule antagonists of MDM2. *Science*, 2004. **303**(5659): p. 844–848.
93. Ding, Q., et al., Discovery of RG7388, a potent and selective p53–MDM2 inhibitor in clinical development. *Journal of Medicinal Chemistry*, 2013. **56**(14): p. 5979–5983.
94. Shangary, S., et al., Temporal activation of p53 by a specific MDM2 inhibitor is selectively toxic to tumors and leads to complete tumor growth inhibition. *Proceedings of the National Academy of Sciences*, 2008. **105**(10): p. 3933–3938.
95. Graves, B., et al., Activation of the p53 pathway by small-molecule-induced MDM2 and MDMX dimerization. *Proceedings of the National Academy of Sciences*, 2012. **109**(29): p. 11788–11793.
96. Mir, M.A., M. Bashir, and N. Jan, The Role of Interleukin (IL)-6/IL-6 Receptor Axis in Cancer, in *Cytokine and Chemokine Networks in Cancer*. 2023, Springer. p. 137–164.
97. Xia, M., et al., Elevated MDM2 boosts the apoptotic activity of p53-MDM2 binding inhibitors by facilitating MDMX degradation. *Cell Cycle*, 2008. **7**(11): p. 1604–1612.
98. Reed, D., et al., Identification and characterization of the first small molecule inhibitor of MDMX. *Journal of Biological Chemistry*, 2010. **285**(14): p. 10786–10796.
99. Wang, H., et al., A small-molecule inhibitor of MDMX activates p53 and induces apoptosis. *Molecular Cancer Therapeutics*, 2011. **10**(1): p. 69–79.
100. Mir, M.A., Sumaya, N. Jan, Implications of Chemokine Heterogenicity in Cancer Metastasis, in *Cytokine and Chemokine Networks in Cancer*. 2023, Springer. p. 115–136.
101. Ding, K., et al., Structure-based design of spiro-oxindoles as potent, specific small-molecule inhibitors of the MDM2– p53 interaction. *Journal of Medicinal Chemistry*, 2006. **49**(12): p. 3432–3435.
102. Islam, M.S., et al., Synthesis, anticancer activity, and molecular modeling of new halogenated spiro [pyrrolidine-thiazolo-oxindoles] derivatives. *Applied Sciences*, 2020. **10**(6): p. 2170.
103. Wang, S., et al., SAR405838: an optimized inhibitor of MDM2–p53 interaction that induces complete and durable tumor regression. *Cancer Research*, 2014. **74**(20): p. 5855–5865.
104. Lu, J., et al., Reactivation of p53 by MDM2 inhibitor MI-77301 for the treatment of endocrine-resistant breast cancer. *Molecular Cancer Therapeutics*, 2016. **15**(12): p. 2887–2893.
105. Saxena, R., et al., Spiro-oxindole derivative 5-chloro-4′, 5′-diphenyl-3′-(4-(2-(piperidin-1-yl) ethoxy) benzoyl) spiro [indoline-3, 2′-pyrrolidin]-2-one triggers apoptosis in breast cancer cells via restoration of p53 function. *The International Journal of Biochemistry & Cell Biology*, 2016. **70**: p. 105–117.
106. Mu, J., et al., Discovery of spirooxindole–ferrocene hybrids as novel MDM2 inhibitors. *Chinese Chemical Letters*, 2021. **32**(6): p. 1897–1901.
107. Kumar, A., et al., Design and synthesis of new bioisosteres of spirooxindoles (MI-63/219) as anti-breast cancer agents. *Bioorganic & Medicinal Chemistry*, 2015. **23**(4): p. 839–848.
108. Liu, S.-J., et al., Design, synthesis, and biological evaluation of nitroisoxazole-containing spiro [pyrrolidin-oxindole] derivatives as novel glutathione peroxidase 4/mouse double minute 2 dual inhibitors that inhibit breast adenocarcinoma cell proliferation. *European Journal of Medicinal Chemistry*, 2021. **217**: p. 113359.
109. Issaeva, N., et al., Small molecule RITA binds to p53, blocks p53–HDM-2 interaction and activates p53 function in tumors. *Nature Medicine*, 2004. **10**(12): p. 1321–1328.
110. Spinnler, C., et al., Abrogation of Wip1 expression by RITA-activated p53 potentiates apoptosis induction via activation of ATM and inhibition of HdmX. *Cell Death & Differentiation*, 2011. **18**(11): p. 1736–1745.
111. Brandão, P., et al., Targeting the MDM2-p53 protein-protein interaction with prenylchalcones: Synthesis of a small library and evaluation of potential antitumor activity. *European Journal of Medicinal Chemistry*, 2018. **156**: p. 711–721.

112. Hsu, Y.-L., et al., Tricetin, a dietary flavonoid, inhibits proliferation of human breast adenocarcinoma mcf-7 cells by blocking cell cycle progression and inducing apoptosis. *Journal of Agricultural and Food Chemistry*, 2009. **57**(18): p. 8688–8695.
113. Portman, N., et al., MDM2 inhibition in combination with endocrine therapy and CDK4/6 inhibition for the treatment of ER-positive breast cancer. *Breast Cancer Research*, 2020. **22**: p. 1–17.
114. Wang, Y., et al., Degradation of proteins by PROTACs and other strategies. *Acta Pharmaceutica Sinica B*, 2020. **10**(2): p. 207–238.
115. Li, Y., et al., Discovery of MD-224 as a first-in-class, highly potent, and efficacious proteolysis targeting chimera murine double minute 2 degrader capable of achieving complete and durable tumor regression. *Journal of Medicinal Chemistry*, 2018. **62**(2): p. 448–466.
116. Qin, J.-J., et al., Identification of a new class of natural product MDM2 inhibitor: In vitro and in vivo anti-breast cancer activities and target validation. *Oncotarget*, 2015. **6**(5): p. 2623.
117. Qin, J.-J., et al., Inulanolide A as a new dual inhibitor of NFAT1-MDM2 pathway for breast cancer therapy. *Oncotarget*, 2016. **7**(22): p. 32566.
118. Qin, J.-J., et al., Identification of lineariifolianoid A as a novel dual NFAT1 and MDM2 inhibitor for human cancer therapy. *Journal of Biomedical Research*, 2016. **30**(4): p. 322.
119. Wang, W., et al., The pyrido [b] indole MDM2 inhibitor SP-141 exerts potent therapeutic effects in breast cancer models. *Nature Communications*, 2014. **5**(1): p. 5086.
120. Singh, A.K., et al., Dual targeting of MDM2 with a novel small-molecule inhibitor overcomes TRAIL resistance in cancer. *Carcinogenesis*, 2016. **37**(11): p. 1027–1040.
121. Mrkvová, Z., et al., Benzimidazoles downregulate Mdm2 and MdmX and activate p53 in MdmX overexpressing tumor cells. *Molecules*, 2019. **24**(11): p. 2152.
122. Dolfi, S.C., et al., Fulvestrant treatment alters MDM2 protein turnover and sensitivity of human breast carcinoma cells to chemotherapeutic drugs. *Cancer Letters*, 2014. **350**(1–2): p. 52–60.
123. Wang, W., et al., In vitro and in vivo anticancer activity of novel synthetic makaluvamine analogues. *Clinical Cancer Research*, 2009. **15**(10): p. 3511–3518.
124. Wang, W., et al., A novel synthetic iminoquinone, BA-TPQ, as an anti-breast cancer agent: in vitro and in vivo activity and mechanisms of action. *Breast Cancer Research and Treatment*, 2010. **123**: p. 321–331.
125. Proietti, S., et al., Melatonin down-regulates MDM 2 gene expression and enhances p53 acetylation in MCF-7 cells. *Journal of Pineal Research*, 2014. **57**(1): p. 120–129.
126. Rong, J.-J., et al., Gambogic acid down-regulates MDM2 oncogene and induces p21Waf1/CIP1 expression independent of p53. *Cancer Letters*, 2009. **284**(1): p. 102–112.
127. Van Poznak, C., et al., Oral gossypol in the treatment of patients with refractory metastatic breast cancer: a phase I/II clinical trial. *Breast Cancer Research and Treatment*, 2001. **66**: p. 239–248.
128. Xiong, J., et al., Gossypol has anti-cancer effects by dual-targeting MDM2 and VEGF in human breast cancer. *Breast Cancer Research*, 2017. **19**: p. 1–10.
129. Lu, T.-L., et al., Hispolon promotes MDM2 downregulation through chaperone-mediated autophagy. *Biochemical and Biophysical Research Communications*, 2010. **398**(1): p. 26–31.
130. Mu, R., et al., Involvement of p53 in oroxylin A-induced apoptosis in cancer cells. *Molecular Carcinogenesis: Published in Cooperation with the University of Texas MD Anderson Cancer Center*, 2009. **48**(12): p. 1159–1169.
131. Kitagaki, J., et al., Targeting tumor cells expressing p53 with a water-soluble inhibitor of Hdm2. *Molecular Cancer Therapeutics*, 2008. **7**(8): p. 2445–2454.
132. Dickens, M.P., et al., 5-Deazaflavin derivatives as inhibitors of p53 ubiquitination by HDM2. *Bioorganic & Medicinal Chemistry*, 2013. **21**(22): p. 6868–6877.
133. Avtanski, D.B., et al., Indolo-pyrido-isoquinolin based alkaloid inhibits growth, invasion and migration of breast cancer cells via activation of p53-miR34a axis. *Molecular Oncology*, 2016. **10**(7): p. 1118–1132.
134. Herman, A.G., et al., Discovery of Mdm2-MdmX E3 ligase inhibitors using a cell-based ubiquitination assay. *Cancer Discovery*, 2011. **1**(4): p. 312–325.
135. Tabernero, J., et al., A phase I first-in-human pharmacokinetic and pharmacodynamic study of serdemetan in patients with advanced solid tumors. *Clinical Cancer Research*, 2011. **17**(19): p. 6313–6321.
136. Kojima, K., et al., The novel tryptamine derivative JNJ-26854165 induces wild-type p53-and E2F1-mediated apoptosis in acute myeloid and lymphoid leukemias. *Molecular Cancer Therapeutics*, 2010. **9**(9): p. 2545–2557.
137. Silwal-Pandit, L., A. Langerød, and A.-L. Børresen-Dale, TP53 mutations in breast and ovarian cancer. *Cold Spring Harbor Perspectives in Medicine*, 2017. **7**(1): p. a026252.

138. Berke, T.P., S.H. Slight, and S.M. Hyder, Role of reactivating mutant p53 protein in suppressing growth and metastasis of triple-negative breast cancer. *OncoTargets and Therapy*, 2022: p. 23–30.
139. Rivlin, N., et al., Mutations in the p53 tumor suppressor gene: important milestones at the various steps of tumorigenesis. *Genes & Cancer*, 2011. **2**(4): p. 466–474.
140. Rangel, L.P., et al., p53 reactivation with induction of massive apoptosis-1 (PRIMA-1) inhibits amyloid aggregation of mutant p53 in cancer cells. *Journal of Biological Chemistry*, 2019. **294**(10): p. 3670–3682.
141. Liang, Y., C. Besch-Williford, and S.M. Hyder, PRIMA-1 inhibits growth of breast cancer cells by re-activating mutant p53 protein. *International Journal of Oncology*, 2009. **35**(5): p. 1015–1023.
142. Synnott, N.C., et al., Mutant p53: a novel target for the treatment of patients with triple-negative breast cancer? *International Journal of Cancer*, 2017. **140**(1): p. 234–246.
143. Zhang, M., et al., WEE1 inhibition by MK1775 as a single-agent therapy inhibits ovarian cancer viability Corrigendum in/10.3892/ol. 2018.8757. *Oncology Letters*, 2017. **14**(3): p. 3580–3586.
144. Ha, D.-H., et al., Antitumor effect of a WEE1 inhibitor and potentiation of olaparib sensitivity by DNA damage response modulation in triple-negative breast cancer. *Scientific Reports*, 2020. **10**(1): p. 9930.
145. Fallah, Y., et al., Targeting WEE1 inhibits growth of breast cancer cells that are resistant to endocrine therapy and CDK4/6 inhibitors. *Frontiers in Oncology*, 2021. **11**: p. 681530.
146. Jones, C.B., et al., UCN-01 and camptothecin induce DNA double-strand breaks in p53 mutant tumor cells, but not in normal or p53 negative epithelial cells. *International Journal of Oncology*, 2000. **17**(5): p. 1043–1094.
147. Ma, C.X., et al., Targeting Chk1 in p53-deficient triple-negative breast cancer is therapeutically beneficial in human-in-mouse tumor models. *The Journal of Clinical Investigation*, 2012. **122**(4): p. 1541–1552.
148. Ma, Z., et al., The Chk1 inhibitor AZD7762 sensitises p53 mutant breast cancer cells to radiation in vitro and in vivo. *Molecular medicine reports*, 2012. **6**(4): p. 897–903.
149. Jabbour-Leung, N.A., et al., Sequential combination therapy of CDK inhibition and doxorubicin is synthetically lethal in p53-mutant triple-negative breast cancer. *Molecular Cancer Therapeutics*, 2016. **15**(4): p. 593–607.
150. Zonneville, J., et al., Selective therapeutic strategy for p53-deficient cancer by targeting dysregulation in DNA repair. *Communications Biology*, 2021. **4**(1): p. 862.
151. Jung, Y., et al., Crosstalk between Plk1, p53, cell cycle, and G2/M DNA damage checkpoint regulation in cancer: computational modeling and analysis. *NPJ Systems Biology and Applications*, 2021. **7**(1): p. 46.
152. Giordano, A., et al., Polo-like kinase 1 inhibitor onvansertib synergizes with paclitaxel in breast cancer carrying p53 mutation. *Annals of Oncology*, 2019. **30**: p. v125–v126.
153. Emerling, B.M., et al., Depletion of a putatively druggable class of phosphatidylinositol kinases inhibits growth of p53-null tumors. *Cell*, 2013. **155**(4): p. 844–857.
154. Valente, J.F.A., J.A. Queiroz, and F. Sousa, p53 as the focus of gene therapy: past, present and future. *Current Drug Targets*, 2018. **19**(15): p. 1801–1817.
155. Wang, X., et al., Ad-p53 enhances the sensitivity of triple-negative breast cancer MDA-MB-468 cells to the EGFR inhibitor gefitinib. *Oncology Reports*, 2015. **33**(2): p. 526–532.
156. Cristofanilli, M., et al., A nonreplicating adenoviral vector that contains the wild-type p53 transgene combined with chemotherapy for primary breast cancer: safety, efficacy, and biologic activity of a novel gene-therapy approach. *Cancer: Interdisciplinary International Journal of the American Cancer Society*, 2006. **107**(5): p. 935–944.
157. Okal, A., et al., Re-engineered p53 activates apoptosis in vivo and causes primary tumor regression in a dominant negative breast cancer xenograft model. *Gene Therapy*, 2014. **21**(10): p. 903–912.
158. Ubby, I., et al., Cancer therapeutic targeting using mutant–p53-specific siRNAs. *Oncogene*, 2019. **38**(18): p. 3415–3427.
159. Komor, A.C., et al., Programmable editing of a target base in genomic DNA without double-stranded DNA cleavage. *Nature*, 2016. **533**(7603): p. 420–424.
160. Chen, X., et al., Mutant p53 in cancer: from molecular mechanism to therapeutic modulation. *Cell Death & Disease*, 2022. **13**(11): p. 974.
161. Shostak, K., et al., MDM2 restrains estrogen-mediated AKT activation by promoting TBK1-dependent HPIP degradation. *Cell Death & Differentiation*, 2014. **21**(5): p. 811–824.

5 p53 and Cell Death Regulation
Managing Apoptosis in Breast Cancer

Arfa Ji[1], Ibtisam Mumtaz[2], Nusrat Jan[3], Shahnaz Anjum[4], Aaqib Rashid[5], Asfer Hamid[6], Ehtisham-ul Haq[1], and Manzoor Ahmad Mir[*3]*

[1]Department of Biotechnology, University of Kashmir, Srinagar,
[2]Department of Nanotechnology, University of Kashmir
[3]Department of Bioresources, School of Biological Sciences, University of Kashmir, Srinagar, J&K, India
[4]Department of Botany, School of Bioengineering and Biosciences, Lovely Professional University, Phagwara, Punjab, India
[5]Department of Physics, National Institute of Technology, Srinagar, India
[6]Division of Soil Science and Agricultural Chemistry, SKUAST, Jammu, India
*drmanzoor@kashmiruniversity.ac.in

5.1 INTRODUCTION

One of the most common malignancies to strike women worldwide is breast cancer [1, 2], for which the p53 gene is largely responsible. Recent studies have focused a great deal of emphasis on this gene. Often called the "gatekeeper" gene, p53 is essential for controlling cell proliferation and preventing the development of malignant cells [3, 4]. As a tumor suppressor, p53 typically detects DNA damage and initiates cellular repair processes. On the other hand, mutations in the p53 gene might cause it to malfunction, which can result in unchecked cell division and perhaps promote the growth of cancer. Notably, p53 mutations are present in up to 30% of breast cancer cases, highlighting the importance of this gene in this illness. Research suggests that those with inherited p53 mutations are significantly more likely to get breast cancer as well as other cancers such as ovarian, pancreatic, and colorectal cancers [5–7]. p53 has several diverse roles, including tissue homeostasis, development, and stem cell maintenance in addition to tumor suppression. Mutant p53 has several carcinogenic characteristics in cell culture models, including enhanced invasion, migration, angiogenesis, and stem cell proliferation, underscoring its complex role in the development of cancer. Even though there is currently no treatment for breast cancer, people who have p53 mutations can greatly reduce their chance of developing the disease by being identified and given access to customized preventive interventions like prophylactic surgery or increased surveillance. Thus, it becomes critical to understand how the p53 gene contributes to the prevention of breast cancer. Research efforts to understand the role of p53 in the initiation and spread of breast cancer are promising in terms of revealing new interventions and cures for this terrible disease [8]. Furthermore, TP53 has a significant impact on the formation of malignancies as it is the gene that is altered in human cancers the most commonly. The p53 protein, which primarily functions as a transcription factor, is involved in the control of

DOI: 10.1201/9781003520771-5

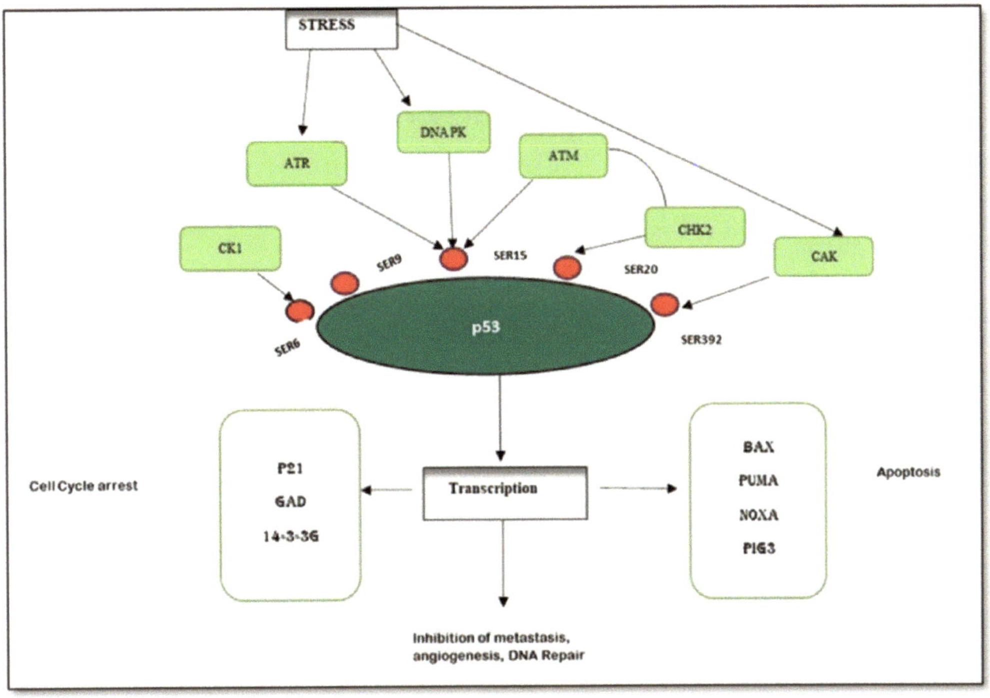

FIGURE 5.1 Components of p53 signaling: p53 is inactive under normal conditions. Activation occurs in response to various stresses such as DNA damage and post-translational modifications such as phosphorylation on serine residues downstream.

several pathways that are essential for deciding the fate of cells under stress. These pathways include cell cycle regulation, DNA repair, apoptosis, and metabolism. Mutations in TP53 can decrease DNA-specific binding and protein conformational stability, hence disrupting the operation of the p53 pathway, despite its deep interconnectedness and intricacy. Researchers are making progress in targeted therapeutics targeting p53, despite the obstacles presented by its complex structure and the difficulties in restoring its function. Novel therapeutic approaches can be made possible by having a thorough understanding of the structural characteristics, signaling pathways, and biological workings of p53. Different upstream regulatory kinases are required for diverse pathways that are involved in the activation of the p53 signaling pathway, which is activated by different cellular stressors. Significantly, p53 activation raises protein levels, decreases degradation, and increases DNA binding affinity, all of which lead to the activation of several genes with various roles that are critical in the fight against cancer. p53 is in pause mode under normal body functions. Under stress conditions, p53 and many other independent pathways are activated that are believed to be dependent on the upstream regulatory kinases (Figure 5.1). These pathways include ATM (ataxia-telangiectasia), the human homolog of the Rad53 (Chk2)-dependent pathway that is activated by DNA double-strand breaks, another pathway that is activated by ultraviolet light and cytotoxic anti-tumor agents but is independent of ATM, Chk2, and p14ARF [9, 10]. The activation of all these pathways results in high levels of p53 because of the mouse double minute 2 (MDM2)-dependent proteolytic degradation and increased affinity of p53 for DNA. The activation of p53 results in its sequence-specific DNA binding activity, and a large number of genes are being recognized as transcriptional targets of wild-type p53 [11]. Table 5.1 illustrates the biochemical modifications of p53.

TABLE 5.1
Biochemical Modifications of p53

Target Residue	Modification	Modifying Protein
Ser 6	Phosphorylation	CHK1
Ser 9	Phosphorylation	CHK1
Ser 15	Phosphorylation	ATM, ATR, CHK1, P38
Thr 18	Phosphorylation	CHK1
Ser 20	Phosphorylation	CHK1, CHK2
Ser 33	Phosphorylation	P38, JNK
Ser 37	Phosphorylation	ATR, DNA PK
Thr 55	Phosphorylation	TAFII, 250, ERK2
Thr 81	Phosphorylation	JNK
Ser 127, Pro 128	*Cis-trans* isomerization	PIN1
Thr 155	Phosphorylation	CK2
Ser 215	Phosphorylation	STK15
Lys 305	Acetylation	P300
Lys 320	Acetylation	PCAF
Ser 371	Phosphorylation	PKC

5.2 p53 AND CANCER PROGRESSION

Mostly missense mutations are believed to occur in around 50% of all malignancies, and p53 is regarded as the most commonly altered gene among many having a role in human cancers [12]. These mutations frequently lead to poor sequence-specific DNA binding, which hinders the ability of the wild-type p53 protein to transactivate genes that are normally elevated. The prevalence of missense mutations in p53 is interesting since it is higher than in other tumor suppressor genes. This suggests that the production of p53 mutants may have selective benefits in addition to eliminating wild-type function [13, 14]. This idea is supported by the fact that a large number of p53 mutations linked to human cancers show characteristics not found in the wild-type protein. A considerable fraction of tumors without mutations have p53 function impaired by other established mechanisms. For example, interaction with virally encoded proteins in malignancies linked with viruses might result in sequestration or increased degradation of p53. MDM2, which attaches to p53 and aids in the ubiquitination of its C-terminus, designating it for destruction, is a crucial component in the control of p53. But by attaching to MDM2, p14ARF shatters this relationship, stopping MDM2 and p53 from interacting and stabilizing p53 [4, 9]. Consequently, conditions like MDM2 overexpression or the deletion or epigenetic silencing of p14ARF may unintentionally promote the degradation of p53. Many common human malignancies have been shown to have lost p14ARF, especially in cases where the p53 gene is still wild type. The cytoplasmic sequestration of the p53 protein, which prevents its nuclear localization and thus reduces its function, is another method of p53 inactivation. These complex mechanisms highlight the variety of tactics cancer cells use to sidestep p53's tumor-suppressive actions, which aid in the spread of the disease and increase resistance to treatment. A thorough comprehension of these pathways is essential for the development of targeted medicines intended to improve or restore p53 function in the treatment of cancer. A common feature of human malignancies is a mutation in the TP53 gene, which is present in about half of cases of skin, breast, colon, lung, liver, prostate, and bladder cancers. The p53 protein in its wild-type form is essential for stopping cell division in response to DNA damage, which stops damaged cells from proliferating and developing into malignant cells. On the other hand, TP53 mutations cause the cell cycle to become unbalanced, which results in unchecked cell division and the spread of damaged

DNA to offspring cells, giving rise to malignant cells. The p53 proteins, which are encoded by the wild-type TP53 gene, act as transcription factors that have a role in a variety of cellular responses vital to halt or reduce the spread of cancer and thereby protect genomic integrity. The nuclear p53 protein, which serves as the "guardian of the genome," controls normal cell proliferation [4, 15]. On the other hand, the buildup of mutant p53 that is not functional in tumor cell nuclei is linked to the initiation and spread of several malignancies, including breast cancer [16]. A key mechanism in tumor suppression, p53 activation causes senescence and cell cycle arrest under extreme oncogenic stress. When oncogenic stimuli concentrate on important signaling nodes, including the mTOR kinase, they can incite cell proliferation by deactivating the p53/p21 CD-interacting protein 1 (Cipl) complex through activation of the Raf/MEK/ERK cascade, which can happen in both Ras-dependently and Ras-independently [17]. Moreover, the pathways p53/p21/p27 and p53/Bcl-2/Bex influence several biological functions, such as cell division, the G2/M phase, and apoptosis. Notably, the inter-alpha-trypsin inhibitor heavy chain 5 protein, which is encoded by the ITIH5 gene, may be regulated by p53 in addition to other tumor suppressor proteins [14, 18]. Furthermore, by inhibiting the expression of transcription factors ZEB1 and ZEB2, p53 prevents the epithelial–mesenchymal transition (EMT). In cultured cells, mutant p53 proteins show carcinogenic properties; in mice models, they encourage metastasis and genomic instability [19]. These mutations, which usually affect the core DNA-binding domain, change the structural stability of p53 and cause phenotypes that either gain or lose function. Through a variety of pathways, such as altered gene expression, interactions with multiple transcription factors, and modification of downstream effector genes, mutant p53 proteins, cause cancer. By directly interacting with DNA sequences or binding to important transcription factors like p63 and p73, they may regulate the expression of certain genes [4]. Furthermore, mutant p53 protein targets regulatory molecules, microRNAs, and signaling pathways that facilitate the development, invasion, and metastasis of cancer. In response to cellular stress, post-translational changes like phosphorylation, acetylation, and methylation further control p53 activity and stability (Figure 5.2). Specific serine and threonine residues on p53 can be phosphorylated to activate or alter its actions, which can affect DNA repair and death in cells [20]. These

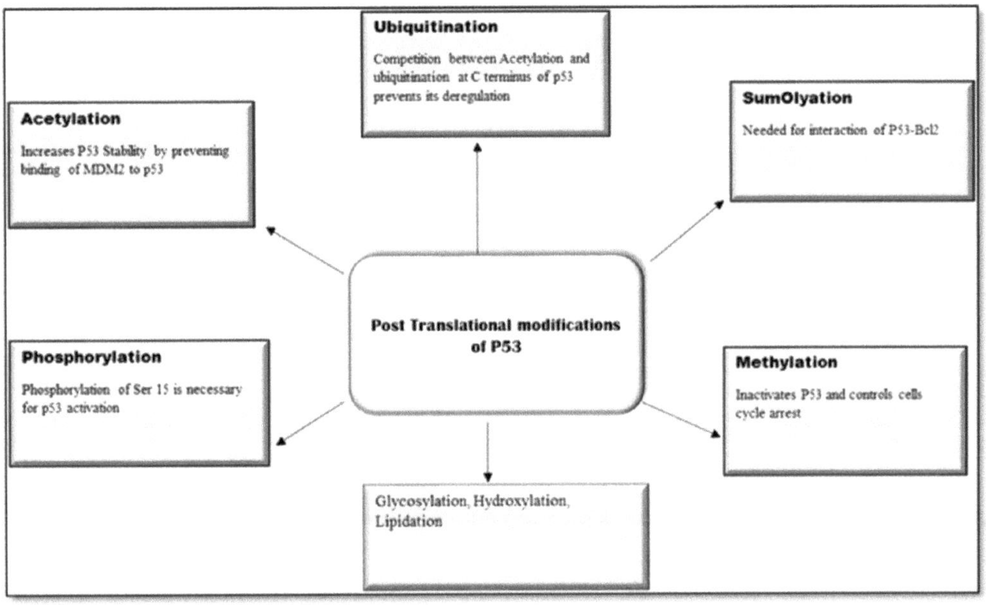

FIGURE 5.2 Ubiquitination, phosphorylation, methylation, and other modifications on p53 protein play a crucial role in regulating p53 stability and localization in response to genotoxic stress.

modifications include phosphorylation, methylation, glycosylation, acetylation, ubiquitination, and sumoylation, which occur in different regions of the p53 protein and are essential in controlling p53 stability and localization, which in turn affects p53's capacity to modulate cell proliferation and cell death [21]. The lysine and arginine residues on p53 are important locations for the modifications of acetylation and methylation, which control the transcriptional activity and stability of the protein. In conclusion, understanding the intricate processes that underlie the activity of mutant p53 is essential for creating tailored treatments that counteract the progression, and mutant p53 protein post-transcriptional modifications have a quick turnover because of ubiquitination, which is mediated by the E3 ubiquitin ligase MDM2 and subsequent proteasomal destruction. Several post translational modifications (PTMs) regulate p53 stability in response to genotoxic stress [22]. There are different phosphorylation sites identified on serine and threonine on p53 proteins. Mostly phosphorylation of serine 15 is very important for the activation of p53. ATM- and ATR-mediated phosphorylation of downstream substrates, including casein kinase (CK1), checkpoint kinase 1 (Chk2), and p53, limits cancer cell viability by modulating many critical biochemical pathways leading to cell cycle arrest, DNA repair, senescence, and death [23]. Mutant p53 becomes a key figure in the pathophysiology of cancer through a variety of interactions and regulatory functions, underscoring its potential as a target for treatment.

Gene p53 encodes the p53 protein, which functions as a transcription factor to prevent abnormal cell division and proliferation. Recent studies have shown that TP53 has a regulatory role in several types of programmed cell death (PCD), including apoptosis, autophagy, pyroptosis, and ferroptosis [20]. TP53 also influences pathways that result in the generation of reactive oxygen species (ROS). For example, p53 increases the expression of proteins involved in apoptosis to support the organism, hence encouraging apoptosis [24]. On PCD, mutant p53 has a contrasting effect. The wild-type p53 protein undergoes rapid degradation. Conversely, when the TP53 gene is modified, p53 builds up in tumor cells, accelerating the initiation and propagation of cancer [17]. Approximately 50% of all cancer cases have been found to contain TP53 mutations. Analysis of the MSK MetTropism database on cBioPortal shows that the prevalence of these mutations varies depending on the type of cancer [25]. The most often altered areas of TP53's DNA binding domain are amino acid residues 102–292, as shown by previous research [26]. These mutations are commonly overexpressed in cancerous cells and lead to three carcinogenic properties: acquisition of new functions that usually promote tumor growth; loss of p53 function, which leads to the inability to activate downstream target genes; and dominant-negative effects (DNEs), which result in blocking the function of normal p53 protein in cells [20]. TP53 mutations result in the loss of tumor suppressor function and the acquisition of oncogenic properties [17]. In recent years, researchers have discovered several new ways in which death occurs, and some studies have provided a clear understanding of the underlying processes of different death modes in cancer. Concurrently, there is a growing body of extensive research on TP53 gene mutations in malignancies. However, the topic of how TP53 mutations regulate programmed cell death is hardly addressed. This study aims to examine the correlation between TP53 mutation and programmed cell death, providing novel insights into tumor therapy [27].

5.3 REGULATION OF TP53 ACTIVATION AND p53-DRIVEN CELLULAR OUTCOMES

In cells that are not under stress and have not undergone any changes, the levels of wild-type p53 protein are usually extremely low, and in certain instances, they may even be impossible to detect, despite the existence of mRNA expression that can be easily detected. An important element in this process is the E3 ligase MDM2, which guides p53 toward proteasomal degradation [28]. Upon exposure to various stressors, such as the activation of oncogenes, DNA damage, or nutritional restriction, there is a substantial elevation in the levels of p53 protein. This effect arises due to the

TABLE 5.2
p53 Target Genes Known to be Altered under Multiple Stress Conditions

Function	Regulated Genes
Cell cycle arrest	CyclinA2, Cyclin B1, Cyclin G1, DDA3, TERT
DNA repair	53PB2, DDB2, P53R2, RECQ4, XPC
Apoptosis and survival	APAF-1, BAI.1, P53AIP1, PIR121, BCL2, BCL2L14, BAK1, BAX, BID, NOXA. SURVIVIN, WIP1
Angiogenesis	BAI1, ENDOSTATIN, KAI1/CD82, MASPIN, MMP2, VEGF
Other effects	BRCA1, CHK1, CHK2, COP1, CSPG2, MDM2, PCAF, PML

activation of many signaling pathways by these stressors, which eventually results in the inhibition of MDM2. Concurrently, certain alterations (such as acetylation and phosphorylation) can take place in the p53 protein itself [29, 30]. Upon activation, p53 forms a homotetramer and selectively binds to certain sequences within the regulatory regions of around 500 target genes. Experiments conducted on cell lines using temperature-sensitive mutants or artificially increased levels of p53 have demonstrated that p53 can initiate a variety of cellular processes, such as programmed cell death, cellular aging, halting of the cell cycle, coordination of different DNA repair pathways, and adjustment of cellular metabolism [31]. These findings have been extensively reviewed by Vousden and Lane (2007), as well as Freed-Pastor and Prives (2012). Gene-targeted mice were employed in gene expression studies and functional assays to precisely identify genes essential for certain p53-activated cellular responses. For instance, the process of p53-mediated G1/S border cell cycle arrest and cell senescence requires the involvement of the cyclin-dependent kinase inhibitor (CDKi) p21, along with other p53 target genes that contribute to this process. Furthermore, research has shown that p53 can directly impact or indirectly regulate several genes involved in distinct DNA repair processes. Ultimately, it was discovered that the direct activation of Mdm2 by p53 at the transcriptional level was essential for the negative feedback loop of p53 signaling. The observation that the elimination of MDM2 leads to increased p53 activation and early embryonic mortality in mice, which may be averted by the concomitant absence of Trp53, is an exceptionally remarkable example [32] (Table 5.2).

5.4 p53-DRIVEN INDUCTION OF APOPTOSIS

If cells are impaired by pathogens or detrimental substances, apoptosis, a form of programmed cell death, functions to reinstate equilibrium [33]. Illustratively, the scientific comprehension of apoptosis in the context of cancer unveils its capacity to eradicate malignant cells and impede the advancement and spread of malignancies. TP53 plays a vital role in regulating apoptosis, which is the process of programmed cell death. Cells can detect external pressure through kinases when they are exposed to stress from cytotoxins or radiation. These kinases proceed to modify the p53 protein by phosphorylating or acetylating it at various sites, resulting in the activation of p53 [34, 35]. An increase in the transcriptional expression of several BH3-only proteins, including Bid, Bim, Bad, Bmf, Bik/Nbk, Blk, Noxa, Bbc3, and DP5, occurs upon p53 activation. Initiated by the increased presence of BH3-only proteins, the formation of oligomers on the mitochondrial membrane results in the direct activation of BAX/BAK. Consequently, the outer mitochondrial membrane becomes more permeable, leading to the liberation of cytochrome c into the cytoplasm. The interaction between cytochrome c and the apoptosis protease activator factor (Apaf)-1 results in the recruitment of procaspase-9 and the subsequent development of apoptotic bodies. Initiating the caspase cascade pathway within the apoptosome is caspase-9 autoproteolytic cleavage [36]. It has been discovered that the TP53R175H mutation influences caspase-dependent apoptosis. Through interaction and inhibition with caspase-8, caspase-9, and caspase-3, it effectively restricts the progression of the process. This is the result of mutant p53 being produced [37]. Scientific research has established that TP53R175H possesses the capability to induce miRNA128-2 expression in non-small cell lung cancer (NSCLC). Following transcription, the E2F5 protein is profoundly influenced by this particular microRNA. Subsequently, the capacity of E2F5 to impede the cytoplasmic transcription of p21 (waf1) is compromised. Cleaving caspase-3 inhibits an anti-apoptotic effect [38]. Specific TP53 mutations, such as TP53P72R, do not significantly impair p53's capacity to induce cell death in ovarian cancer, according to another study. An intriguing finding was reported by Thomas et al. in their investigation of the P72R p53 mutant. They discovered that this mutant is structurally similar to the wild type and has the same affinity for the DNA sequence that p53 recognizes [39]. Furthermore, variations in Arg72 and Pro72 may result from TP53 gene single-nucleotide polymorphisms. Nevertheless, research has demonstrated that the Arg72 variant induces apoptosis more efficiently. Furthermore, it has been discovered that p53 mutations contribute to the coordination of the miRNA network, thereby conferring resistance to doxorubicin, 5-fluorouracil, and cisplatin-induced apoptosis. Furthermore, specific pharmaceutical agents function by impeding MDM2, a critical negative regulator of TP53, or by reinstating the regular activity of mutant cells [37]. An investigation was undertaken to examine the impacts of a temperature-sensitive conditionally active mutant of p53 on a myeloid leukemia cell line. At 37°C, this mutant protein exhibits mutant characteristics; however, at 32°C, it assumes the structure and function of wild-type p53. The research outcomes unveiled the prospective function of p53 as an inducer of apoptotic cell death. Additional research has corroborated and expanded upon the finding that p53 is capable of inducing apoptosis. A multitude of cell lines were utilized in these investigations, including Burkitt lymphoma cells, erythroleukemia cells, and colon cancer cell lines, in addition to temperature-sensitive and wild-type p53 [40]. Two distinct mechanisms emerge within mammalian cells, which ultimately converge and lead to apoptosis. The death receptor pathway, alternatively referred to as the extrinsic pathway, is initiated when specific tumor necrosis factor receptor family members containing an intracellular death domain bind [37]. Conversely, the BCL-2-regulated pathway, which is alternatively known as the intrinsic, mitochondrial, or stress pathway, becomes active in response to a range of stressors including DNA damage, cytokine deprivation, and endoplasmic reticulum stress. Through transcriptional and post-transcriptional processes, specific pro-apoptotic BH3-only members of the BCL-2 protein family are elevated; this initiates cell death along the apoptotic pathway that is regulated by BCL-2. BCL-2 proteins that promote survival (BCL-2, BCLXL, MCL-1, BCL-W, and A1/BFL1) are subject to regulation by BH3-only proteins that inhibit their activity. These two proteins, BAX and BAK, are members of the BCL-2 family. In addition to their involvement in cell death, they might also contain a protein known as BOK. BH3-only proteins have been shown to possess the capability of directly activating BAX/BAK, according to research cited in numerous scientific reviews. The cell disassembly process is initiated in the pathway delineated by caspase-939 and its activator APAF-142. Once the point of no return in apoptosis signaling, mitochondrial outer membrane permeabilization (MOMP) is triggered by the activation of BAX/BAK. On the contrary, the activation of caspase-8 occurs via the death receptor pathway, wherein adaptors FADD and, in specific instances, TRADD bind to death receptors located in the plasma membrane. The result is cellular demise. To effectively induce apoptosis in type 1 cells, including thymocytes, activation of caspase-8 followed by activation of effector caspases (caspase-3 and caspase-7), is adequate. On the contrary, the activation of the BCL-2-regulated apoptotic pathway is necessary for the caspase cascade to be amplified in type 2 cells, such as hepatocytes, to induce cell death. This amplification is accomplished via caspase-8-mediated proteolytic activation of the inactive BH3-only protein BID. Research conducted on cell lines containing forced-expression or temperature-sensitive wild-type p53 has shown that elevated concentrations of anti-apoptotic BCL-2 have the potential to impede p53-induced apoptosis [41]. It is noteworthy that the implementation of BCL-2 prevented p53-induced cell mortality while permitting cell cycle arrest. This indicates that p53 continues to operate at full capacity, given that BCL-2 does not entirely impede all of its functions. As a result,

BCL-2 (or other members of the pro-survival BCL-2 family) inhibits apoptosis induced by p53 at a subsequent phase of the signaling pathway; p53 itself must employ unique mechanisms to induce cell cycle arrest and death [42]. It is critical to emphasize that the p53 concentrations utilized in the aforementioned experiments were exceedingly high, resulting in apoptosis. Thus, the ability of p53 to induce apoptosis under typical physiological circumstances remains unknown. Thymocytes and other subsets of lymphoid cells derived from Trp53 mutant rodents were discovered to be resistant to apoptosis induced by γ-radiation and chemotherapy treatments that damage DNA (e.g., cisplatin, cyclophosphamide, etoposide) [43].

5.5 HOW p53-RELATED PROTEINS TRIGGER APOPTOSIS

A substantial duration of time was devoted to the scientific community's conviction that p53 lacked any identifiable relatives. It is noteworthy that two proteins, p6381 and p73,82, were promptly identified. Considering the resemblances in DNA-binding and transactivation domains between p63 and p73 and p53, it is generally acknowledged that p63 and p73 possess the capability to regulate a multitude of firmly established p53 target genes as well as the associated cellular processes [44]. Preliminary inquiries revealed that elevated concentrations of p63 or p73 are capable of inducing cellular demise characterized by apoptosis characteristics, even at levels that are atypical under typical circumstances. Initial evidence that p63 might induce apoptosis under natural conditions was obtained through meticulous experiments conducted in the mouse ovary. Fetal viability is impaired in rodents at the five-day age mark following exposure to a comparatively modest dose of γ-radiation (0.5 Gy); this leads to the destruction of all primordial follicles. In the absence of p63, cellular demise is averted; conversely, p53 lacks any protective effect. The primary follicles in the ovary were protected from γ-radiation to the same extent as when PUMA and NOXA were both absent [45] (Figure 5.3). It is evident that p63 and p53 both initiate apoptosis. It is interesting to note that female mice that were exposed to radiation, whether as pups or adults, showed no negative effects on their fertility. This was observed in both PUMA/NOXA double knockout

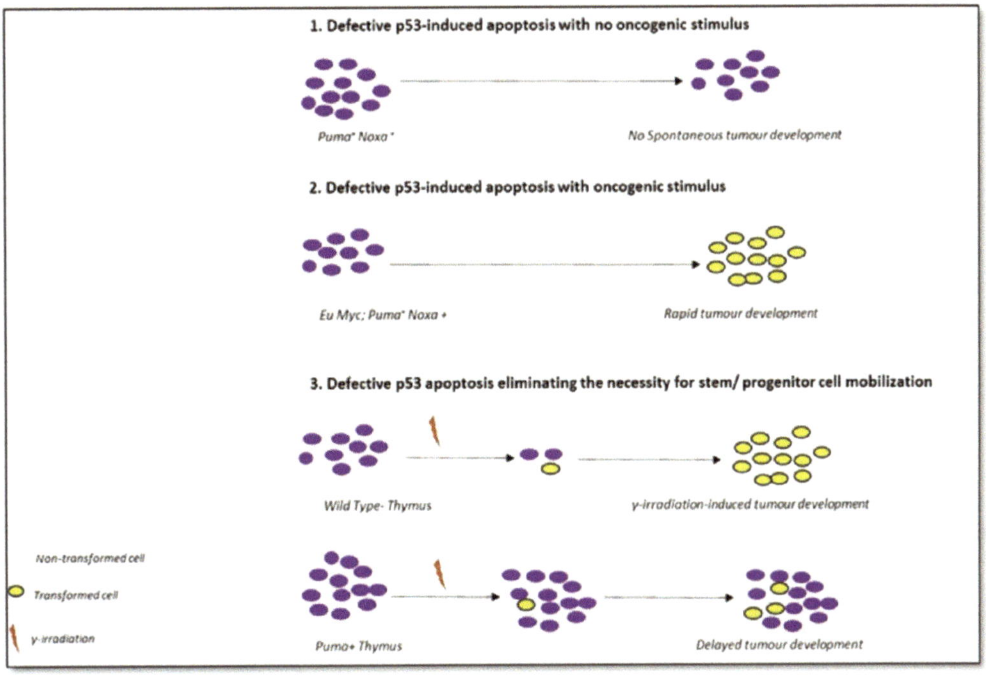

FIGURE 5.3 Impact of p53-induced apoptosis on cancer development.

and PUMA single knockout females. It is worth mentioning that none of the numerous children born to Puma–/–Noxa–/– or Puma–/– mothers who were exposed to radiation showed any signs of developmental defects or an increased risk of cancer [1, 14, 45]. Therefore, primordial follicles that do not have PUMA or PUMA plus NOXA and are protected from apoptosis caused by γ-radiation require a significantly rapid DNA lesion repair rate. It is worth mentioning that the worm *C. elegans* counterpart of p53/p63/p73 also plays a part in the demise of female germ cells resulting from DNA damage. It also triggers a pathway that leads to cell death, which can be prevented by a protein called CED-9 [46] that promotes cell survival. Another protein known as EGL-1 initiates this process by promoting cell demise. The high conservation of the p63-induced, DNA damage induced apoptosis process in female reproductive cells across species is indisputable. It is highly probable that this mechanism, which is controlled by BCL-2, is essential for preserving the genetic material's integrity in the germline.

5.6 p53 AND DEATH RECEPTOR APOPTOTIC PATHWAY

It is worth noting that p53 is also responsible for tuning the expression of constituents in the extrinsic apoptotic pathway. Transcriptional induction of the FAS gene, also referred to as APO-1 and CD95, and potentially other genes encoding similar death receptors, can be attributed to the p53 protein [10, 47, 48]. Based on scientific research, certain medications like cyclophosphamide and etoposide, as well as γ-radiation, have been found to potentially induce apoptosis in leukemia cells via the death receptor pathway [49, 50]. Nevertheless, research using a group of genetically modified mice has demonstrated that both γ-radiation and certain cancer drugs, which induce DNA damage, can eliminate both healthy and mutated cells by switching on the p53-dependent BCL-2-regulated apoptotic pathway [51, 52]. However, these medications are unable to protect these cells if the death receptor apoptotic pathway is completely disrupted, such as when caspase-8 or its activator FADD is no longer functional. Overexpression of death receptors by p53 may enhance cell sensitivity to death ligands produced by neighboring cells. This sensitization process may not be essential for cell death but has a part to play in the response to these ligands. By harnessing the power of cytotoxic T cells or natural killer cells, there is potential to enhance the effectiveness of cancer treatment for certain types of cancer. This could lead to the destruction of paracrine targets and ultimately improve patient outcomes [53].

5.7 THE ROLE OF p53-INDUCED APOPTOSIS IN p53-MEDIATED TUMOR SUPPRESSION

The discovery that p53 has the potential to initiate apoptosis led to the widespread acceptance of the idea that this is the major, if not the only, biological mechanism by which p53 inhibits the development of tumors. If cells that are in the early stages of neoplastic transformation are removed by p53-induced apoptosis, then it is reasonable to infer that this clone will not produce any cells that have fully changed into malignant cells. It is important to note that the issue is not as clear as it may appear. It is fair to assume that animals lacking both Puma and Noxa will demonstrate a similar sensitivity to the growth of tumors as mice without Trp53. This would imply that apoptosis plays a significant part in the process of p53-mediated tumor suppression [2, 54]. Surprisingly, a sizable fraction of mice that lacked the Puma and Noxa genes did not grow tumors, contrary to what was initially anticipated. The idea that cell senescence and the promotion of G1/S border cell cycle arrest play a significant role in the suppression of p53 tumors is broadly acknowledged across the scientific community. In addition to its significance in the mechanism of cell cycle arrest, the CDK inhibitor p21 also has a significant influence on the process of cellular senescence. The fact that animals with Trp53 mutations that inhibit the gene's capacity to activate Puma, Noxa, and p21, as well as mice that are completely devoid of these genes (Puma–/–Noxa–/–p21–/– mice), cannot grow tumors on their own is an intriguing observation [55, 56]. It is worth mentioning that after p53 activation, the cells from all of these mutant animals lose the ability to undergo apoptosis, cell cycle arrest, or senescence. After p53 is activated, the cells of all of these mutant animals lose the capacity to undergo apoptosis, cell cycle arrest, or senescence. This is an important fact that should be mentioned. Even in situations in which it is unable to produce cell senescence, G1/S cell cycle arrest, or apoptosis, it is clear that p53 possesses the capacity to prevent cancer from developing on its own. Additionally, the evolution of c-MYC-driven lymphoma and mutant RAS-driven lung cancer is accelerated by variations in the two transactivation domains of p53, which play a vital role in the activation of Puma, Noxa, and p21 at the transcriptional level. Variations in these domains, as well as the concomitant lack of PUMA and p21, quicken the progression of both cancers. The impact, on the other hand, is not quite as dramatic as the lack of p53 itself. It has been found that the lack of PUMA (or the absence of both PUMA and NOXA, or the absence of PUMA and p21 combined) might hasten the advancement of c-MYC-driven cancer. This is a discovery that was made throughout research. On the other hand, studies have demonstrated that the process of p53-mediated apoptosis, more especially through the activation of PUMA and NOXA, can have a significant influence on the battle against malignancies. The amount to which apoptotic induction contributes to overall TP53-mediated tumor suppression is likely to vary significantly, depending on the particular type of cell that is undergoing neoplastic transformation as well as the nature of the oncogenic lesions that lead to carcinogenesis. Researchers were able to acquire important insights into the mechanisms involved in TP53-mediated tumor suppression by employing a highly sophisticated genetically engineered mouse model. This model was used to study the mechanisms. With the use of this model, they were able to control the activity of p53 as required, which resulted in key discoveries [57]. A model of thymic T-cell lymphoma that was produced by radiation was utilized by the researchers in these investigational trials. As a result of the observations, it was discovered that tumor suppression might potentially occur even in the absence of p53, particularly during the early reaction to DNA damage. This reaction is characterized by the death of a large variety of hematopoietic cells in a widespread manner. On the other hand, the function of p53 was extremely important in the subsequent stage of the healing process. Instead of being initiated by the detection of DNA damage, p53-mediated tumor suppression was activated through p19/ARF114, which was activated by the presence of oncogenes (such as dysregulated c-MYC expression). This results in the suppression of tumors. The P19/ARF pathway is responsible for blocking MDM2, which is the primary inhibitor of p53. Through the utilization of this scenario, it is hypothesized that thymic T-cell lymphomas are produced by stem/progenitor cells that have DNA lesions that have the potential to induce cancer. The lymphomas are then triggered to heal the hematopoietic system, which has been injured as a result of exposure to γ-radiation. It is possible for the fast proliferation of progenitor cells that have oncogenic lesions to enhance the acquisition of mutations in oncogenes or suppressor genes, which ultimately results in the transition of the tumor into a neoplastic state. There is a high probability that this process accounts for the development of several different cancers. These findings are consistent with several scientific discoveries that, at first glance, can appear to be paradoxical. According to the findings of the research conducted on the animal model that was discussed before, the growth of tumors may be entirely halted by either boosting the levels of pro-survival BCL-2 or decreasing the levels of pro-apoptotic PUMA. This is because of the overexpression of PR survival BCL-2 or the deletion of pro-apoptotic PUMA, both of which successfully averted the mortality of several leukocyte populations that were triggered by γ-radiation. With this concept, there is no longer a requirement for the bone marrow to mobilize and proliferate an excessive quantity of hematopoietic stem/progenitor cells. These cells are believed to be the cancer stem cells that are responsible for the development of lymphoma and leukemia [58, 59]. The development of liver cancer is accelerated when pro-survival MCL-1 disappears from the body. It is interesting to note that the overexpression of the pro-survival BCL-2 protein inhibits its growth [2]. This finding has the potential to be relevant to a variety of different types of cancers, including epithelial cancers [37, 54, 60].

5.8 PROSPECTS OF TARGETING p53 SIGNALING FOR CANCER TREATMENT

Reactivating the wild-type traits of p53 mutants, which are frequently overexpressed in cancer, has gained attention as a possible therapeutic approach since wild-type p53 is effective in inducing senescence and apoptosis in tumor cells [61]. Gene therapy strategies aiming at reinforcing normal p53 expression and function may be promising in the treatment of cancer since several studies have shown that apoptosis and/or growth arrest can be activated by transfection of cancer cells with plasmids expressing wild-type p53. Many clinical research projects have been conducted to deliver p53 genes, either alone or in conjunction with other treatments, utilizing viral and non-viral vectors [57]. There may be structural reversibility because certain point mutations that result in the loss of function of wild-type p53 can be counteracted by other point mutations that stabilize the p53 protein [62, 63]. It has been discovered that tiny compounds such as PK7088 and PhiKan083 bind to p53, stabilizing certain mutations like Y220C and increasing the amounts of functioning wild-type p53. In addition, structures such as CP-31398, SCH29074, PRIMA-1, and PRIMAmet/APR-246 interact with mutant p53 proteins to support appropriate protein folding and p53 function recovery. The correct folding of wild-type p53 depends on the zinc-binding domain (ZBD) at residues 367–369; hence, the finding that zinc supplementation can restore wild-type folding raises the possibility of regaining chemosensitivity in cells containing mutant p53 proteins [1, 7, 64]. In mutant cell lines, the thiourea metal chelator NSC31926 has demonstrated potential in regaining wild-type p53 activity, presumably by increasing p53 mutants' zinc bioavailability. Many chemicals can interact with and inhibit various members of the p53 family, including p63 and p73, even though some are specifically intended to inhibit mutant p53. For example, the link between mutant p73 and p53 is disrupted by a drug called RETRA, which inhibits the growth of xenograft tumors and tumor cell survival. Treatments such as APR-246 and COTI-2, which show promise, are being investigated for triple-negative breast cancers with p53 mutations [65]. Preclinical models expressing mutant p53 have shown antitumor activity in response to these medicines. Individuals with advanced serous ovarian cancer are being investigated for APR-246, which has demonstrated low adverse effects in clinical studies; individuals with advanced gynecological cancers are being tested for COTI-2 [66, 67]. The China Food and Drug Administration (CFDA) has authorized Gendicine, a recombinant human p53 adenovirus manufactured by Shenzhen SiBiono GeneTech Co. Ltd., as a gene therapy treatment for head and neck cancer. More than 30,000 people have used it successfully, demonstrating a history of safety and effectiveness, especially when paired with radiation and chemotherapy. Published studies have shown that, despite the high frequency of p53 mutations in human malignancies, these mutations did not appear to have an impact on the effectiveness or long-term survival of patients treated with Gendicine [1, 68].

5.9 IMMUNOTHERAPY APPROACHES: TARGETING MUTANT p53 AND BEYOND

Even though accumulating mutant p53 (mutp53) frequently avoids MDM2-mediated degradation, it can nonetheless be broken down via proteasome-dependent, MDM2-independent mechanisms. This mechanism produces peptides that are then displayed by class I major histocompatibility complex molecules on the surface of tumor cells (MHC). As a result, mutp53 and the mutant peptide–MHC complexes produced from p53 may both be used as therapeutic targets for immunotherapies [41, 69]. Because of limitations in MHC binding, peptides with mutp53 sequences are rare; nevertheless, P1C1TM, an engineered T-cell receptor-like (TCRL) antibody, has been produced. The HLA-A24:02 (HLA-24) MHC allele presents the wild-type p53 peptide (p53125–134), which is the particular target of this antibody [70, 71]. Notably, P1C1TM has proven to be able to differentiate between cells expressing wild-type and mutant p53 according to the amounts of antigen expression. Targetable cell surface peptide–MHC complexes and intracellular mutp53 precisely interact to enable efficient antibody-dependent cellular cytotoxicity against mutp53-expressing cells in both lab and animal models [1, 72]. In the future, it will be important to investigate the discovery of new cell surface peptides that are particularly generated from mutp53, since this might improve the effectiveness of targeted immunotherapies.

5.10 CONCLUSION

Programmed cell death is a very important biological process that helps to maintain the balance in organisms and remove cancerous cells. The vital gene involved in programmed cell death is TP53, a tumor suppressor gene that works by activating an array of pathways that lead to cell cycle arrest, DNA repair, and initiation of apoptosis, therefore acting as a guardian against oncogenes. Mutations in TP53 represent the major challenge in cancer biology because these mutations lead to the loss of its normal tumor-suppressing function and cells with mutated TP53 evade natural cell death, which leads to uncontrolled cell growth, tumor proliferation and survival, and finally metastasis. Therefore, advancing our understanding of the role of mutant genes in the development and progression of cancer can potentially help to devise more effective strategies to counteract tumor growth. This understanding is important for the development of targeted therapies, thereby improving the efficacy of treatments and patient outcomes in cancer therapy.

REFERENCES

1. Mir, M.A., M. Rashid, and N. Jan, Cytokines and Chemokines in Tumor Growth and Progression, in *Cytokine and Chemokine Networks in Cancer.* 2023, Springer. p. 33–77.
2. Sofi, S., et al., A comprehensive analysis of notch signaling genes in breast cancer: expression pattern and prognostic significance. *Advances in Cancer Biology-Metastasis*, 2023. **7**: p. 100104.
3. Kastenhuber, E.R. and S.W. Lowe, Putting p53 in context. *Cell*, 2017. **170**(6): p. 1062–1078.
4. Mir, M.A., N. Jan, and S. Sofi, Introduction to Metronomic Chemotherapy, in *Novel Approaches in Metronomic Chemotherapy for Breast Cancer Treatment.* 2024, CRC Press. p. 1–14.
5. Chen, D., et al., Overexpression of integrin-linked kinase correlates with malignant phenotype in non-small cell lung cancer and promotes lung cancer cell invasion and migration via regulating epithelial–mesenchymal transition (EMT)-related genes. *Acta Histochemica*, 2013. **115**(2): p. 128–136.
6. Farhadieh, R.D., et al., Down-regulation of KAI1/CD82 protein expression in oral cancer correlates with reduced disease free survival and overall patient survival. *Cancer letters*, 2004. **213**(1): p. 91–98.
7. Mir, M.A., M. Bashir, and N. Jan, The Role of Interleukin (IL)-6/IL-6 Receptor Axis in Cancer, in *Cytokine and Chemokine Networks in Cancer.* 2023, Springer. p. 137–164.
8. Liu, J., et al., Tumor suppressor p53 and its mutants in cancer metabolism. *Cancer Letters*, 2015. **356**(2): p. 197–203.
9. Vogelstein, B., D. Lane, and A.J. Levine, Surfing the p53 network. *Nature*, 2000. **408**(6810): p. 307–310.
10. Mir, M.A., A. Shabir, and N. Jan, Metronomic Chemotherapy in Breast Cancer, in *Novel Approaches in Metronomic Chemotherapy for Breast Cancer Treatment.* CRC Press. p. 72–86.
11. El-Deiry, W.S. *Regulation ofp53downstream Genes.* Elsevier.
12. Haq, B.U., et al., Targeting p53 misfolding conundrum by stabilizing agents and their analogs in breast cancer therapy: a comprehensive computational analysis. *Frontiers in Pharmacology*, 2024. **14**: p. 1333447.
13. Hussain, S.P. and C.C. Harris, Molecular epidemiology and carcinogenesis: endogenous and exogenous carcinogens. *Mutation Research/Reviews in Mutation Research*, 2000. **462**(2–3): p. 311–322.
14. Sofi, S., et al., Clinicopathological and prognostic significance of Bcl2 in breast cancer: a comprehensive in silico and in vitro study. *Saudi Journal of Biological Sciences*, 2023. **31**(2): p. 103916.
15. George, P., p53 how crucial is its role in cancer. *International Journal of Current Pharmaceutical Research*, 2011. **3**(2): p. 19–25.
16. Allred, D.C., et al., Association of p53 protein expression with tumor cell proliferation rate and clinical outcome in node-negative breast cancer. *JNCI: Journal of the National Cancer Institute*, 1993. **85**(3): p. 200–206.
17. Loayza-Puch, F., et al., p53 induces transcriptional and translational programs to suppress cell proliferation and growth. *Genome Biology*, 2013. **14**: p. 1–12.

18. Drosten, M., et al., Loss of p53 induces cell proliferation via Ras-independent activation of the Raf/Mek/Erk signaling pathway. *Proceedings of the National Academy of Sciences*, 2014. **111**(42): p. 15155–15160.
19. Olive, K.P., et al., Mutant p53 gain of function in two mouse models of Li-Fraumeni syndrome. *Cell*, 2004. **119**(6): p. 847–860.
20. Kim, T., et al., p53 regulates epithelial-mesenchymal transition through microRNAs targeting ZEB1 and ZEB2. *Journal of Experimental Medicine*, 2011. **208**(5): p. 875–83.
21. Weisz, L., M. Oren, and V. Rotter, Transcription regulation by mutant p53. *Oncogene*, 2007. **26**(15): p. 2202–2211.
22. Meek, D.W. and C.W. Anderson, Posttranslational modification of p53: cooperative integrators of function. *Cold Spring Harbor Perspectives in Biology*, 2009. **1**(6): p. a000950.
23. Dahl, E.S. and K.M. Aird, Ataxia-telangiectasia mutated modulation of carbon metabolism in cancer. *Frontiers in Oncology*, 2017. **7**: p. 291.
24. Suh, Y.-A., et al., Multiple stress signals activate mutant p53 in vivo. *Cancer Research*, 2011. **71**(23): p. 7168–7175.
25. Qiu, L., et al., FKBP11 promotes cell proliferation and tumorigenesis via p53-related pathways in oral squamous cell carcinoma. *Biochemical and Biophysical Research Communications*, 2021. **559**: p. 183–190.
26. Liu, J., et al., ITIH5, a p53-responsive gene, inhibits the growth and metastasis of melanoma cells by downregulating the transcriptional activity of KLF4. *Cell Death & Disease*, 2021. **12**(5): p. 438.
27. Marei, H.E., et al., p53 signaling in cancer progression and therapy. *Cancer Cell Int*, 2021. **21**(1): p. 703.
28. Haupt, Y., et al., Mdm2 promotes the rapid degradation of p53. *Nature*, 1997. **387**(6630): p. 296–299.
29. Freed-Pastor, W.A. and C. Prives, Mutant p53: one name, many proteins. *Genes & Development*, 2012. **26**(12): p. 1268–1286.
30. Menendez, D., A. Inga, and M.A. Resnick, The expanding universe of p53 targets. *Nature Reviews Cancer*, 2009. **9**(10): p. 724–737.
31. Kamada, R., et al., Tetramer formation of tumor suppressor protein p53: Structure, function, and applications. *Peptide Science*, 2016. **106**(4): p. 598–612.
32. Michael, D. and M. Oren, The p53 and Mdm2 families in cancer. *Current Opinion in Genetics & Development*, 2002. **12**(1): p. 53–59.
33. O'Connor, L., et al., Bim: a novel member of the Bcl-2 family that promotes apoptosis. *The EMBO Journal*, 1998. https://doi.org/10.1093/emboj/17.2.384
34. Li, M., et al., Distinct regulatory mechanisms and functions for p53-activated and p53-repressed DNA damage response genes in embryonic stem cells. *Molecular Cell*, 2012. **46**(1): p. 30–42.
35. Broz, D.K., et al., Global genomic profiling reveals an extensive p53-regulated autophagy program contributing to key p53 responses. *Genes & Development*, 2013. **27**(9): p. 1016–1031.
36. Tonelli, C., et al., Genome-wide analysis of p53 transcriptional programs in B cells upon exposure to genotoxic stress in vivo. *Oncotarget*, 2015. **6**(28): p. 24611.
37. Aubrey, B.J., et al., How does p53 induce apoptosis and how does this relate to p53-mediated tumour suppression? *Cell Death & Differentiation*, 2018. **25**(1): p. 104–113.
38. Rathmell, J.C., et al., Deficiency in Bak and Bax perturbs thymic selection and lymphoid homeostasis. *Nature Immunology*, 2002. **3**(10): p. 932–939.
39. Sarosiek, K.A., et al., Developmental regulation of mitochondrial apoptosis by c-Myc governs age-and tissue-specific sensitivity to cancer therapeutics. *Cancer Cell*, 2017. **31**(1): p. 142–156.
40. Montazersaheb, S., et al., Investigation the apoptotic effect of silver nanoparticles (Ag-NPs) on MDA-MB 231 breast cancer epithelial cells via signaling pathways. *Heliyon*, 2024. **10**(5): p. e26959.
41. Sobhani, N., et al., Mutant p53 as an antigen in cancer immunotherapy. *International Journal of Molecular Sciences*, 2020. **21**(11): p. 4087.
42. Wang, Y., et al., Wild-type p53-triggered apoptosis is inhibited by bcl-2 in a v-myc-induced T-cell lymphoma line. *Oncogene-Basingstoke*, 1993. **8**: p. 3427–3427.
43. Clarke, A.R., et al., Thymocyte apoptosis induced by p53-dependent and independent pathways. *Nature*, 1993. **362**(6423): p. 849–852.
44. Kaghad, M., et al., Monoallelically expressed gene related to p53 at 1p36, a region frequently deleted in neuroblastoma and other human cancers. *Cell*, 1997. **90**(4): p. 809–819.
45. Kerr, J.B., et al., DNA damage-induced primordial follicle oocyte apoptosis and loss of fertility require TAp63-mediated induction of Puma and Noxa. *Molecular Cell*, 2012. **48**(3): p. 343–352.
46. Hofmann, E.R., et al., Caenorhabditis elegans HUS-1 is a DNA damage checkpoint protein required for genome stability and EGL-1-mediated apoptosis. *Current Biology*, 2002. **12**(22): p. 1908–18.

47. Müller, M., et al., p53 activates the CD95 (APO-1/Fas) gene in response to DNA damage by anticancer drugs. *Journal of Experimental Medicine*, 1998. **188**(11): p. 2033–2045.
48. Mir, M.A., A. Manzoor, and N. Jan, *CCL5/CCR5 Axis in Cancer, in Cytokine and Chemokine Networks in Cancer.* 2023, Springer. p. 219–240.
49. Friesen, C., et al., Involvement of the CD95 (APO-1/FAS) receptor/ligand system in drug-induced apoptosis in leukemia cells. *Nature Medicine*, 1996. **2**(5): p. 574–577.
50. Mir, M.A., N. Jan, and I. Noor, Therapeutic Implications of Cytokines and Chemokines Network in Cancer, in *Cytokine and Chemokine Networks in Cancer.* 2023, Springer. p. 385–414.
51. Strasser, A., A.W. Harris, and S. Cory, bcl-2 transgene inhibits T cell death and perturbs thymic self-censorship. *Cell*, 1991. **67**(5): p. 889–899.
52. Miyashita, T. and J.C. Reed, bcl-2 gene transfer increases relative resistance of S49.1 and WEHI7.2 lymphoid cells to cell death and DNA fragmentation induced by glucocorticoids and multiple chemotherapeutic drugs. *Cancer Research*, 1992. **52**(19): p. 5407–511.
53. Marvalim, C., A. Datta, and S.C. Lee, Role of p53 in breast cancer progression: An insight into p53 targeted therapy. *Theranostics*, 2023. **13**(4): p. 1421–1442.
54. Michalak, E.M., et al., Apoptosis-promoted tumorigenesis: gamma-irradiation-induced thymic lymphomagenesis requires Puma-driven leukocyte death. *Genes & Development*, 2010. **24**(15): p. 1608–13.
55. Valente, L.J., et al., p53 efficiently suppresses tumor development in the complete absence of its cell-cycle inhibitory and proapoptotic effectors p21, Puma, and Noxa. *Cell Reports*, 2013. **3**(5): p. 1339–1345.
56. Sofi, S., et al., Elucidation of interleukin-19 as a therapeutic target for breast cancer by computational analysis and experimental validation. *Saudi Journal of Biological Sciences*, 2023. **30**(9): p. 103774–103774.
57. Valente, J.F.A., J.A. Queiroz, and F. Sousa, p53 as the focus of gene therapy: past, present and future. *Current Drug Targets*, 2018. **19**(15): p. 1801–1817.
58. Christophorou, M.A., et al., The pathological response to DNA damage does not contribute to p53-mediated tumour suppression. *Nature*, 2006. **443**(7108): p. 214–217.
59. Jan, N., et al., Metronomic chemotherapy and drug repurposing: a paradigm shift in oncology. *Heliyon*, 2024. https://doi.org/10.1016/j.heliyon.2024.e24670
60. Jan, N., et al., Exploring the role of trifarotene against RAR-α: an investigation of expression pattern and clinicopathological significance of RAR-α in breast cancer. *Frontiers in Pharmacology*, 2024. **15**: p. 1361679.
61. Mir, M.A., et al., Proteomics: Application of Next-Generation Proteomics in Cancer Research, in *Proteomics.* 2023, Elsevier. p. 55–76.
62. Joerger, A.C. and A.R. Fersht, Structural biology of the tumor suppressor p53 and cancer-associated mutants. *Advances in Cancer Research*, 2007. **97**: p. 1–23.
63. Mir, M.A., Sumaya, N. Jan, Implications of Chemokine Heterogenicity in Cancer Metastasis, in *Cytokine and Chemokine Networks in Cancer.* 2023, Springer. p. 115–136.
64. Pintus, S.S., et al., The substitutions G245C and G245D in the Zn(2+)-binding pocket of the p53 protein result in differences of conformational flexibility of the DNA-binding domain. *Journal of Biomolecular Structure and Dynamics*, 2013. **31**(1): p. 78–86.
65. Duffy, M.J., N.C. Synnott, and J. Crown, Mutant p53 in breast cancer: potential as a therapeutic target and biomarker. *Breast Cancer Research and Treatment*, 2018. **170**(2): p. 213–219.
66. Duffy, M.J., N.C. Synnott, and J. Crown, Mutant p53 as a target for cancer treatment. *European Journal of Cancer*, 2017. **83**: p. 258–265.
67. Mir, M.A., et al., Metronomics: toward personalized chemotherapy. *Novel Approaches in Metronomic Chemotherapy for Breast Cancer Treatment*, 2024. p. 99–119. https://doi.org/10.1201/9781032632674-8
68. Zhang, W.W., et al., The First Approved Gene Therapy Product for Cancer Ad-p53 (Gendicine): 12 Years in the Clinic. *Human Gene Therapy*, 2018. **29**(2): p. 160–179.
69. Mir, M.A., M. Rashid, and N. Jan, The Interleukin-8 Pathway in Cancer, in *Cytokine and Chemokine Networks in Cancer.* 2023, Springer. p. 165–190.
70. Zhang, J., et al., Engineering and targeting neutrophils for cancer therapy. *Advanced Materials*, 2024. **36**(19): p. e2310318.
71. Mir, M.A., et al., Proteomics: A Groundbreaking Development in Cancer Biology, in *Proteomics.* 2023, Elsevier. p. 31–53.
72. Low, L., et al., Targeting mutant p53-expressing tumours with a T cell receptor-like antibody specific for a wild-type antigen. *Nature Communications*, 2019. **10**(1): p. 5382.

6 The Contribution of p53 in DNA Repair and Genomic Stability in Breast Cancer

*Iqra Jan, Asma Jan, Alia Jabar, and Manzoor Ahmad Mir**

Department of Bioresources, School of Biological Sciences, University of Kashmir, Srinagar, J&K, India
*drmanzoor@kashmiruniversity.ac.in

6.1 INTRODUCTION

Breast cancer is characterized by genomic instability, which gives rise to multiple etiologies for this diverse illness and increases the propensity to modify the genome [1]. Since these systems are recognized for maintaining the integrity of the human genome, any modification to any of them—such as telomere maintenance, DNA repair machinery, cell-cycle checkpoints, or mitotic checkpoints—results in genomic instability [2]. Genomic instability is the primary characteristic that gives cancer cells their maximum functional potential. It is known to cause inadvertent genetic alterations and chromosomal rearrangements enabling them to survive, proliferate, and spread through multiple mechanisms at various points during the tumorigenesis process. Sometimes accumulating mistakes caused by a weak DNA repair mechanism result in the functional loss of tumor-suppressor genes; other times, it might stimulate the function of oncogenes, which ultimately promotes the growth and development of cancer [3]. One important transcription factor that controls a few biological processes is the tumor suppressor p53. In cancer, p53 stops cancer cells from growing in response to certain stimuli. including food deprivation, hypoxia, hyperproliferative signals, and damage to DNA, which stops tumor formation (Figure 6.1) [4]. Its moniker, "guardian of the genome," is thus fitting. MDM2, an E3 ligase, strictly controls the amount of p53 under normal physiological settings. It does this by inducing p53 degradation via the ubiquitin–proteasome-dependent route. Through connecting to MDM2's promoter, p53 can also cause the gene to express. Consequently, a negative feedback loop is established, promoting the degradation of p53 and maintaining its cellular levels [5, 6]. Low p53 changes post-translationally in response to cellular stressors. Phosphorylation is one kind of alteration that stabilizes p53 by interfering with its two primary processes of transactivation and sequence-specific DNA binding. Genes are targeted for their role in controlling the cell cycle, repairing DNA damage, and initiating senescence, and apoptosis can be activated or repressed by p53 through a process known as transactivation. A fundamental characteristic shared by all human cancer forms is genome instability. It has been demonstrated that mutant p53's gain-of-function (GOF) activity encourages genomic instability. Mutant p53 is linked to aberrant copy numbers in breast cancer samples [7]. A study shows that mutant p53 can bind to and upregulate the expression of genes related to chromatin regulation, such as MLL1 and MLL2, which are methyltransferases. These enzymes contribute to genomic instability and the advancement of cancer by increasing histone methylation and acetylation [8, 9]. Breast cancer (BC) is a multifaceted disease that mostly affects the breast tissues and strikes seldom. It is the most common cancer in

DOI: 10.1201/9781003520771-6

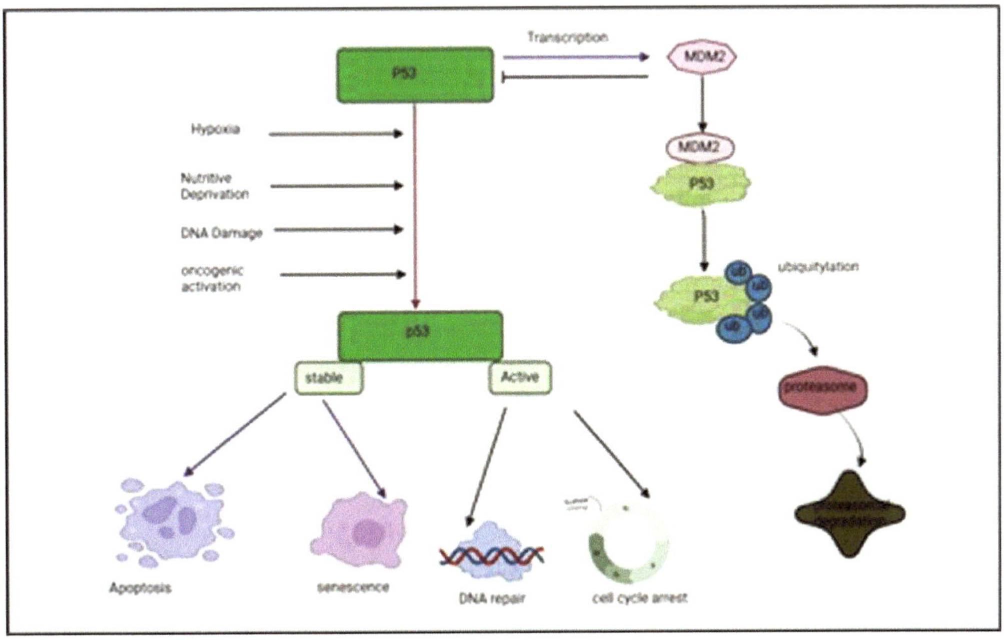

FIGURE 6.1 Normal circumstances result in MDM2 controlling the p53 protein. To control the cell cycle, apoptosis, DNA repair, and senescence, p53 is activated by circumstances such as hypoxia, oncogene activation, DNA damage, and starvation.

women globally, affecting women from all countries and ethnicities. Lung cancer has recently been eclipsed by breast cancer, stands as the most frequently diagnosed illness globally, and currently ranks as the leading cause of cancer-related deaths among women. Though less prevalent, BC can also strike men [6, 10].

Genomic instability is a key characteristic of breast cancer, which greatly increases the functional competence of malignant cells. During cancer, this instability enables the cells to endure, multiply, and disseminate via a variety of pathways. Owing to a weak DNA repair system, the tendency for accidental mutations and chromosomal rearrangements frequently leads to accumulated mistakes. This may result in the tumor suppressor's functional loss or it might stimulate the function of oncogenes, which ultimately promotes the growth and development of cancer [3, 11].

6.2 p53 PROTEIN STRUCTURE AND FUNCTION

More than half of all human cancers involve mutations in the p53 gene, while the rest result from the biological inactivation of the pathway. It is not surprising that the mutant form of p53 is present in many cancer tissues considering that it was mistakenly identified as an oncogene when it was first discovered in 1979. The p53 gene, found at position 13.1 on chromosome 17, was first connected to the large T antigen simian virus 40 (SV40), which caused cancerous cells to undergo metamorphosis, consisting of 11 exons, the first of which is encoding and spans 20kb. Region 17p is frequently decreased to homozygosity in cancer tissue [12, 13]. The extraordinary conservation of the DNA-binding domain across vertebrate species is indicative of its crucial function in cellular processes and gene regulation. This conservation includes not only the gene's general structure but also the sequences of certain domains that are essential to preserving the integrity and functionality of the protein [14], which exhibits the highest homology (around 60%) and is the most similar. With 393 residues arranged in five structural and functional domains, the protein p53 is an oligomeric transcription factor. These regions include an N-terminal or transcriptional activation domain (TA), an oligomerization domain or nuclear localization signal (NLS), a sequence-specific DNA-binding domain (DBD), a proline-rich regulatory domain (PRD), and a flexible carboxy-terminal domain (CTD) that is crucial for the regulation of DNA binding. Furthermore, the TA region is the site of the interaction between the MDM2 protein and TATA-binding protein (TBP) associated factor (TAF). The core DNA-binding domain is the primary factor influencing the protein's shape. The DBD is where most mutations linked to tumors originate. When the large T antigen of the simian virus 40 (SV40) attaches to this area, the p53 protein is rendered inactive. The p53 protein's oligomerization domain (NLS), which is crucial for DNA binding, oligomerizes the protein into dimers and tetramers. CTD is regarded as the primary allosteric and the sequences required for dimerization and tetramerization are found in CTD, which is thought to be the primary allosteric regulatory domain of p53 action. Additionally, it is in charge of keeping the p53 protein dormant. When some antibodies neutralize this domain, the p53 protein undergoes structural alteration enabling DNA binding [4, 15, 16]. There are several levels at which the p53 protein is strictly regulated. Numerous positive and negative regulators, frequently resulting in feedback loops, accomplish this. It is known that there are three main levels of regulation: subcellular distribution, protein activity, and protein stability. The proto-oncogene mdm2 serves as a principal adversary to p53, exerting significant influence over its regulatory pathways both under normal physiological conditions and in times of stress. Recent advancements in research have significantly enhanced our understanding of how p53 is governed, shedding light on the intricate molecular mechanisms orchestrating these regulatory dynamics [17–20], because p53 transcriptionally induces Mdm2. After p53 causes DNA damage, it starts a negative feedback loop that eventually leads to its degeneration. Oscillations are brought about in the levels of p53 and the proteins that are linked to it by this feedback loop [21]. The deadly effect of mdm2 mutant mice during early developmental stages highlights the critical role of Mdm2 in negatively controlling embryonic development. These mice are effectively saved from early death by the simultaneous reduction of p53, highlighting the complex balance that Mdm2 maintains in this regulatory process [22, 23]. In numerous cancers, the upregulation of Mdm2 is often adequate to incapacitate p53 without additional genetic alterations. Similar to this, p53-mediated apoptosis can be induced in vivo simply by losing Mdm2 [24, 25]. Consequently, Mdm2 is essential. The revelation that Mdm2 triggers the degradation of p53 through the ubiquitin–proteasome pathway was crucial in clarifying the regulation of p53 stability [5, 26]. It also assisted in explaining why cancer cells express more p53 mutant proteins than normal because they are unable to stimulate the expression of mdm2 [27]. This result could be attributed to p53 mutants' decreased affinity for Mdm2 [28]. Even without the HECT (homologous to E6AP carboxy terminus) domain, Mdm2 operates as an E3 ubiquitin ligase, crucial for promoting the degradation of p53. This functionality hinges on its RING-finger domain, which is indispensable for its E3 activity [13, 29, 30]. The oligomerization of p53 appears to be a crucial step for its degradation facilitated by Mdm2 [26, 30]. Moving the final 30–40 amino acids from p53's C-terminal hinders Mdm2's ability to degrade p53, but it has no effect on how much p53 is ubiquitinated. Numerous lysines in this area have the potential to be ubiquitination sites. When the six lysines between residues 370–386 are substituted, Mdm2's ubiquitination of p53 and its vulnerability to Mdm2-mediated destruction is significantly reduced [31–33]. Furthermore, it has recently been demonstrated that two N-terminal areas influence p53's vulnerability to Mdm2 instability. Residues 62–91 in the polyproline region of p53 may shield the protein from Mdm2. When p53 lacks this area, it becomes overly susceptible to Mdm2's inhibition and instability [34]. However, it seems that the neighboring area (residues 92–112) is necessary for Mdm2 to degrade p53 [35]. These results imply that other proteins are most likely involved in Mdm2's in vivo ubiquitination of p53. JNK, which binds p53 between residues 97 and 116 and has been linked to the ubiquitination and destruction of p53 in unstressed cells, is one potential candidate [36].

6.2.1 Post-Translational Modifications

p53 degradation requires the Mdm2–p53 interaction [26, 34]. It is sufficient to stop this interaction to shield p53 from deterioration [37, 38]. This connection is disrupted in response to γ-IR and UV stress stimuli, among others. How is the regulation of this connection affected by stress? The Mdm2 binding domain's serine 20 (Ser-20) phosphorylation of p53 decreases Mdm2's affinity for p53 and improves p53's stability in response to γ-IR and UV radiation [39, 40]. It was discovered that checkpoint kinase 2 (Chk2) is the kinase in charge of phosphorylating Ser-20 [41], without which p53's ability to stabilize in response to DNA damage is negated [42]. Thus, the accumulation of p53 is caused by a series of DNA damage signaling events, ranging from ATM to Chk2 to p53 phosphorylation. A CKI-like kinase also phosphorylates p53 on Thr-18 in response to γ-IR, which lowers the binding affinity of p53 with Mdm2 [43, 44]. The latter modification's physiological significance has not yet been investigated, though. Apart from these alterations, p53 undergoes phosphorylation at both its N- and C-termini. Although phosphorylation of Ser-15 or Ser-37 does not seem to control p53 stability, it does control p53 transcriptional activity and p53 binding to DNA [45, 46]. Comparably, p53's transcriptional activity is increased when lysine residues in its C-terminus are acetylated. Lastly, p53 experiences simulation, a change that marginally increases its activity without changing the stability of p53 [33, 47]. Additionally, changes are made to the Mdm2 protein that might have an impact on its capacity to control p53. For instance, Mdm2's reduced sumoylation in response to DNA damage improves p53's ubiquitination capacity [48]. Furthermore, in vivo, Mdm2 is rapidly phosphorylated by ATM in response to medicines that mimic radioactivity or γ-IR [49]. It's still unknown how this change will affect the autoregulatory cycle. DNA-PK also phosphorylates Mdm2 at several locations in reaction to damage to the DNA. Although the p53–Mdm2 interaction is hindered by this phosphorylation, its significance in vivo is now uncertain. In response to stress signals, the simultaneous alteration of p53 and Mdm2 may have synergistic effects on the autoregulatory loop.

6.3 p53 IN DNA REPAIR MECHANISM

The activation of p53 is caused by several cellular stresses, including hypoxia, nucleotide shortage, and damage to DNA. Studies have demonstrated that many DNA damage pathways, such as those brought on by ionizing radiation (IR), radiomimetic medications, ultraviolet light (UV), and substances like methyl methane sulfonate (MMS), can activate p53. Under normal circumstances, p53 levels are normally kept at low levels because of its relatively short half-life. Furthermore, p53 seldom stops being largely quiescent and is not very good at attaching to DNA or starting transcription. When DNA damage triggers p53 activation, its levels rise quickly and it becomes more capable of binding DNA and facilitating transcription. As a consequence, this triggers the activation of numerous genes whose functions entail DNA repair, apoptosis, or halting of the cell cycle. According to recent research, DNA damage is primarily responsible for this regulation, as it sets off a sequence of phosphorylation, de-phosphorylation, and acetylation processes on the p53 polypeptide. Here, we go over the characteristics of these modifications, the enzymes responsible for causing them, and how alterations in p53 modification result in p53 activation.

6.3.1 Types of DNA Lesions and Their Repair Mechanisms

Physical DNA lesions come in various forms and are acquired throughout life through previously mentioned mechanisms. Chromosomal abnormalities include a variety of DNA problems, such as chromosomal fusion and single- and double-strand breaks. Mutations in DNA, such as insertions, deletions, and erroneous repeats, are also included in this category. Other aberrations include hypermethylation of promoter regions. Following are techniques for repairing DNA damage that are being studied in clinical trials; these processes primarily concern the BRCA1, BRIT1, and PARP-1 proteins. Single-nucleotide alterations, insertions, deletions, and repetitive errors can be caused by environmental variables or errors in DNA polymerase. Nucleotide excision repair, base excision repair, or mismatch repair processes are usually used to fix such damage.

6.3.1.1 Nucleotide Excision Repair (NER)

Nucleotide excision repair (NER) corrects large adducts and bulky lesions that cause the double-strand helix to be distorted when only one of the two DNA strands is impacted; examples of such damage include exposure to UV radiation and chemical mutagens. These mutagens cause intra-strand adducts and cross-link nearby purine and pyrimidine bases. This damage prevents fundamental biological processes including transcription and DNA replication [50]. The two mechanisms involved in NER, a vital mechanism for preserving genomic integrity, are succinctly summarized here. The reason transcription-coupled repair (TC-NER) is so intriguing is that it targets lesions that specifically impede RNA polymerase's progression during active transcription. This makes sure that DNA damage doesn't affect genes that are essential for cell activity. Global genome repair (GG-NER), on the other hand, is a more comprehensive method that works throughout the cell cycle to detect and fix damage to the entire genome, independent of transcriptional status. When these pathways are combined, NER becomes a very effective and adaptable mechanism for repairing DNA damage [51]. Prior to ligating the DNA, NER must first identify the damage, collect the complex that is linked to it, and unwind it at a specific location in the DNA. A precise cut is made at both ends to excise damaged portions. These damaged segments are then removed. New nucleotides are synthesized to fill the gap, utilizing a separate DNA strand as a guide/template for accurate replication [52]. Several proteins cooperate during the repair process. The DNA helix is first unwound by a complex known as transcription factor IIH (TFIIH), which consists of nine units and includes the helicases XPB and XPD in addition to the proteins XPA and RPA. After that, ERCC1 and endonucleases XPG and XPF carefully cleave one side of the broken strand. This procedure preserves the integrity of the DNA. Replication factor C (RFC) then attaches itself to the removed area and helps to load proliferating cell nuclear antigen (PCNA), which ties together DNA polymerases δ and ε to keep them from disengaging during repair. Ligase I seals the repaired strands to the original ones at the end [53]. RPA facilitates the formation of a secondary repair complex following the initial step.

6.3.1.2 Base Excision Repair (BER)

Base mispairings are frequently caused by mutations that affect a small number of bases and result in little harm. Usually, the base excision repair (BER) pathway is used to heal this damage. Damage brought on by oxidation, alkylation, deamination, and ionizing radiation, among other sources, is handled via the BER pathway [54]. In this case, mutagens are usually endogenous—they're agents from within that induce mutations. Here, when a nucleoside is damaged, leaving behind a basic (AP) site, it's because the compromised nucleoside is removed by cleaving its glycosidic bond [55]. APE1/Ref1, also known as AP endonuclease/redox factor 1, modifies the loose DNA ends to create precise termini that can accommodate a new base. This process is a key mechanism ensuring the specificity of BER. To ensure that the sensitive AP site is always covered, the 11 lesion-detecting glycosylases remain attached to the site [56]. XRCC1 stabilizes the injured area in addition to managing the sequential binding and release of proteins. The PCNA sliding clamp facilitates the interaction between RFC and the newly produced nucleotides, and XRCC1, another stabilizer, also serves as a helicase [57]. Proofreading polymerases occasionally might miss mistakes made by DNA polymerase during DNA replication. In this case, faults are cleared and the system uses the parental strand as a template for mismatched repair (MMR), a post-replicative repair technique, to fix mistakes in the freshly synthesized DNA strand. MMR's damage sensors are good at identifying the difference between the original DNA strand and the newly synthesized DNA strand. The integrity of the original parental DNA strand is preserved since this capability makes sure that only the mismatches in the freshly synthesized strand are found and fixed [58]. MSH2 and MSH2 are two damage recognition complexes used by the MMR mechanism to fix short insertion/deletion loops and single-base mismatches. In particular, the MSH2 complex detects insertion/deletion loops involving up to ten nucleotides, whereas it only recognizes single-base changes and the smallest insertion/deletion loops [59]. They then enlist a complex that includes MSH–MLH complexes, increased proteins 1 or 2 (PMS1 or PMS2), and replication factor A, which serves as a marker at the compromised site. These combine to generate a sliding clamp that tracks the DNA strand until it comes across a gap in the single strand of DNA. A DNA exonuclease (Exol) can penetrate the DNA structure when the Mutl complex comes into contact with the cluster. DNA polymerase Pol delta synthesizes new DNA at the excision sites while Exol removes the damaged segment and a few extra nucleotides under the guidance of the MLH– MSH complex. Ligase 1 then reunites the freshly created DNA with the original daughter strand [60].

6.3.1.3 Double-Strand Breaks (DSBs)

Double-strand breaks (DSBs), though infrequent, are extremely hazardous and challenging to repair. They are predominantly caused by external factors such as ionizing radiation and disruptions in replication forks due to polymerase stalling at unrepaired base lesions. Radiation therapy and chemotherapy are two anticancer treatments that can also cause various types of double-stranded DNA damage [61]. Fixing DSBs is a difficult task. When it comes to DSBs, there is no template for new strand synthesis, in contrast to single-strand damage, where the complementary strand offers one for repair. Human cells use two main mechanisms to deal with this: homologous recombination repair (HRR) and non-homologous end joining (NHEJ). Cell-cycle checkpoints impact the repair process by assessing the level of end processing necessary [62]. The process is somewhat complex because HRR is operational during the S and G2 phases, which occur after DNA replication. In contrast, NHEJ operates throughout all cell-cycle phases but is most active during the G0 and G1 phases, which occur before DNA replication. Homologous replication is also more accurate because it is template-based, which increases its fidelity. The damage sensor complex Mre11-Rad50-Nbs1 (MRN) is shared by both NHEJ and HRR. The functioning of MRN is just one of the many puzzles surrounding DSB repair.

6.3.1.4 Non-Homologous End Joining (NHEJ)

To reunite DSB ends without the need for a template, NHEJ does not look for or make use of a sizable portion of DNA to determine which bases existed before the damage and where the fracture ends. As a result, repair proceeds rapidly despite the possibility of nucleotide loss from either side of the double-strand break, modification of base pair sequences at the breakpoint, or, in the event of many breaks, attachment to an end that is not part of the sequence. Consequently, NHEJ can lead to a significant quantity of mutation, yet the cell prefers it [63]. The main difficulty in NHEJ is to enclose the two free DNA ends and prevent nucleolytic degradation from occurring. This defense is offered by the Ku heterodimer, which also recruits more proteins for completion processing and functions as a damaged sensor and lyase. Then, DNA-PKcs, a catalytic subunit of DNA-dependent protein kinase, binds to Ku to create the DNA-PK complex, which acts as a docking site for different enzymes that digest DNA. Ligase IV ligates the processed DNA ends across gaps to form the XRCC4, ligase IV, and XLF complex, which bridges the ends of the DNA. Even with our growing knowledge, there are still a lot of unanswered questions concerning NHEJ. For example, we don't know if its processes are sequential, iterative, or adaptable based on how complicated the injury is. Only occurring in T and U, V(D)J recombination is the most researched form of NHEJ [64].

6.3.1.5 Homologous Recombination Repair

In the cell cycle's replication phase (S phase), HRR, a sophisticated repair mechanism, is triggered when DNA damage occurs. Before cell division (M phase), HRR ensures that the two DNA strands remain connected by the cohesion complex. This arrangement enables HRR to utilize an intact copy of neighboring DNA for repair. By locating a similar region, HRR can utilize it as a template on the sister chromatid to repair the broken DNA strand. In the initial step, a complex comprising MRN generates single-stranded DNA at the site of the DSB. This single-stranded DNA extends beyond the original break, facilitating the binding of Rad51 to the 3′ end. Meanwhile, RPA binds to the exposed DNA stretch, assisting Rad51 in identifying DNA sequences resembling the 3′ overhang. HRR plays a crucial role in preserving the stability of the genome. Rad51 initiates its action by infiltrating the double-stranded DNA, particularly drawn to regions abundant in homology. This infiltration leads to the formation of a heteroduplex. Once engaged, Rad51 promotes homology-bearing

DNA sequences to interchange within the sister chromatid. Through its ability to draw additional repair proteins to the location, Nbsl plays a critical part in this process. Rad50 acts as a tether in the meantime, helping to stabilize the DNA helix. As the repair progresses, the overhang at the site gradually extends with the creation of new nucleotides beyond the initial breakage point. Additionally, MRE11 plays a multifaceted role, possessing both exonuclease and endonuclease functions essential for the repair process [65]. When the loop is compressed during DNA synthesis, an X-shaped structure known as a Holliday junction is created. The junction is resolved and the ends are linked together at the conclusion of this process. Numerous homologous recombination-related genes, including BRCA1 and BRCA2, are connected to both cancer prevention and genomic stability. This demonstrates how intricate a cell's DNA repair machinery is. Cancer, however, can take advantage of and alter this system in several ways.

6.4 p53 AND GENOMIC STABILITY: MECHANISMS BY WHICH p53 MAINTAINS GENOME STABILITY

The ability of p53 to trigger cell-cycle arrest and death (Figure 6.2) is largely attributed to its role as a transcription factor. These mechanisms serve to protect both the individual cell and the organism from DNA damage, thus preventing potential genomic instability [66]. One typical reaction of cells to different types of stress or damage to their DNA is to stop going through the cell cycle. The tumor-suppressor protein p53 controls the increased production of the cell-cycle inhibitor p21 (Cdkn1a), which causes this stop [67]. Furthermore, p53 upregulates additional genes like Gadd45a

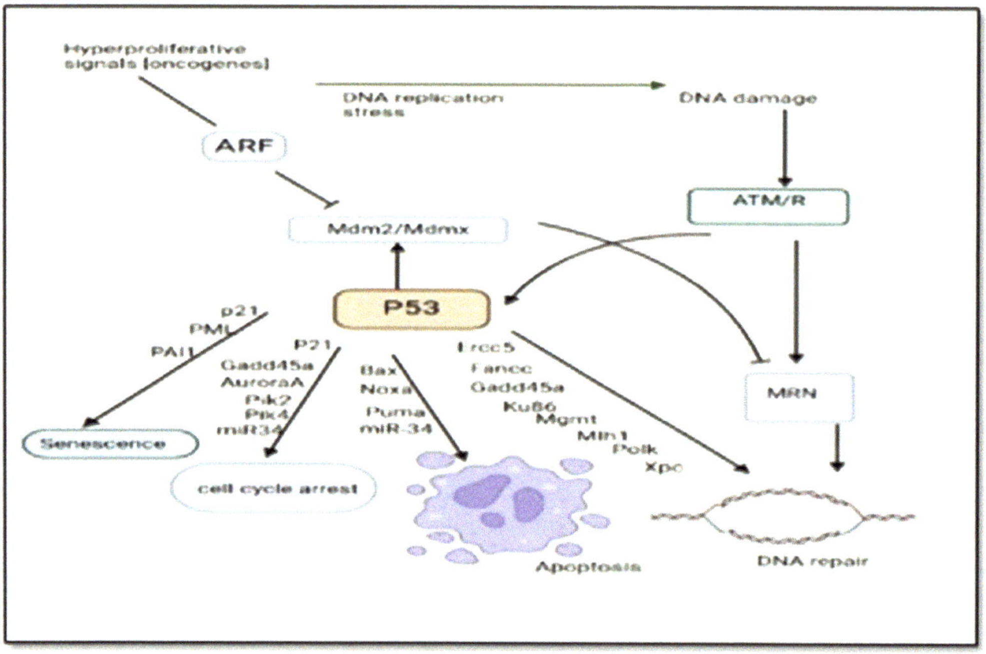

FIGURE 6.2 When DNA damage occurs, various pathways are activated to regulate the activity of p53, a key tumor suppressor protein. Activation of p53 can be triggered by multiple upstream regulators such as Arf, Mdm2, ATM, and ATR kinases. Arf activation induces hyperproliferation, while Mdm2 regulation and activation of ATM and ATR kinases signal DNA damage. These events converge to activate p53. Once activated, p53 initiates the transcription of specific target genes, leading to various biological outcomes. These outcomes include cell-cycle arrest, apoptosis, or DNA repair. The DNA damage response pathway involves molecules including Mre11, Rad50, and Nbs1 (MRN complex), which participate in DNA repair processes. In cases where DNA damage is severe and irreparable, or when checkpoint activation persists, p53-mediated cell-cycle arrest can ultimately lead to programmed cell death, known as apoptosis.

that obstruct cell-cycle progression. According to research, p53 not only transcriptionally upregulates these genes but also prevents the translation of genes linked to the cell cycle, such as CDK4, stopping the cell cycle in its G1 phase [68]. Moreover, p53 is linked to cellular senescence, a condition in which cells stop proliferating permanently. Senescence, a result of p53 activity that is still not fully understood, is seen in cells that have experienced oxidative damage, telomere shortening, overexpression, or hyperactivation of an oncogene [69]. Although p21 has been implicated in senescence mediated by p53 (Figure 6.2), this involvement is insufficient in and of itself [70]. Other p53 target genes (e.g., promyelocytic leukemia (*PML*) and plasminogen activator inhibitor-1(*PAI-1*)) have also been linked to senescence [71].

To destroy cells with damaged DNA, p53 can potentially trigger apoptosis in addition to cell-cycle arrest. Even though p53-mediated apoptosis has been thoroughly investigated, many things are still unknown. Following various forms of DNA damage, p53 triggers the transcriptional activation of proapoptotic genes such as Bax, Noxa, and Puma. This activation leads to the inhibition of antiapoptotic Bcl-2 proteins by p53, ultimately resulting in apoptosis [72]. Additionally, it is suggested that p53 functions within the mitochondria, where it directly blocks anti-apoptotic members of the Bcl-2 family, leading to apoptosis [73]. Determining the factors influencing localization to mitochondria or the specific proapoptotic gene(s) to transcribe remains uncertain. To make matters more complicated, p53 has also been connected to autophagy and necrosis. Whether a cell-cycle block is required for cellular repair to occur or whether the damage is too severe or persistent for apoptosis to take place in its place, p53 is categorized as a gatekeeper or hub protein. There is much research being done on how p53 determines which path—cell-cycle arrest, senescence, or apoptosis—to take. It is likely influenced by several factors, including the intensity of the signal, the extent and kind of cellular damage, and the transcriptional cofactors and epigenetic modulators that are recruited [74]. Whether p53 induces senescence, cell-cycle arrest, or apoptosis, the result is that a damaged cell shouldn't be permitted to multiply.

6.4.1 BRCA1

BRCA1, encoded by the 17q21 gene, serves as both a tumor suppressor and a DNA damage response protein. It's a nuclear phosphoprotein consisting of 1863 amino acids. Mutations in BRCA1 can lead to uncontrolled cell proliferation and tumorigenesis. The protein features three primary domains: a RING domain with ubiquitin-conjugating activity located at the N-terminus, a BRCT domain at the C-terminus, which acts as a transcriptional activation domain; and a large unstructured region located in the center that is encoded by exons 11–13 [34]. Breast cancer is associated with mutations in BRCT and RING, two proteins that are implicated in the interaction between BRCA1 and other proteins [75, 76].

BRCA1-deficient cells displayed genomic instability, including chromosomal abnormalities, according to early research on BRCA1 functions [77–79]. These reports raised the possibility that BRCA1 was implicated in DDR brought on by DSBs. DSBs cause BRCA1 to become phosphorylated. The phosphorylated Abraxas 1 protein then attracts BRCA1 to the DSB sites, where it can form several, mutually exclusive complexes that function at different stages of the cell cycle and different periods during DDR [18, 80]. The exact role that BRCA1 plays in DDR is unknown. However, it binds to the primary human recombinase, RAD51 (RAD51 recombinase), suggesting a crucial function in HRR for DSB repair [81]. This points to BRCA1's involvement in HRR-mediated DSB repair. BRCA1 may also play a part in NHEJ. The other major DSB repair mechanism, albeit this function, is far less well understood than BRCA1's role in HRR. Moreover, BRCA1 is involved in the resolution of DNA replication inhibition caused by DNA damage as well as DNA damage-responsive checkpoint regulation [82]. BRCA1 also has a role in DNA repair activities in addition to HRR. According to Saha et al., BRCA1 transcriptionally increased the number of BER-related genes, such as APEX1 (apurinic/apyrimidinic end deoxyribonuclease 1), NTHL1 (Nth-like DNA glycosylase 1), and OGG1 (8-oxoguanine DNA glycosylase) [83, 84]. In doing so, BRCA1 increased the activity of the transcription factor Oct-1 (octamer-binding transcription factor 1).

6.4.2 GADD45A and Its Role in Breast Cancer

The GADD45A gene plays a crucial function in controlling cellular stress responses by becoming more active in response to circumstances that cause growth arrest or DNA damage. It accomplishes this by assisting in the activation of the p38/JNK pathway via MTK1/MEKK4, launching a series of actions intended to support the cell's ability to repair damage and adapt to stress. Kinase, the protein produced by this gene responds to environmental stressors. This gene has been reported to contain alternatively spliced transcript variants that encode different isoforms [85]. The GADD45A protein, which has a length of 165 amino acids and is found in the nucleus of most healthy tissues, is produced by the GADD45A gene. GADD45A levels are correlated with the cell cycle, peaking in the G1 phase when S is significantly reduced [86, 87]. When ubiquitination occurs, it is broken down by the proteasome; however, GADD55A can be shielded from degradation by PKC delta activation, which deubiquitinates the protein [88]. Inhibiting cell development, inducing cell death (apoptosis), controlling the cell cycle by stopping it at the G2/M phase, and interacting with important proteins like p53, CDK1 (also called cyclin-dependent kinase 1 or Cdc2), and cyclin B1 are just a few of the critical roles that GADD45A performs in the cell [89]. These activities highlight how crucial GADD45A is to preserving genomic integrity, DDR, and cancer transformation. Indeed, one of the primary biological roles of GADD45A that has been shown thus far is its protective role against DNA damage-induced carcinogenesis (Figure 6.3) [90–92]. The exact molecular mechanisms behind GADD45A's cancer-prevention function are unknown, nevertheless.

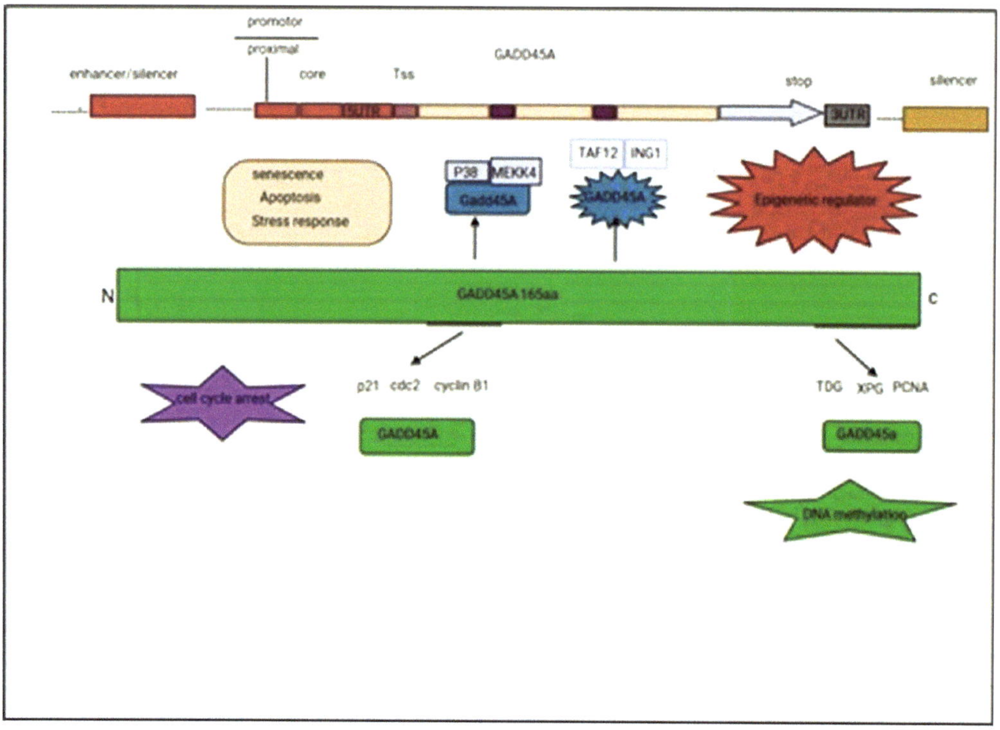

FIGURE 6.3 The growth arrest and DNA damage-inducible 45 alpha gene, or GADD45A for short, is located at 1p31.3 and has four exons. Numerous physiological activities, including stress signaling, DNA repair, cell survival, control of the cell cycle, senescence, and apoptosis, depend on it. For these purposes, the GADD45 protein interacts with several other proteins, including ING1 (inhibitor of growth family member 1), TAF12 (TATA-box binding protein associated factor 12), cdc2 (cyclin-dependent kinase 2), TDG (thymine DNA glycosylase), XPG (xerodermatic pigmentosum group G), and PCNA (proliferating cell nuclear antigen).

In Figure 6.3, the regions of the DNA that are not essential for the GADD45A gene are depicted by dashed lines. It has also been demonstrated that GADD45A plays a significant role in the transformation of breast cancer. When comparing breast cancer samples to nearby non-cancerous tissues, a greater expression of GADD45A was seen [83]. Tront et al. noted that animals with mammary tumors induced by Ras activation were more likely to develop when GADD45A was lost, and these tumors exhibited more aggressive behavior and grew more quickly [93]. Furthermore, they observed a reduction in Ras-triggered cellular aging, attributed to lower activity of p38. They also noted a decline in cell death, associated with increased activation of mitogen-activated protein kinase 8 (MAPK8). Additionally, mutant p53 proteins can develop oncogenic characteristics that foster genetic instability and advancement of tumors.

6.5 IMPACT OF TP53 MUTATIONS ON CLINICAL RESULTS FOR BREAST CANCER

The gene most frequently mutated in cancer is TP53 [94]. When the body faces stressors like radiation or chemotherapy, the TP53 gene produces a protein called p53. This protein triggers the activation of various genes responsible for actions such as halting cell division, inducing cell death (apoptosis), regulating metabolism, repairing DNA damage, and promoting cellular aging (senescence) [23, 95]. Mutations predominantly occur in the DNA-binding domain of the TP53 gene, leading to the production of a mutant p53 protein that lacks its transcriptional activity in response to stress [96]. Although p53 induction levels and the precise targets that p53 transactivates differ depending on the kind of tumor and cell, wild-type p53 activity is generally associated with a better prognosis for cancer patients [97]. Mutations in the TP53 gene occur most commonly in breast cancer, affecting approximately 30% of cases [94]. Numerous studies, both in preclinical and clinical settings, have sought to understand the role of p53 in breast cancer due to the consistent presence of tumors harboring mutated TP53 across all molecular subtypes of the disease [94]. However, conflicting research has shown that TP53 mutations are linked to either good, neutral, or negative outcomes misinterpreting the clinical relevance of the presence or absence of TP53 mutations in breast cancer [98, 99]. Receptor 2 for human epidermal growth factor (HER2)-targeting medicines, hormonal therapies, surgery, and chemotherapy treatment are only a few of the several treatment choices available for breast cancer, which is a diverse illness [100, 101]. Within each of these categories are also other choices. The presence or lack of molecular markers for HER2 and steroid hormone receptors—the estrogenic receptor (ER) or progesterone receptor—determines the best course of treatment [13, 102]. Chemotherapies based on anthracyclines and non-anthracyclines that damage DNA are frequently utilized in breast cancer clinics. Doxorubicin and epirubicin are two examples of anthracycline-based medications that cause cytotoxicity interfering with the DNA-topoisomerase II complex and impeding the process of DNA synthesis [103, 104]. DNA-damaging treatments that don't involve anthracyclines have a broader mechanism of action. This category includes drugs like antimetabolites such as 5-fluorouracil, which disrupt DNA synthesis, and DNA-alkylating agents like cyclophosphamide, which modify DNA by attaching alkyl groups [105]. In a similar vein, radiation therapy damages DNA by producing strand breaks [105]. Non-DNA-damaging taxanes, which disrupt microtubule activity to obstruct mitotic cell division, are also used to treat breast cancer [37]. The fate of cells under stress due to DNA damage [106] or mitotic failure [107] is greatly influenced by p53 activity. Chemotherapy can be used as a therapeutic adjuvant or neoadjuvant [108, 109]. Therapies administered following the main course of treatment are known as adjuvants (i.e., surgical excision of tumors). Therapies administered before the main course of treatment are known as neoadjuvant therapies. Whether residual disease is present or not can be evaluated using these criteria: (i) complete response, (ii) partial response, (iii) stable disease, and (iv) progressive disease. Pathologists can ascertain how successful the treatment is in shrinking the tumor [110]. HRTs that block the HR-signaling pathways that fuel HR-positive breast tumors are frequently used in their treatment. Hormone replacement therapies (HRTs) encompass several pharmacological categories, including selective estrogen receptor modulators (SERMs), selective estrogen receptor degraders

(SERDs), and aromatase inhibitors [111, 112]. Breast cancer treatment can differ from patient to patient in addition to biological considerations because of institutional guidelines, insurance coverage, access to healthcare, physician and patient preferences, and reimbursement incentives [113, 114]. In short, breast cancer is a complicated disease that is treated with a range of approaches based on numerous biological and nonbiological variables.

6.6 TECHNIQUES FOR ASSESSING TP53 MUTATION STATUS IN BREAST CANCER

Researchers and medical professionals have examined how TP53 mutations correlate with patient outcomes due to p53's significant involvement in cancer initiation and advancement, notably in breast cancer [115]. Various techniques like DNA sequencing, immunohistochemistry staining, and yeast-based functional assays have been employed to assess TP53 mutation status.

6.6.1 Immunohistochemistry Staining

In many prior studies, researchers have used affirmative immunohistochemistry (IHC) staining as a substitute indicator to detect p53 mutations. Robust nuclear IHC staining serves as an indicator of heightened stability of the p53 protein, often attributable to missense mutations occurring within the DNA-binding domain of the TP53 gene. These mutations predominantly constitute the majority of alterations observed in the TP53 gene [116]. Nevertheless, not all truncating changes, splice variants, frameshift mutations, or point mutations in TP53 will be produced. Using IHC to evaluate p53 status in such cases will erroneously categorize these tumors as having a normal TP53 gene [116, 117]. This finding is significant because, based on recent research using advanced detection methods, approximately 40% of TP53 mutations identified in breast cancer cases won't lead to the creation of a functional protein [118]. Furthermore, IHC analysis of tumor tissues can reveal the presence of wild-type p53 protein [119]. It is estimated that in breast cancer, there is less than 75% connection between TP53 mutations found through DNA sequencing and p53 accumulation assessed by IHC [120]. Because of these methodological constraints, certain patients whose tumors are assumed to be the interpretation of TP53 status through IHC might not always accurately reflect the true genetic status. Tumors labeled as TP53 wild type via IHC could potentially harbor TP53.

6.6.2 Functional Assay Using Yeast as the Model System

A functional test based on yeast can also be used to determine the status of TP53 mutations. Tumor biopsies from patients are used to extract RNA, which is then reverse-transcribed into cDNA. After being amplified using PCR, the TP53 transcripts are transfected into yeast cells that have a p53 transcription reporter plasmid incorporated into them. Red colonies are produced by yeast transfected with mutant p53, which lacks transcriptional activity, whereas white colonies are produced by yeast colonies transfected with wild-type p53 [121].

6.6.3 DNA Sequencing

DNA sequencing serves as an alternative approach for detecting TP53 mutations in breast cancer [14]. Early studies indicate that mutations are predominantly located within exons 5–8 of the TP53 gene [122]. Conversely, this is the area that has been sequenced the most, if not entirely [123]. Next-generation sequencing has enabled the detection of TP53 mutations beyond exons 5–8, which might have been missed in studies focusing solely on this region. As a result, patients with TP53 mutations occurring elsewhere may mistakenly be categorized as wild type in such studies [124]. The most reliable method for determining TP53 mutations is DNA sequencing mutations, while tumors marked as mutants based on positive IHC staining might possess TP53 wild-type genes [125].

6.7 INNOVATIVE TREATMENTS TARGETING MUTANT p53 IN BREAST CANCER

Tumor development, progression, and metastasis are driven by mutant p53, which is commonly detected in TNBC and HER2-enriched subtypes [126]. This makes it a desirable target for breast cancer therapy. In TNBC, p53 mutation is also most often clonal, offering a unique homogeneity characteristic in a heterogenic malignancy such as breast cancer [127, 128]. Targeting mutant p53 is therapeutically valuable, as evidenced by the intrinsic aggressiveness of TNBC and the relative absence of targeted treatments available. Targeted therapies for p53-mutant tumors aim to (1) reinstate or revive mutant p53 to its normal functions, (2) prompt degradation, (3) induce synthetic lethality, (4) obstruct interactors or pathways associated with its altered functionality, (5) utilize immunotherapies, and (6) apply gene therapies employing vectors to introduce the wild-type p53 gene into tumor cells. Numerous investigations have looked into the possibility that mutant p53/protein status is probably complicated by this error (Table 6.1) [129].

Numerous investigations have looked into the possibility that mutant p53/protein overexpression in breast cancer could be a predictor of therapy and/or prognosis. Since the p53 protein is stabilized and accumulates in cancer cells due to mutations, immunohistochemistry was utilized in the majority of early clinical investigations to identify p53. There are several possible explanations for the mutant p53's increased stability over the wild-type protein, including interactions with stabilizing proteins like HSP90, the mutant p53's inability to activate MDM2, which destroys p53, and post-translational changes such as Thr180 and Ser20 phosphorylation. The mutant p53 protein was found by immunochemistry, and its presence was taken as a sign of a mutation because it tends to concentrate in tumor cells. Nonetheless, it is now understood that some mutations, just like the truncating mutation found in p53, other alterations in this protein don't necessarily lead to instability. Even without mutation, natural p53 can become more stable under various stresses. Initial studies noted a link between immunohistochemically detected p53 and negative prognosis, even though not all

TABLE 6.1
Compounds and Genes or Immunotherapies against Mutant p53 Tumors That Have Been Evaluated in Breast Cancer Models or Patients

Compound Name	Mode of Action	Phase of Development	Reference
PRIMA-1APR-246	Michael addition: prevent mutant p53 from aggregating; target cysteine residue to restore p53's capacity to bind DNA	Early-stage breast cancer research through to phase III clinical trials for myelodysplastic syndrome (NCT03745716) using APR-246 in combination with azacitidine.	[130, 131, 132]
PK11007	Targeted alkylation of two cysteine residues, increasing the p53 Y220C DNA-binding domain's heat stability	Preclinical	[133, 134]
COTI-2	Zn2+ chelator, restore p53's capacity to bind DNA	Phase I clinical trial for multiple diseases, including preclinical in breast cancer (NCT02433626)	[135]
PC14586	Binds to the Y220C mutant's fissures, increasing the DNA-binding domain of p53 Y220C's heat stability	Phase I/II in TP53 Y220C mutation, malignant solid tumors including breast cancer (NCT04585750)	[136]
Chemotin	Restores wild-type function via attaching to Hsp40 and improving binding to p53 R175H	Preclinical	[137]

mutant genes lead to stabilized protein. Similarly, the presence of direct p53 mutations often correlates with poor patient outcomes.

6.8 MUTANT p53 DRIVES CANCER PROGRESSION

6.8.1 Triggering Genetic Instability

The primary function of p53 as the "guardian of the genome" is to ensure genetic stability by blocking the passage of genetic mutations to future cell generations [138, 139]. Cells harboring mutated p53 proteins exhibit significantly heightened chromosomal instability, manifesting as intrachromosomal rearrangement and aneusomy. This underscores the tumorigenic GOF potential of p53 mutants. Interestingly, even in the lack of functional p53, cells still possess residual checkpoint mechanisms and DNA repair capabilities [140–142]. These differences play a pivotal role in the genetic variety that accelerates the growth of malignant tumors. Common p53 mutations can interact with the nuclease Mre11 to disrupt the DNA DSB damage response in its early stages. The main detector of DNA DSB damage, ATM, is rendered inactive as a result of this interaction, which prevents the recruitment of the Mre11/Rad50/NBS1 (MRN) complex to the DSB site. As a result, this causes the G2/M checkpoint to be compromised [143, 144]. Because they prevent DNA replication, mutant p53 (mutp53) proteins can be involved in genomic disorders. Certain mutp53 proteins stimulate the checkpoint kinase 1, which helps to maintain replication fork integrity, and cyclin A, which encourages the creation of DNA replication origins, to aid in the duplication of these aberrant genomic DNase [145].

6.8.2 Accelerating Proliferation

A wealth of research suggests that mutp53 facilitates two important "hallmarks of cancer": the unbridled capacity for replication and when normal cells undergo malignant transformation, they become unresponsive to signals that normally hinder their growth [146, 147]. Mutp53 has been demonstrated to directly engage nuclear factor Y, a crucial regulator of the cell cycle, and oversees pivotal genes involved in progressing through different phases of the cell cycle, such as cyclin A, cyclin B, cdk1, and cdc25C, which are activated by p300's acetyltransferase or by YAP, the principal effector of the Hippo pathway [148, 149]. Furthermore, research indicates that TEAD collaborates with mutant p53 and YAP to form a trimeric transcriptional complex, resulting in the production of circular RNA (circPVT1) and the activation of genes associated with cell proliferation, such as mki67 and aurka [13, 139, 150]. MicroRNA miR-27a plays an essential part in sustaining the activation of ERK1/2 induced by EGF, which in turn stimulates cellular proliferation and contributes to carcinogenesis. Its expression is regulated by mutp53, a mutated variant of the p53 protein. This mutated protein changes gene expression patterns, including the upregulation of miR-27a, thereby aiding in cancer progression [151, 152]. Furthermore, methyltransferases mixed lineage leukemia 1 and mixed lineage leukemia 2 as well as acetylase are important chromatin regulators that are targeted by p53 mutants. This leads to an increase in epigenetic activation marks, specifically histone 3 lysine 4 tri-methylation and histone 3 lysine 9 acetylation, throughout the genome, which in turn stimulates cell proliferation. Additionally, TP53 R249S mutants, commonly found in HBV-positive human hepatocellular carcinoma (HCC), exhibit a unique GOF. This GOF mechanism sustains the growth and survival of HCC cells by enhancing c-Myc-mediated transcription of ribosomal DNA (rDNA), crucial for ribosome synthesis [32, 153].

6.8.3 Promoting Metastasis

Another "hallmark of cancer" is metastasis, leading to more than 90% of fatalities in cancer cases [146, 154]. Reports suggest that mutp53 can increase the expression of several key transcription factors associated with the epithelial-to-mesenchymal transition (EMT), such as ZEB1, SLUG, and TWIST1, through various mechanisms including transcriptional, post-translational, and epigenetic processes. This enhances the ability of cells to alter their morphology, facilitating invasion and migration, thus marking the earliest and most crucial phase of metastasis. According to reports, mutp53 may enhance the regulation of multiple important transcription factors associated with EMT, such as ZEB1, SLUG, and TWIST1, which occurs through mechanisms involving transcriptional, post-translational, and epigenetic processes, mechanisms that only provide a paraphrasing and not an explanation [10, 155]. ZEB1 is negatively regulated by miR-130b, whose expression is suppressed by mutp53 in endometrial cancer tissues. Mutp53 inhibits MDM2-mediated SLUG degradation in non-small cell lung cancers (NSCLCs), which leads to elevated SLUG and decreased E-cadherin expression. Mutp53, on the other hand, causes the TWIST1 promoter's H3K27me3 repression mark to decrease in prostate cells. Furthermore, it has been shown by a numerous indication that p63 mediates the metastasis mediated by mutant p53. When TGF-β signaling is active, mutp53 interacts with p63, leading to the formation of a ternary complex alongside phosphorylated Smad2. This complex effectively suppresses the activation of downstream metastasis suppressor genes such as cyclin G2 and Sharp-1, thereby impeding their function. Additionally, mutp53 blocks the inactivation of Rab-coupling protein (RCP) mediated by p63, which leads to increased trafficking of EGFR and α5β1 integrin to the plasma membrane. This also activates EGFR/integrin signaling constitutively and its subsequent pro-metastatic act pathway activation. Additionally, the mutp53-induced activation of RCP boosts HSP90α production, which in turn promotes cell motility by interacting with the extracellular matrix (ECM). Mutp53-induced metastasis also involves reprogramming of metabolism. Xiong et al. used a model of p53R172H/+ mice (R175H in humans). When mutant p53 and ETS2 interact, it triggers the activation of Pla2g16. This gene produces a phospholipase enzyme that facilitates the transformation of phosphatidic acid into lysophosphatidic acid and free fatty acids. In simpler terms, this interaction leads to the production of a specific enzyme that plays a role in converting one type of lipid into another. These two products have been linked to the promotion of metastasis and migration. Furthermore, the frequent mutp53 polymorphism Pro72Arg increases tumor migration and metastasis by binding and controlling PGC-1α target genes, an important regulator of mitochondrial biogenesis and oxidative phosphorylation.

6.9 CONCLUSION

The contribution of p53 in DNA restoration and genomic stability in the domain of breast cancer represents a complex and intricate area of research that holds significant implications for both understanding the underlying mechanisms of tumorigenesis and developing novel therapeutic approaches. In this chapter, we have extensively explored the pivotal role of p53, a cornerstone tumor-suppressor protein, in safeguarding genomic integrity through its intricate participation in DNA repair mechanisms, precise orchestration of cell-cycle progression, and decisive induction of apoptosis. Particularly in breast cancer, where genomic instability is a hallmark feature, elucidating the interplay between p53 and DNA repair mechanisms is crucial for advancing our understanding of disease progression and improving patient outcomes. First and foremost, it's crucial to understand the central importance of p53 in protecting genetic material. Acting as a transcription factor, p53 oversees a wide range of cellular reactions triggered by different stress signals, notably DNA damage. When it detects abnormalities in DNA, p53 coordinates the activation of various DNA repair mechanisms, including nucleotide excision repair (NER), base excision repair (BER), homologous recombination (HR), and non-homologous end joining (NHEJ). Through its role in facilitating the repair of damaged DNA, p53 significantly contributes to preventing the accumulation of mutations that might otherwise promote the development of tumors. In breast cancer, alterations in p53 are frequently observed, contributing to genomic instability and disease progression. Mutations in the TP53 gene, responsible for encoding the p53 protein, are prevalent in a considerable portion of breast tumors, especially those categorized as aggressive subtypes. When the wild-type p53 function is lost due to mutations, it hampers its capacity to efficiently regulate DNA repair mechanisms, ultimately heightening genomic instability and fostering the progression of tumors. Moreover, aberrant expression of upstream regulators or downstream effectors of p53 can perturb its activity, further disrupting DNA repair processes and exacerbating genomic instability in breast cancer. Interestingly, recent studies have uncovered additional layers of the relationship between p53 and DNA repair mechanisms, with recent findings indicating that p53's actions can influence the selection of various repair pathways depending on the type and context of DNA damage. In certain situations, p53 might favor the activation of error-prone repair methods like non-homologous end joining, particularly when cells face intense genomic stress. This preference could potentially result in the buildup of genetic changes and the development of more aggressive characteristics in breast cancer cells. Additionally, the interplay between p53 and other fundamental cellular processes like cell-cycle control and programmed cell death adds another layer of complexity to this dynamic interaction, significantly influencing the maintenance of genomic stability in breast cancer. Dysregulation of these interconnected pathways can tip the balance toward unchecked cell proliferation, genomic instability, and tumor progression. Consequently, targeting p53 and its associated pathways has surfaced as a promising strategy for developing novel therapeutics aimed at restoring genomic integrity and suppressing the proliferation of breast cancer cells. In conclusion, the contribution of p53 in DNA repair and genomic stability in breast cancer is a multifaceted and dynamic process that holds significant implications for both basic research and clinical practice. By unraveling the intricate mechanisms underlying p53 function and dysregulation in breast cancer, we can uncover the factors that drive the development of tumors and identify new targets for treatment. Moving forward, continued exploration of the interplay between p53 and DNA repair pathways promises to yield novel insights into breast cancer biology and lay the foundation for the creation of more effective treatments tailored to individual patient's genomic profiles.

REFERENCES

1. Levitt, N.C. and I.D. Hickson, Caretaker tumour suppressor genes that defend genome integrity. *Trends in Molecular Medicine*, 2002. **8**(4): p. 179–186.
2. Eroles, P., et al., Molecular biology in breast cancer: intrinsic subtypes and signaling pathways. *Cancer Treatment Reviews*, 2012. **38**(6): p. 698–707.
3. Cheng, N., et al., Transforming growth factor-β signaling–deficient fibroblasts enhance hepatocyte growth factor signaling in mammary carcinoma cells to promote scattering and invasion. *Molecular Cancer Research*, 2008. **6**(10): p. 1521–1533.
4. Pitolli, C., et al., Do mutations turn p53 into an oncogene? *International Journal of Molecular Sciences*, 2019. **20**(24): p. 6241.
5. Haupt, Y., et al., Mdm2 promotes the rapid degradation of p53. *Nature*, 1997. **387**(6630): p. 296–299.
6. Mir, M.A., et al., Metronomics: toward personalized chemotherapy. *Novel Approaches in Metronomic Chemotherapy for Breast Cancer Treatment*, 2024. p. 99–119. https://doi.org/10.1201/9781032632674-8
7. Jain, A.N., et al., Quantitative analysis of chromosomal CGH in human breast tumors associates copy number abnormalities with p53 status and patient survival. *Proceedings of the National Academy of Sciences*, 2001. **98**(14): p. 7952–7957.
8. Zhu, J., et al., Gain-of-function p53 mutants co-opt chromatin pathways to drive cancer growth. *Nature*, 2015. **525**(7568): p. 206–211.
9. Jan, N., et al., Targeting breast cancer stem cells through retinoids: a new hope for treatment. *Critical Reviews in Oncology/Hematology*, 2023: p. 104156.
10. Mir, M.A., M. Bashir, and N. Jan, The Role of Interleukin (IL)-6/IL-6 Receptor Axis in Cancer, in *Cytokine and Chemokine Networks in Cancer*. 2023, Springer. p. 137–164.
11. Mir, M.A., N. Jan, and S. Sofi, Introduction to Metronomic Chemotherapy, in *Novel Approaches in Metronomic Chemotherapy for Breast Cancer Treatment*. 2024, CRC Press. p. 1–14.
12. D'Errico, M. and E. Dogliotti, The role of p53 mutations in skin cancer. *Chronica Dermatologica*, 1996. **6**: p. 27–36.
13. Mir, M.A., M. Rashid, and N. Jan, Cytokines and Chemokines in Tumor Growth and Progression, in *Cytokine and Chemokine Networks in Cancer*. 2023, Springer. p. 33–77.

14. Hainaut, P. and M. Hollstein, p53 and human cancer: the first ten thousand mutations. *Advances in Cancer Research*, 1999. **77**: p. 81–137.
15. Harris, C.C. and M. Hollstein, Clinical implications of the p53 tumor-suppressor gene. *New England Journal of Medicine*, 1993. **329**(18): p. 1318–1327.
16. Lane, D.P. and L.V. Crawford, T antigen is bound to a host protein in SY40-transformed cells. *Nature*, 1979. **278**(5701): p. 261–263.
17. Momand, J., H.-H. Wu, and G. Dasgupta, MDM2—master regulator of the p53 tumor suppressor protein. *Gene*, 2000. **242**(1–2): p. 15–29.
18. Sofi, S., et al., Clinicopathological and prognostic significance of Bcl2 in breast cancer: a comprehensive in silico and in vitro study. *Saudi Journal of Biological Sciences*, 2023. **31**(2): p. 103916.
19. Freedman, D., L. Wu, and A. Levine, Functions of the MDM2 oncoprotein. *Cellular and Molecular Life Sciences CMLS*, 1999. **55**: p. 96–107.
20. Juven-Gershon, T. and M. Oren, Mdm2: the ups and downs. *Molecular Medicine*, 1999. **5**: p. 71–83.
21. Lev Bar-Or, R., et al., Generation of oscillations by the p53-Mdm2 feedback loop: a theoretical and experimental study. *Proceedings of the National Academy of Sciences*, 2000. **97**(21): p. 11250–11255.
22. Jones, S.N., et al., Rescue of embryonic lethality in Mdm2-deficient mice by absence of p53. *Nature*, 1995. **378**(6553): p. 206–208.
23. de Oca Luna, R.M., D.S. Wagner, and G. Lozano, Rescue of early embryonic lethality in mdm2-deficient mice by deletion of p53. *Nature*, 1995. **378**(6553): p. 203–206.
24. De Rozieres, S., et al., The loss of mdm2 induces p53 mediated apoptosis. *Oncogene*, 2000. **19**(13): p. 1691–1697.
25. Sofi, S., et al., A comprehensive analysis of notch signaling genes in breast cancer: expression pattern and prognostic significance. *Advances in Cancer Biology-Metastasis*, 2023. **7**: p. 100104.
26. Kubbutat, M.H., S.N. Jones, and K.H. Vousden, Regulation of p53 stability by Mdm2. *Nature*, 1997. **387**(6630): p. 299–303.
27. Blagosklonny, M.V., p53 from complexity to simplicity: mutant p53 stabilization, gain-of-function, and dominant-negative effect. *The FASEB Journal*, 2000. **14**(13): p. 1901–1907.
28. Buschmann, T., et al., Analysis of JNK, Mdm2 and p14ARF contribution to the regulation of mutant p53 stability. *Journal of Molecular Biology*, 2000. **295**(4): p. 1009–1021.
29. Fang, S., et al., Mdm2 is a RING finger-dependent ubiquitin protein ligase for itself and p53. *Journal of Biological Chemistry*, 2000. **275**(12): p. 8945–8951.
30. Honda, R. and H. Yasuda, Activity of MDM2, a ubiquitin ligase, toward p53 or itself is dependent on the RING finger domain of the ligase. *Oncogene*, 2000. **19**(11): p. 1473–1476.
31. Nakamura, S., J.A. Roth, and T. Mukhopadhyay, Multiple lysine mutations in the C-terminal domain of p53 interfere with MDM2-dependent protein degradation and ubiquitination. *Molecular and Cellular Biology*, 2000. **20**(24): p. 9391–9398.
32. Mir, M.A., Sumaya, N. Jan, Implications of Chemokine Heterogenicity in Cancer Metastasis, in *Cytokine and Chemokine Networks in Cancer.* 2023, Springer. p. 115–136.
33. Rodriguez, M.S., et al., Multiple C-terminal lysine residues target p53 for ubiquitin-proteasome-mediated degradation. *Molecular and Cellular Biology*, 2000. **20**(22): p. 8458–8467.
34. Berger, M., et al., A role for the polyproline domain of p53 in its regulation by Mdm2. *Journal of Biological Chemistry*, 2001. **276**(6): p. 3785–3790.
35. Gu, J., et al., Identification of a sequence element from p53 that signals for Mdm2-targeted degradation. *Molecular and Cellular Biology*, 2000. https://doi.org/10.1128/mcb.20.4.1243-1253.2000
36. Fuchs, S.Y., et al., JNK targets p53 ubiquitination and degradation in nonstressed cells. *Genes & Development*, 1998. **12**(17): p. 2658–2663.
37. Böttger, A., et al., Design of a synthetic Mdm2-binding mini protein that activates the p53 response in vivo. *Current Biology*, 1997. **7**(11): p. 860–869.
38. Wasylyk, C., et al., p53 mediated death of cells overexpressing MDM2 by an inhibitor of MDM2 interaction with p53. *Oncogene*, 1999. **18**(11): p. 1921–1934.
39. Chehab, N.H., et al., Phosphorylation of Ser-20 mediates stabilization of human p53 in response to DNA damage. *Proceedings of the National Academy of Sciences*, 1999. **96**(24): p. 13777–13782.
40. Shieh, S.Y., Y. Taya, and C. Prives, DNA damage-inducible phosphorylation of p53 at N-terminal sites including a novel site, Ser20, requires tetramerization. *The EMBO Journal*, 1999. https://doi.org/10.1093/emboj/18.7.1815
41. Chehab, N.H., et al., Chk2/hCds1 functions as a DNA damage checkpoint in G1 by stabilizing p53. *Genes & Development*, 2000. **14**(3): p. 278–288.
42. Hirao, A., et al., DNA damage-induced activation of p53 by the checkpoint kinase Chk2. *Science*, 2000. **287**(5459): p. 1824–1827.

43. BoÈttger, V., et al., Comparative study of the p53-mdm2 and p53-MDMX interfaces. *Oncogene*, 1999. **18**(1): p. 189–199.
44. Sakaguchi, K., et al., Damage-mediated phosphorylation of human p53 threonine 18 through a cascade mediated by a casein 1-like kinase: Effect on Mdm2 binding. *Journal of Biological Chemistry*, 2000. **275**(13): p. 9278–9283.
45. Dumaz, N. and D.W. Meek, Serine 15 phosphorylation stimulates p53 transactivation but does not directly influence interaction with HDM2. *The EMBO Journal*, 1999. **18**(24): p. 7002–7010.
46. Gostissa, M., et al., Activation of p53 by conjugation to the ubiquitin-like protein SUMO-1. *The EMBO Journal*, 1999. https://doi.org/10.1093/emboj/18.22.6462
47. Buschmann, T., et al., SUMO-1 modification of Mdm2 prevents its self-ubiquitination and increases Mdm2 ability to ubiquitinate p53. *Cell*, 2000. **101**(7): p. 753–762.
48. Khosravi, R., et al., Rapid ATM-dependent phosphorylation of MDM2 precedes p53 accumulation in response to DNA damage. *Proceedings of the National Academy of Sciences*, 1999. **96**(26): p. 14973–14977.
49. Mayo, L.D., J.J. Turchi, and S.J. Berberich, Mdm-2 phosphorylation by DNA-dependent protein kinase prevents interaction with p53. *Cancer Research*, 1997. **57**(22): p. 5013–5016.
50. Chatterjee, N. and G.C. Walker, Mechanisms of DNA damage, repair, and mutagenesis. *Environmental and Molecular Mutagenesis*, 2017. **58**(5): p. 235–263.
51. Kowalczykowski, S.C., An overview of the molecular mechanisms of recombinational DNA repair. *Cold Spring Harbor Perspectives in Biology*, 2015. **7**(11): p. a016410.
52. Shuck, S.C., E.A. Short, and J.J. Turchi, Eukaryotic nucleotide excision repair: from understanding mechanisms to influencing biology. *Cell Research*, 2008. **18**(1): p. 64–72.
53. Dip, R., U. Camenisch, and H. Naegeli, Mechanisms of DNA damage recognition and strand discrimination in human nucleotide excision repair. *DNA Repair*, 2004. **3**(11): p. 1409–1423.
54. Khanna, A., DNA damage in cancer therapeutics: a boon or a curse? *Cancer research*, 2015. **75**(11): p. 2133–2138.
55. Sancar, A., et al., Molecular mechanisms of mammalian DNA repair and the DNA damage checkpoints. *Annual Review of Biochemistry*, 2004. **73**(1): p. 39–85.
56. Hegde, M.L., T.K. Hazra, and S. Mitra, Functions of disordered regions in mammalian early base excision repair proteins. *Cellular and Molecular Life Sciences*, 2010. **67**: p. 3573–3587.
57. Kelley, M. and M. Fishel, Overview of DNA repair pathways, current targets, and clinical trials bench to clinic. *DNA Repair in Cancer Therapy*, 2016: p. 1–54.
58. Bai, P., Biology of poly (ADP-ribose) polymerases: the factotums of cell maintenance. *Molecular Cell*, 2015. **58**(6): p. 947–958.
59. Lazzaro, F., et al., Checkpoint mechanisms at the intersection between DNA damage and repair. *DNA Repair*, 2009. **8**(9): p. 1055–1067.
60. Curtin, N.J., DNA repair dysregulation from cancer driver to therapeutic target. *Nature Reviews Cancer*, 2012. **12**(12): p. 801–817.
61. Mehta, A. and J.E. Haber, Sources of DNA double-strand breaks and models of recombinational DNA repair. *Cold Spring Harbor Perspectives in Biology*, 2014. **6**(9): p. a016428.
62. Aparicio, T., R. Baer, and J. Gautier, DNA double-strand break repair pathway choice and cancer. *DNA Repair*, 2014. **19**: p. 169–175.
63. Srivastava, M. and S.C. Raghavan, DNA double-strand break repair inhibitors as cancer therapeutics. *Chemistry & Biology*, 2015. **22**(1): p. 17–29.
64. Grundy, G.J., et al., One ring to bring them all—the role of Ku in mammalian non-homologous end joining. *DNA Repair*, 2014. **17**: p. 30–38.
65. Daley, J.M., et al., Regulation of DNA pairing in homologous recombination. *Cold Spring Harbor Perspectives in Biology*, 2014. **6**(11): p. a017954.
66. Eischen, C.M. and G. Lozano, The M dm network and its regulation of p53 activities: a rheostat of cancer risk. *Human Mutation*, 2014. **35**(6): p. 728–737.
67. Harper, J.W., et al., The p21 Cdk-interacting protein Cip1 is a potent inhibitor of G1 cyclin-dependent kinases. *Cell*, 1993. **75**(4): p. 805–816.
68. Ewen, M.E., et al., p53-dependent repression of CDK4 translation in TGF-beta-induced G1 cell-cycle arrest. *Genes & Development*, 1995. **9**(2): p. 204–217.
69. Campisi, J., Senescent cells, tumor suppression, and organismal aging: good citizens, bad neighbors. *Cell*, 2005. **120**(4): p. 513–522.
70. Pantoja, C. and M. Serrano, Murine fibroblasts lacking p21 undergo senescence and are resistant to transformation by oncogenic Ras. *Oncogene*, 1999. **18**(35): p. 4974–4982.
71. Mir, M.A., et al., Proteomics: Application of Next-Generation Proteomics in Cancer Research, in *Proteomics*. 2023, Elsevier. p. 55–76.

72. Czabotar, P.E., et al., Control of apoptosis by the BCL-2 protein family: implications for physiology and therapy. *Nature Reviews Molecular Cell Biology*, 2014. **15**(1): p. 49–63.
73. Galluzzi, L., et al., Mitochondrial liaisons of p53. *Antioxidants & Redox Signaling*, 2011. **15**(6): p. 1691–1714.
74. Xu, X., et al., Centrosome amplification and a defective G2–M cell cycle checkpoint induce genetic instability in BRCA1 exon 11 isoform–deficient cells. *Molecular Cell*, 1999. **3**(3): p. 389–395.
75. Brzovic, P.S., et al., BRCA1 RING domain cancer-predisposing mutations: structural consequences and effects on protein-protein interactions. *Journal of Biological Chemistry*, 2001. **276**(44): p. 41399–41406.
76. Brzovic, P.S., et al., Structure of a BRCA1–BARD1 heterodimeric RING–RING complex. *Nature Structural Biology*, 2001. **8**(10): p. 833–837.
77. Tirkkonen, M., et al., Distinct somatic genetic changes associated with tumor progression in carriers of BRCA1 and BRCA2 germ-line mutations. *Cancer Research*, 1997. **57**(7): p. 1222–1227.
78. Tirkkonen, M., et al., Somatic genetic alterations in BRCA2-associated and sporadic male breast cancer. *Genes, Chromosomes and Cancer*, 1999. **24**(1): p. 56–61.
79. Weaver, Z., et al., Mammary tumors in mice conditionally mutant for Brca1 exhibit gross genomic instability and centrosome amplification yet display a recurring distribution of genomic imbalances that is similar to human breast cancer. *Oncogene*, 2002. **21**(33): p. 5097–5107.
80. Castillo, A., et al., The BRCA1-interacting protein Abraxas is required for genomic stability and tumor suppression. *Cell Reports*, 2014. **8**(3): p. 807–817.
81. Son, M.Y. and P. Hasty, Homologous recombination defects and how they affect replication fork maintenance. *AIMS Genetics*, 2018. **5**(04): p. 192–211.
82. You, Z. and J.M. Bailis, DNA damage and decisions: CtIP coordinates DNA repair and cell cycle checkpoints. *Trends in Cell Biology*, 2010. **20**(7): p. 402–409.
83. Bochar, D.A., et al., BRCA1 is associated with a human SWI/SNF-related complex: linking chromatin remodeling to breast cancer. *Cell*, 2000. **102**(2): p. 257–265.
84. Saha, J. and A.J. Davis, Unsolved mystery: the role of BRCA1 in DNA end-joining. *Journal of radiation research*, 2016. **57**(S1): p. i18–i24.
85. Zhang, Y., et al., Nucleolin links to arsenic-induced stabilization of GADD45α mRNA. *Nucleic Acids Research*, 2006. **34**(2): p. 485–495.
86. Kearsey, J.M., et al., Gadd45 is a nuclear cell cycle regulated protein which interacts with p21Cip1. *Oncogene*, 1995. **11**(9): p. 1675–1683.
87. Bykov, V.J., et al., Restoration of the tumor suppressor function to mutant p53 by a low-molecular-weight compound. *Nature Medicine*, 2002. **8**(3): p. 282–288.
88. Leung, C.-H., et al., PKCδ-dependent deubiquitination and stabilization of Gadd45 in A431 cells overexposed to EGF. *Biochemical and Biophysical Research Communications*, 2001. **285**(2): p. 283–288.
89. Salvador, J.M., J.D. Brown-Clay, and A.J. Fornace Jr, Gadd45 in stress signaling, cell cycle control, and apoptosis. *Gadd45 Stress Sensor Genes*, 2013: p. 1–19.
90. Hildesheim, J., et al., Gadd45a protects against UV irradiation-induced skin tumors, and promotes apoptosis and stress signaling via MAPK and p53. *Cancer Research*, 2002. **62**(24): p. 7305–7315.
91. Hollander, M.C., et al., Dimethylbenzanthracene carcinogenesis in Gadd45a-null mice is associated with decreased DNA repair and increased mutation frequency. *Cancer Research*, 2001. **61**(6): p. 2487–2491.
92. Hollander, M.C., et al., Genomic instability in Gadd45a-deficient mice. *Nature Genetics*, 1999. **23**(2): p. 176–184.
93. Tront, J.S., B. Hoffman, and D.A. Liebermann, Gadd45a suppresses Ras-driven mammary tumorigenesis by activation of c-Jun NH2-terminal kinase and p38 stress signaling resulting in apoptosis and senescence. *Cancer Research*, 2006. **66**(17): p. 8448–8454.
94. Belizario, J.E. and A.F. Loggulo, Insights into breast cancer phenotying through molecular omics approaches and therapy response. *Cancer Drug Resistance*, 2019. **2**(3): p. 527.
95. Kastenhuber, E.R. and S.W. Lowe, Putting p53 in context. *Cell*, 2017. **170**(6): p. 1062–1078.
96. Soussi, T., TP53 mutations in human cancer: database reassessment and prospects for the next decade. *Advances in Cancer Research*, 2011. **110**: p. 107–139.
97. Soussi, T. and C. Béroud, Assessing TP53 status in human tumours to evaluate clinical outcome. *Nature Reviews Cancer*, 2001. **1**(3): p. 233–239.
98. Berns, E.M., et al., Complete sequencing of TP53 predicts poor response to systemic therapy of advanced breast cancer. *Cancer Research*, 2000. **60**(8): p. 2155–2162.
99. Chen, M.-B., et al., Value of TP53 status for predicting response to neoadjuvant chemotherapy in breast cancer: a meta-analysis. *PloS One*, 2012. **7**(6): p. e39655.
100. Gonzalez-Angulo, A.M., F. Morales-Vasquez, and G.N. Hortobagyi, Overview of resistance to systemic therapy in patients with breast cancer. *Breast Cancer Chemosensitivity*, 2007: p. 1–22. https://doi.org/10.1093/annonc/mdq612

101. Waks, A.G. and E.P. Winer, Breast cancer treatment: a review. *Jama*, 2019. **321**(3): p. 288–300.
102. Jan, N., et al., Metronomic chemotherapy and drug repurposing: a paradigm shift in oncology. *Heliyon*, 2024. https://doi.org/10.1016/j.heliyon.2024.e24670
103. Roninson, I.B., E.V. Broude, and B.-D. Chang, If not apoptosis, then what? Treatment-induced senescence and mitotic catastrophe in tumor cells. *Drug Resistance Updates*, 2001. **4**(5): p. 303–313.
104. Gianni, L., et al., Role of anthracyclines in the treatment of early breast cancer. *Journal of Clinical Oncology*, 2009. **27**(28): p. 4798–4808.
105. Fu, D., J.A. Calvo, and L.D. Samson, Balancing repair and tolerance of DNA damage caused by alkylating agents. *Nature Reviews Cancer*, 2012. **12**(2): p. 104–120.
106. Gudkov, A.V. and E.A. Komarova, The role of p53 in determining sensitivity to radiotherapy. *Nature Reviews Cancer*, 2003. **3**(2): p. 117–129.
107. Meek, D., The role of p53 in the response to mitotic spindle damage. *Pathologie-Biologie*, 2000. **48**(3): p. 246–254.
108. Buchholz, T.A., et al., Neoadjuvant chemotherapy for breast carcinoma: multidisciplinary considerations of benefits and risks. *Cancer: Interdisciplinary International Journal of the American Cancer Society*, 2003. **98**(6): p. 1150–1160.
109. Jan, N., et al., Exploring the role of trifarotene against RAR-α: an investigation of expression pattern and clinicopathological significance of RAR-α in breast cancer. *Frontiers in Pharmacology*, 2024. **15**: p. 1361679.
110. Eisenhauer, E., et al., 32 INVITED New response evaluation criteria in solid tumors: revised RECIST guideline version 1.1. *European Journal of Cancer Supplements*, 2008. **6**(12): p. 13.
111. Osborne, C.K., H. Zhao, and S.A. Fuqua, Selective estrogen receptor modulators: structure, function, and clinical use. *Journal of Clinical Oncology*, 2000. **18**(17): p. 3172–3186.
112. Fabian, C.J., The what, why and how of aromatase inhibitors: hormonal agents for treatment and prevention of breast cancer. *International Journal of Clinical Practice*, 2007. **61**(12): p. 2051–2063.
113. Mitchell, A.P., et al., Association between reimbursement incentives and physician practice in oncology: a systematic review. *JAMA Oncology*, 2019. **5**(6): p. 893–899.
114. Hadley, J., et al., Medicare breast surgery fees and treatment received by older women with localized breast cancer. *Health Services Research*, 2003. **38**(2): p. 553–573.
115. Haq, B.U., et al., Targeting p53 misfolding conundrum by stabilizing agents and their analogs in breast cancer therapy: a comprehensive computational analysis. *Frontiers in Pharmacology*, 2024. **14**: p. 1333447.
116. Murnyák, B. and T. Hortobágyi, Immunohistochemical correlates of TP53 somatic mutations in cancer. *Oncotarget*, 2016. **7**(40): p. 64910.
117. Slebos, R., et al., Clinical and pathological associations with p53 tumour-suppressor gene mutations and expression of p21WAF1/Cip1 in colorectal carcinoma. *British Journal of Cancer*, 1996. **74**(2): p. 165–171.
118. Curtis, C., et al., The genomic and transcriptomic architecture of 2,000 breast tumours reveals novel subgroups. *Nature*, 2012. **486**(7403): p. 346–352.
119. Barrow, T.M., et al., Aberrant methylation of imprinted genes is associated with negative hormone receptor status in invasive breast cancer. *International Journal of Cancer*, 2015. **137**(3): p. 537–547.
120. Norberg, T., et al., Comparison between p53 protein measurements using the luminometric immunoassay and immunohistochemistry with detection of p53 gene mutations using cDNA sequencing in human breast tumors. *International Journal of Cancer*, 1998. **79**(4): p. 376–383.
121. Flaman, J., et al., A simple p53 functional assay for screening cell lines, blood, and tumors. *Proceedings of the National Academy of Sciences*, 1995. **92**(9): p. 3963–3967.
122. Hollstein, M., et al., New approaches to understanding p53 gene tumor mutation spectra. *Mutation Research/Fundamental and Molecular Mechanisms of Mutagenesis*, 1999. **431**(2): p. 199–209.
123. Hartmann, A., et al., p53 gene mutations inside and outside of exons 5–8: the patterns differ in breast and other cancers. *Oncogene*, 1995. **10**(4): p. 681–688.
124. Hainaut, P. and G.P. Pfeifer, Somatic TP53 mutations in the era of genome sequencing. *Cold Spring Harbor Perspectives in Medicine*, 2016. **6**(11): p. a026179.
125. Robles, A.I. and C.C. Harris, Clinical outcomes and correlates of TP53 mutations and cancer. *Cold Spring Harbor Perspectives in Biology*, 2010. **2**(3): p. a001016.
126. Silwal-Pandit, L., A. Langerød, and A.-L. Børresen-Dale, TP53 mutations in breast and ovarian cancer. *Cold Spring Harbor Perspectives in Medicine*, 2017. **7**(1): p. a026252.
127. Berke, T.P., S.H. Slight, and S.M. Hyder, Role of reactivating mutant p53 protein in suppressing growth and metastasis of triple-negative breast cancer. *OncoTargets and Therapy*, 2022: p. 23–30.

128. Sofi, S., et al., Elucidation of interleukin-19 as a therapeutic target for breast cancer by computational analysis and experimental validation. *Saudi Journal of Biological Sciences*, 2023. **30**(9): p. 103774–103774.
129. Bertheau, P., et al., TP53 status and response to chemotherapy in breast cancer. *Pathobiology*, 2008. **75**(2): p. 132–139.
130. Rangel, L.P., et al., p53 reactivation with induction of massive apoptosis-1 (PRIMA-1) inhibits amyloid aggregation of mutant p53 in cancer cells. *Journal of Biological Chemistry*, 2019. **294**(10): p. 3670–3682.
131. Liang, Y., C. Besch-Williford, and S.M. Hyder, PRIMA-1 inhibits growth of breast cancer cells by re-activating mutant p53 protein. *International Journal of Oncology*, 2009. **35**(5): p. 1015–1023.
132. Sallman, D.A., et al., Eprenetapopt (APR-246) and azacitidine in TP53-mutant myelodysplastic syndromes. *Journal of Clinical Oncology*, 2021. **39**(14): p. 1584.
133. Bauer, M.R., A.C. Joerger, and A.R. Fersht, 2-Sulfonylpyrimidines: Mild alkylating agents with anticancer activity toward p53-compromised cells. *Proceedings of the National Academy of Sciences*, 2016. **113**(36): p. E5271–E5280.
134. Synnott, N.C., et al., Mutant p53 as a therapeutic target for the treatment of triple-negative breast cancer: Preclinical investigation with the anti-p53 drug, PK11007. *Cancer Letters*, 2018. **414**: p. 99–106.
135. Synnott, N.C., et al., COTI-2 reactivates mutant p53 and inhibits growth of triple-negative breast cancer cells. *Breast Cancer Research and Treatment*, 2020. **179**: p. 47–56.
136. Dumbrava, E.E., et al., First-in-human study of PC14586, a small molecule structural corrector of Y220C mutant p53, in patients with advanced solid tumors harboring a TP53 Y220C mutation. *Journal of Clinical Oncology*, 2022. **40**(16): p. 3003.
137. Hiraki, M., et al., Small-molecule reactivation of mutant p53 to wild-type-like p53 through the p53-Hsp40 regulatory axis. *Chemistry & Biology*, 2015. **22**(9): p. 1206–1216.
138. Lane, D.P., p53, guardian of the genome. *Nature*, 1992. **358**(6381): p. 15–16.
139. Mir, M.A., A. Manzoor, and N. Jan, CCL5/CCR5 Axis in Cancer, in *Cytokine and Chemokine Networks in Cancer*. 2023, Springer. p. 219–240.
140. Chen, S., et al., Arsenic trioxide rescues structural p53 mutations through a cryptic allosteric site. *Cancer Cell*, 2021. **39**(2): p. 225–239.
141. Liu, D., H. Song, and Y. Xu, A common gain of function of p53 cancer mutants in inducing genetic instability. *Oncogene*, 2010. **29**(7): p. 949–956.
142. Hanel, W. and U.M. Moll, Links between mutant p53 and genomic instability. *Journal of Cellular Biochemistry*, 2012. **113**(2): p. 433–439.
143. Andreopoulou, E., et al., Feasibility and cardiac safety of pegylated liposomal doxorubicin plus trastuzumab in heavily pretreated patients with recurrent HER2-overexpressing metastatic breast cancer. *Clinical Breast Cancer*, 2007. **7**(9): p. 690–696.
144. Mir, M.A., N. Jan, and I. Noor, Therapeutic Implications of Cytokines and Chemokines Network in Cancer, in *Cytokine and Chemokine Networks in Cancer*. 2023, Springer. p. 385–414.
145. Singh, S., et al., Mutant p53 establishes targetable tumor dependency by promoting unscheduled replication. *The Journal of Clinical Investigation*, 2017. **127**(5): p. 1839–1855.
146. Hanahan, D. and R.A. Weinberg, The hallmarks of cancer. *Cell*, 2000. **100**(1): p. 57–70.
147. Hanahan, D. and R.A. Weinberg, Hallmarks of cancer: the next generation. *Cell*, 2011. **144**(5): p. 646–674.
148. Di Agostino, S., et al., Gain of function of mutant p53: the mutant p53/NF-Y protein complex reveals an aberrant transcriptional mechanism of cell cycle regulation. *Cancer Cell*, 2006. **10**(3): p. 191–202.
149. Di Agostino, S., et al., YAP enhances the pro-proliferative transcriptional activity of mutant p53 proteins. *EMBO Reports*, 2016. **17**(2): p. 188–201.
150. Verduci, L., et al., The oncogenic role of circPVT1 in head and neck squamous cell carcinoma is mediated through the mutant p53/YAP/TEAD transcription-competent complex. *Genome Biology*, 2017. **18**: p. 1–24.
151. Wang, W., et al., Mutant p53-R273H gains new function in sustained activation of EGFR signaling via suppressing miR-27a expression. *Cell Death & Disease*, 2013. **4**(4): p. e574–e574.
152. Mir, M.A., M. Rashid, and N. Jan, The Interleukin-8 Pathway in Cancer, in *Cytokine and Chemokine Networks in Cancer*. 2023, Springer. p. 165–190.
153. Liao, P., et al., Mutant p53 gains its function via c-Myc activation upon CDK4 phosphorylation at serine 249 and consequent PIN1 binding. *Molecular Cell*, 2017. **68**(6): p. 1134–1146.e6.
154. Gupta, G.P. and J. Massagué, Cancer metastasis: building a framework. *Cell*, 2006. **127**(4): p. 679–695.
155. Dong, P., et al., Mutant p53 gain-of-function induces epithelial–mesenchymal transition through modulation of the miR-130b–ZEB1 axis. *Oncogene*, 2013. **32**(27): p. 3286–3295.

7 Interaction of Mutant p53 with Transcription Factors and DNA Repair Enzymes

Adeeba Farooq, Nusrat Jan[2], and Manzoor Ahmad Mir[2]*

[1]Department of Biotechnology, School of Life Sciences, Central University of Kashmir Nunar Campus, Ganderbal, J&K, India
[2]Department of Bioresources, School of Biological Sciences, University of Kashmir, Srinagar, J&K, India
*drmanzoor@kashmiruniversity.ac.in

7.1 INTRODUCTION

p53 (protein 53) is activated during cell stress conditions, including damage in genetic material, hypoxia, or when an oncogene gets stimulated. All of these results in processes that work to repair DNA, cell cycle arrest, cell death, and autophagy, which don't allow the development of a tumor. To inhibit transcription in such cells, and enhance protein stability and nuclear localization, MDM2 (HDM2 in humans) acts as the central regulator [1, 2]. p53 binding proteins reported so far are more than 30 and include MDM2, MDM4, p300, BRCA½, ATM, ABL, and 53 BP-1/2. Most of these proteins are nuclear [3, 4]. When it comes to the activities of mutant p53, the abnormal regulation of transcription has a crucial role in the oncogenic effects of certain mutant forms of p53 proteins [5, 6]. Studies have found that these mutant proteins, which usually differ from the normal p53 by just one amino acid, are highly stable and abundant in tumor cells. It's important to note that these mutant proteins not only lose the normal p53 function but also gain oncogenic properties that significantly add to the development, maintenance, and spread of tumors. Research suggests that the specific mutations in p53 lead to different cellular responses, which are not like those triggered by the wild-type p53, and can differ between different mutant p53 proteins [7, 8]. These mutations in p53 affect key molecules and pathways involved in tumor growth and progression, including immune system evasion, metabolic changes, and stem cell characteristics. This provides potential targets for therapeutic approaches [9–11].

7.2 p53 AND TRANSCRIPTION FACTORS: UNVEILING THE MOLECULAR CROSS-TALK

The MDM2 gene is activated by p53, which is a protein that helps control cell growth and stops the development of tumors. When p53 binds to a specific region called the p53 response element within the P2 promoter, it triggers the activation of the MDM2 gene [2, 12, 13]. Now, here's where things get interesting. In about 50% of cancers, there are mutations in the p53 gene [3]. These mutations disrupt the normal function of p53, leading to an imbalance in cell growth and an increased risk of tumor development. But wait, there's more! In cases of oncogenic stress, a protein called p19arf (or p14arf in humans) steps in to regulate MDM2 [1, 14, 15]. It directly binds to MDM2, which

 DOI: 10.1201/9781003520771-7

stabilizes and activates p53. This activation of p53 is crucial in controlling the cell cycle, inducing cell cycle arrest, promoting apoptosis (cell death), and even triggering autophagy (a process where cells break down and recycle their components) [16, 17]. In early-stage cancer cells, the induction of Arf (p19arf) occurs. This leads to both p53-dependent and p53-independent responses. The responses dependent on p53 involve cell cycle arrest, cell death, and autophagy, as mentioned earlier. On the other hand, p53-independent responses refer to additional mechanisms that help control tumor growth and prevent further progression [7, 18, 19]. Interestingly, studies have shown that mice lacking the Arf protein are extremely susceptible to tumorigenesis. This highlights the important role that Arf plays in suppressing tumor formation. Lastly, other transcription factors that directly interact with both p53 and MDM2 include Dmpl, E2F1, YB-1, and YY-1. Dmpl and YB-1 particularly bind to p53, while E2F1 and YY-1 have the ability to bind to both p53 and MDM2 [1, 3, 18].

7.2.1 Dmp1

Dmpl, also known as Dmtf1, has a secondary mechanism for suppressing tumors in cells that lack Arf. It inhibits the functions of MDM2 and activates p53. The gene product of Arf, p19arf, stabilizes p53 by binding to MDM2, preventing MDM2 from tagging p53 for degradation [2]. This keeps p53 levels high and active. Dmpl is deleted in about 35% of human lung carcinomas and 42% of breast cancers. Activation of Ras35 and Her2/neu can increase the activity of the Dmpl promoter, while NFkB can inhibit it [1, 20]. Dmpl physically binds to p53, not MDM2, and by interacting with each other, they neutralize the effect of HDM2 on p53. It's worth noting that Dmpl variants b and y lack most of the amino acids needed for p53 interaction [1, 6, 21].

7.2.2 E2Fs

E2Fs are a group of proteins that control important processes in the cell, like cell division, DNA repair, and energy production. They work by forming partnerships with other proteins called DPs. There are two types of E2Fs: activators and repressors. Activators, such as E2F1, E2F2, and E2F3a, help promote cell division. Repressors, like E2F3b, E2F4, E2F5, E2F6, E2F7, and E2F8, slow down cell division [1, 22]. The activator E2Fs specifically activate genes that are important for the DNA replication phase of the cell cycle [23, 24]. Some of these genes include DNA polymerase alpha, dihydrofolate reductase, and thymidine kinase. Additionally, E2F1 activators are thought to reduce the activity of a gene called hTERT, which is involved in maintaining telomere length [1, 25, 26]. E2F1, E2F2, and E2F3a interact with another important protein called p53. This interaction helps keep p53 in the nucleus of the cell, where it can carry out its functions. Specifically, the amino acid terminal domain of E2F1 binds to a specific region of p53, preventing it from being exported out of the nucleus. This allows p53 to activate other genes like p21, PIG3, and Bax, which are involved in controlling cell growth and preventing cancer. When p53 is phosphorylated at a specific site called Ser315, it can be destabilized and moved out of the nucleus. However, E2Fs can bind to phosphorylated p53 and prevent its degradation in the cytoplasm. This leads to the activation of p53 and its ability to regulate gene expression. The p53–E2F1 complex can also inhibit the expression of PLK1, a gene involved in cell division, and promote apoptosis, which is programmed cell death [27, 28].

7.2.3 YB-1

YB-1, also called NSEP1, is a protein that binds to nucleic acids and is comparable to the CCAAT box [1]. It plays a role in various cellular processes like RNA chaperoning, RNA splicing, translation, DNA repair, and transcription. YB-1 interacts with p53 and affects its binding to specific sequences. To become active, YB-1 needs to move from the cytoplasm to the nucleus. This translocation can be triggered by factors like ultraviolet (UV) exposure, DNA damage, heat, and cytokines. YB-1 is cleaved, and only the N-terminal portion moves to the nucleus during the G1S phase, leading to an increase in cyclin A/B1 [10, 29]. YB-1 is also found in the promoters of genes involved in cell division, such as EGFR, c-ErbB2, PCNA, DNA pol alpha, thymidine kinase, and topoisomerase II [1, 8]. By binding to Y-Box sequences, YB-1 can inhibit the transcription of cell death-promoting genes like FAS and p53. It is often found at high levels in drug-resistant tumors. YB-1 interacts with p53 through three distinct domains, while a specific 14-amino acid sequence at the C-terminal of p53 is necessary for this interaction. YB-1 can inhibit p53's ability to induce apoptosis and its activation of pro-apoptotic molecules like Apaf-1, Noxa, and Bax [10, 30].

7.2.4 YY-1

YY-1, also known as Yin Yang-1, is a protein that is found in the nucleus of cells. It is widely present in different organisms, from *Xenopus* to humans, and it is highly conserved across species. YY-1 belongs to a group of transcriptional factors called the GLI-Kruppel class of Zn finger proteins. These proteins can activate or repress genes by interacting with other proteins involved in modifying histones and remodeling chromatin structure. In particular, YY-1 can bind to Arf and MDM2, which leads to the ubiquitination and subsequent degradation of p53. As a result, YY-1 acts as a negative regulator of p53, influencing its activity. The connection between purified Dmpla and p53 requires changes in the structure of the proteins after they are made. On the other hand, when E2F1, YB-1, or YY-1 bind to p53/Mdm2, these changes are not necessary. Even though all four of these transcription factors (TFs) directly attach to p53, the way they interact and the effects they have on the body are quite different. Dmpl and YB-1 only bind to p53, while E2F1 and YY-1 bind to both p53 and Mdm2 [1]. When Dmpl and p53 bind together, it stops Mdm2 from doing its usual job of inhibiting p53, which helps suppress tumors. E2F1 and p53 binding together act as a checkpoint to control overactive E2F1. On the other hand, when YB-1 or YY-1 interacts with p53, it interferes with p53's activity, leading to cell cycle progression and the development of tumors. Since many human cancers have high levels of YB-1 and/or YY-1, which inhibit p53 and make cells resistant to drugs, scientists are exploring ways to block or speed up the breakdown of these proteins using small chemicals as a potential new strategy for cancer treatment [1, 25, 31] (Figure 7.1).

7.3 MUTANT p53: TRANSCRIPTIONAL INSIGHTS

Mutations in the p53 gene, known as missense mutations, are very common in cancer cells [5, 32]. These mutations are often associated with resistance to anticancer drugs and a poor prognosis for patients. When p53 is mutated, it gains new functions, referred to as gain-of-function (GOF) activities, that promote various aspects of cancer progression [9, 12]. These activities include stimulating cancer cell growth, facilitating their movement and invasion into surrounding tissues, altering cellular metabolism, and promoting resistance to drugs used in the treatment of tumors [33]. One of the effects of mutant p53 is the increase in intracellular reactive oxygen species (ROS) levels. This increase in ROS contributes to the survival of cancer cells and aids in the progression of tumors. Mutant p53 can also act as a transcription factor, meaning it can regulate the expression of other genes. It does this by interacting with different proteins involved in transcriptional processes, such as transcription factors, acetylases, deacetylases, and scaffold proteins. Through these interactions, mutant p53 can affect the expression of specific genes that are crucial for tumor development [5, 34].

Furthermore, mutant p53 can physically interact with and deactivate other tumor suppressor proteins, such as p73 and p63, which are part of the p53 family. This interaction further contributes to the oncogenic effects of mutant p53. Additionally, the PML gene, which is associated with acute promyelocytic leukemia (APL), codes a protein that acts as a growth and tumor suppressor. PML can enhance the transcriptional activity of mutant p53, suggesting that the decrease in PML expression might have an important impact on the build-up of mutant p53 and its oncogenic effects. Various transcription factors interacting with mutant p53 have also been found, including NF-Y, VDR, ETS1, SP1, ZEB-1, and E2F-1 [35, 36]. These interactions may lead to the abnormal

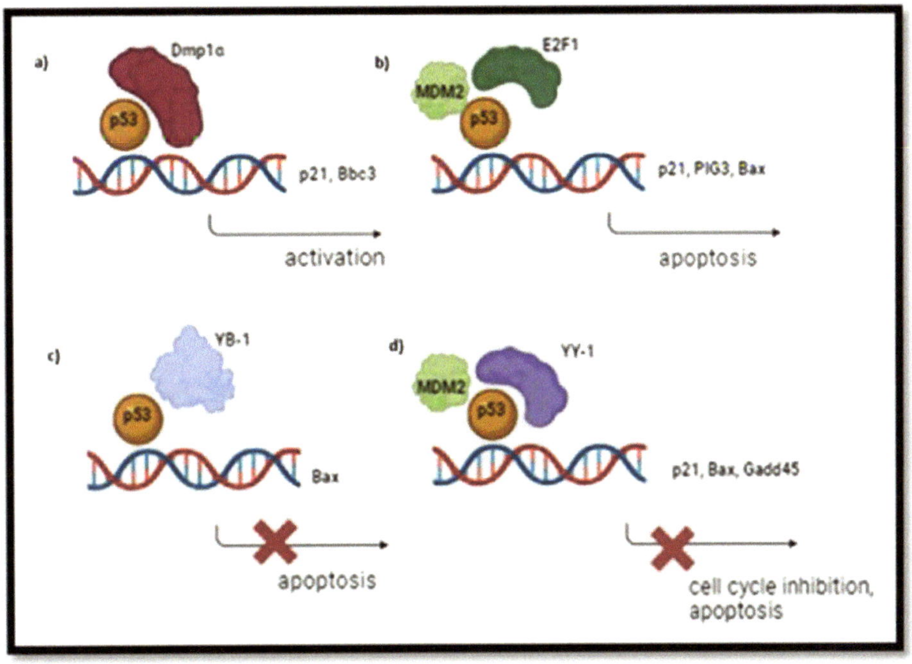

FIGURE 7.1 Schematic presentation of wt p53 and TF interactions and their biological consequences. (a) The Dmpl–p53 interaction happens when Dmpla directly binds to the end part of p53, counteracting the effects of MDM2 on p53. This doesn't depend on Arf. (b) The E2F1–p53/MdDM2 interaction occurs when E2F1 binds to the end part of p53 using its front part. This interaction serves as a checkpoint to prevent abnormal E2F1 signaling and apoptosis, which can lead to cancer. (c) The YB-1–p53 interaction takes place when YB-1, excluding its cold-shock domain, binds to the end part of p53, preventing it from activating genes related to apoptosis. (d) The YY-1–p53/Hdm2 interaction involves YY-1 binding to both Hdm2 and p53, which speeds up the process of p53 being marked for degradation. This interaction doesn't have a checkpoint function and allows YY-1's oncogenic activity to continue [1, 12].

expression of specific genes that are engaged in driving the formation of certain kinds of human tumors. Researchers are still actively studying mutant p53 and how it interacts with other proteins and transcription factors. Scientists are working to uncover the precise mechanisms by which these interactions occur and how they contribute to the development and progression of cancer [37]. Mutant p53 in cancer cells hampers the expression of important downstream targets like PUMA and p21, which leads to resistance to chemotherapy in colon cancer cells. Unlike the normal p53, mutant p53 fails to bind to the promoter of PUMA and activate its transcription [32, 34]. In epithelial ovarian cancer, mutant p53 has varied effects, promoting invasion, and metastasis, and reducing the activity of TP53 [7]. In mice studies, mutant p53 has been found to regulate ovarian cancer progression, differentiation, and response to steroid hormones. In pancreatic ductal adenocarcinoma (PDAC), mutant p53 collaborates with oncogenic KRAS effectors to overactivate transcriptional networks that promote metastasis. The p53-R175H mutation, commonly found in various cancers, has gain-of-function properties that contribute to cancer development [37]. Therapeutic approaches for p53-R175H include reactivating it with small molecules, promoting its degradation, and developing immunotherapies. TP53 missense mutations result in a mutant p53 protein that lacks tumor-suppressing abilities and accumulates at high levels in cells [5]. This mutant protein demonstrates pro-oncogenic activities, such as heightened pro-growth signaling and facilitation of metastasis [9, 38]. Mutant p53 also interacts with several transcription factors, including p63, p73, Spl, Smad2, Smad3, NF-Y, E2F1, Etsl, Ets-2, and Medl of the Mediator complex. Scientists think that these interactions play a role in controlling the transcription of many genes, which contributes to the gain-of-function effects of mutant p53 [38]. When we dive a bit deeper into the world of mutant p53, we get to know it's a protein that plays a crucial role in regulating various genes and signaling pathways within our cells [12]. When the p53 gene gets mutated, it can lead to the production of a faulty or altered version of the p53 protein, known as mutant p53. Now, this mutant p53 protein can have some interesting effects on gene expression. It can directly impact the expression of different genes, including ABCB1 (also known as MDR), GRO1 chemokine, ID2 and ID4 transcription regulators, and hsMAD1 protein, among others. These genes participate in a wide range of cellular activities, including developing resistance to drugs, promoting cell growth, and facilitating cell differentiation. Mutant p53 can also influence signaling pathways by stimulating the expression of certain receptor tyrosine kinases. These include EGFR (epidermal growth factor receptor), IGF1R (insulin-like growth factor 1 receptor), Axl, MET, PDGFRb (platelet-derived growth factor receptor beta), and VEGFR2 (vascular endothelial growth factor receptor 2) [39]. These receptors are involved in cell division, viability, and vascularization, which is the formation of new blood vessels. Interestingly, mutant p53 can even enhance the recycling of receptors like EGFR and MET through a protein called Rab coupling protein. This amplifies their signaling and can further contribute to the dedifferentiation of tumor cells, which is when they become less specialized and more aggressive [39]. So, in a nutshell, mutant p53 might have an important effect on gene expression as well as signaling pathways within our cells. These changes might add to the formation and advancement of tumors [38]. It's truly fascinating how molecular alterations like mutant p53 can influence our health and the behavior of our cells.

These discoveries, combined with the observation that mutant p53 does not attach to the p53 response element, could potentially clarify the reason why wild-type p53 and mutant p53 produce distinct impacts on gene expression, despite their shared interaction with certain TFs. Mutant p53 may also result in opposite results in gene expression, despite interacting with coactivators that also work with wild-type p53, like p300 [38]. For example, when mutant p53 is present on loci that wild-type p53 normally switches on, such as p21, GADD45, PERP, and PTEN, it suppresses their expression [9, 39]. It's not immediately clear why wild-type p53 and mutant p53 result in opposite gene expression results, even though they are associated with the same factors and coactivators. A reason could be that when wild-type p53 is overexpressed or activated, it still prefers to bind to its response element, whereas mutant p53 is directed to distinct gene promoters (or different parts of the promoter for wild-type p53-regulated genes), resulting in gene dysregulation. Mutant p53 probably controls gene expression by using a mix of TFs to kickstart gene activation at the TF's position, since the TF is already bound to DNA. Coactivators brought in by the TF or mutant p53 then boost gene expression. However, it's not clear how much mutant p53 relies on specific TFs or other chromatin modifiers to activate target genes. This might depend on the particular p53 mutation and the active signaling pathways in the cell that determine which TFs are active. It's also possible that after being recruited by a TF or chromatin modifier, mutant p53 brings in more factors that stimulate the role of the starting recruiting factor. There might be other mechanisms at play too, but a lot of study still needs to be done [36, 38].

Mutant p53 and SWI/SNF work together to either decrease or increase gene transcription in about half of the mutant p53 target genes [39]. Since mutant p53 and wild-type p53 have opposite impacts on their associates, it's possible that mutant p53 disrupts the normal functions of SWI/SNF that wild-type p53 needs for transcription. This could happen by impacting its role, interactions with other proteins, or how it's positioned on chromosomes. Mutant p53 is thought to enable changes in gene expression, and its interaction with SWI/SNF, a chromatin-remodeling complex found throughout the genome, might explain how mutant p53 can affect gene expression at multiple places. Nucleosome positioning, which affects access to DNA-binding proteins, is important for gene regulation. So, mutant p53's interaction with SWI/SNF could either activate or repress gene transcription [39]. It's important to note that we don't fully understand how mutant p53 interacts with transcription factors and coactivators, but these interactions likely have a great effect on the gain-of-function effects of mutant p53. To better understand these effects, we need to figure out how mutant p53 interacts with transcription factors, coactivators, and other chromatin regulators [38].

We also need to identify new coactivators and corepressors that could explain the transcriptional changes caused by mutant p53. If factors that are necessary for mutant p53 to activate genes, like a new coactivator, are found, potential drugs that specifically target the mutant p53-coactivator complex can be developed.

7.4 EXPLORING DNA TOPOLOGY-DRIVEN INTERACTIONS

The interaction between mutated p53 and DNA is mostly influenced by the structure of the DNA rather than specific sequences. Mutated p53 proteins have a strong affinity for MAR elements, which are important for organizing chromatin, enhancing gene function, and maintaining chromatin modifications [9, 35]. Interestingly, the binding of mutp53 to MAR elements doesn't rely on specific consensus motifs, but rather on the length of the DNA. In contrast, the normal p53 protein has the ability to interact with DNA in various ways. It can bind to DNA in a specific sequence or a non-specific manner. Non-specific interactions include attaching to double-stranded or single-stranded DNA, secondary DNA structures, and abnormal DNA sites [2]. Mutp53 proteins have a preference for attaching to DNA structures that are not straight. This is why they strongly bind to MAR elements. Unlike the normal p53, the DNA binding specificity of mutp53 is determined only by the shape of the DNA. When there are mutations in the core domain of mutp53, it affects its ability to recognize specific DNA sequences [9].

7.5 UNLOCKING MUTp53: THE COLLABORATIVE ROLE OF TRANSCRIPTION FACTORS IN BINDING

It's really fascinating to see that most studies on p53 mutations have focused on specific "hot-spot" mutations, like R248, R273, R175, and R249 [7, 35]. These mutations have different effects on p53's ability to bind to DNA. Some mutations, like R175 and R249, completely lose their DNA binding ability, while others, like R282, G245, and Y220, may still retain partial DNA binding abilities [7, 9]. Interestingly, the interaction between mutated p53 and the intermediary TFs doesn't depend on the specific mutation type. These interactions can regulate various pathways, such as upregulating genes involved in G2-M transition, modifying chromatin, signaling through growth factors like EGFR, stimulating glycoprotein folding, reducing apoptosis in breast cancer cells, and promoting neo-angiogenesis in tumor cells. What's cool is that the same TFs that bind to mutated p53 associate with wild-type p53 too, but the outcomes of these interactions can be different and sometimes even opposite. This is because different cofactors are recruited when transcription is carried out by either wild-type p53 or mutated p53 from the same promoter. This has been observed in the interaction between p53 and the transcription factor NF-Y [7]. When there's damage in DNA, the mutp53/NF-Y complex brings in a histone acetyltransferase called p300, while the WTp53/NF-Y complex recruits a histone deacetylase. First, this leads to abnormal control of the cell cycle and then it ensures the appropriate cell-cycle checkpoint. In case of no DNA damage, a contrary scenario is observed. It was once thought that WTp53 controlled genes involved in the cell cycle without physically attaching to DNA. Rather, the DNA's unique binding site is where the partner TF makes contact with it. This shows that WTp53 functions independently of its own DNA binding as a repressor of target genes, acting through intermediate transcription factors such as NFY. However, since certain genes that are listed as repressed are active or because WTp53 does not bind to their promoters, it's possible that this is not a universal mechanism for transcriptional repression by WTp53. Alternatively, it is also possible that both proteins in the WTp53/TF complex interact with DNA at adjacent specific locations. The DNA connections to p53 are broken in the instance of mutp53. WTp53 and at least one other generic TF need to share particular areas in the same promoter area for this to function. For NF-Y, E2F1, and SP1, this appears to be the case. It has been demonstrated that certain TFs present in mutp53/TF complexes on GOF binding sites may bend the DNA helix when creating particular complexes, including SP1, NF-Y, Ets, and E2F [7]. Thus, the complex including WTp53 may possess a bent DNA structure that allows for the accommodation of both WTp53 and the second TF. They both establish contact with their respective zones in this complex. When p53 is mutated, the normal p53 response element (RE) becomes ineffective in stabilizing mutp53–TF complexes. Instead, the accumulation of mutp53 can lead to its binding to promoters that specifically interact with the second TF and are not bound by normal p53 at normal expression levels. Because p53-interacting TFs are universal transcription factors that bind to many promoters, mutp53 GOF can influence a wide variety of genes [40]. It is yet unclear, though, if this mechanism is unique to mutp53 and what prerequisites must be met for actual GOF effects. This process could only apply to mutp53 proteins that have lost their capacity to bind DNA, according to certain theories. Although in diverse ways, mutp53 proteins with limited DNA binding capacity can nonetheless display GOF activity. For instance, it's thought that the partially DNA-binding R282W mutant interacts with other TFs to behave in a GOF manner [40]. Additionally, mutp53 can bind to non-B-DNA structures, similar to normal p53, but through its non-mutated C-terminal domain (CTD) instead of sequence-specific binding. One example of deleterious GOF effects through structure-specific interactions is the association of mutp53 with MAR/SAR DNA elements, which are attached to the nuclear matrix.

For example, p53R273H, a particular p53 mutation, is coupled to recurrent intergenic DNA sequences in U251 human glioma cells [41]. These components give DNA its non-B structure and serve as binding sites for regulatory proteins that can detect the conformation of DNA. It was demonstrated that the expression of two genes, PPARGC1A and FRMD5, was mutp53-dependent, suggesting that these structure-specific interactions may have an impact on gene expression [35, 41]. A tiling array of genes that were thought to be mutp53 target genes was used in another research, and the results showed that most mutp53 binding areas matched with CpG islands at transcription start sites. Around 20 bp long, the binding motif was rich in G nucleobases, which can occur in non-B-DNA conformations, especially as G4-quadruplexes. Both the normal p53 and mutated p53 (R273H, R248W, and G245S) were found to bind the intramolecular quadruplex structure in vitro, with the mutants forming higher molecular weight complexes [9]. It was ruled out that the SP1 and Ets-1 transcription factors were involved in producing complexes with mutp53 on the G, C-rich regions [7, 41].

The presence of certain double-stranded DNA binding sites that exclusively bind to mutant p53 and not to wild-type p53 is not well supported by the available data. In one investigation, the K120R mutant was specifically bound and transactivated at the TNFAIP8 locus; however, the binding site that was found matched a conventional p53 binding site, casting doubt on the site's specificity to mutant p53. Another option is that the K120R–DNA complex contains unique protein–protein interactions not seen in the WTp53–DNA complex, or the two species differ in their patterns of acetylation at the K120 residue, which may have an impact on the affinity of DNA binding. Additionally,

TABLE 7.1
Genes Activated by Mutp53 and the Associated Cancerous Phenotype

Gene Activated	Resultant Cancerous Phenotype
MDR-1	Chemoresistance of cancer cells
IGF-I-R	Blocks cell death
IGF-II P3/P4	Blocks cell death
BAG-1	Blocks cell death
Hsp70	Protein chaperone inhibiting apoptosis
c-myc	Enhances cell division
c-fos	Enhances cell division
PCNA	Enhances cell division
EGF-R	Vascularization

Source: Kim and Deppert [35].

the study found that mutant p53 can indirectly bind to certain gene promoters through the Ets-2 transcription factor, activating genes involved in chromatin remodeling and histone modification [41]. This leads to an overall increase in the expression of genes throughout the genome, which is reported to promote the development of tumors. Another way that mutant p53 can have an impact is by displacing nucleosomes. For example, at the VEGFR2 promoter, mutant p53 recruits SWI/SNF, which then brings in other transcription factors and chromatin modifiers. Together, they remodel the promoter region and create an environment that allows for the activation of VEGFR2 gene transcription. Same chromatin remodeling events involving SWI/SNF, facilitated by mutant p53 binding nearby, have been observed at many other gene promoters. SWI/SNF proteins are known to have tumor suppressor functions in certain contexts, but mutant p53 may interfere with these functions, resulting in genetic instability [41]. By targeting mutant p53, we may be able to restore the tumor suppressor capabilities of SWI/SNF proteins, offering a potential cancer therapy specifically for p53 hot-spot mutants.

Mutations in the p53 protein, particularly in its DNA-binding domain, are a strong indication of cancer and can impact how the protein interacts with our genetic material. For instance, certain alterations in the β-sandwich region of the DNA-binding domain have been demonstrated to diminish p53's capacity to bind to DNA and make the DNA-binding groove less stable. It's pretty remarkable how these variations can affect the protein's functionality [41]. These mutations can disturb the interactions between p53 and DNA, causing problems with the stability of the genome and influencing the development of cancer. Additionally, mutations in specific positions where p53 contacts DNA, like R273, have been found to have different stability and aggregation patterns, which could play a role in how cancer develops in the body.

7.6 MUTANT p53: A DISRUPTED DIALOGUE WITH DNA REPAIR ENZYMES

p53 plays a significant role in coordinating the body's response to DNA damage. It helps with things like repairing the DNA, stopping the cell cycle to give the repair mechanisms time to work, and even triggering cell death if needed. It acts as a tumor suppressor, that is it assists in preventing the development of cancer by promoting repair of DNA and establishes genome stability. p53 also has a role in repairing DNA damage caused by UV radiation by relaxing the chromatin structure and initiating the repair process. It interacts with different DNA repair systems and influences the activity of factors involved in DNA repair. Additionally, p53 interacts with proteins and kinases such as CHK1, CHK2, ATM, and DNA-PK to regulate the DNA repair process [42]. Lastly, p53's involvement in the p53 network's oscillations after DNA damage highlights its role in controlling the repair process.

When DNA damage occurs and there are problems with DNA repair, it can mess up the integrity of our genes. This, along with issues in maintaining telomeres (the protective caps on our chromosomes), is a big deal in the growth of different kinds of solid cancers. The TP53 gene, which is super important for regulating how cells respond to damage, can be affected by changes called somatic mutations. These mutations in TP53 have a major impact on how our cells handle DNA damage. The specific mutations in TP53 can also affect the ability of cells to repair DNA, which then influences the risk of developing cancer, how the cancer progresses, and even how it responds to treatment. It's also worth noting that the engagements between DNA repair, telomere maintenance, and the mutational status of TP53 have important implications for colorectal cancer, including how it starts, progresses, and how it might behave in the long run [42, 43]. So, when it comes to cancer, there are a bunch of things that can go wrong in our cells. One important player in all of this is a gene called p53. It's like the superhero of our cells, keeping an eye on things and making sure everything is in order. When our DNA can get damaged sometimes, p53 comes to the rescue! It's part of a system called the DNA damage response, which helps detect and repair any damage to our DNA. It's like a repair crew for our genetic material. But here's the thing: if p53 isn't working properly, it can lead to trouble. Mutations in the p53 gene can mess up the DNA damage response, making it harder for our cells to fix any problems. And when our cells can't fix the damage, it can increase the risk of cancer.

Now, telomeres, which are like the protective caps at the ends of our chromosomes, play a role in keeping our DNA stable and preventing it from getting damaged, and p53 is involved in telomere homeostasis too [40]. So, when we talk about the interactions between DNA repair, telomere homeostasis, and p53 mutations, we're looking at how all these factors come together and affect the development and progression of cancer. It's a complex puzzle, but understanding it can help us find new ways to fight this disease. Our cells have these amazing mechanisms called DNA repair machinery that can fix different types of DNA damage caused by both internal and external factors and p53 is involved in many of these repair processes.

There's this repair process called nucleotide excision repair (NER) that helps get rid of those helix-distorting issues caused by UV radiation. And then there's another repair mechanism called base excision repair (BER) that specifically targets and fixes oxidative changes to the DNA bases [38]. Mismatch repair (MMR) is another process that scans for errors in replicated DNA and fixes them. When it comes to more severe damage like DNA double-strand breaks (DSBs) caused by things such as ionizing radiation (IR), our cells have two main ways to repair them. Non-homologous end joining (NHEJ) and homologous recombination (HR) are the two pathways involved in fixing DSBs [40]. Further, RecQ helicases, play important roles in maintaining genome stability during recombination repair and replication [38, 44]. It's incredible how our cells have all these intricate mechanisms to keep our DNA in check and prevent cancer. And p53 plays an important role in coordinating repair processes. It's like the conductor of an orchestra, making sure everything runs smoothly.

7.6.1 p53 in Nucleotide Excision Repair

p53 has been connected to fixing DNA damage caused by UV rays for over 20 years! It seems like p53 plays multiple roles in this process, both by controlling gene activity (transactivation and transrepression) and by doing other things not directly related to gene control. Studies have shown that p53 can attach to DNA in different ways, depending on the DNA sequence, which suggests that it might recognize certain structures associated with DNA damage. One early study showed how p53 is linked to NER. They discovered that human cells with impaired p53 didn't do as well and had lower survival rates after being exposed to UV radiation [45]. Additionally, they demonstrated that UV-induced DNA damage could not be tolerated by extracts from these p53-defective cells. This work set the stage for further investigation into the roles of p53 in NER, even if it was unable to ascertain whether p53 directly contributed to UV resistance or whether other p53-associated variables were also involved. Subsequent research appears to have further limited the function of p53 in the NER pathway in UV-induced DNA damage repair. Studies have shown that whereas p53 is less important for transcription-coupled NER (TC-NER), it is critical for controlling the global genome NER (GG-NER) [38]. In one of the studies, the functions of p53 in fibroblasts from individuals with Li–Fraumeni syndrome who had either one or two copies of the p53 gene were reported. It was found that fibroblasts with two copies of the mutated p53 gene, which had lost the normal p53 allele during culturing, had a defect in removing cyclobutene pyrimidine dimers (CPDs) from the entire genomic DNA compared to fibroblasts with one copy of the mutated p53 gene. This implied that GG-NER was lost. Furthermore, it was established that p53 participates in DNA polymerases δ and ε-mediated repair, which are significant enzymes in the NER pathway. This suggests that p53 is essential for repairing UV-induced damage to DNA. p53 affects UV-induced DNA damage repair more broadly [45]. Furthermore, a noteworthy finding between p53 and NER was found. The capacity of p53 to directly interact with XPC, XBP, and CSB, among other NER pathway components, has been shown [38, 45]. This interaction suggests that p53 has a crucial role in coordinating and regulating the NER process.

All things considered, these investigations have shed important light on the complex interaction between p53 and NER, particularly as it relates to UV-induced DNA damage repair. How these discoveries advance our knowledge of the systems that protect the integrity of our DNA is very interesting. While p53's significance in the GG-NER pathway has usually been verified by consistent studies, its involvement in TC-NER is primarily the subject of dispute [38]. It has been noted that p53 loss decreases TC-NER following exposure to broad-spectrum UV light (290–324 nm), but not following narrow-band UV radiation (254 nm) [38]. This observation suggests that p53 may have a more specific role in TC-NER when exposed to certain types of UV radiation. It's interesting to note that the spectrum of light from the sun that reaches Earth virtually completely lacks UV at 254 nm. This suggests that since p53 is triggered by the broad-spectrum UV radiation seen in sunshine; it is probably implicated in the response to natural damage in both the transcribed and non-transcribed DNA strands [45]. Considering the different types of UV sources and their effects on p53's involvement in GG-NER and TC-NER can help explain the discrepancies in the research findings. It highlights the complexity of studying DNA repair mechanisms and the need for further investigation to fully understand the role of p53 in UV-induced damage repair.

The early studies did establish that p53 plays a role in the NER pathway, but they didn't provide much insight into the specific mechanisms by which p53 is involved in DNA repair. It appears that p53 acts through both its transactivation activity and its direct involvement in DNA-associated transactions during repair. While its role as a transcriptional regulator in NER seems limited, p53 does have known regulatory targets, such as the genes encoding the DDB2 protein (p48) and the XPC protein (XPC) [45]. DDB2 forms a complex with DDB1 to create the UV-DDB heterodimer, which binds to specific types of DNA damage to help recruit XPC during the early stages of NER [46]. When DNA damage occurs due to UV exposure, activated p53 induces the expression of p48 and XPC, thereby enhancing the cell's ability to locate and target the damaged DNA for repair [45]. There are a couple of observations that support the requirement of p53's transactivation activity in regulating NER. First, the presence of endogenous DDB2 in p53-deficient cells improves the efficiency of GG-NER [46]. Second, while XPC and DDB2 are recruited to sites of DNA damage, p53 is not. NER is a vital mechanism that cells use to fix DNA damage caused by various factors like UV radiation or certain chemicals. It involves a series of steps to identify and remove the damaged DNA segment and replace it with a new, undamaged sequence. Now, p53 is well-known for its role as a transcriptional activator, meaning it helps regulate gene expression by promoting the production of specific proteins. However, it turns out that p53 also has other functions in NER that are not directly related to its transcriptional activity. One of these functions is the modulation of helicase activities. Helicases are enzymes that unwind the DNA double helix during DNA repair processes. In NER, the TFIIH protein complex plays a crucial role by locally relaxing the DNA, allowing other repair proteins to access and fix the damaged site. XPB and XPD are subunits of TFIIH that possess helicase activity. Studies have shown that p53 can interact with XPB and XPD, leading to a decrease in their helicase activity [45, 47]. This interaction suggests that p53 can regulate the unwinding of DNA during NER, potentially influencing the efficiency and accuracy of the repair process [47].

Additionally, p53 can also modulate chromatin accessibility. Chromatin refers to the complex structure of DNA and proteins in the nucleus. By altering the accessibility of the DNA within the chromatin, p53 can affect how easily DNA lesions, or damaged areas, can be recognized and repaired by the NER machinery. These transcription-independent functions of p53 in NER provide additional layers of regulation and coordination to ensure effective DNA repair. Understanding these mechanisms helps us appreciate the intricate ways in which cells maintain genomic integrity and protect against potential mutations. The chromatin relaxation function of p53 is indeed associated with TFIIH during NER in both space and time [45]. When a DNA lesion is recognized by the TC-NER branch, the chromatin throughout the genome is relaxed. This global relaxation is thought to enhance the detection of lesions across the entire genome.

Researchers have hypothesized that this global relaxation facilitated by p53 leads to improved lesion detection. They proposed that p53 recruits the p300 histone acetylase to the damaged sites. The p300 histone acetylase then acetylates the histone H3 subunit, which helps in making the DNA more accessible for repair. By increasing lesion detection across the entire genome, p53 may contribute to maintaining genome stability and preventing the accumulation of mutations. Moreover, p53 has another function in regulating NER during chronic exposure to aflatoxin B1 (AFB1), a potent genotoxin [45]. In mice with normal p53 levels, when they were exposed to AFB1 through their diet, there was an increase in NER activity as measured by an in vitro assay. However, this upregulation of NER was not observed in mice with reduced levels of p53. Interestingly, this effect was independent of the levels of the NER proteins XPA and XPB. The exact mechanism behind this regulation is still unknown and requires further investigation.

7.6.2 p53 in Base Excision Repair

Just like in NER, p53 has roles in both transcription-dependent and transcription-independent processes in BER. In BER, AP endonucleases are key players that step in after DNA glycosylases (like OGG1) remove damaged bases and help repair the resulting AP sites. It's interesting to note that there are connections between AP endonucleases and p53. Early studies found an interaction between the dual-function AP endonuclease APE1/Ref-1 and p53 [38, 48]. Researchers observed that APE1/Ref-1 can regulate p53 through redox-dependent and redox-independent pathways [48]. Subsequent research revealed that Ref-1 improves p53's in vitro DNA binding capacity, and this modulation has consequences in vivo as well. APE1/Ref-1 can control the transactivation and pro-apoptotic properties of p53 through these interactions. According to research, p53 tetramerization is facilitated by APE1/Ref-1 and is essential for the protein's correct operation. It's interesting to note that APE1/Ref-1 was shown to have a redox-dependent mechanism for modulating the DNA-binding activity of mutant p53 [38]. These findings highlight the intricate and dynamic nature of p53's involvement in DNA repair pathways like BER. It's fascinating how these interactions contribute to the regulation of p53's functions and its impact on cellular processes. There appear to be even more levels in the relationship between p53 and APE1/Ref-1. Moreover, it was shown that p53 may be activated by selenomethionine (SeMet) in a Ref-1-dependent manner [48]. It's interesting to note the relationship between the dietary mineral selenium and the control of DNA repair. In actuality, selenomethionine demonstrated some ionizing radiation protection. Researchers have extensively studied the effects of selenomethionine on p53 and BER because it can stimulate p53's genome protective functions without causing genotoxic effects [49]. This suggests that selenomethionine could be used as a chemotherapeutic agent. It's amazing how a dietary nutrient can have such an impact on DNA repair and p53 activation. Furthermore, it appears that p53 directly inhibits the APE1 gene's transcription. At first, this function of p53 could appear paradoxical. When cells encounter DNA damage, why would they inhibit a gene that repairs damaged DNA? On the other hand, this function could support p53's tumor suppressor role. In order to assist in removing severely damaged genomes, p53 can drive the DNA damage response toward apoptosis by downregulating DNA repair activities.

BER is a crucial DNA repair pathway that fixes damaged bases in DNA. The question was whether p53, a well-known tumor suppressor protein, could also regulate BER. A variant of p53 called p53-22-23, which lacks transactivation ability, was more proficient in regulating BER than the wild-type p53. This finding suggested that p53's role in BER is not solely dependent on its ability to regulate gene expression. Instead, it appears that p53 has a transcription-independent function in BER, that could give a better immediate reaction to DNA damage. Subsequent research examined the impact of DNA damage severity on the p53–BER pathway. A dose-dependent connection was found, indicating that p53's control over BER activity was influenced by the degree of DNA damage. When DNA-damaging treatments such as γ-irradiation or cisplatin were used at modest dosages, BER activity increased right away. This suggests that p53 enhances BER as a response to mild DNA damage, potentially helping to repair the DNA before it accumulates further damage. However, at higher doses of DNA damage, the researchers observed a reduction in BER activity and an induction of p53-dependent apoptosis. This indicates that p53, in this context, promotes cell death (apoptosis) instead of repairing the damaged DNA. Additionally, the researchers found that p53's role in BER is dependent on the cell cycle stage. During the G0–G1 stages of the cell cycle (when cells are not actively dividing), p53 enhances BER activity [45]. In contrast, during the G2–M stages (when cells are preparing to divide), p53 reduces BER activity and promotes apoptosis.

All things considered, our results imply that p53 regulates BER activity during the cell cycle, enhancing repair during non-dividing stages and promoting cell death during dividing stages. This dynamic regulation by p53 helps maintain genome stability and prevents the propagation of DNA damage. An essential component of the BER pathway, 3-methyladenine (3-MeAde) DNA glycosylase, has its activity controlled by p53 as well. The activity of 3-MeAde rises as predicted in the presence of nitric oxide therapy. But as a transcriptional regulator, wild-type p53 inhibits this rise by suppressing the glycosylase mRNA. This indicates that p53 regulates gene expression to control the amount of the enzyme produced. Interestingly, the study found that the activity of the AP endonuclease protein, another component of BER, was not affected by p53 under these conditions. This suggests that p53 specifically targets the glycosylase enzyme without altering the overall activity of the repair pathway. Without p53, the increased glycosylase activity could result in a greater number of AP sites (abasic sites) in DNA. However, if there isn't a corresponding increase in AP endonuclease activity to repair these sites, it could result in genome instability and weakened DNA repair. These findings highlight the important role of p53 in maintaining the balance of the BER pathway and limiting the mutagenic effects of certain genotoxins. Besides regulating the glycosylase mRNA, p53 controls the expression of two other BER genes at the transcriptional level: OGG1 (8-oxo guanine glycosylase) and MUTYH (adenine DNA glycosylase). The interaction between p53 and MUTYH is especially fascinating because MUTYH has been the focus of research nowadays due to its connection to hereditary colorectal cancer [45]. This suggests that p53 might play an important role in maintaining genomic stability and preventing cancer. It's incredible how p53, as a transcriptional regulator, can have such a broad impact on the BER pathway and potentially influence the development of diseases like colorectal cancer. After exposure to cadmium, p53 has an impact on BER by regulating the expression of OGG1 and APE1. Interestingly, p53 directly regulates the expression of APE1, but its effect on OGG1 seems to be indirect [44, 45].

Another intriguing finding is the relationship between p53 and chronic exposure to low doses of AFB1. It was discovered that in p53-proficient mouse livers, BER activity was decreased, while in p53-heterozygous knockouts, it remained unchanged. The information provided by the same group about p53's control of NER following exposure to AFB1 is completely different from this [38, 45]. These studies highlight the complex and multifaceted role of p53 in response to different carcinogen exposures. It's fascinating how p53 can exhibit different effects on different components of DNA repair pathways depending on the specific circumstances. It seems that p53 can indeed be directly involved at repair sites. There have been studies showing direct interactions between p53 and several BER components, both proteins and DNA. Wild-type p53 has been shown to enhance the activity of OGG1, a key enzyme in BER, both in laboratory experiments and in living organisms. When cells were exposed to ROS, which can cause DNA damage, cells with wild-type p53 were able to remove the resulting lesions (specifically, 8-oxoG) from the DNA more quickly compared to cells lacking functional p53. As p53 linked to DNA with OGG1 and AP endonuclease, there was an improvement in DNA repair [45]. It was proposed that p53 may increase the joint activity of OGG1 and AP endonuclease, improving the efficiency of repairing DNA damage brought on by ROS. It appears that p53 is involved in BER in more ways than merely upregulating OGG1 and AP endonuclease activity. Zhou et al.'s work indicates that p53 may also induce BER by direct interaction with DNA polymerase β (DNA pol β), the primary DNA polymerase that causes short patch BER [45, 49].

The investigation demonstrated that p53-induced BER stimulation was seen in both live things and lab settings. The degree of BER activation was linked with the p53 level. Even more intriguing is the fact that this impact required direct p53 interaction with DNA pol β. Mutant p53 variants were unable to activate BER because they were unable to bind with DNA pol β. The possibility that the stability of the polymerase is influenced by the interaction between p53 and DNA pol β is one explanation for this phenomenon. DNA pol β levels were markedly reduced in p53-deficient cells. Therefore, by keeping DNA pol β stable, the direct connection between p53 and DNA pol β may be essential for maintaining appropriate BER function.

7.6.3 p53 in Mismatch Repair

The relationships between p53 and DNA MMR, one of the three conventional DNA repair pathways, have not been as well investigated as those between the protein and the other routes. That does not imply, however, that these interactions are not significant. MSH2, the central component of MMR, appears to be at the center of the link between p53 and MMR. Not to be overlooked is the fact that MSH2 is somewhat involved in other DNA repair pathways as well, such as BER, HR, and NER. So, any p53-dependent effects on MSH2 may also have implications for these other repair pathways [45]. It's fascinating how interconnected these DNA repair mechanisms are and how p53's influence can potentially extend beyond MMR. The more we learn about these intricate interactions, the better we can understand the complex network of DNA repair and its regulation.

In research, it was shown that in mice lacking the p53 and MSH2 genes, the females were arrested as embryos and, while the males lived, they rapidly developed tumors in comparison to the animals with a single mutation. This implies that p53 and MMR have a synergistic role that is essential for the development of embryos and the suppression of tumors. Furthermore, it was shown that MMR and p53 can work together to control a colon cancer cell line that lacks MMR in terms of how sensitive the cell is to the genotoxic chemical cisplatin. This highlights the intricate relationship between MMR and p53 in modulating the response to DNA damage. These studies provide valuable insights into the cross-talk between p53 and MMR, shedding light on their combined roles in development, tumor suppression, and response to genotoxic stress. It's interesting to note how, following DNA damage, the MMR proteins hMutL and PMS1/2 are stabilized by the DNA damage response checkpoint protein ATM, which increases p53 activation. Interestingly, the MSH2–MSH6 complex can improve p53 binding to DNA substrates with topological abnormalities, at least in vitro [38, 50]. This seems to depend on the phosphorylation state of p53. This suggests that there may be a connection between MMR and p53 in dealing with DNA damage and maintaining genomic stability. Furthermore, there are indications that p53 and MSH2 can colocalize to early recombination intermediates, suggesting that p53 may be involved in recombination through a non-MMR function of MSH2. Additionally, recent studies reported that p53 signaling is suppressed in MSH2-deficient cells, and MUTS3 has been found to play a significant role in p53-dependent tumor formation [50].

These findings highlight the intricate relationship between p53 and MMR, as well as their involvement in DNA damage response, recombination, and tumorigenesis. It's truly remarkable how interconnected these processes are. It seems that the transcriptional function of p53 can also play a role in regulating MMR. It's interesting to know that p53, along with the transcription factor c-Jun, can interact with motifs in the promoter region of hMSH2 [45]. This binding leads to an upregulation of hMSH2 after UV exposure. This suggests that p53 may have a direct impact on the expression of MMR genes. The literature has a wealth of clinically significant associations between p53 and MMR. However, in many cases, the exact mechanisms behind these observations are still not fully understood. It's an area that requires further research and exploration to uncover the intricacies of the relationship between MMR and p53.

7.6.4 p53 in DNA Double-Strand Break Repair and Recombination

There are two primary methods for repairing DNA DSBs: HR and NHEJ. Depending on where the cell cycle is, one can choose between different paths [45, 51]. Although it is active at all stages of the cell cycle, NHEJ is especially significant during the G1 phase. It involves directly joining the broken ends of DNA, which can sometimes lead to inaccuracies and genomic instability. However, it's worth noting that opinions on the accuracy of NHEJ repair are evolving. On the other hand, HR is most active during the late S phase and G2 phase. It utilizes a homologous DNA template to accurately repair DSBs. HR-dependent repair is generally considered to be error-free and helps maintain genomic stability [45].

In each of these pathways, p53 plays diverse roles. It can regulate the choice between NHEJ and HR repair mechanisms based on the cell cycle stage and the severity of DNA damage. An additional level of control is provided by p53's ability to affect the expression of genes related to cell cycle arrest and DNA repair.

7.6.5 p53 in Non-Homologous End Joining

It seems that under certain conditions, the functions of p53 can intersect with NHEJ, but the biological outcome appears to be linked to apoptosis, which is programmed cell death. For instance, in mice that lack NHEJ due to defects in XRCC4 and DNA ligase IV, DNA DSBs are not repaired, leading to activation of p53-dependent apoptosis and ultimately embryonic lethality [40]. In this context, the loss of p53 can rescue the embryonic lethality, but it may come at the cost of genome stability. It's a delicate balance between the protective role of p53 in preventing damaged cells from proliferating and the potential consequences of impaired DNA repair. The intricate relationship between p53, NHEJ, and apoptosis highlights the complexity of cellular processes and the interconnectedness of different pathways. It's been reported that mice deficient in both p53 and NHEJ can develop various pathologies, including progenitor B-cell lymphomas. However, the work from Fred Alt's group sheds light on the role of the Artemis endonuclease in suppressing the development of these lymphomas in cooperation with p53. Artemis not only has a DNA repair function within the NHEJ pathway but also plays a role in p53 regulation independently of DNA repair. When Artemis is depleted in U2-OS cells, p53 accumulates, leading to cell cycle arrest and apoptosis [45]. This suggests that a component of NHEJ, such as Artemis, can also have a regulatory effect on p53. The intricate interplay between NHEJ, p53, and Artemis highlights the complexity of these cellular processes and how they can influence each other. It seems that there are several connections between p53 and the repair of DSBs through NHEJ, although some of these connections may be more circumstantial. For example, in one study, it was found that wild-type p53 inhibited NHEJ that utilized microhomologies near the cut site. In the second study, pharmacological inhibition of p53 using pifithrin-α had little effect on overall end joining, but it did diminish high-fidelity end joining. This suggests that p53 may have another important function in protecting the genome by minimizing genome instability caused by low-fidelity NHEJ. These findings highlight the multifaceted role of p53 in maintaining genome stability and its potential involvement in different aspects of DSB repair. It's fascinating to see how p53 can influence NHEJ and contribute to the overall integrity of the genome. The roles of p53 in NHEJ are still not fully understood. It's clear that p53 has genetic interactions with components of the NHEJ pathway, and these interactions have downstream effects on cellular survival, cell-cycle control, and DNA repair. However, the specific molecular mechanisms of these interactions are still poorly understood or not understood at all. It can be challenging to unravel the intricate details of these molecular interactions and pathways. Scientists are continually studying and researching to gain a better understanding of how p53 influences NHEJ and its impact on cellular processes. As more research is conducted, hopefully, more about the molecular mechanisms behind these interactions will be uncovered.

7.6.6 p53 in Homologous Recombination

The roles of p53 in HR are indeed clearer compared to its roles in NHEJ. Studies have shown that p53 has both transactivation-dependent and transactivation-independent functions in regulating HR, separate from its functions in cell-cycle checkpoint control. Interestingly, most of the roles of p53 in HR are independent of its transcriptional activity [52]. However, some studies have revealed potential transactivation functions for p53 in the regulation of HR, which could turn out to be important. These findings suggest that p53 has multifaceted roles in maintaining genome stability and influencing different aspects of DNA repair. It's fascinating to see how p53 can have diverse functions in HR, both dependent and independent of its transcriptional activity. Many experiments shed light on the role of p53 in the repair of I-SceI DSBs [40]. They found that p53 regulates HR-dependent repair of induced DSBs through its transactivation function. However, they also discovered that p53's role in HR repair of replication-associated DSBs is independent of its transactivation function [52].

It's fascinating to see how p53 can regulate DSB repair transcriptionally. Several studies have shown direct interactions between p53 and the Rad51 promoter, resulting in changes in RAD51 expression. Recent research confirmed that p53 can directly regulate RAD51, although its contribution was relatively small compared to other transcription factors. Additionally, the p53 isoform Δ133p53, which is expressed from an internal promoter in the p53 gene, has been shown to upregulate several DNA repair genes, including RAD51 [45, 53]. These findings highlight the complexity of p53's involvement in DNA repair and the various mechanisms it employs to ensure genome stability. HR is a crucial process in DNA repair, where damaged DNA is repaired using an undamaged copy of the same DNA sequence as a template. p53, a tumor suppressor protein, plays a role in regulating HR by interacting with RAD51 and RAD54 proteins. One-way p53 modulates HR is by regulating the expression of Rad51. Rad51 is a key protein involved in the HR process [45]. When p53 is inhibited, either through mutation or other means, the frequency of both spontaneous and damage-induced HR between repetitive DNA sequences increases. This suggests that p53 normally acts to suppress HR in these contexts. A study conducted later confirmed the role of p53 in HR regulation by examining the interaction between p53 and RAD51. They overexpressed a mutant form of RAD51 that couldn't interact with p53. Interestingly, this overexpression resulted in a two- to threefold increase in HR, similar to what was observed when p53 was inhibited. This suggests that the interaction between p53 and RAD51 is important for suppressing HR and maintaining genome stability. Additionally, the study also found an interaction between p53 and RAD54, another protein involved in HR. This interaction occurs through the carboxy-terminal domain of p53. It is believed that p53's interaction with RAD54 further contributes to the inhibition of illegitimate recombination, providing an additional mechanism by which p53 can prevent genome instability. It's worth noting that the relationship between RAD51 and p53 is bidirectional. RAD51 can stimulate the 5′ to 3′ exonuclease activity of p53 during the production of strand transfer intermediates. This suggests that RAD51 and p53 can influence each other's functions in HR.

Overall, these findings highlight the intricate regulatory network involved in HR and the diverse ways in which p53 maintains genome stability. Understanding these interactions can provide valuable insights into the mechanisms of DNA repair and the role of p53 in preventing genomic instability and cancer development. One study found that even when the transactivation domain of p53 was deactivated, p53 could still regulate HR. This is quite interesting because it contradicts the earlier findings we discussed. Another important finding was that p53 can both repress and stimulate HR, depending on the specific sequence of the DNA involved. It was also discovered that interactions between p53 and DNA topoisomerase I could influence these effects. This highlights the complexity of p53's role in HR regulation. In a later study, it was demonstrated that p53 stimulates HR specifically in the ribosomal gene cluster repeat. They speculate that this function of p53 helps maintain the integrity of rDNA sequences, which are important for proper cell function. Overall, these studies suggest that p53 promotes genome stability through various mechanisms. It interacts with topoisomerase I, represses mutant genetic strand exchange, and promotes specific recombination events to safeguard the integrity of important DNA sequences [45]. It's amazing how p53 is involved in regulating replication-related recombination and the ATM/ATR checkpoint kinases. When there's replication stress caused by inhibitors or DNA cross-linking agents, p53 suppresses HR.

What's interesting is that this activity requires phosphorylation of p53 and a direct interaction with the ssDNA binding protein RPA. Further, it was clarified by showing that the anti-recombinogenic activity of p53 relies on its phosphorylation by ATR. This allows p53 to modulate the frequency of HR during the S phase replication stress checkpoint without affecting the cell's ability to use HR for repairing exogenously generated DSBs. In another study, it was found that the checkpoint components ATM, ATR, and DNA-dependent protein kinase (DNA-PK) can influence the physical interaction between p53 and RPA [54]. When DNA is damaged, p53 is phosphorylated by

DNA-PK, and RPA is phosphorylated by both ATM and ATR at specific sites. These phosphorylation events work together to disrupt the p53–RPA interaction, allowing both proteins to carry out their functions related to DNA damage. It's fascinating how this pathway also shows some crosstalk between p53's regulation of HR and another DNA repair pathway called NHEJ, as DNA-PK is involved in both.

7.7 p53 AND RECQ HELICASES

There are five DNA helicases in the RecQ helicase family in the human genome [55]. Each of these helicases performs a distinct recombination function that contributes significantly to the stability of the genome. It is known that deficiencies in three of these helicases—BLM, WRN, and RECQL4—cause heritable human illnesses such as Rothmund–Thomson syndrome, Werner syndrome, and Bloom syndrome [45]. Numerous symptoms, such as immunological and developmental abnormalities, genomic instability, a higher risk of cancer, and accelerated aging in the case of WRN, might result from these illnesses [38]. Remarkably, connections between the p53 protein and various disease-related helicases have been discovered. BLM raises the risk of getting cancers of the breast, colon, and lung; and lymphomas, leukemias, sarcomas, and embryonic tumors, among other malignancies. Researchers noticed that variations in p53 levels following DNA damage were contingent upon the presence of BLM, and this observation led to the identification of the relationship between BLM and p53. Subsequent research demonstrated that BLM and p53 directly interact and cooperate to control transcription and cell division. Through p53 location and Holliday junction processing regulation, BLM also contributes to the control of homologous recombination at halted replication forks. Additionally, BLM can impact apoptosis and has important interactions with p53 in various clinical situations.

As previously mentioned, one of the significant clinical characteristics associated with WRN is premature aging. Similar to BLM, a deficiency in WRN also leads to an increased, albeit more limited, risk of developing cancer. Numerous studies have shed light on the crucial connections between WRN activity and the tumor suppressor protein p53. Just like BLM, WRN has a role in p53-dependent apoptosis, the process of programmed cell death. WRN and p53 physically interact with each other, and this interaction can impact the transactivation functions of p53, which is crucial for regulating gene expression. Interestingly, when cells lacking WRN are exposed to DNA damage, they fail to activate the p53 gene, a critical response that helps protect against cancer development. This impaired function of p53 in WRN-deficient cells may partially explain the increased susceptibility to cancer observed in individuals with WRN mutations. Additionally, insights into the molecular mechanisms underlying premature aging in WRN patients have emerged from studies conducted on mouse models. These studies revealed that WRN deficiency can enhance the aging process even when p53 is not present. Furthermore, subsequent research demonstrated that p53 can manage the biochemical activities of WRN. Specifically, p53 has the ability to regulate WRN's role in processing Holliday junctions, which are critical DNA structures involved in genetic recombination.

In summary, the relationship between WRN, premature aging, and cancer risk is complex and multifaceted. WRN and p53 mutually influence each other's functions, with WRN deficiency impacting p53 activation and p53 modulating WRN's biochemical activities. These findings add to our understanding of the underlying mechanisms associated with premature aging and the elevated cancer risk observed in individuals with WRN deficiency.

Scientists have recently discovered that RECQL4 and p53 interact with each other. It appears that RECQL4 has a function related to p53 that doesn't depend on DNA damage [45]. Specifically, RECQL4 plays a crucial role in helping p53 move to the mitochondria in normal, unstressed human cells. It's interesting to note that p53 appears to inhibit RECQL4 expression; this observation may indicate that p53 controls its position inside cells, but this theory is still tentative. Research on the relationship between p53 and RECQL4 is ongoing, thus further discoveries should be made in the near future [56]. DDR and processes including cellular senescence, cell cycle arrest, and programmed cell death that are regulated by the wild-type (wt) p53 protein can be significantly impacted by the status of TP53 mutations [40, 45]. To maintain stability, wt p53 is dependent on posttranslational alterations brought about by DNA damage, including acetylation of its DNA-binding domain and phosphorylation by kinases such as ATM, ATR, and DNA protein kinase. Stabilized and active wt p53 triggers several reactions and processes, such as controlled cell death and cellular senescence. Activated wild-type p53 performs its tumor suppressor role by binding to particular DNA areas of target genes such as p21, Wip1, Noxa, and PUMA. However, because the Hsp90 complex prevents MDM2 from acting on mutant p53, mutated p53 in the core domain—which is susceptible to conformational changes—accumulates in cancer cells [1].

Though wt p53 is mostly recognized for its transcription-associated functions, it is also capable of transcription-independent action. In the nucleus, p53 functions as a transcription factor that can activate the transcription of genes that cause or control regulated cell death (RCD) in response to the degree and duration of DNA damage. Among the important genes that wt p53 activates to induce apoptosis are the BH3-only proteins Puma/BBC3 and Noxa/PMAIP1 [45, 57]. Furthermore, p53 stimulates the activation of other pro-apoptotic genes, including TRAIL-R2/DR540, Apaf1, Bax, Bim, and Fas/CD95. Conversely, p53 has the ability to suppress apoptosis through the indirect upregulation of microRNA miR-34a, which specifically targets the anti-apoptotic protein Bcl-2. Another interesting finding is that p53 may interact with Bcl-XL, an anti-apoptotic protein, to stop it from sequestering Bak1 or Bax proteins. The variety of ways that p53 affects apoptosis is amazing.

In the mitochondria, p53 interacts with a protein called cyclophilin D, which helps open pores and cause a type of cell death called necrosis. p53 is also involved in regulating other types of cell death like ferroptosis and autophagic cell death. It indirectly enhances ferroptosis by suppressing the expression of a specific protein. It also contributes to autophagic cell death by increasing the activity of certain proteins. Additionally, p53 plays a role in cellular senescence, which is important in the early stages of cancer prevention. However, in advanced stages, senescent cells may promote cancer growth and resistance. p53 also controls the cell cycle by increasing the expression of a protein that stops cell division. This protein can make cancer cells more resistant to cell death. Overall, p53 is a versatile factor that responds to various cellular stresses and plays a complex role in cancer development.

7.8 GENETIC SAFEGUARDING: EXPLORING DNA DAMAGE, REPAIR, AND THE ROLE OF TP53

In addition to cell cycle arrest, apoptosis, and senescence, DNA damage repair is a component of the p53-induced cellular response. The BER pathway is mostly in charge of repairing DNA damage caused by ROS, which is a significant contributor to DNA damage. The interaction between the p53R175H mutant p53 and NRF2, a crucial regulator of the cell's antioxidant response, was recently found. Because of this connection, cancer cells are better equipped to withstand high levels of ROS inside the cell and can mount a defensive response against oxidative stress [17, 45].

As we've seen before, p53 is involved in repairing single-strand breaks (SSBs) through the BER process. The normal form of p53, unlike the mutated versions, can boost BER activity in lab experiments. Researchers have discovered that p53 interacts with a protein called APE1/Ref-1, which is important for BER. p53 can directly inhibit the production of APE1, and studies have shown that higher levels of normal p53 are associated with increased BER activity. Additionally, normal p53 can enhance BER activity both in lab settings and within living organisms. It seems that p53's ability to enhance BER is also linked to another protein called DNA pol β. The core part of p53 has its built-in ability to remove damaged DNA, while the C-terminus of p53 can detect abnormal DNA structures. Throughout the cell cycle, p53 can influence BER activity in response to DNA damage. On the other hand, certain p53 mutations commonly found in tumors don't have the same ability to enhance BER, which suggests their involvement in tumorigenesis.

TABLE 7.2
Impact of Tp53 on Various DNA Repair Pathways

TP53 Variant	Repair Pathway	Effect
TP53 missense mutation	BER	APE1 regulation
Hot-spot tumor-derived T53 mutants	BER	It doesn't increase the activity of the repair pathway as compared to wt p53
Arg273 His mutant TP53	NER	XPD (Rad3) and XPB DNA helicase activities are not stopped as wt p53 does
p53 knock out	NER	Facilitates chromosomal abnormalities
R248W and R273H mutant TP53	HR	Engages with MRE11; interchromosomal translocations

Source: Stiewe and Haran [9].

p53 performs both transcription-dependent and transcription-independent roles during NER. GG-NER and TC-NER are the two forms of NER that it regulates. p53 interacts with XPC, XPB, and CSB proteins, among other NER pathway constituents [45, 58]. The XPD (Rad3) and XPB DNA helicases can be inhibited by the normal version of p53, but not by the Arg273His mutant p53. Furthermore, compared to cells with normal p53, cells with heterozygous p53 mutations repair UV-induced DNA damage more slowly. Studies conducted in vivo on p53 knockout mice have demonstrated that GG-NER is compromised, which increases the frequency of chromosomal aberrations. Additionally, via activating genes linked to DNA repair and interacting with machinery involved in repair and recombination, p53 also plays a critical role in mending DSBs [40, 45, 58].

Mutations in p53 that cause R248W and R273H may interact with MRE11, a component of the MRN complex that is involved in homologous recombination repair [9]. Due to this interaction, MRE11 is unable to attract ATM to DNA DSBs, which leads to faulty cell-cycle checkpoints and interchromosomal translocations. Additionally, p53 interacts with RAD51 to prevent HR and RAD51 polymerization. Additional research has demonstrated that p53 interacts with BRCA1, BRCA2, BLM, RAD54, RPA, and WRN, among other HR components [10, 45, 57]. While the exact function of p53 in NHEJ remains unclear, XRCC4 and ligase IV knockout experiments have shown that in the absence of NHEJ, DSBs remain unrepaired and ultimately cause p53-dependent cell death. Hypermutation and microsatellite instability are caused by inadequate or deficient MMR activity, namely in MLH1 and MSH2 in some cancers such as colorectal and ovarian cancer. The interaction between p53 and MMR may affect how sensitive MMR-defective colorectal cancer cells are to cisplatin [26, 45].

7.9 DECIPHERING CANCER COMPLEXITY: DNA REPAIR DYNAMICS AND THE IMPACT OF p53 MUTATIONS

Researchers hypothesized that gastrointestinal (GI) tumors may be associated with a drop in SOD, an enzyme involved in DNA damage, and an increase in p53, a protein connected to tissue change, in a study that employed markers to evaluate telomere dysfunction [59]. The degree of GI cancer in patients was shown to be significantly correlated with indicators of telomere disruption, p53, oxidative stress, and these conditions. Another intriguing study examined the relationship between particular genetic polymorphisms and telomere alterations in blood cells and the risk of juvenile solid tumors. According to the findings, kids who had longer telomeres were more likely to get solid tumors. However, it was discovered that the MDM2 rs2279744 GG genotype greatly reduced the incidence of juvenile solid tumors. A study on TP53 gene mutations and oxidative DNA damage in colorectal adenoma and adenocarcinoma was carried out to investigate this relationship. The mucosa of cancer patients with non-cancerous tissues had greater levels of TP53 than the mucosa of healthy persons. In comparison to non-cancerous cells, tumor tissues also showed much greater oxidative DNA damage and increased TP53 levels. The authors concluded that TP53 mutation and oxidative DNA damage are linked in all samples and that these variables are important in the progression of colorectal adenoma to cancer. Germline variations of the TP53 gene, such as single nucleotide polymorphisms, can also affect the gene's function in addition to somatic mutations. Specifically, rs35514263 in ATR, rs492510 and rs558351 in CHEK1, rs189037 in ATM, and rs2236141, rs5762748, rs2236142, and rs9620817 in CHEK2 that are involved in DNA damage response were examined by Wang and colleagues along with their associations with colorectal cancer risk in a Chinese population [45]. Compared to people with the G allele of rs189037, individuals with the A allele exhibited a noticeably increased risk of colorectal cancer. Older patients who had rectal cancer, had early-stage tumors, and had higher-grade tumors were more at risk. According to a bioinformatic investigation, rs189037 could change the secondary structure of the protein [25, 45, 57].

REFERENCES

1. Inoue, K., E.A. Fry, and D.P. Frazier, Transcription factors that interact with p53 and Mdm2. *International Journal of Cancer*, 2016. **138**(7): p. 1577–1585.
2. Wang, H., et al., Targeting p53 pathways: mechanisms, structures, and advances in therapy. *Signal Transduction and Targeted Therapy*, 2023. **8**(1): p. 92.
3. Vaughan, C., I. Pearsall, A. Yeudallet, S.P. Deb, and S. Deb, p53: its mutations and their impact on transcription. *Subcellular Biochemistry*, 2014: p. 71–90.
4. Marvalim, C., A. Datta, and S.C. Lee, Role of p53 in breast cancer progression: An insight into p53 targeted therapy. *Theranostics*, 2023. **13**(4): p. 1421–1442.
5. Asl, E.R., et al., Mutant P53 in the formation and progression of the tumor microenvironment: friend or foe. *Life Sciences*, 2023. **315**: p. 121361.
6. Mir, M.A., A. Shabir, and N. Jan, Metronomic Chemotherapy in Breast Cancer, in *Novel Approaches in Metronomic Chemotherapy for Breast Cancer Treatment*. CRC Press. p. 72–86.
7. Kim, M.P. and G. Lozano, Mutant p53 partners in crime. *Cell Death & Differentiation*, 2018. **25**(1): p. 161–168.
8. Mir, M.A., Sumaya, N. Jan, Implications of Chemokine Heterogenicity in Cancer Metastasis, in *Cytokine and Chemokine Networks in Cancer*. 2023, Springer. p. 115–136.
9. Stiewe, T. and T.E. Haran, How mutations shape p53 interactions with the genome to promote tumorigenesis and drug resistance. *Drug Resistance Updates*, 2018. **38**: p. 27–43.
10. Mir, M.A., N. Jan, and S. Sofi, Introduction to Metronomic Chemotherapy, in *Novel Approaches in Metronomic Chemotherapy for Breast Cancer Treatment*. 2024, CRC Press. p. 1–14.
11. Mir, M.A., et al., Proteomics: A Groundbreaking Development in Cancer Biology, in *Proteomics*. 2023, Elsevier. p. 31–53.
12. Weisz, L., M. Oren, and V. Rotter, Transcription regulation by mutant p53. *Oncogene*, 2007. **26**(15): p. 2202–2211.
13. Jan, N., et al., Metronomic chemotherapy and drug repurposing: a paradigm shift in oncology. *Heliyon*, 2024. https://doi.org/10.1016/j.heliyon.2024.e24670
14. Maggi Jr, L.B., et al., ARF tumor suppression in the nucleolus. *Biochimica et Biophysica Acta (BBA)-Molecular Basis of Disease*, 2014. **1842**(6): p. 831–839.
15. Sofi, S., et al., Elucidation of interleukin-19 as a therapeutic target for breast cancer by computational analysis and experimental validation. *Saudi Journal of Biological Sciences*, 2023. **30**(9): p. 103774–103774.
16. Vaughan, C., et al., p53: its mutations and their impact on transcription. *Subcellular Biochemistry*, 2014. **85**: p. 71–90.
17. Mir, M.A., et al., Proteomics: Application of Next-Generation Proteomics in Cancer Research, in *Proteomics*. 2023, Elsevier. p. 55–76.
18. Jan, N., et al., Exploring the role of trifarotene against RAR-α: an investigation of expression pattern and clinicopathological significance of RAR-α in breast cancer. *Frontiers in Pharmacology*, 2024. **15**: p. 1361679.

19. Mir, M.A., A. Manzoor, and N. Jan, CCL5/CCR5 Axis in Cancer, in *Cytokine and Chemokine Networks in Cancer.* 2023, Springer. p. 219–240.
20. Mir, M.A., et al., Imaging Techniques, Biomarkers, and Methods for Metronomic Chemotherapy, in *Novel Approaches in Metronomic Chemotherapy for Breast Cancer Treatment.* CRC Press. p. 58–71.
21. Mir, M.A., N. Jan, and H. Qayoom, Conventional Chemotherapy vs. Metronomic Chemotherapy, in *Novel Approaches in Metronomic Chemotherapy for Breast Cancer Treatment.* CRC Press. p. 27–42.
22. Mir, M.A., M. Rashid, and N. Jan, Cytokines and Chemokines in Tumor Growth and Progression, in *Cytokine and Chemokine Networks in Cancer.* 2023, Springer. p. 33–77.
23. Kurimchak, A. and X. Graña, PP2A: more than a reset switch to activate pRB proteins during the cell cycle and in response to signaling cues. *Cell Cycle*, 2015. **14**(1): p. 18–30.
24. Mir, M.A., N. Jan, and I. Noor, Therapeutic Implications of Cytokines and Chemokines Network in Cancer, in *Cytokine and Chemokine Networks in Cancer.* 2023, Springer. p. 385–414.
25. Sofi, S., et al., Clinicopathological and prognostic significance of Bcl2 in breast cancer: a comprehensive in silico and in vitro study. *Saudi Journal of Biological Sciences*, 2023. **31**(2): p. 103916.
26. Mir, M.A., M. Bashir, and N. Jan, The Role of Interleukin (IL)-6/IL-6 Receptor Axis in Cancer, in *Cytokine and Chemokine Networks in Cancer.* 2023, Springer. p. 137–164.
27. Zhou, Z., et al., p53 Suppresses E2F1-dependent PLK1 expression upon DNA damage by forming p53–E2F1–DNA complex. *Experimental Cell Research*, 2013. **319**(20): p. 3104–3115.
28. Kasim, V., et al., Synergistic cooperation of MDM2 and E2F1 contributes to TAp73 transcriptional activity. *Biochemical and Biophysical Research Communications*, 2014. **449**(3): p. 319–326.
29. van Roeyen, C.R., et al., Cold shock Y-box protein-1 proteolysis autoregulates its transcriptional activities. *Cell Communication and Signaling*, 2013. **11**: p. 1–16.
30. Lasham, A., et al., The Y-box-binding protein, YB1, is a potential negative regulator of the p53 tumor suppressor. *Journal of Biological Chemistry*, 2003. **278**(37): p. 35516–35523.
31. Ramkumar, C., et al., Smurf2 suppresses B-cell proliferation and lymphomagenesis by mediating ubiquitination and degradation of YY1. *Nature Communications*, 2013. **4**(1): p. 2598.
32. Sofi, S., et al., A comprehensive analysis of notch signaling genes in breast cancer: expression pattern and prognostic significance. *Advances in Cancer Biology-Metastasis*, 2023. **7**: p. 100104.
33. Metcalf, S. and P. Hollenhorst, Investigating the interaction between ETS family members and mutant p53. *Cancer Research*, 2024. **84**(6_Supplement): p. 1706–1706.
34. Sullivan, K.D., et al., Mechanisms of transcriptional regulation by p53. *Cell Death & Differentiation*, 2018. **25**(1): p. 133–143.
35. Kim, E. and W. Deppert, Transcriptional activities of mutant p53: when mutations are more than a loss. *Journal of Cellular Biochemistry*, 2004. **93**(5): p. 878–886.
36. Strano, S., et al., Mutant p53: an oncogenic transcription factor. *Oncogene*, 2007. **26**(15): p. 2212–2219.
37. Bellazzo, A., et al., Complexes formed by mutant p53 and their roles in breast cancer. *Breast Cancer (Dove Med Press)*, 2018. **10**: p. 101–112.
38. Pfister, N.T. and C. Prives, Transcriptional regulation by wild-type and cancer-related mutant forms of p53. *Cold Spring Harbor Perspectives in Medicine*, 2017. **7**(2): p. a026054.
39. Vodicka, P., et al., The interactions of DNA repair, telomere homeostasis, and p53 mutational status in solid cancers: risk, prognosis, and prediction. *Cancers*, 2021. **13**(3): p. 479.
40. Stiewe, T. and T.E. Haran, How mutations shape p53 interactions with the genome to promote tumorigenesis and drug resistance. *Drug Resistance Updates*, 2018. **38**: p. 27–43.
41. Vodicka, P., et al., DNA damage and repair measured by comet assay in cancer patients. *Mutation Research, Genetic Toxicology and Environmental Mutagenesis*, 2019. **843**: p. 95–110.
42. Goldstein, M. and M.B. Kastan, The DNA damage response: implications for tumor responses to radiation and chemotherapy. *Annual Review of Medicine*, 2015. **66**: p. 129–43.
43. Williams, A.B. and B. Schumacher, p53 in the DNA-damage-repair process. *Cold Spring Harbor Perspectives in Medicine*, 2016. **6**(5): p. a026070.
44. Hastak, K., et al., Identification of a functional in vivo p53 response element in the coding sequence of the xeroderma pigmentosum group C gene. *Genes & Cancer*, 2012. **3**(2): p. 131–140.
45. Wang, S., et al., Association of genetic variants in ATR-CHEK1 and ATM-CHEK2 pathway genes with risk of colorectal cancer in a Chinese population. *Oncotarget*, 2018. **9**(42): p. 26616.
46. Cun, Y., et al., APE1/Ref-1 enhances DNA binding activity of mutant p53 in a redox-dependent manner. *Oncology Reports*, 2014. **31**(2): p. 901–909.
47. Jung, H.J., et al., A novel chemopreventive mechanism of selenomethionine: enhancement of APE1 enzyme activity via a Gadd45a, PCNA and APE1 protein complex that regulates p53-mediated base excision repair. *Oncology Reports*, 2013. **30**(4): p. 1581–1586.

48. van Oers, J.M., et al., The MutSβ complex is a modulator of p53-driven tumorigenesis through its functions in both DNA double-strand break repair and mismatch repair. *Oncogene*, 2014. **33**(30): p. 3939–3946.
49. Deriano, L. and D.B. Roth, Modernizing the nonhomologous end-joining repertoire: alternative and classical NHEJ share the stage. *Annual Review of Genetics*, 2013. **47**: p. 433–455.
50. Rieckmann, T., et al., p53 modulates homologous recombination at I-SceI-induced double-strand breaks through cell-cycle regulation. *Oncogene*, 2013. **32**(8): p. 968–975.
51. Gong, L., et al., p53 isoform Δ113p53/Δ133p53 promotes DNA double-strand break repair to protect cell from death and senescence in response to DNA damage. *Cell Research*, 2015. **25**(3): p. 351–369.
52. Serrano, M.A., et al., DNA-PK, ATM and ATR collaboratively regulate p53–RPA interaction to facilitate homologous recombination DNA repair. *Oncogene*, 2013. **32**(19): p. 2452–2462.
53. Croteau, D.L., et al., Human RecQ helicases in DNA repair, recombination, and replication. *Annual Review of Biochemistry*, 2014. **83**: p. 519–552.
54. Lu, L., et al., RECQL4 regulates p53 function in vivo during skeletogenesis. *Journal of Bone and Mineral Research*, 2015. **30**(6): p. 1077–1089.
55. Jan, N., et al., Targeting breast cancer stem cells through retinoids: a new hope for treatment. *Critical Reviews in Oncology/Hematology*, 2023: p. 104156.
56. Mir, M.A., et al., Metronomics: toward personalized chemotherapy. *Novel Approaches in Metronomic Chemotherapy for Breast Cancer Treatment*, 2024. p. 99–119. https://doi.org/10.1201/9781032632674-8
57. Haq, B.U., et al., Targeting p53 misfolding conundrum by stabilizing agents and their analogs in breast cancer therapy: a comprehensive computational analysis. *Frontiers in Pharmacology*, 2024. **14**: p. 1333447.

8 p53 Control of Cell Cycle Dynamics in Breast Cancer
Maintaining a Balance between Arrest and Proliferation

*Mehvish Feroz, Asma Jan, Janifar Yasin, and Manzoor Ahmad Mir**

Department of Bioresources, School of Biological Sciences, University of Kashmir, Srinagar, J&K, India
*drmanzoor@kashmiruniversity.ac.in

8.1 INTRODUCTION

Breast carcinoma stands out as the predominantly identified cancer and primary cause of cancer-associated deaths among women worldwide. Around 1.7 million cases were identified in 2014, representing a quarter of all female cancer diagnoses [1–3]. One in every eight women will develop breast cancer at some point in their lives [4, 5]. After being diagnosed, breast cancers are classified into different subtypes determined by their advancement stage, the level of intrusiveness, and the presence of hormonal receptors [6, 7]. In breast cancer, there are three main groups based on hormone receptor status that often show high levels and cause significant disturbances. These groups are estrogen receptor (ERα)/progesterone receptor (PR), human epidermal growth factor receptor 2 (HER2), and triple-negative breast cancer (TNBC), which do not have these three receptors [8–11]. Breast carcinoma presents as a diverse condition with numerous biologic subtypes, each possessing distinct traits and varying responses to treatments [12]. In breast cancer, the TP53 gene is commonly changed, affecting about a third of all cases [13]. In breast cancer, the majority of mutations in the p53 gene happen within its DNA binding region stem from precise point mutations that interfere with its capacity to control gene expression. These mutations are strongly linked to various kinds of tumors [14, 15]. These mutations are linked to lower survival rates in breast cancer patients [16, 17]. Often referred to as the "guardian of the genome," p53 (created by the TP53 gene) is regarded as the most extensively studied and intricate anti-cancer protein identified to date [18, 19]. p53 extends its influence beyond tumor suppression, emerging as a vital controller of metabolic balance, intricately involved in numerous fundamental cellular activities [20–22]. In breast tissue, p53 is crucial for keeping cells balanced by regulating metabolic activities during pregnancy and protecting against hidden breast cancer [23]. Also, its conventional functions involve safeguarding breast tissue, as p53 is essential for managing the genetic material, fixing DNA, and coordinating controlled cell death [24]. Frequent mutations in the TP53 gene play a pivotal role in advancing cancer in various types of cancer. Nevertheless, the majority of breast cancers retain the wild-type p53 (wt-p53) gene, yet the p53 protein frequently loses functionality. This impairment is attributed, in part, to the absence of upstream regulators within the p53 pathway [15, 25, 26]. Traditional views suggest that reactivating the p53 pathway could be a more effective approach to treating breast cancer. This is because activating p53 can trigger programmed cell death pathways, which may help eliminate cancer cells.

DOI: 10.1201/9781003520771-8

This concept could be problematic because of the insufficient understanding of the involvement of p53 in cellular metabolic processes. Initially, altered metabolism in cancer was thought to be just a by-product, not integral to cancer's development and maintenance. Over the past decade, however, research into cancer metabolism has surged. Now, cancer metabolism is recognized as a succession of crucial metabolic changes and adaptations in pathways involved in the synthesis of biomolecules and energy production, essential for supporting cancer cell growth and survival [27–29]. The recent resurgence of interest in the metabolic processes in cancer has highlighted p53 as a pivotal controller of metabolic pathways and metabolic alterations within cancer cells [30–32]. The p53 protein functions as a transcription factor, becoming stabilized within the nucleus, and reactions are triggered in response to DNA damage or signals indicating oncogenic activity. It oversees the activation of genes responsible for inducing the halting of the cell cycle. Cell apoptosis (cellular demise), DNA restoration, and senescence are all aimed at thwarting tumor formation and progression [33–35]. One of the primary roles initially recognized for p53 is to hinder the buildup of damaged DNA, thereby enhancing genomic stability and impeding the onset of tumorigenesis [36]. This is accomplished by halting cell growth for a brief period to allow for the repair of DNA damage before DNA replication restarts. Within cases where the DNA damage is beyond repair, p53 initiates cellular apoptosis to eliminate altered cells. The conventional method by which p53 initiates DNA restoration is by activating the process of transcribing the cell cycle suppressor p21 located downstream, thus activating mechanisms to repair DNA damage [7, 37, 38, 39]. Predictably, the regulatory checkpoint machinery involving p21 is frequently bypassed in cancer [40]. When halting of cell division occurs, methods for repairing DNA are often activated to fix the genetic injury before the cell can resume cellular division. Specifically, p53 has a confirmed function in transcriptionally regulating genes associated with DNA excision repair and glycosylase-mediated repair pathways [40–42]. The repair pathways facilitated by p53 manage DNA repair tasks such as single-stranded break repair and addressing various DNA abnormalities to prevent instability in the genetic material. Ironically, mutations within the p53 gene itself are the very cause of tumor development. A significant portion of p53 research focuses on its well-known tumor suppressor functions, which are usually compromised when p53 is mutated or deleted. This impairment often results in the formation of various oncogenic versions of p53 [30, 43–45]. Approximately half of all human cancers show changes in the cancer-causing form of the p53 gene, which modify how it works, making it one of the most frequently changed proteins in cancer [44, 46, 47]. Due to its broad gene regulator function, p53 has the capability to initiate the activation of genes involved in halting cell proliferation and promoting apoptosis, DNA repair, and cell dormancy. This response is triggered by various stress-induced p53 activation signals after translation [34, 48–50].

8.2 p53 AND CELL CYCLE ARREST IN BREAST CANCER

p53, acting as a transcription factor, can be significantly stimulated by different stressor alerts such as genome disruption, activation of oncogenes, and lack of nutrients. The first outcomes of p53 activation are cellular division halting and programmed cell death. The main way p53 causes cellular division to halt is by activating the transcription of p21/WAF [51, 52]. p53 binds to two locations situated 2.4 kb and 1.4 kb upstream of the p21 promoter, the region located 5′ of the p21 promoter is one of the most potent p53-responsive elements studied, with an equilibrium constant of approximately 5 nM [53–55]. Following p53 activation, p21 mRNA is significantly upregulated and was the initial p53-regulated gene recognized through an impartial differential screening method [51]. p21 stops the cell cycle in the G1 phase by binding to and inhibiting the function of E/cdk2 and D/cdk4 complexes [56]. p21 hinders the phosphorylation of pRb by blocking Cdk2 and Cdk4, enabling the association of pRb with E2F1. This interaction results in the suppression of transcription for genes targeted by E2F1, which are crucial for DNA duplication and cellular division advancement. Additionally, p21's binding with proliferating cell nuclear antigen disrupts DNA duplication in laboratory settings, reinforcing its effectiveness in halting the cell cycle [57]. In mouse embryonic fibroblasts (MEFs) without p21, there is an observed impairment in halting the cell cycle after genomic injury, underscoring p21's role as a crucial intermediary in p53-triggered cell cycle halt [58]. However, cells lacking p21 are not completely deficient in the G1 phase halt, indicating that additional genes targeted at p53 also play a role in controlling cell cycle arrest [59]. p53 activation also halts cells in the late stages of the cell cycle (G2/M phase and S). While p21 can block cyclin B/Cdc2 to hinder advancement via genetic alterations, it's probable that additional p53-regulated genes, such as 14-3-3σ, also contribute to obstructing the transition from the G2 to the M phase [60, 61]. When DNA damage occurs, p53 blocks the cdc25C promoter, aiding in the initiation of the G2/M phase halt [62]. Recent research indicates that the upregulation of the presence of microRNA mir34a helps with the growth arrest that p53 initiates, likely through the transcriptional suppression of multiple target genes [63–65]. Mice with a disrupted mir34 gene family did not affect p53-induced cell cycle arrest and programmed cell death, suggesting that the role of mir34 in organisms might be restricted or counterbalanced by other mechanisms [66, 67]. In breast cancer, p53 is curtailed for halting the cell cycle by responding to genetic injury and alternative stress stimuli. When activated, p53 becomes stable and acts as a transcription factor, boosting the levels of genes such as p21. This gene, in turn, hinders cyclin-dependent kinases (CDKs) necessary for progressing through the cell cycle. By preventing the retinoblastoma protein (Rb) phosphate addition, this action results in G1 phase arrest. Additionally, p53 promotes genes such as growth arrest and DNA damage (GADD45) and 14-3-3σ that are activated by p53 to control the G2/M checkpoint, pausing the cell cycle before mitosis. If DNA damage is severe, p53 triggers apoptosis by activating pro-apoptotic genes such as BAX and PUMA. Mutations in TP53, often found in breast cancer, disrupt these processes, leading to uncontrolled cell growth and tumor formation. p53 acts as a nuclear regulatory protein that triggers the transcription of various target genes, playing a role in stopping the cell cycle and promoting programmed cell death [43, 68]. Under typical circumstances, p53 exists in minimal quantities because it undergoes breakdown by the proteasome, primarily mediated by the MDM2, a type of E3 ubiquitin ligase with a RING-finger structure [69, 70]. In its normal state, p53 remains non-functional in response to DNA damage. p53 levels increase within the cellular nucleus due to protein modifications such as the addition of phosphate and acetyl groups. These changes activate p53, possibly by causing MDM2 to dissociate from it [68, 71]. When p53 becomes functionally active, it activates specific genes targeted to initiate cellular division halt or cell death, depending upon the type and severity of the genomic injury [15, 68, 71, 72]. p53-triggered cell cycle halt allows cells the chance to mend DNA damage. After the repair is finished, cells return to their typical cell cycle. However, if the DNA damage is severe, p53 triggers apoptosis to remove these damaged cells, preventing the transmission of defective DNA to daughter cells. This ability of p53 helps maintain genomic integrity.

8.3 p53-MEDIATED CONTROL OF CELL PROLIFERATION BALANCE OF CELL CYCLE

The p53 protein, often termed the "guardian of the genome," plays a vital role in controlling cell growth and preserving genetic stability. p53 can induce G/S phase halt, by stimulating the production of p21, which blocks CDK. p21 puts the brakes on CDKs essential for moving from the G1 to the S phase, stopping cell growth when DNA damage is identified. Thus preventing cell proliferation when DNA damage is detected [55, 73]. When DNA damage occurs due to factors like UV radiation, ionizing radiation, or chemical agents, p53 undergoes stabilization and activation. The stabilization occurs due to the phosphorylation of p53 by enzymes like ATM and ATR, which prevent its breakdown by MDM2, an E3 ubiquitin ligase [74]. Once activated, p53 functions as a regulatory protein and increases the production of p21 (also known as CDKN1A), a potent inhibitor of cyclin-dependent kinase. p21 attaches to and blocks the function of cyclin-dependent kinase 2 (CDK2) or cyclin-dependent kinase 4 (CDK4) complexes, resulting in a cell cycle halt in phase [73]. p21 suppresses the function of cyclin-CDK2 and cyclin-CDK4 complexes, pivotal for the phosphorylated state of Rb protein. When Rb undergoes phosphorylation, it frees the E2F regulatory protein, which plays a crucial role in facilitating the shift from the G1 phase to the S phase of the cell cycle. By suppressing the activity of CDK complexes, p21 prevents Rb phosphorylation, thereby blocking the G1/S transit [56]. p53 is also involved in regulating the G2/M phase transition control point. It can induce the expression of HME1 or stratifin (14-3-3σ), which sequesters the cytoplasmic CDC2/cyclin B1 complex, stopping it from entering the nucleus and thus blocking the initiation of mitosis. p21 also plays a role in G2 phase halt by inhibiting the cyclin B1/CDC2 complex [75]. Besides arresting the cell cycle, p53 increases the activity of genes that handle DNA repair tasks, such as GADD45, which plays a role in fixing DNA and safeguarding the genome. This gives the cell a chance to mend DNA issues before progressing through the cell cycle [76]. If the injury is too significant to be rectified, p53 can shift the balance toward apoptosis. This ensures that severely damaged cells, which might otherwise become cancerous, are eliminated. This decision-making process is vital for sustaining tissue equilibrium and preventing tumorigenesis [77]. p53-induced cell cycle halt is a multifaceted process involving the enhancing and triggering of p53 upon genetic injury, upregulation of target gene expression like p21 and 14-3-3σ, inhibition of cyclin-CDK complexes, and induction of DNA repair mechanisms. This intricate network guarantees that cells do not proliferate with impaired DNA, thereby maintaining genetic stability and preventing the development of cancer.

8.3.1 Activation of DNA Repair Mechanisms

p53 stimulates DNA to get repaired by increasing the activity of genes responsible for nucleotide excision repair (NER) and base excision repair (BER). This ensures that cells do not proliferate with damaged DNA, reducing the risk of mutations and cancer development [78]. p53 triggers the activation of GADD45, a crucial gene involved in NER and BER. It contributes to the preservation of genomic integrity by enhancing DNA-maintaining processes and interacting with other repair proteins [76]. p53 upregulates the activation of the XPC gene and produces a protein crucial for identifying genetic injury within the NER pathway. XPC binds to damaged DNA and initiates the repair process by recruiting other NER factors to excise and replace damaged nucleotides [79]. p53 enhances the expression and activity of APE1 (apurimac/pyrimidine endonuclease 1), a crucial enzyme in the BER pathway. APE1 processes basic sites in DNA, which are common forms of damage resulting from oxidative stress and other insults [80]. p53 can influence the activation of genes associated with the mismatch repair (MMR) process, such as MSH2 and MSH6. These proteins form a complex that identifies and fixes mismatches between bases and loop insertions or deletions that arise during DNA duplication [73]. p53 boosts the non-homologous end joining (NHEJ) method for fixing double-strand breaks by increasing DNA-PKcs (DNA-dependent protein kinase catalytic subunits), an essential enzyme in NHEJ. p53 also influences homologous recombination repair (HRR) by modulating the expression of RAD51, a protein critical for HRR [81, 82]. p53 also directly interfaces with ERCC1, a protein participating in the NER pathway, enhancing its recruitment to sites of genetic injury and promoting efficient repair [76]. p53 plays an integral function in maintaining genomic stability by activating and regulating various DNA repair mechanisms. It ensures that cells can effectively repair DNA damage and prevent the propagation of mutations. This multifaceted role underscores p53's importance as a guardian of the genome and its participation in protecting against cancer development (Table 8.1).

8.3.2 Apoptosis

When the DNA damage is irreparable, p53 can initiate cell death, known as apoptosis (programmed cell death process), to eliminate potentially cancerous cells. It does so by upregulating apoptosis-promoting genes like Bcl-2-associated X (often abbreviated as BAX), and p53 upregulated modulator of apoptosis (PUMA) while reducing the expression of apoptosis-suppressing genes like B-cell lymphoma 2 (BCL-2) [83]. TP53 is essential in controlling apoptosis, which is a programmed cell death process that eliminates damaged or abnormal cells. Upon DNA genomic injury or cellular strain, p53 is stabilized and induced by activated phosphorylation by kinases including ATM, ATR, Chk1, and Chk2. This modification prevents MDM2-triggered ubiquitination and breakdown of p53 leading to

TABLE 8.1
DNA Repair Genes Directly Regulated by TP53 and Whose Knock-Out Can Promote Spontaneous, UV-B-Induced, or γ-Radiation-Induced Tumor Development in Mice

Gene	DNA Damage Repair Pathway	Gene Knockout	Treatment	Outcome
Xpc	NER	–/–	UV-B irradiation	Skin squamous cell carcinoma
Gadd45a	NER	–/–	Ionizing radiation	Lymphoma
Ddb2	NER	–/–	UV-B irradiation	Skin carcinoma
Mlh1	MMR	–/–	—	Lymphoma and gastrointestinal tumors
Msh2	MMR	–/–	—	Colon carcinoma and lymphoid tumors

its accumulation within the cell [74]. p53 triggers the expression of the BAX gene, which produces a protein that supports apoptosis and belongs to the Bcl-2 family. BAX aids apoptosis by aiding in the movement of cytochrome c from the mitochondria to the cytoplasm, a critical process in the intrinsic pathway of apoptosis [83]. p53 also boosts the levels of PUMA and NOXA, which are both BH3-only proteins. PUMA and NOXA can counteract anti-apoptotic Bcl-2 family members, causing mitochondrial outer membrane remobilization (MOMP) and ultimately leading to apoptosis [84, 85]. When p53 activates BAX and BH3-only proteins like PUMA and NOXA, it causes the mitochondrial outer membrane to open, enabling cytochrome c to move into the cytoplasm. Afterward, cytochrome c joins with Apaf-1 (apoptotic protease activating factor 1) to form the protostome complex [86]. The protostome brings in and triggers initiator caspase-9, which then activates executioner caspases like caspase-3 and caspase-7. These executioner caspases cut different cellular targets, causing characteristic changes in cell structure and function during apoptosis [87]. p53 can also boost the external (death receptor) pathway of apoptosis by increasing the levels of death receptors like FAS (CD95) and TRAIL (TNF-related apoptosis-inducing ligand) receptors DR4 and DR5. When their ligands bind, it triggers the creation of the death-inducing signaling complex (DISC) and the activation of initiator caspases such as caspase-8 [88, 89]. p53 can also cause cell death without involving gene transcription by directly engaging with Bcl-2 family proteins at the mitochondria. p53 can attach to and deactivate anti-apoptotic proteins such as Bcl-2 and Bcl-xL, encouraging the permeabilization of the mitochondrial membrane [90]. p53 triggers cell death through different methods, such as activating genes that promote apoptosis, starting intrinsic and extrinsic apoptotic pathways, and directly interacting with mitochondrial proteins. By efficiently removing unhealthy or potentially cancerous cells, p53 plays a vital role as a tumor suppressor and protector of genetic stability.

8.3.3 Control of p53 Function

The role of p53 is related and controlled by the MDM2 protein, which binds to TP53 and marks it for ubiquitin-mediated breakdown. Under adverse circumstances, like genomic injury, p53 is phosphorylated and stabilized, resulting in its buildup and initiation [84]. The regulation of p53 activity is closely monitored to guarantee that it can respond appropriately to cellular stress and DNA damage while avoiding unnecessary apoptosis or halt in cell division when lacking such signals. The regulation of p53 involves multiple layers of control, including modifications after protein synthesis connections with other proteins, and feedback mechanisms. The MDM2 protein acts as a key inhibitor of TP53. Additionally, murine double minute 2 acts as an E3 ubiquitin ligase, tagging p53 with ubiquitin molecules, targeting it for proteasome breakdown. This keeps p53 levels low under normal conditions [91, 92]. When DNA damage occurs, p53 undergoes phosphorylation at multiple serine and threonine sites by enzymes such as ATM, ATR, Chk1, and Chk2. These phosphorylation events stabilize p53 by preventing its association with MDM2, resulting in its accumulation and stimulation [74, 93]. When p53 gets acetylated by acetyltransferases like p300/CBP and PCAF, it becomes more stable and active in gene expression. Acetylation occurs at the lysine parts at the end of p53 and stops ubiquitination and breakdown [94, 95]. The alternative reading frame protein, encoded by the CDKN2A locus, interacts with MDM2 and inhibits its E3 ubiquitin ligase mechanism. This leads to stabilization and expression of p53, particularly in response to oncogenic signals [96]. Besides MDM2, other E3 ligases such as COP1 and Pirh2 also ubiquitinate p53, leading to its degradation. This provides additional layers of regulation to ensure precise control over p53 levels [97, 98]. Several microRNAs (miRNAs) regulate p53 activity either directly by targeting p53 mRNA for degradation or indirectly by modulating the expression of p53 regulators such as MDM2 and other interacting proteins [99]. A crucial regulatory cycle entails p53 triggering the production of MDM2. Increased MDM2 levels, in turn, ubiquitinate and degrade p53, creating a tightly controlled feedback loop to maintain p53 activity at optimal levels [100]. Additional changes after protein creation, like sumoylation (attaching a small ubiquitin-like modifier) and neddylation (attaching neural precursor cell-expressed developmentally downregulated protein 8) can also influence p53's stability, localization, and activity [101, 102]. The control of p53 function is an intricate and precisely orchestrated mechanism that guarantees suitable cellular reactions to stress while avoiding unnecessary cell death or excessive proliferation. This regulation is achieved through multiple methods involving engagement with MDM2, alterations after protein synthesis, feedback loops, and the influence of microRNAs.

8.3.4 p53 and Cellular Senescence

p53 can trigger cellular senescence, which is a condition where cells permanently stop dividing in reaction to different stress signals. This acts as a barrier to uncontrolled cell proliferation and tumor development. The senescence process is mediated by increasing p21 through p53 [74]. Cellular senescence is a vital mechanism for preventing tumors and contributing to aging and tissue repair. p53 is essential for regulating this process. p53 becomes active when there is DNA damage, oxidative stress, or oncogenic signals. Once activated, p53 causes cells to permanently stop dividing, leading to senescence. This is achieved by turning on specific genes that inhibit the cell cycle and promote senescence-related secretions [91]. A key player in p53-triggered senescence is p21 (CDKN1A), a blocker of cyclin-dependent kinases. p21 stops cyclin-CDK pairs, causing the activation of Rb through dephosphorylation. This leads to cell cycle halt at the G1/S phase boundary, a characteristic of senescence [63]. Besides p21, p53 can also indirectly influence the p16INK4a/Rb pathway. Senescence is often associated with the upregulation of p16INK4a, which inhibits CDK4/6, leading to hypophosphorylation and activation of Rb. The active Rb protein represses genes targeted by E2F that are necessary for advancing through the cell cycle [103]. It impacts the formation of the SASP, which is a type of pro-inflammatory state marked by the release of cytokines, chemokines, growth factors, and proteases. The SASP reinforces the senescence growth arrest, alters the tissue microenvironment, and can have paracrine effects on neighboring cells [104]. p53 has several isoforms generated through alternative splicing and promoter usage, such as Δ133p53, which can act as a dominant-negative inhibitor of total length p53. Δ133p53 antagonizes p53-enhanced senescence and cell death, highlighting the complexity of p53 regulation in senescence [105]. Telomere shortening due to repeated cell divisions or dysfunction activates p53, leading to senescence. Dysfunctional telomeres are recognized as DNA damage, activating the ATM/ATR pathway and subsequently p53, which enforces a permanent cell cycle arrest [106]. p53 activity and the induction of senescence are also controlled by changes in epigenetics, such as alterations in histones, and DNA methylation can influence the expression of p53 target genes involved in senescence. For example, histone deacetylases (HDACs) can suppress p53 activity, and their inhibition can promote p53-mediated senescence (Figure 8.1) [107]. p53 is crucial in controlling cellular senescence through the activation of p21 and the p16INK4a/Rb pathway, the modulation of the SASP, and the response to telomere dysfunction and genetic injury. The control of p53 itself is intricate, encompassing multiple isoforms, feedback mechanisms, and epigenetic modifications.

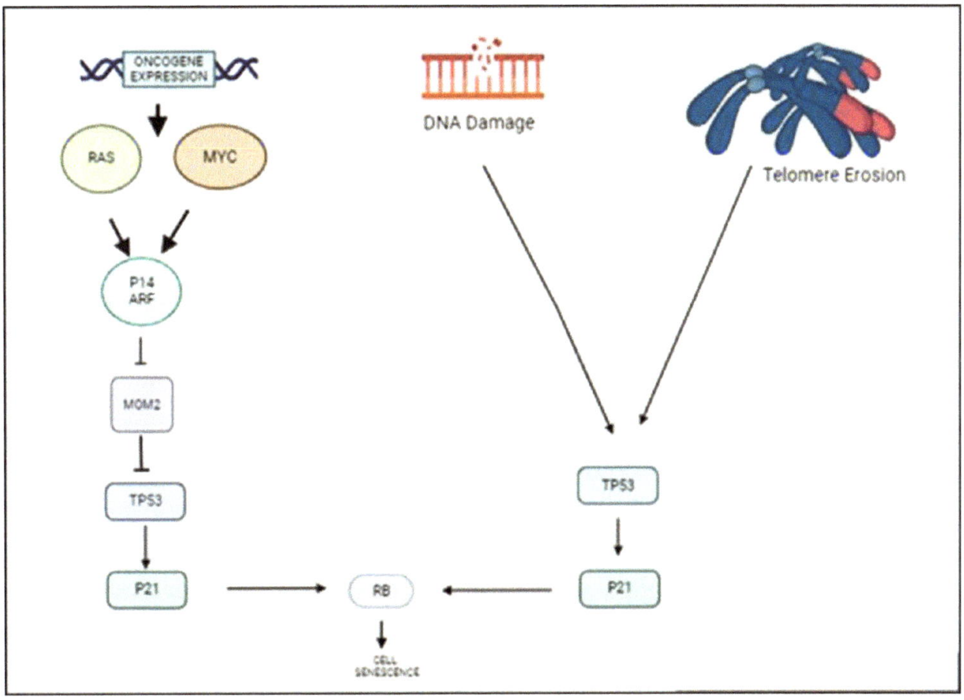

FIGURE 8.1 Cellular senescence can be induced by TP53 in response to various factors like oxidative damage, DNA damage, shortened telomeres, and stress from oncogenes. TP53 helps by increasing the expression of the p21 gene and other elements. During senescence, the RB tumor suppressor protein is activated, blocking the expression of genes needed for cell cycle advancement.

8.3.5 Tumor Suppression

When p53 stops working correctly, it often happens in various cancers, highlighting its importance as a tumor suppressor. Changes in the TP53 gene, responsible for p53 production, result in the loss of its ability to control cell growth, promoting the formation of tumors [108, 109]. p53, known as the "guardian of the genome," is crucial for preventing tumor formation. It carries out its anti-tumor functions through different methods like DNA repair, halting the cell cycle, inducing cell death, and promoting senescence. p53 becomes active in response to various DNA damage like breaks and base damage. Kinases like ATM, ATR, Chk1, and Chk2 trigger p53's activation by adding phosphate groups, which shield it from degradation [74, 93]. p53 helps activate genes that play a role in repairing DNA, like p53R2, which is part of ribonucleotide reductase for fixing nucleotides, and DDB2 for overall genomic repair [110, 111]. p53 causes cells to stop at the G1/S checkpoint by activating p21 (CDKN1A). p21 blocks CDKs, stopping the phosphorylation of Rb, which pauses cell cycle advancement [73]. p53 is also involved in controlling the G2/M checkpoint by activating genes such as 14-3-3σ. This gene works by trapping CDK1-cyclin B1 complexes in the cytoplasm, blocking them from triggering cell division [75]. p53 triggers cell death through the intrinsic (mitochondrial) pathway by increasing the expression of pro-apoptotic genes like BAX, PUMA, and NOXA. These proteins help release cytochrome c from mitochondria, activating caspases and causing cell demise [83, 84]. p53 can also kick-start the extrinsic (death receptor) pathway by boosting death receptors like FAS (CD95) and TRAIL receptors (DR4 and DR5), which triggers caspase-8 activation [84, 85, 88, 89]. p53 can cause cellular senescence, a lasting halt in the cell cycle, by using pathways that involve p21 and p16INK4a/Rb. Senescent cells stop dividing, which helps stop the spread of possible cancer cells [103]. p53 controls cell metabolism by impacting the activity of genes related to glycolysis, oxidative phosphorylation, and antioxidant defense. For example, p53 boosts TIGAR

(TP53-induced glycolysis and apoptosis regulator), which decreases glycolysis and reduces levels of reactive oxygen species (ROS) inside cells [112]. p53 also strengthens the body's defense against antioxidants by increasing the activity of genes like Sestrin1/2 and GPX1. These genes help combat oxidative stress, which in turn protects against DNA damage and the development of tumors [113]. p53 blocks angiogenesis and the creation of new blood vessels, which is vital for tumor expansion and spread. p53 reduces the expression of pro-antigenic elements like VEGF (vascular endothelial growth factor) and increases anti-angiogenic factors such as TSP-1 (thrombospondin-1) [114, 115]. p53 plays a role in shaping the epigenetic environment by controlling the activity of genes linked to chromatin modification. p53 can adjust histone acetylation, methylation, and DNA methylation levels, which in turn impact gene expression patterns associated with tumor prevention [116]. p53, the tumor suppressor, has a complex role in stopping tumor formation by engaging in activities such as DNA repair, halting the cell cycle, triggering cell death, inducing senescence, controlling metabolism, blocking blood vessel formation, and adjusting epigenetic factors. These varied functions highlight p53's crucial role in protecting cells against cancer.

8.4 p53 CONTROL OF CELLULAR METABOLISM

p53, known as the genome protector, plays a crucial role in preventing tumors in humans by controlling cell growth, aging, DNA repair, and cell death in cancer through various activities, including gene regulation and other processes [77]. p53 is the gene that is most frequently mutated in human cancer, yet the precise mechanisms by which its genetic alteration or loss results in the development of tumors remain unclear [117]. Increasing evidence has highlighted p53's crucial role in regulating cellular function helping with metabolism and supporting the body during times of limited nutrients [118]. On the other hand, altered p53 proteins, particularly those with specific mutations, show completely different functions compared to normal p53 [119]. The tumor-inhibiting protein p53 first identified in 1979 [35], is the predominantly acknowledged genetic element to carcinoma [120]. At the moment, clinical trials are assessing a minimum of eight compounds that activate p53. Two primary drug discovery approaches include targeting the interaction between TP53 and MDM2 and restoring normal functions in mutant p53 [121]. p53 reacts to a variety of external and internal threats, including DNA damage, activation of oncogenes, hypoxia, exposure to extreme temperatures, protein stress, lack of nutrients, whole genome duplication, and shortened telomeres [122]. Through both its ability to control gene expression and other activities beyond transcription, TP53 is essential in responding to various stimuli, influencing cell growth, aging, genome maintenance, and apoptosis. Nevertheless, recent research challenges the traditional perception of TP53 solely as an inhibitor of tumorigenesis. Mounting indications propose that p53 also influences cellular metabolism regulation, affecting processes such as glucose metabolism, citric acid cycle, electron transport chain, glutamine metabolism, hexose monophosphate shunt, lipid processing, nucleotide production, iron processing, and polyamine synthesis pathway [123]. The control of metabolism seems pivotal to the tumor suppression role of p53. Furthermore, unlike the normal form of p53, mutated versions of p53 have entirely distinct roles in regulating oncogenic metabolism. Grasping these distinctions could supply a valuable understanding of the mechanisms through which p53 combats tumors. Metabolic regulation appears integral to the tumor-inhibiting role of TP53 [124].

8.4.1 The Evolving Significance of p53 in Metabolism

p53 plays a critical role in regulating metabolic homeostasis by directing metabolic processes from anabolism toward catabolism. It influences key pathways, such as the core carbon pathway, lipid and amino acid processing, ion processing, ammonia elimination, and polyamine synthesis pathway. During nutrient scarcity, p53 ensures the maintenance of energy levels necessary for cell viability and fundamental life tasks, in addition to the synthesis of essential biological macromolecules (Figure 8.2) [125].

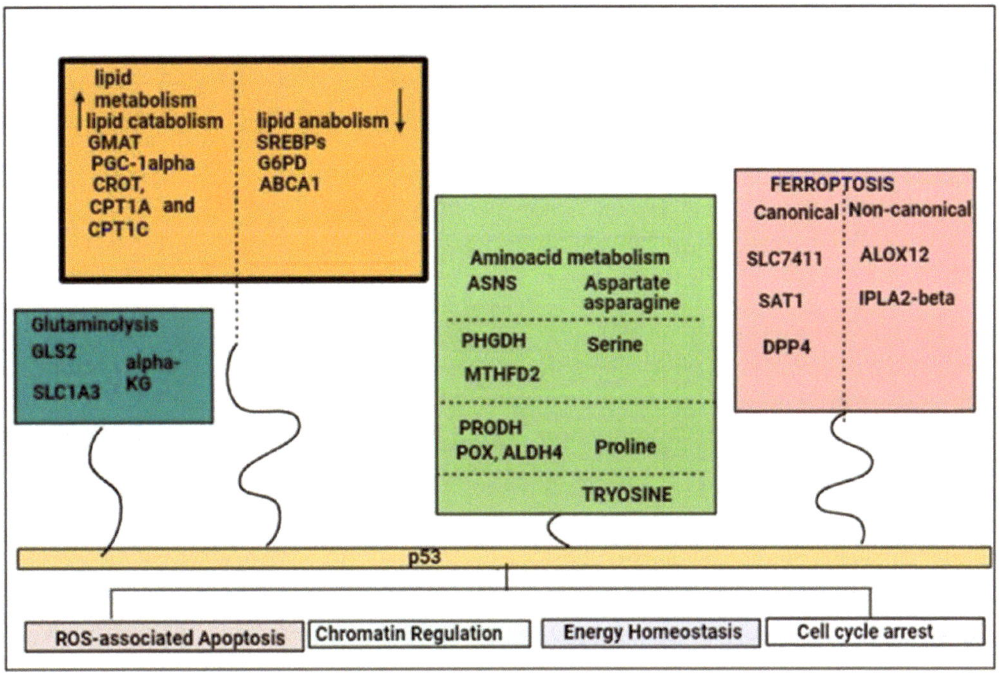

FIGURE 8.2 The important function of p53 in controlling anabolism and catabolism is crucial. p53 is a key regulator of processes such as glutaminolysis, lipid metabolism, amino acid metabolism, and ferroptosis, which are essential for managing ROS-related cell death, chromatin control, maintaining energy balance, and halting the cell cycle.

8.4.2 p53 and Glutaminolysis

Glutamine, the most prevalent plasma amino acid, serves as a key energy source for both the citric acid cycle and the malate shuttle system [126]. Glutamine is crucial for sustaining cellular energy production, neutralizing ROS, synthesizing nucleotides and proteins, and activating cell signaling pathways. The process of converting glutamine to glutamate is referred to as glutaminolysis [127]. A crucial enzyme in this process is mitochondria glutamine synthesis (GLS), which transforms glutamine to glutamate and participates in regulating glutathione (GSH) production thereby supporting oxidative stress protection and energy generation. Glutamic acid is subsequently transformed into 2-oxoglutarate (α-KG) through the action of glutamate dehydrogenase (GLUD) or the action of transaminases such as glutamate oxaloacetate transaminase (GOT), glutamate pyruvate transaminase (GPT), and phosphoserine transaminase (PSAT) [128]. Some tumor cells exhibit increased levels of activity in glutamine syntheses (GS), an enzyme responsible for converting glutamic acid to 2-aminoglutaramic acid [129].

In cancer, the glutamine metabolic pathway is modified, featuring enhanced uptake and breakdown of 2-aminoglutaramic acid to generate adenosine triphosphate and lactic acid [130]. p53 regulates glutamine catabolism by controlling GLS2, which decreases cellular susceptibility to ROS-induced cell death in a manner regulated by p53 [131]. p53 modulates TCA cycle activity by inhibiting malic enzymes, which results in accelerated cell senescence [132]. In breast cancer tissue, SIRT4 expression is elevated in samples that are p53-positive [133], and the loss of SIRT4 enhances glutamine catabolism by promoting ADP-ribosylation and repressing GLUD [134, 135]. In pancreatic ductal adenocarcinoma (PDAC), inhibiting SIRT4 promotes the phosphorylation of p53, thereby decreasing tumor development [136].

p53 alters carbohydrate and amino acid metabolism to prioritize the buildup of alpha-ketoglutarate (α-KG) over succinate. Reintroducing p53 in PDAC cells with KRAS mutations boosts α-KG levels, enhancing the chromatin's 5-hydroxymethylcytosine (5-hmC) [137]. p53 triggers transcriptional patterns associated with premalignant differentiation and supplementing with α-KG can partially mimic this effect. The absence of p53 hinders these metabolic changes, resulting in more aggressive carcinomas with diminished α-KG-dependent functions [138]. Maintaining genomic stability relies on the collaboration between p53 and SIRT1, where SIRT1-mediated deacetylation of p53 governs cell destiny during oxidative stress [139, 140]. Therefore, p53 connects cancer cell metabolism, chromatin control, and the destiny of tumor cells.

Cancer cells frequently encounter shortages of nutrients and oxygen, like the diminished levels of glutamine observed in tumors. p53 mobilizes proteins to bolster its physiological role, resulting in variations in cell responses to glutamine depletion based on p53 activity [141]. p53 aids cancer cells in adjusting to glutamine deficiency, as cells lacking p53 fail to sustain the TCA cycle when faced with such circumstances. Additionally, p53 ensures the utilization of aspartate during glutamine scarcity by boosting SLC1A3, a transporter for aspartate and glutamate [142], essential for sustaining the electron transport chain and TCA cycle function, which supports de novo synthesis of glutamate, glutamine, and nucleotides to restore cell viability. Depleting TP53-regulated inhibitor of apoptosis, results in strong p53-regulated resilience to physiological pressure when glutamine is scarce [143]. Therefore, p53 exhibits dual roles in glutaminolysis, functioning as both a facilitator and an inhibitor depending on context.

8.4.3 p53 Controls Lipid Metabolism

Lipids, which include fatty acids, phospholipids, sterols, and glycolipids, serve crucial functions as components of cell membranes, sources of energy, and signaling molecules [144, 145]. To support their rapid proliferation, cancer cells boost the production of new lipids and uptake more lipids [120, 146]. However, p53 can counteract these effects by activating important proteins involved in lipid breakdown, thus leading to the deprivation of essential lipids for cancer cells. In patients diagnosed with breast cancer, those with normal p53 exhibited increased amounts of fatty acid binding protein 4 (FABP4), perilipin 1 (PLIN1), and monoglyceroid lipase (MGLL), and lower levels of fatty acid binding protein 5 (FABP5) compared to patients with altered p53 [147]. p53 modulates lipid metabolism by triggering the activity of guanidinoacetate methyltransferase (GAMT), thus amplifying fatty acid oxidation (FAO) and the synthesis of creatine, essential for sustaining energy equilibrium during glucose deficiency [148]. During malnutrition, the activation of GAMT by p53 leads to increased energy usage and induces programmed cell death. Peroxisome proliferator-activated receptor-gamma coactivator (PGC)-1 alpha, a controller of lipid metabolism, attaches to the p53 gene regulatory region, facilitating cell cycle arrest and the scavenging of oxygen radicals during glucose deprivation [149]. Furthermore, p53 enhances the expression of carnitine acyltransferases (CROT, CPT1A, and CPT1C) and malonyl-CoA decarboxylase (MCD) [150], and lipid 1 (LPIN1) in response to nutrient scarcity, aiding in the transport of fatty acids into mitochondria [151]. In colorectal cancer, p53 enhances paroxysmal fatty acid β-oxidation, which raises cytosolic acetyl-CoA levels and increases the acetylation of ATIC, an enzyme involved in purine synthesis. In colorectal cancer, p53 boosts paroxysmal fatty acid β-oxidation, leading to higher cytosolic acetyl-CoA levels and greater ATIC acetylation processes, an enzyme critical for purine synthesis [152].

p53 indirectly hinders lipid production by transcriptionally suppressing sterol regulatory element-binding proteins (SREBPs), which are crucial transcription factors regulating genes involved in lipogenesis [153]. It restrains the synthesis of new fatty acids by lowering NADPH levels, which occurs through the inhibition of glucose-6-phosphate dehydrogenase (G6PD) [154]. p53 regulates cholesterol metabolism via the mevalonate pathway by increasing the expression of ABCA1. ABCA1 facilitates the movement of sterols from the cell surface to the endoplasmic reticulum and inhibits the maturation of SREBP-2 [155, 156].

Considering the significant role and common changes in lipid processing in malignant cells, focusing on the lipogenesis pathway could be essential for cancer detection, therapy, and prevention. The connection between p53 and lipid regulation might contribute to tumor inhibition by preserving the equilibrium between glycolysis and respiration and counteracting the metabolic alterations associated with tumorigenesis.

8.4.4 p53 in Amino Acid Metabolism

Human body utilizes 20 fundamental amino acids as the building blocks of peptides. Here, we focus on the amino acid residues influenced by TP53, including aspartic acid, asparagic acid, hydroxymethyl amino acid, 4-hydroxyphenylalanine, and proline. Asparagic acid can be generated from aspartate through the action of asparagine synthetase (ASNS), which is responsible for changing aspartate and glutamine into asparagine and glutamate. Blocking ASNS makes cancer cells more prone to apoptosis induced by glutamine deficiency, an intermediate condition that can be reversed by supplementing with asparagine, irrespective of TCA cycle anaplerosis [157]. In mice lacking p53, there is a notable elevation in asparagine levels, which promotes the proliferation of lymphomas. p53 directly regulates the expression of ASNS, and its absence disturbs the balance between aspartate and asparagine, resulting in the buildup of asparagine [158]. This describes why mice lacking p53 primarily develop lymphomas [25]. Cells that multiply quickly require abundant serine levels for protein synthesis and various building processes such as sphingolipid, nucleotide, NADPH, and GSH production [159]. Vousden and her collaborators [160] linked p53 to serine metabolism, showing that p53 supports cell survival during serine starvation by causing cell cycle arrest mediated by p21. This implies possible therapeutic strategies for treating p53-deficient tumors through serine depletion. Additionally, in melanoma cells cultured in a full medium, p53 suppresses PHGDH, a crucial enzyme involved in serine production [161]. Serine metabolism facilitates the production of purines through a metabolic pathway involving one-carbon units, with methylenetetrahydrofolate dehydrogenase (MTHFD2) frequently overexpressed in cancers. MTHFD2 is an enzyme found in the mitochondria that uses NAD(P)+ to convert 5,10-methylene tetrahydrofolate into 10-formyltetrahydrofolate, which is essential for purine biosynthesis [162]. The expression of MTHFD2 is strongly linked to the absence or alteration of p53, and MTHFD2 is directly controlled by p53 at the transcriptional level. Blocking MTHFD2 limits the production of NADPH and DNA, leading to DNA harm and programmed cell death in tumor cells lacking functional p53 or with p53 mutations [163]. Changes in tyrosine metabolism due to the absence of p53 affect the tumor microenvironment. In oral cavity squamous cell carcinomas (OCSCCs) carrying mutated p53, there is a higher density of adrenergic fibers, which contain tyrosine hydroxylase (TH), compared to tumors with normal p53. Changes in tyrosine metabolism due to the absence of p53 affect the tumor microenvironment. In OCSCCs carrying mutated p53, there is a higher density of adrenergic fibers, which contain TH, compared to tumors with normal p53 [164].

p53 governs proline metabolism, influencing the regeneration of NAD/NADP [165]. p53 activates proline dehydrogenase (PRODH)/proline oxidase (POX) and aldehyde dehydrogenase 4 (ALDH4), initiating the first and second steps of proline degradation, respectively [166]. This control affects cell redox status and p53-driven reactions. Consequently, p53 closely manages amino acid metabolism, influencing tumor growth by altering the tumor's surroundings, redox condition, and nutrient access.

8.4.5 p53 and Ferroptosis

Ferroptosis is an iron-mediated non-programmed cell demise that was discovered in 2012 through treatment with erastin, causing overoxidation of polyunsaturated fatty acids and oxidative stress [167, 168]. In the context of tumorigenesis, developmental processes, and resistance to drugs, glutathione peroxidase 4 (GPX4) and radical trapping antioxidants (RTAs) are instrumental in mediating this crucial mechanism [169, 170]. GPX4 inhibition is a proposed cancer therapy, though its effectiveness varies across cancer cells, exhibits resistance to ferroptosis, indicating the potential involvement of additional factors in mediating this process. p53 has a dual impact on ferroptosis, exerting both positive and negative influences through specific metabolic factors.

p53 enhances cellular susceptibility to ferroptosis. The p533KR mutant induces ferroptosis via SLC7A11 upon ROS-induced stress but fails to trigger cell cycle cessation, cell aging, and programmed cell death [35]. A mutant p53 lacking a functional transactivation domain fails to inhibit SLC7A11 and instead encourages ferroptosis [171]. p53 influences ferroptosis through epigenetic means, reducing SLC7A11 protein levels by modifying histone H2B at a specific location (lysine 120), known as H2Bub1, and facilitating the movement of USP7 into the cell nucleus [172]. Additionally, p53 triggers the activation of spermidine N1-acetyltransferase 1 (SAT1), a biocatalyst pivotal in polyamine metabolism. This activation results in lipid peroxidation, making cells more susceptible to ferroptosis, a process that inhibits tumor development in xenograft models [173]. Conversely, p53 can suppress ferroptosis. In colorectal cancer, p53 blocks the activity of dipeptidyl peptidase-4 (DPP4), which decreases the occurrence of ferroptosis [174]. p53 prompts the movement of DPP4 into the cell nucleus, where it functions as a partner in transcriptional processes [175]. Boosting p53 stability using the MDM2 inhibitor nutlin-3 delays the onset of ferroptosis in HT-1080 cells with normal p53 expression. However, its effectiveness is diminished in mitigating erastin2-triggered ferroptosis in p53-deficient H1299 cells and p53-altered T98G cells [176]. Dysfunctional p53, controlled by RRM1 and MDM2, hampers GPX4 activity and expression through the suppression of p21 protein [177]. In epithelial ovarian cancer, MEX3A aids in maintaining p53 stability, which suppresses ferroptosis and facilitates tumor growth [178], while CUL9 interacts with p53 to hinder erastin-triggered ferroptosis [179]. The diverse range of cell types and treatments investigated, combined with the dual nature of p53's roles, may account for the conflicting findings regarding p53's involvement in ferroptosis regulation. Fresh perspectives on ferroptosis are emerging, moving beyond traditional models. While classical ferroptosis relies on the activity of acyl-CoA synthetizes long-chain family member 4 (ACSL4) for GPX4 suppression, p53 activation influences ferroptosis independently of GPX4. Knocking down ALOX12 reduces ROS-induced stress, thereby diminishing p53-mediated ferroptosis and impeding p53-driven tumor growth in animal models, highlighting ALOX12's significance in p53-mediated ferroptosis. Notably, ALOX12 is not essential for ferroptosis induced by GPX4 inhibitors or erastin, suggesting that p53-mediated ferroptosis hinges on ALOX12 rather than ACSL4 [180]. The detoxification of peroxidized lipids by iPLA2β also hampers p53-induced ferroptosis independently of GPX4. Tumor cells lacking iPLA2β are vulnerable to p53-mediated ferroptosis, thereby enhancing p53-dependent tumor suppression in animal models. iPLA2β decreases levels of peroxidized membrane lipids by restraining ALOX12 protein levels. Targeting iPLA2β could offer a potential treatment approach for cancers with minimal toxicity concerns, as its absence doesn't impact normal tissue development or cell viability but is crucial for ROS-induced ferroptosis in tumor cells [181]. The intricate metabolic influences on ferroptosis highlight the importance of uncovering additional metabolic and non-metabolic pathways regulated by p53 that impact ferroptosis.

8.5 CONCLUSION

p53, the guardian tumor suppressor protein, plays a crucial role in the complex realm of controlling the cell cycle, especially concerning breast cancer. Its multifaceted role encompasses not only the orchestration of halting the cell cycle when faced with genetic damage, but also the modulation of pathways governing proliferation, apoptosis, and senescence. Through its diverse array of downstream effectors and interaction partners, p53 exerts a profound influence on the fate of mammary carcinoma cells, dictating whether they undergo growth arrest, repair, or apoptosis. However, the balance between p53 causing cells to stop dividing and grow in breast cancer is a nuanced interplay affected by a wide range of factors, including the cellular context, genetic alterations, and environmental cues. At the heart of p53's function lies its ability to integrate signals from both intrinsic and extrinsic sources, enabling it to make context-specific decisions regarding cell fate. Upon encountering cellular tension, such as genetic injury or tumorigenic signaling, p53 is triggered, starting a series of successive actions aimed at restoring genetic integrity and preventing aberrant cell proliferation. p53 mainly stops cell division at specific points in the cell cycle to prevent tumor growth. This pause allows for DNA repair or cell death if the damage is severe. In breast cancer, p53's control over cell cycle progression is vital due to the frequent p53 mutations and disruptions found in breast tumors. When p53 is normal, it helps prevent tumors by stopping cell growth and encouraging cell death. However, if there are mutations in the p53 gene, it can't function properly, leading to uncontrolled cell growth and genetic changes. Indeed, mutations in the p53 gene are frequently found among the gene alterations seen in mammary carcinoma, with a significant proportion of tumors harboring missense mutations that impair p53's tumor-suppressive functions. Despite the frequency of p53 gene changes in breast cancer, emerging evidence suggests that the impact of these mutations on cell cycle regulation is complex and context dependent. While some p53 mutants exhibit loss of function and promote tumor growth by abrogating cell cycle checkpoints, others acquire gain-of-function properties that confer pro-oncogenic effects, such as increased proliferation, invasion, and metastasis. Additionally, the cellular context, including the presence of other genetic alterations and the tumor microenvironment, can modulate the effects of p53 mutations on cell cycle dynamics in breast cancer. Furthermore, the regulation of p53 activity in breast cancer extends beyond genetic alterations to encompass a diverse array of protein modifications, protein associations, and regulatory pathways. For instance, the stability and activity of p53 are tightly controlled by an intricate network of ubiquitin ligases and deubiquitinases, which govern its proteasomal degradation and nuclear localization. Moreover, p53 interacts with numerous cofactors and signaling molecules, including Rb, p21, MDM2, and ATM, forming a complex regulatory network that fine-tunes its response to various stimuli. In light of the complexity surrounding p53 regulation in breast cancer, therapeutic strategies aimed at restoring p53 function or targeting its downstream effectors hold promise for the treatment of this disease. Several approaches have been explored, including small-molecule inhibitors of MDM2, which disrupt the interaction between MDM2 and p53, leading to the stabilization and activation of p53. Additionally, efforts to develop p53-reactivating compounds, such as PRIMA-1 and its derivatives, offer potential avenues for restoring p53 function in tumors harboring mutant p53. However, the clinical translation of p53-targeted therapies in breast cancer faces several challenges, including the need to select patients who are most likely to benefit from these treatments based on their p53 status and the development of resistance mechanisms. Moreover, the potential for off-target effects and toxicity remains a concern, highlighting the importance of carefully evaluating the efficacy and safety of p53-targeted therapies in clinical trials. In conclusion, the intricate interplay between p53 and cell cycle dynamics in breast cancer underscores the complexity of tumor biology and the challenges associated with developing effective therapeutic strategies. While p53 serves as a critical guardian of genomic integrity and a potent barrier against cancer development, its dysregulation in breast cancer can lead to diverse outcomes, ranging from tumor suppression to promotion. Understanding the molecular mechanisms governing p53 function and its regulation in breast cancer is essential for the development of targeted therapies that aim to restore p53's tumor-suppressive functions while minimizing potential adverse effects.

REFERENCES

1. Stewart, B.W. and P. Kleihues, *World cancer report*. Vol. 57. 2003. IARC press Lyon.
2. Sofi, S., et al., A comprehensive analysis of notch signaling genes in breast cancer: expression pattern and prognostic significance. *Advances in Cancer Biology-Metastasis*, 2023. **7**: p. 100104.
3. Mir, M.A., N. Jan, and S. Sofi, Introduction to Metronomic Chemotherapy, in *Novel Approaches in Metronomic Chemotherapy for Breast Cancer Treatment*. 2024, CRC Press. p. 1–14.
4. Jemal, A., et al., Annual report to the nation on the status of cancer, 1975–2014, featuring survival. *JNCI: Journal of the National Cancer Institute*, 2017. **109**(9): p. djx030.
5. Ghoncheh, M., Z. Pournamdar, and H. Salehiniya, Incidence and mortality and epidemiology of breast cancer in the world. *Asian Pacific Journal of Cancer Prevention*, 2016. **17**(sup3): p. 43–46.
6. Clarke, R., J.J. Tyson, and J.M. Dixon, Endocrine resistance in breast cancer–an overview and update. *Molecular and Cellular Endocrinology*, 2015. **418**: p. 220–234.
7. Mir, M.A., et al., Metronomics: toward personalized chemotherapy. *Novel Approaches in Metronomic Chemotherapy for Breast Cancer Treatment*, 2024. p. 99–119. https://doi.org/10.1201/9781032632674-8

8. Althuis, M.D., et al., Etiology of hormone receptor–defined breast cancer: a systematic review of the literature. *Cancer Epidemiology Biomarkers & Prevention*, 2004. **13**(10): p. 1558–1568.
9. Jan, N., et al., Metronomic chemotherapy and drug repurposing: a paradigm shift in oncology. *Heliyon*, 2024. https://doi.org/10.1016/j.heliyon.2024.e24670
10. Mir, M.A., et al., *Proteomics: Application of Next-Generation Proteomics in Cancer Research, in Proteomics*. 2023, Elsevier. p. 55–76.
11. Allred, D.C., Issues and updates: evaluating estrogen receptor-α, progesterone receptor, and HER2 in breast cancer. *Modern Pathology*, 2010. **23**: p. S52–S59.
12. Yersal, O. and S. Barutca, Biological subtypes of breast cancer: Prognostic and therapeutic implications. *World Journal of Clinical Oncology*, 2014. **5**(3): p. 412.
13. Ungerleider, N.A., et al., Breast cancer survival predicted by TP53 mutation status differs markedly depending on treatment. *Breast Cancer Research*, 2018. **20**: p. 1–8.
14. Desmedt, C., et al., Next-generation sequencing in breast cancer: first take home messages. *Current Opinion in Oncology*, 2012. **24**(6): p. 597–604.
15. Jan, N., et al., Targeting breast cancer stem cells through retinoids: a new hope for treatment. *Critical Reviews in Oncology/Hematology*, 2023: p. 104156.
16. Lai, H., et al., Spectrum of p53 tumor suppressor gene mutations and breast cancer survival. *Breast Cancer Research and Treatment*, 2004. **83**: p. 57–66.
17. Haq, B.U., et al., Targeting p53 misfolding conundrum by stabilizing agents and their analogs in breast cancer therapy: a comprehensive computational analysis. *Frontiers in Pharmacology*, 2024. **14**: p. 1333447.
18. Vousden, K.H. and K.M. Ryan, p53 and metabolism. *Nature Reviews Cancer*, 2009. **9**(10): p. 691–700.
19. Vousden, K.H. and C. Prives, Blinded by the light: the growing complexity of p53. *Cell*, 2009. **137**(3): p. 413–431.
20. Itahana, Y. and K. Itahana, Emerging roles of p53 family members in glucose metabolism. *International Journal of Molecular Sciences*, 2018. **19**(3): p. 776.
21. Gnanapradeepan, K., et al., The p53 tumor suppressor in the control of metabolism and ferroptosis. *Frontiers in Endocrinology*, 2018. **9**: p. 355592.
22. Vousden, K.H., Functions of p53 in metabolism and invasion. *Biochemical Society Transactions*, 2009. **37**(3): p. 511–517.
23. McGowan, E.M., Y. Lin, and D. Hatoum, Good guy or bad guy? The duality of wild-type p53 in hormone-dependent breast cancer origin, treatment, and recurrence. *Cancers*, 2018. **10**(6): p. 172.
24. Kruiswijk, F., C.F. Labuschagne, and K.H. Vousden, p53 in survival, death and metabolic health: a lifeguard with a licence to kill. *Nature Reviews Molecular Cell Biology*, 2015. **16**(7): p. 393–405.
25. Balint, E. and K. Vousden, Activation and activities of the p53 tumour suppressor protein. *British Journal of Cancer*, 2001. **85**(12): p. 1813–1823.
26. Jan, N., et al., Exploring the role of trifarotene against RAR-α: an investigation of expression pattern and clinicopathological significance of RAR-α in breast cancer. *Frontiers in Pharmacology*, 2024. **15**: p. 1361679.
27. Cairns, R.A., I.S. Harris, and T.W. Mak, Regulation of cancer cell metabolism. *Nature Reviews Cancer*, 2011. **11**(2): p. 85–95.
28. DeBerardinis, R.J., et al., The biology of cancer: metabolic reprogramming fuels cell growth and proliferation. *Cell Metabolism*, 2008. **7**(1): p. 11–20.
29. Cairns, R.A. and T.W. Mak, The current state of cancer metabolism. *Nature Reviews Cancer*, 2016. **16**(10): p. 613–614.
30. Liu, J., et al., Tumor suppressor p53 and its mutants in cancer metabolism. *Cancer Letters*, 2015. **356**(2): p. 197–203.
31. Berkers, C.R., et al., Metabolic regulation by p53 family members. *Cell Metabolism*, 2013. **18**(5): p. 617–633.
32. Matoba, S., et al., p53 regulates mitochondrial respiration. *Science*, 2006. **312**(5780): p. 1650–1653.
33. Vousden, K.H. and X. Lu, Live or let die: the cell's response to p53. *Nature Reviews Cancer*, 2002. **2**(8): p. 594–604.
34. Bieging, K.T., S.S. Mello, and L.D. Attardi, Unravelling mechanisms of p53-mediated tumour suppression. *Nature Reviews Cancer*, 2014. **14**(5): p. 359–370.
35. Khoo, K.H., C.S. Verma, and D.P. Lane, Drugging the p53 pathway: understanding the route to clinical efficacy. *Nature Reviews Drug discovery*, 2014. **13**(3): p. 217–236.
36. Lakin, N.D. and S.P. Jackson, Regulation of p53 in response to DNA damage. *Oncogene*, 1999. **18**(53): p. 7644–7655.
37. He, G., et al., Induction of p21 by p53 following DNA damage inhibits both Cdk4 and Cdk2 activities. *Oncogene*, 2005. **24**(18): p. 2929–2943.

38. Brooks, C.L. and W. Gu, New insights into p53 activation. *Cell Research*, 2010. **20**(6): p. 614–621.
39. Abbas, T. and A. Dutta, p21 in cancer: intricate networks and multiple activities. *Nature Reviews Cancer*, 2009. **9**(6): p. 400–414.
40. Musgrove, E.A., et al., Cyclin D as a therapeutic target in cancer. *Nature Reviews Cancer*, 2011. **11**(8): p. 558–572.
41. Poletto, M., et al., p53 coordinates base excision repair to prevent genomic instability. *Nucleic Acids Research*, 2016. **44**(7): p. 3165–3175.
42. Smith, M.L. and Y.R. Seo, p53 regulation of DNA excision repair pathways. *Mutagenesis*, 2002. **17**(2): p. 149–156.
43. Mir, M.A., M. Bashir, and N. Jan, The Role of Interleukin (IL)-6/IL-6 Receptor Axis in Cancer, in *Cytokine and Chemokine Networks in Cancer*. 2023, Springer. p. 137–164.
44. Muller, P.A. and K.H. Vousden, p53 mutations in cancer. *Nature Cell Biology*, 2013. **15**(1): p. 2–8.
45. Freed-Pastor, W.A. and C. Prives, Mutant p53: one name, many proteins. *Genes & Development*, 2012. **26**(12): p. 1268–1286.
46. Mir, M.A., et al., Imaging Techniques, Biomarkers, and Methods for Metronomic Chemotherapy, in *Novel Approaches in Metronomic Chemotherapy for Breast Cancer Treatment*. CRC Press. p. 58–71.
47. Bykov, V.J., et al., Restoration of the tumor suppressor function to mutant p53 by a low-molecular-weight compound. *Nature Medicine*, 2002. **8**(3): p. 282–288.
48. Green, D.R. and G. Kroemer, Cytoplasmic functions of the tumour suppressor p53. *Nature*, 2009. **458**(7242): p. 1127–1130.
49. Riley, T., et al., Transcriptional control of human p53-regulated genes. *Nature Reviews Molecular Cell Biology*, 2008. **9**(5): p. 402–412.
50. Menendez, D., A. Inga, and M.A. Resnick, The expanding universe of p53 targets. *Nature Reviews Cancer*, 2009. **9**(10): p. 724–737.
51. El-Deiry, W.S., et al., WAF1, a potential mediator of p53 tumor suppression. *Cell*, 1993. **75**(4): p. 817–825.
52. Mir, M.A., M. Rashid, and N. Jan, Cytokines and Chemokines in Tumor Growth and Progression, in *Cytokine and Chemokine Networks in Cancer*. 2023, Springer. p. 33–77.
53. Weinberg, R.L., et al., Comparative binding of p53 to its promoter and DNA recognition elements. *Journal of Molecular Biology*, 2005. **348**(3): p. 589–596.
54. Sofi, S., et al., Clinicopathological and prognostic significance of Bcl2 in breast cancer: a comprehensive in silico and in vitro study. *Saudi Journal of Biological Sciences*, 2023. **31**(2): p. 103916.
55. Mir, M.A., Sumaya, N. Jan, Implications of Chemokine Heterogenicity in Cancer Metastasis, in *Cytokine and Chemokine Networks in Cancer*. 2023, Springer. p. 115–136.
56. Harper, J.W., et al., The p21 Cdk-interacting protein Cip1 is a potent inhibitor of G1 cyclin-dependent kinases. *Cell*, 1993. **75**(4): p. 805–816.
57. Luo, Y., J. Hurwitz, and J. Massagué, Cell-cycle inhibition by independent CDK and PCNA binding domains in p21Cip1. *Nature*, 1995. **375**(6527): p. 159–161.
58. Deng, C., et al., Mice lacking p21CIP1/WAF1 undergo normal development, but are defective in G1 checkpoint control. *Cell*, 1995. **82**(4): p. 675–684.
59. Brugarolas, J., et al., Radiation-induced cell cycle arrest compromised by p21 deficiency. *Nature*, 1995. **377**(6549): p. 552–557.
60. Martín-Caballero, J., et al., Tumor susceptibility of p21 Waf1/Cip1-deficient mice. *Cancer Research*, 2001. **61**(16): p. 6234–6238.
61. Mir, M.A., A. Shabir, and N. Jan, Metronomic Chemotherapy in Breast Cancer, in *Novel Approaches in Metronomic Chemotherapy for Breast Cancer Treatment*. CRC Press. p. 72–86.
62. Clair, S.S., et al., DNA damage-induced downregulation of Cdc25C is mediated by p53 via two independent mechanisms: one involves direct binding to the cdc25C promoter. *Molecular Cell*, 2004. **16**(5): p. 725–736.
63. Chang, B.-D., et al., A senescence-like phenotype distinguishes tumor cells that undergo terminal proliferation arrest after exposure to anticancer agents. *Cancer Research*, 1999. **59**(15): p. 3761–3767.
64. He, L., et al., A microRNA component of the p53 tumour suppressor network. *Nature*, 2007. **447**(7148): p. 1130–1134.
65. Tarasov, V., et al., Differential regulation of microRNAs by p53 revealed by massively parallel sequencing: miR-34a is a p53 target that induces apoptosis and G1-arrest. *Cell Cycle*, 2007. **6**(13): p. 1586–1593.
66. Concepcion, C.P., et al., Intact p53-dependent responses in miR-34–deficient mice. *PLoS Genetics*, 2012. **8**(7): p. e1002797.
67. Jain, A.K. and M.C. Barton, Unmet expectations: miR-34 plays no role in p53-mediated tumor suppression in vivo. *PLoS Genetics*, 2012. https://doi.org/10.1371/journal.pgen.1002859

68. Sionov, R.V. and Y. Haupt, The cellular response to p53: the decision between life and death. *Oncogene*, 1999. **18**(45): p. 6145–6157.
69. Kubbutat, M.H., S.N. Jones, and K.H. Vousden, Regulation of p53 stability by Mdm2. *Nature*, 1997. **387**(6630): p. 299–303.
70. Honda, R., H. Tanaka, and H. Yasuda, Oncoprotein MDM2 is a ubiquitin ligase E3 for tumor suppressor p53. *FEBS Letters*, 1997. **420**(1): p. 25–27.
71. Lacroix, M., R.-A. Toillon, and G. Leclercq, p53 and breast cancer, an update. *Endocrine-Related Cancer*, 2006. **13**(2): p. 293–325.
72. El-Deiry, W.S., The role of p53 in chemosensitivity and radiosensitivity. *Oncogene*, 2003. **22**(47): p. 7486–7495.
73. Ws, E.-D., WAF1, a potential mediator of p53 tumor suppression. *Cell*, 1993. **75**: p. 817–825.
74. Shieh, S.-Y., et al., DNA damage-induced phosphorylation of p53 alleviates inhibition by MDM2. *Cell*, 1997. **91**(3): p. 325–334.
75. Hermeking, H., et al., 14–3-3σ is a p53-regulated inhibitor of G2/M progression. *Molecular Cell*, 1997. **1**(1): p. 3–11.
76. Smith, M.L., et al., Involvement of the p53 tumor suppressor in repair of uv-type DNA damage. *Oncogene*, 1995. **10**(6): p. 1053–1059.
77. Kh, V., Blinded by the light: the growing complexity of p53. *Cell.*, 2009. **137**: p. 413–431.
78. Mirzayans, R., et al., New insights into p53 signaling and cancer cell response to DNA damage: implications for cancer therapy. *BioMed Research International*, 2012. **2012**. https://doi.org/10.1155/2012/170325
79. Adimoolam, S. and J.M. Ford, p53 and regulation of DNA damage recognition during nucleotide excision repair. *DNA Repair*, 2003. **2**(9): p. 947–954.
80. Offer, H., et al., Direct involvement of p53 in the base excision repair pathway of the DNA repair machinery. *FEBS Letters*, 1999. **450**(3): p. 197–204.
81. Smith, G.C. and S.P. Jackson, The DNA-dependent protein kinase. *Genes & Development*, 1999. **13**(8): p. 916–934.
82. Sengupta, S., et al., Functional interaction between BLM helicase and 53BP1 in a Chk1-mediated pathway during S-phase arrest. *The Journal of Cell Biology*, 2004. **166**(6): p. 801–813.
83. Toshiyuki, M. and J.C. Reed, Tumor suppressor p53 is a direct transcriptional activator of the human bax gene. *Cell*, 1995. **80**(2): p. 293–299.
84. Nakano, K. and K.H. Vousden, PUMA, a novel proapoptotic gene, is induced by p53. *Molecular Cell*, 2001. **7**(3): p. 683–694.
85. Oda, E., et al., Noxa, a BH3-only member of the Bcl-2 family and candidate mediator of p53-induced apoptosis. *Science*, 2000. **288**(5468): p. 1053–1058.
86. Green, D.R. and G. Kroemer, The pathophysiology of mitochondrial cell death. *Science*, 2004. **305**(5684): p. 626–629.
87. Li, P., et al., Cytochrome c and dATP-dependent formation of Apaf-1/caspase-9 complex initiates an apoptotic protease cascade. *Cell*, 1997. **91**(4): p. 479–489.
88. Müller, M., et al., Drug-induced apoptosis in hepatoma cells is mediated by the CD95 (APO-1/Fas) receptor/ligand system and involves activation of wild-type p53. *The Journal of Clinical Investigation*, 1997. **99**(3): p. 403–413.
89. Sheikh, M.S. and A.J. Fornace, Death and decoy receptors and p53-mediated apoptosis. *Leukemia*, 2000. **14**(8): p. 1509–1513.
90. Chipuk, J.E., et al., Direct activation of Bax by p53 mediates mitochondrial membrane permeabilization and apoptosis. *Science*, 2004. **303**(5660): p. 1010–1014.
91. Haupt, Y., et al., Mdm2 promotes the rapid degradation of p53. *Nature*, 1997. **387**(6630): p. 296–299.
92. MH, K., Regulation of p53 stability by Mdm2. *Nature*, 1997. **387**: p. 299–303.
93. Canman, C.E., et al., Activation of the ATM kinase by ionizing radiation and phosphorylation of p53. *Science*, 1998. **281**(5383): p. 1677–1679.
94. Gu, W. and R.G. Roeder, Activation of p53 sequence-specific DNA binding by acetylation of the p53 C-terminal domain. *Cell*, 1997. **90**(4): p. 595–606.
95. Liu, L., et al., p53 sites acetylated in vitro by PCAF and p300 are acetylated in vivo in response to DNA damage. *Molecular and Cellular Biology*, 1999. **19**(2): p. 1202–1209.
96. Zhang, Y., Y. Xiong, and W.G. Yarbrough, ARF promotes MDM2 degradation and stabilizes p53: ARF-INK4a locus deletion impairs both the Rb and p53 tumor suppression pathways. *Cell*, 1998. **92**(6): p. 725–734.

97. Dornan, D., et al., The ubiquitin ligase COP1 is a critical negative regulator of p53. *Nature*, 2004. **429**(6987): p. 86–92.
98. Leng, R.P., et al., Pirh2, a p53-induced ubiquitin-protein ligase, promotes p53 degradation. *Cell*, 2003. **112**(6): p. 779–791.
99. He, L., et al., microRNAs join the p53 network—another piece in the tumour-suppression puzzle. *Nature Reviews Cancer*, 2007. 7(11): p. 819–822.
100. Barak, Y., et al., mdm2 expression is induced by wild type p53 activity. *The EMBO Journal*, 1993. **12**(2): p. 461–468.
101. Rodriguez, M.S., et al., SUMO-1 modification activates the transcriptional response of p53. *The EMBO Journal*, 1999. 18: p. 6455–6461.
102. Xirodimas, D.P., et al., Mdm2-mediated NEDD8 conjugation of p53 inhibits its transcriptional activity. *Cell*, 2004. **118**(1): p. 83–97.
103. Serrano, M., et al., Oncogenic ras provokes premature cell senescence associated with accumulation of p53 and p16INK4a. *Cell*, 1997. **88**(5): p. 593–602.
104. Campisi, J., Senescent cells, tumor suppression, and organismal aging: good citizens, bad neighbors. *Cell*, 2005. **120**(4): p. 513–522.
105. Coppé, J., et al., Senescence-associated secretory phenotypes reveal cell-nonautonomous functions of oncogenic RAS. *PLoS Biology*, 2008. https://doi.org/10.1371/journal.pbio.0060301
106. Fujita, K., et al., Positive feedback between p53 and TRF2 during telomere-damage signalling and cellular senescence. *Nature Cell Biology*, 2010. **12**(12): p. 1205–1212.
107. Fagagna, F.d.A.d., et al., A DNA damage checkpoint response in telomere-initiated senescence. *Nature*, 2003. **426**(6963): p. 194–198.
108. Krizhanovsky, V., et al., Senescence of activated stellate cells limits liver fibrosis. *Cell*, 2008. **134**(4): p. 657–667.
109. Hollstein, M., et al., p53 mutations in human cancers. *Science*, 1991. **253**(5015): p. 49–53.
110. Levine, A.J. and M. Oren, The first 30 years of p53: growing ever more complex. *Nature Reviews Cancer*, 2009. **9**(10): p. 749–758.
111. Tanaka, H., et al., A ribonucleotide reductase gene involved in a p53-dependent cell-cycle checkpoint for DNA damage. *Nature*, 2000. **404**(6773): p. 42–49.
112. Tan, T. and G. Chu, p53 Binds and activates the xeroderma pigmentosum DDB2 gene in humans but not mice. *Molecular and Cellular Biology*, 2002. **22**: p. 3247–3254.
113. Bensaad, K., et al., TIGAR, a p53-inducible regulator of glycolysis and apoptosis. *Cell*, 2006. **126**(1): p. 107–120.
114. Budanov, A.V., et al., Regeneration of peroxiredoxins by p53-regulated sestrins, homologs of bacterial AhpD. *Science*, 2004. **304**(5670): p. 596–600.
115. Mukhopadhyay, D., et al., Hypoxic induction of human vascular endothelial growth factor expression through c-Src activation. *Nature*, 1995. **375**(6532): p. 577–581.
116. Dameron, K., et al. *The p53 Tumor Suppressor Gene Inhibits Angiogenesis by Stimulating the Production of Thrombospondin in Cold Spring Harbor Symposia on Quantitative Biology*. 1994. Cold Spring Harbor Laboratory Press.
117. Mao, Y. and P. Jiang, The crisscross between p53 and metabolism in cancer: The crisscross between p53 and metabolism in cancer. *Acta Biochimica et Biophysica Sinica*, 2023. **55**(6): p. 914.
118. Linzer, D. and A. Levine, Characterization of a 54K dalton cellular SV40 tumour antigen present in SV40 transformed cells and uninfected embryonal carcinoma cells. *Cell*, 1979. **17**: p. 43–52.
119. Dolgin, E., The most popular genes in the human genome. *Nature*, 2017. **551**(7681): p. 427–432.
120. Zeng, J., et al., Cyclin E-induced replicative stress drives p53-dependent whole-genome duplication. *Cell*, 2023. **186**(3): p. 528–542.e14.
121. Li, L., et al., p53 regulation of ammonia metabolism through urea cycle controls polyamine biosynthesis. *Nature*, 2019. **567**(7747): p. 253–256.
122. Kamphorst, J.J., et al., Human pancreatic cancer tumors are nutrient poor and tumor cells actively scavenge extracellular protein. *Cancer Research*, 2015. **75**(3): p. 544–553.
123. Moreadith, R., and A. Lehninger, The pathways of glutamate and glutamine oxidation by tumor cell mitochondria. Role of mitochondrial NAD (P)+-dependent malic enzyme. *Journal of Biological Chemistry*, 1984. **259**(10): p. 6215–6221.
124. Yang, L., S. Venneti, and D. Nagrath, Glutaminolysis: a hallmark of cancer metabolism. *Annual Review of Biomedical Engineering*, 2017. **19**: p. 163–194.
125. Tardito, S., et al., Glutamine synthetase activity fuels nucleotide biosynthesis and supports growth of glutamine-restricted glioblastoma. *Nature Cell Biology*, 2015. **17**(12): p. 1556–1568.

126. Reitzer, L.J., W. BM, and D. Kennel, Evidence that glutamine, not sugar, is the major energy source for cultured HeLa cells. *Journal of Biological Chemistry*, 1979. **254**: p. 2569–2676.
127. Suzuki, S., et al., Phosphate-activated glutaminase (GLS2), a p53-inducible regulator of glutamine metabolism and reactive oxygen species. *Proceedings of the National Academy of Sciences*, 2010. **107**(16): p. 7461–7466.
128. Jiang, P., et al., Reciprocal regulation of p53 and malic enzymes modulates metabolism and senescence. *Nature*, 2013. **493**(7434): p. 689–693.
129. Shi, Q., et al., Decreased sirtuin 4 expression is associated with poor prognosis in patients with invasive breast cancer. *Oncology Letters*, 2016. **12**(4): p. 2606–2612.
130. Csibi, A., et al., The mTORC1 pathway stimulates glutamine metabolism and cell proliferation by repressing SIRT4. *Cell*, 2013. **153**(4): p. 840–854.
131. Jeong, S.M., et al., SIRT4 has tumor-suppressive activity and regulates the cellular metabolic response to DNA damage by inhibiting mitochondrial glutamine metabolism. *Cancer Cell*, 2013. **23**(4): p. 450–463.
132. Li, J., et al., Sirtuin 4 activates autophagy and inhibits tumorigenesis by upregulating the p53 signaling pathway. *Cell Death & Differentiation*, 2023. **30**(2): p. 313–326.
133. Xiao, M., et al., Inhibition of α-KG-dependent histone and DNA demethylases by fumarate and succinate that are accumulated in mutations of FH and SDH tumor suppressors. *Genes & Development*, 2012. **26**(12): p. 1326–1338.
134. Wong, J., C. Gambrah-Sampaney, and L. Adang, Teaching NeuroImages: Cranial neuropathies following clival infarction. *Neurology*, 2019. **93**(10): p. e1031–e1031.
135. Wang, R.-H., et al., Impaired DNA damage response, genome instability, and tumorigenesis in SIRT1 mutant mice. *Cancer Cell*, 2008. **14**(4): p. 312–323.
136. Yi, J. and J. Luo, SIRT1 and p53, effect on cancer, senescence and beyond. *Biochimica et Biophysica Acta (BBA)-Proteins and Proteomics*, 2010. **1804**(8): p. 1684–1689.
137. Cetinbas, N.M., et al., Glucose-dependent anaplerosis in cancer cells is required for cellular redox balance in the absence of glutamine. *Scientific Reports*, 2016. **6**(1): p. 32606.
138. Tajan, M., et al., A role for p53 in the adaptation to glutamine starvation through the expression of SLC1A3. *Cell Metabolism*, 2018. **28**(5): p. 721–736.e6.
139. Nedara, K., et al., Relevance of the TRIAP1/p53 axis in colon cancer cell proliferation and adaptation to glutamine deprivation. *Frontiers in Oncology*, 2022. **12**: p. 958155.
140. Parrales, A. and T. Iwakuma, p53 as a regulator of lipid metabolism in cancer. *International journal of Molecular Sciences*, 2016. **17**(12): p. 2074.
141. Chen, Y. and P. Li, 脂肪酸代谢与癌症发生. *Science Bulletin*, 2016. **61**: p. 1473–1479.
142. Roingeard, P. and R.C. Melo, Lipid droplet hijacking by intracellular pathogens. *Cellular Microbiology*, 2017. **19**(1): p. e12688.
143. Koundouros, N. and G. Poulogiannis, Reprogramming of fatty acid metabolism in cancer. *British Journal of Cancer*, 2020. **122**(1): p. 4–22.
144. Yousuf, U., et al., Identification and analysis of dysregulated fatty acid metabolism genes in breast cancer subtypes. *Medical Oncology*, 2022. **39**(12): p. 256.
145. Borude, P., et al., Pleiotropic role of p53 in injury and liver regeneration after acetaminophen overdose. *The American Journal of Pathology*, 2018. **188**(6): p. 1406–1418.
146. Sen, N., Y.K. Satija, and S. Das, PGC-1α, a key modulator of p53, promotes cell survival upon metabolic stress. *Molecular Cell*, 2011. **44**(4): p. 621–634.
147. Sanchez-Macedo, N., et al., Depletion of the novel p53-target gene carnitine palmitoyltransferase 1C delays tumor growth in the neurofibromatosis type I tumor model. *Cell Death & Differentiation*, 2013. **20**(4): p. 659–668.
148. Liu, Y., et al., Ribosomal protein–Mdm2–p53 pathway coordinates nutrient stress with lipid metabolism by regulating MCD and promoting fatty acid oxidation. *Proceedings of the National Academy of Sciences*, 2014. **111**(23): p. E2414–E2422.
149. Zhao, J., et al., p53 promotes peroxisomal fatty acid β-oxidation to repress purine biosynthesis and mediate tumor suppression. *Cell Death & Disease*, 2023. **14**(2): p. 87.
150. Yahagi, N., et al., p53 Activation in adipocytes of obese mice. *Journal of Biological Chemistry*, 2003. **278**(28): p. 25395–25400.
151. Jiang, P., et al., p53 regulates biosynthesis through direct inactivation of glucose-6-phosphate dehydrogenase. *Nature Cell Biology*, 2011. **13**(3): p. 310–316.
152. Moon, S.-H., et al., p53 represses the mevalonate pathway to mediate tumor suppression. *Cell*, 2019. **176**(3): p. 564–580.e19.
153. Panatta, E., et al., Understanding p53 tumour suppressor network. *Biology Direct*, 2021. **16**(1): p. 14.

154. Zhang, J., et al., Asparagine plays a critical role in regulating cellular adaptation to glutamine depletion. *Molecular Cell*, 2014. **56**(2): p. 205–218.
155. Deng, L., et al., p53-mediated control of aspartate-asparagine homeostasis dictates LKB1 activity and modulates cell survival. *Nature Communications*, 2020. **11**(1): p. 1755.
156. Harvey, M., et al., Spontaneous and carcinogen–induced tumorigenesis in p53–deficient mice. *Nature Genetics*, 1993. **5**(3): p. 225–229.
157. Labuschagne, C.F., et al., Serine, but not glycine, supports one-carbon metabolism and proliferation of cancer cells. *Cell Reports*, 2014. **7**(4): p. 1248–1258.
158. Maddocks, O.D., et al., Serine starvation induces stress and p53-dependent metabolic remodelling in cancer cells. *Nature*, 2013. **493**(7433): p. 542–546.
159. Christensen, K.E. and R.E. MacKenzie, Mitochondrial methylenetetrahydrofolate dehydrogenase, methenyltetrahydrofolate cyclohydrolase, and formyltetrahydrofolate synthetases. *Vitamins & Hormones*, 2008. **79**: p. 393–410.
160. Maddocks, O.D., et al., Serine starvation induces stress and p53-dependent metabolic remodelling in cancer cells. *Nature*, 2013. **493**(7433): p. 542–546.
161. Amit, M., et al., Loss of p53 drives neuron reprogramming in head and neck cancer. *Nature*, 2020. **578**(7795): p. 449–454.
162. Phang, J.M., Proline metabolism in cell regulation and cancer biology: recent advances and hypotheses. *Antioxidants & Redox Signaling*, 2019. **30**(4): p. 635–649.
163. Lacroix, M., et al., Metabolic functions of the tumor suppressor p53: Implications in normal physiology, metabolic disorders, and cancer. *Molecular Metabolism*, 2020. **33**: p. 2–22.
164. Dixon, S.J., et al., Ferroptosis: an iron-dependent form of nonapoptotic cell death. *Cell*, 2012. **149**(5): p. 1060–1072.
165. Hassannia, B., P. Vandenabeele, and T.V. Berghe, Targeting ferroptosis to iron out cancer. *Cancer cell*, 2019. **35**(6): p. 830–849.
166. Yang, W.S., et al., Regulation of ferroptotic cancer cell death by GPX4. *Cell*, 2014. **156**(1): p. 317–331.
167. Shah, R., M.S. Shchepinov, and D.A. Pratt, Resolving the role of lipoxygenases in the initiation and execution of ferroptosis. *ACS Central Science*, 2018. **4**(3): p. 387–396.
168. Zou, Y., et al., A GPX4-dependent cancer cell state underlies the clear-cell morphology and confers sensitivity to ferroptosis. *Nature Communications*, 2019. **10**(1): p. 1617.
169. Jiang, L., et al., Dynamic roles of p53-mediated metabolic activities in ROS-induced stress responses. *Cell Cycle*, 2015. **14**(18): p. 2881–2885.
170. Wang, Y., et al., Epigenetic regulation of ferroptosis by H2B monoubiquitination and p53. *EMBO Reports*, 2019. **20**(7): p. e47563.
171. Ou, Y., et al., Activation of SAT1 engages polyamine metabolism with p53-mediated ferroptotic responses. *Proceedings of the National Academy of Sciences*, 2016. **113**(44): p. E6806–E6812.
172. Yamada, K., et al., Nuclear localization of CD26 induced by a humanized monoclonal antibody inhibits tumor cell growth by modulating of POLR2A transcription. *PloS One*, 2013. **8**(4): p. e62304.
173. Xie, Y., et al., The tumor suppressor p53 limits ferroptosis by blocking DPP4 activity. *Cell Reports*, 2017. **20**(7): p. 1692–1704.
174. Tarangelo, A., et al., p53 suppresses metabolic stress-induced ferroptosis in cancer cells. *Cell Reports*, 2018. **22**(3): p. 569–575.
175. Gao, Y., et al., Knockdown of RRM1 in tumor cells promotes radio-/chemotherapy induced ferroptosis by regulating p53 ubiquitination and p21-GPX4 signaling axis. *Cell Death Discovery*, 2022. **8**(1): p. 343.
176. Wang, C.-K., et al., MEX3A mediates p53 degradation to suppress ferroptosis and facilitate ovarian cancer tumorigenesis. *Cancer Research*, 2023. **83**(2): p. 251–263.
177. Yang, L., et al., Cullin-9/p53 mediates HNRNPC degradation to inhibit erastin-induced ferroptosis and is blocked by MDM2 inhibition in colorectal cancer. *Oncogene*, 2022. **41**(23): p. 3210–3221.
178. Chu, B., et al., ALOX12 is required for p53-mediated tumour suppression through a distinct ferroptosis pathway. *Nature Cell Biology*, 2019. **21**(5): p. 579–591.
179. Chen, D., et al., iPLA2β-mediated lipid detoxification controls p53-driven ferroptosis independent of GPX4. *Nature Communications*, 2021. **12**(1): p. 3644.
180. Newman, A.C. and O.D. Maddocks, One-carbon metabolism in cancer. *British Journal of Cancer*, 2017. **116**(12): p. 1499–1504.
181. Chen, S., et al., Arsenic trioxide rescues structural p53 mutations through a cryptic allosteric site. *Cancer Cell*, 2021. **39**(2): p. 225–239.

9 The Complex Interplay between Mutant p53, p63, and p73 and Their Effects on the Cellular Process

*Saima Gul, Nusrat Jan, Sadaf Qadir, and Manzoor Ahmad Mir**

Department of Bioresources, School of Biological Sciences, University of Kashmir, Srinagar, J&K, India
*drmanzoor@kashmiruniversity.ac.in

9.1 INTRODUCTION

Genes are like little pieces of information that get passed down from parents to children. They are made up of DNA and are located on chromosomes in our cells. Genes contain instructions for making proteins that determine functions like hair color or eye color. Then we talk about the tumor suppressor gene. The two homologs of the tumor-suppressing transcription factor p53 are p73 and p63. Because the p53 family members share a high degree of structural similarity, most p53-responsive promoters can be bound by p73 and p63 to activate transcription. In addition to having similar activities to p53 (inducing apoptosis in response to cellular stress), p63 and p73 have distinct responsibilities due to the wide structural heterogeneity within the family. The p63 and p73 knockout mice phenotypes serve as excellent examples of their unique and vital roles in regulating development and differentiation. We're going to talk about how p63 and p73 play a role in human diseases, especially in how tumors form and spread. Let's dive into how these proteins impact the development and spread of cancer. Related to the tumor suppressor p53 are p73 and p63. These transcription factors, which have a longer evolutionary history, mostly aid development but can also aid in the formation of tumors [1]. So, p63 and p73 are like cousins to the tumor-suppressing transcription factor p53. They have similar structures and functions, which means they can do a lot of the same stuff as p53. They can form groups, attach to DNA, activate genes that p53 responds to, and help with things like stopping the cell cycle, aging cells, and causing cell death when there's DNA damage [2]. So, because of some fancy splicing stuff happening at the last of p63 and p73, and thanks to this special promoter thing in the middle, they come in different versions with similar or even opposite effects. The full-length versions, called Tap63 and Tap73, have this cool transactivation part that makes them act a lot like p53, with similar targets and functions. But wait, there's more! These proteins can also be spliced in different ways, creating versions without the transactivation part, called ΔN isoforms. These can't activate genes themselves, but they can stop the active versions from doing their thing. So, because of all this complexity, p63 and p73 have different structures and can do different stuff, which makes them super flexible and diverse in what they can do [3]. When it comes to p63 and p73, they have similar functions to p53 in controlling cancer development. But when not under stress, their main job is to regulate differentiation and growth. Specifically, p63 is crucial for the development of certain types of tissues, while p73 is essential for neuronal differentiation and

DOI: 10.1201/9781003520771-9

building the nervous and olfactory systems. If mice lack p63 and p73, they can have serious developmental issues like missing limbs, skin, hair, teeth, and various glands and complex abnormalities in neural development [3]. The disruption within the p53 protein family can have a big impact on the development of humans [4, 5]. When there's an imbalance in the levels or functions of p63, p73, and p53, it can contribute to a large number of congenital developmental abnormalities. These abnormalities can affect various aspects of human development. For example, if there's an issue with p63, which is responsible for the development of squamous epithelia and its derivatives, it can lead to problems with the formation of skin, hair, teeth, and other related structures. Conversely, p73 plays a critical role in neuronal differentiation and is essential for the development of the nervous and olfactory systems. If affected, it can result in issues with the development of the brain, nerves, and sense of smell. The imbalances within the p53 protein family can have far-reaching consequences. These factors can lead to significant limb shortening and the lack of skin, hair, and teeth, and even the malfunctioning of important glands like the mammary, lachrymal, and salivary glands. These developmental abnormalities highlight the critical roles that p63, p73, and p53 play in shaping our bodies during embryonic development [6].

The transcription factor p53 is often called the "guardian of the genome" because of its crucial role in preventing the formation and progression of tumors. It acts as a powerful tumor suppressor, working hard to maintain the integrity and stability of our genetic material. By regulating the expression of various genes, p53 helps to prevent the accumulation of DNA damage and the development of abnormal cells that could potentially lead to cancer. So, you can think of p53 as a superhero safeguarding our genetic information and keeping our cells in check [7, 8]. When our cells encounter various types of stress, p53 springs into action! It responds to a wide array of cellular stresses, which can include DNA damage, oxidative stress, nutrient deprivation, and even viral infections. Whenever our cells are faced with something that could potentially harm our DNA or disrupt normal cellular processes, p53 steps up to protect us. It's like having a vigilant guardian who constantly monitors the health of our cells and activates appropriate responses to maintain their well-being. So, whether it's a physical or chemical stressor, p53 is always on the lookout and ready to defend our genome [9, 10]. When cells are permanently injured, p53 either induces cell cycle arrest and DNA repair to maintain the genome or leads them to apoptosis [11–13]. It's not shocking that the most frequent genetic change in human tumors is when p53 gets turned off due to mutations [14]. Scientists believed that p53 was unique, but then they discovered p63 and p73, two other important proteins with similar functions [15, 16]. p63 and p73 are pretty interesting because they have modular structures that are quite similar to p53. They also have a high degree of homology with each other, which means they share common features in their genetic sequences [17–19]. Both p63 and p73 have a significant overlap with p53 when it comes to their target genes. They share common genes involved in important cellular processes like apoptosis (programmed cell death) and cell cycle arrest. While their primary functions may not be identical to p53, their ability to regulate these genes makes them potent tumor suppressor genes as well [20, 21]. TP53, TP63, and TP73 genes produce various isoforms with different N-terminal (TA, FL, ΔN) and C-terminal (α, β, γ) sequences. These alternative combinations give rise to a wide range of protein variants, each with its unique functions and characteristics [6]. The function of TP53, TP63, and TP73 in determining cell fate is carefully coordinated. Their functions are influenced by factors like where they are located in specific tissues, how much they are expressed, and the precise timing of their regulation. This intricate orchestration ensures that these proteins play their roles effectively in different cellular contexts [22–24]. Unlike many other tumor suppressor genes that are often lost during the development of tumors, p53 is interestingly still expressed. However, it is frequently affected by missense mutations, which can alter its function. Scientists have pinpointed seven particular mutation hotspots that are closely associated with a negative outlook for patients [25–27]. Some mutations in p53 are called "dominant-negative" because they can disrupt the cancer-fighting ability of the regular, wild-type p53 gene that's there. These mutations essentially hinder the ability of the remaining p53 to carry out its protective role against tumor development [28–30]. Various theories have been suggested to explain how p53 dominant-negative mutations can impact WT (wild-type) p53 function, such as (i) a situation where mutations or different forms decrease the number of spots where the regular protein can attach or the helpers it needs to work properly [31], (ii) when you have these mixed groups with both normal and mutant p53 proteins that are inactive together, or (iii) it's similar to a prion-like scenario where a changed p53 protein causes the normal one to change shape and become inactive [32, 33] Despite the rarity of p63 and p73 mutations in malignancies [32], the expression pattern of these isoforms is drastically dysregulated. It appears that the various isoforms' ratio of expression levels determines how tumor-suppressive they are [34]. Even though TA/FL isoforms are generally thought of as tumor suppressors, some research has indicated that these factors contribute to cancer causing effects through dominant-negative actions, while other studies have shown they remain active in transcription. Their ΔN counterparts, like ΔN-p63 crucial for skin development or ΔN-p73 for neural development, are linked to tumorigenesis. Although the exact role of these isoforms in cancer formation is still unclear, the ongoing discovery of these variations has shown a new level of complexity in the p53 family [23, 35, 36]. Yeast is being used a lot to study p53 family members because of FASAY, which lets scientists check how well human p53 works in yeast [37]. FASAY uses altered yeast strains with a gene regulated by a specific p53 response element to evaluate the functionality of human p53 within yeast cells, aiding in studying how p53 interacts with DNA. Furthermore, due to the absence of a p53 orthologue, yeast is a naive eukaryotic system with regard to p53. Thus, FASAY has made it possible to identify p53 mutations that cause tumor-derived loss of function [38], and afterward the identification of p53 dominant-negative mutations [13, 39]. Yeast is a popular choice for studying p53 family members due to FASAY, enabling human p53 evaluation in yeast. FASAY has successfully assessed p63 and p73 transactivity, leveraging the shared DNA-binding domains of p53, p63, and p73 for these studies [29]. Using FASAY strains, we looked into how seven common p53 mutations and 24 different forms of p53, p63, and p73 affect each other. We found that only inactive p53 mutations and isoforms that can group together in tetramers can weaken the normal p53-WT activity. This weakening happens because these mutants disrupt the tetramer formation. Our study indicates that the inhibitory effects of the examined p53 and p73 proteins are not related to a prion-like process. We also discovered that the mutant p53-R175H gains the ability to interact with p63 and p73, mainly through tetramerization [40].

9.2 MUTATION IN THE p53 GENE

The transformation of a healthy cell into a cancerous one is an intricate process. It encompasses various genetic and epigenetic modifications that provide the mutated cells with specific benefits. These changes allow the evolving tumor to grow independently, ignore signals that would normally stop its growth, evade programmed cell death, replicate endlessly, stimulate the formation of new blood vessels, and eventually invade other tissues and spread throughout the body. It's like the tumor gains special abilities along the way [41]. Even with extensive research and remarkable advancements, the biomedical community still faces a significant challenge in fully comprehending the molecular complexities of cancer. In 1947, Isaac Berenblum and Philippe Shubik made a pivotal discovery regarding chemical carcinogenesis, identifying two distinct stages: initiation and promotion. Initiation refers to the initial genetic alterations that set the stage for cancer development, while promotion involves the subsequent growth and progression of the tumor. This groundbreaking finding shed light on the multistep nature of cancer formation and has paved the way for further investigations into understanding and combating this complex disease [42]. Around 20 years back, a scientist named Knudson put forth a theory called the "Knudson two-hit hypothesis" to explain tumor development. This theory focused on retinoblastoma and suggested a genetic model. It proposed that the first "hit" is an inherited mutation in the RB gene, while the second "hit" is a mutation specific to the tumor. The model was broadened to integrate more genetic changes, such as deactivating tumor suppressor genes and activating oncogenes, as extra factors in the progression. This theory offered a valuable understanding of the genetic elements influencing the onset of specific cancer types [43, 44]. Out of all the genes involved in the development of tumors, one particular gene called TP53, which encodes the p53 transcription factor, plays a crucial role. It functions as a crucial suppressor of tumors and acts as the primary controller for various signaling pathways related to this mechanism. The p53 protein plays a role in inhibiting the development and advancement of tumors by overseeing the DNA's integrity and triggering suitable reactions to any irregularities [12, 45]. p53, as a tumor suppressor, has a wide range of important functions. It can cause cells to stop dividing, repair damaged DNA, trigger senescence (cellular aging), and even initiate apoptosis (cell death). These are just a few examples of the many roles that p53 plays in safeguarding against cancer. Its versatility and ability to regulate various cellular processes make it an essential player in maintaining the health and integrity of our cells [9, 46]. Mutations in the TP53 gene have been observed in nearly all types of cancer, with the frequency varying from around 10% in certain blood-related cancers to nearly 100% in aggressive ovarian cancer known as high-grade serous carcinoma. These mutations in TP53 are quite common and highlight the significant role this gene plays in the development and progression of various cancers [47]. The importance of p53 in guarding against cancer is underscored by a rare disorder known as Li–Fraumeni syndrome. This condition is linked to genetic changes in the TP53 gene that are inherited and raise the chances of getting different cancers. Unlike other genes such as RB, APC, or BRCA1 that are usually turned off by deletions or mutations during cancer development, TP53 mutations in human tumors often happen through a specific type of genetic change called missense mutations involving a single DNA building block substitution. These specific genetic alterations further underscore the importance of TP53 in cancer development [13, 48–50]. When TP53 mutations occur in cancer, they can cause a full-length p53 protein to be made with just one amino acid change. These mutations can appear in different parts of the p53 gene sequence and affect how stable the p53 protein is. However, most of these mutations lead to p53 losing its ability to attach to DNA in a specific way and activate crucial p53 target genes. This disturbance in p53's normal role can play a part in cancer development and advancement [51, 52]. Mutations in the TP53 gene can be found throughout its coding regions, with a concentration of mutations in exons 4–9, which contain the DNA-binding part of the p53 protein. Interestingly, within this area, around 30% of mutations occur at six specific "hotspot" locations: R175, G245, R248, R249, R273, and R282. These hotspot mutations are common and appear in nearly all cancer types [5, 53]. The existence of these hotspot locations can be understood in two main ways. First, certain codons may be more susceptible to alterations caused by carcinogens, leading to mutations in those specific residues. Second, the presence of these hotspot locations can be explained in two ways. One reason is that mutations in these specific areas may provide cells with growth and survival advantages, leading to the prevalence of these hotspot mutations. Additionally, apart from the loss of function caused by TP53 mutations, many p53 mutants can support tumor growth through different mechanisms. When both the normal (WT) and mutant alleles are present together, the mutant p53 can impede the tumor-suppressing actions of the normal p53 in a dominant-negative manner. This occurs because the normal p53's transcriptional activity depends on forming tetramers, and the mutant p53's presence can disrupt this process and hinder its DNA-binding ability [54, 55]. The heterozygous state, where both mutant and wild-type TP53 alleles exist, doesn't tend to last long in cancer progression. It is common to see a phenomenon called loss of heterozygosity (LOH) occur. LOH occurs when the wild-type allele at a specific gene locus is either deleted or mutated, leaving only the mutant allele. In the case of TP53, located on chromosome 17's short arm, LOH frequently occurs. This suggests a selective pressure driving the inactivation of the remaining wild-type allele. This observation is intriguing because it indicates that the dominant-negative effect of the mutant p53 alone is insufficient to fully deactivate the wild-type p53. Other factors must be involved in contributing to the inactivation of the wild-type allele [46, 56]. More and more research is showing that mutant p53 isoforms can gain additional oncogenic functions through a mechanism called gain-of-function. This means that the mutant protein not only loses its normal function but also acquires new properties that promote tumor growth, rather than just being inactive. Both the dominant-negative effects, where the mutant p53 interferes with the wild-type p53, and the gain-of-function effects can contribute to the positive selection of missense mutations

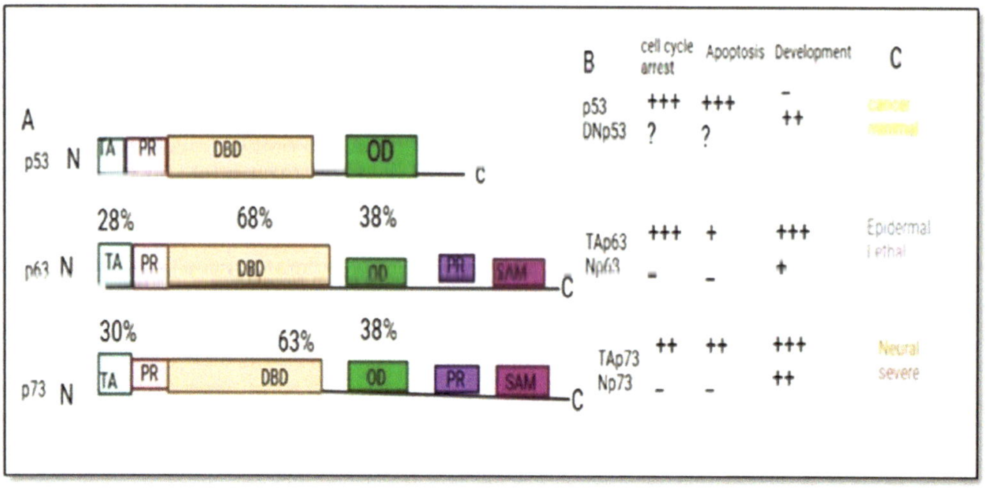

FIGURE 9.1 A diagram illustrating the modular structure of proteins in the p53 family. (A) The genes encoding p53, p73, and p63 are part of the p53 family. These proteins share a conserved domain structure, which includes an amino-terminal transactivation domain (TAD), a central DNA binding domain (DBD), and a carboxy-terminal oligomerization domain (OD). The longest α isoforms of p73 and p63 also feature a sterile alpha motif (SAM), a domain involved in protein–protein interactions found in many signaling proteins and transcription factors. The common identity among p53, p73, and p63 is illustrated. (B) The genes of the p53 family, including p53, p73, and p63, are involved in various cellular processes. Specifically, p63 and p73 are key in regulating cell differentiation and development. Research involving knockout mice has demonstrated that the absence of either p63 or p73 results in developmental abnormalities, emphasizing their crucial roles in proper cell differentiation and development. Although each family member has unique functions, the primary involvement of p63 and p73 in these processes underscores their significance in normal developmental pathways. (C) p63 and p73 exemplify their essential and unique roles in regulating development and differentiation. Knockout mouse studies reveal that the absence of p63 or p73 leads to significant developmental issues, highlighting their importance in ensuring proper development and cell specialization.

in TP53 during the development of tumors. It's fascinating to see how these different mechanisms work together to drive tumorigenesis. The complex interplay between mutant and wild-type p53 is an area of active research and holds great potential for understanding and targeting cancer [57, 58].

The deactivation of the normal p53 can differ significantly based on the mutation type and location, the specific cancer types affected, the timing of mutations in tumor development, and how it influences various stages of cancer advancement. The wide range of p53 mutations offers numerous possibilities for how a mutation can arise during cancer development. Various factors such as oncogenic stress, specific cancer-causing agents, loss of one allele (LOH), dominant-negative effects, gain-of-function advantages, and more can influence this selection process. The research findings in this review indicate that the accumulation of genetic abnormalities, rather than their sequence of appearance, dictates the advancement and severity of tumors. Therefore, knowing the p53 status in a tumor doesn't necessarily indicate the tumor stage. Evaluating the status of p53 can help detect tumors early and monitor their recurrence by detecting p53 antibodies and mutant p53 DNA (Figure 9.1). Additionally, assessing p53 status can help predict suitable treatment approaches, as mutant p53 could serve as a target for cancer therapy [59, 60].

9.3 MUTANT P63 GENE

p63, belonging to the same family as the p53 tumor suppressor, has been discovered in mouse studies to have a distinct role from the typical tumor suppressor function. Instead, it plays a vital part in developmental processes. Mutations in the p63 gene can result in various developmental anomalies in humans, such as limb deformities, cleft lip/palate, and ectodermal dysplasia. The p63 gene is essential for skin development and ensuring the well-being of egg cells. Its significance lies in orchestrating proper development and cell specialization, highlighting its crucial role in human biology. The intricate functions of p63 underscore its importance beyond traditional tumor suppression, shaping our understanding of how genetic variations can impact various aspects of human development and health. If there are mutations in p63, it can mess up how genes are checked in egg cells or even make the cells die early [58].

Maintaining a balanced and healthy cellular environment is crucial for preventing diseases like cancer and neurodegeneration, as well as for proper aging, immune function, and metabolism. The quality control systems act as the first line of defense by detecting potentially harmful conditions and providing the cell with information to initiate an appropriate response. In addition, cells need to respond properly to environmental cues and stress to make correct decisions for development and maintaining tissue and organ balance. When cells encounter stress, they can trigger processes like repairing damaged DNA and pausing the cell cycle to cope with challenging conditions, producing chaperones, inhibiting translation, or triggering an inflammatory action. If the cell can't handle the stress and fix things, it might go into self-destruct mode and activate pathways that lead to cell death. p53, the tumor suppressor, plays a crucial role in coordinating the cellular response to stress pathways. It helps coordinate these responses and ensures that the cell takes appropriate actions to maintain its health. Knowing how p53 contributes to the cell's reaction to stress is essential for researching illnesses and creating new treatment possibilities [61, 62]. When our DNA is harmed or there's a nucleotide imbalance, specific pathways are triggered to maintain low levels of p53 in healthy cells. E3 ligases, such as Mdm2 and Mdm4, are involved in this mechanism [63–65]. When p53 becomes stable, it attaches to specific gene regions. This triggers the activation of genes that manage DNA repair, control the cell cycle, regulate aging, and control programmed cell death. This helps maintain the health and integrity of our cells [14, 66–68]. When cells face different types of stress and how bad it is, they can either hit the pause button on their growth or go into a long-term state known as senescence. When cells experience significant damage, they can initiate a process known as apoptosis, which results in cell death [69, 70]. Due to its crucial function in overseeing cells, p53 is widely recognized as the most significant tumor suppressor and is frequently changed in cancer cells. This underscores its significance in stopping tumor development [15, 71]. p53 is often referred to as the "guardian of the genome" because of its essential role in protecting the integrity of our genetic material. It acts as a diligent guardian, continuously watching over and reacting to possible dangers to our DNA [9].

Scientists have found two close relatives of p53, known as p63 and p73 [16, 17]. When researchers discovered p63, it led to the idea that tumor suppression might involve all three family members working together. However, when they deactivated each gene in mice, they observed distinct differences in the resulting characteristics. For example, the p73–/– mouse showed problems with hippocampus development, hydrocephalus, persistent infections, inflammation, and anomalies in pheromone sensory pathways [6]. The p63 knockout mouse demonstrates a really poor condition. Even though it is born, it does not live very long. It has several defects, including missing limbs, partial skin, and structural problems. These findings contrast sharply with the p53–/– mouse, which mainly displays milder developmental defects like ocular abnormalities, tooth formation issues, and the loss of around 20% of female embryos and baby mice have issues with the closure of their neural tubes [72, 73]. These mouse experiments have shown how important p63 and p73 are in how creatures grow. They've given strong proof of the role these genes play in development. In-depth studies have revealed that p73 plays a role in regulating the communication between developing sperm cells and Sertoli cells. These interactions are crucial for the correct maturation of sperm cells [74, 75]. But male mice lacking p73 are unable to father offspring because they don't have fully mature sperm cells. Moreover, p73 is essential for the formation of multiciliated cells located in areas such as the trachea [76]. The chronic infections observed in p73–/– mice can be attributed to the absence of these multiciliated cells. Without these cells, the mice's respiratory system is compromised, making them more susceptible to infections [6]. This happens because the mucus transport isn't working well, which leads to issues in getting rid of pathogens and foreign substances from the airways. Scientists have identified two main jobs for p63. The initial point is that it aids in the formation and upkeep of layered epithelial tissues, like the skin [1, 3, 77]. It acts as the main quality control factor that monitors the genetic integrity of oocytes [78, 79]. Even evolutionary remote species like *Caenorhabditis elegans* appear to have evolved this quality control role as the initial evolutionary role of the entire p53 protein family [80, 81]. The *Drosophila melanogaster* [82] and *Ciona intestinalis* (or sea squirts) [18] have a protein similar to p63 in their germ cells [83]. In mammals, a particular isoform known as Tap63α is responsible for carrying out genetic quality control [78, 84]. After homologous recombination is completed, this specific form is generated following the repair of DNA double-strand breaks in oocytes induced by the type II topoisomerase-like DNA enzyme Spo11 [85, 86]. If DNA double-strand breaks continue, Tap63α initiates a series of cell death events by activating PUMA and NOXA [87]. It gets rid of harmed eggs. Oocytes proceed to dictyate arrest after reaching this checkpoint, and they stay arrested during the pause of the first stage of cell division until they are chosen for the release of eggs. Tap63α is highly expressed during the duration, which in humans can reach around 50 years. In healthy egg cells, Tap63α stays closed and inactive in a dimer form to prevent apoptosis from starting [88, 89]. When DNA damage is detected, the kinase Chk2 phosphorylates S582 of Tap63α [90]. Although Tap63α is not activated by this alteration, it does attract CK1, another kinase [91], which usually needs substrates that have already been phosphorylated. Adding four extra phosphate groups makes Tap63α shift into its active, tetrameric form [92]. Taking off phosphate groups does not cause the protein to return to its inactive dimer form; this activation is irreversible. Radiation and chemotherapy are two examples of treatments that might cause oocyte destruction and eventually lead to premature ovarian insufficiency (POI) [93] either by p63 mutations or as a therapy for cancer patients [94]. That stops the C-terminal transactivation inhibitory domain from working [95].

p63's work in developing skin tissues relies on a different version called ΔNp63α. When a mouse model lacking the ΔNp63 isoforms exhibits similar skin problems as the p63−/− mouse, and when the p63−/− traits are fixed by adding ΔNp63α with the K5 promoter, it highlights how crucial this isoform is for skin development [96, 97]. In intron 3, there's a different promoter that gets switched on to make ΔNp63. The transactivation section in p63, located in the first 24 amino acids forming a single helix (unlike the divided transactivation domains in p53 and p73), is absent in ΔNp63α [98, 99]. Instead, the N-terminal of ΔNp63α contains 14 unique amino acids [16]. ΔNp63α doesn't function effectively as a transcriptional activator on promoter regions that are usually targeted by p53, like the p21 or Mdm2 promoters [16]. Studies utilizing RNA sequencing (RNAseq) and chromatin immunoprecipitation DNA-sequencing (ChIPseq) have revealed that this isoform plays a role in structuring chromatin and regulating a distinct transcriptional program specific to epithelial cells [96, 100]. Our understanding of how this isoform works in developing epithelial tissues and related structures has increased. This knowledge has enhanced our grasp of how p63 mutations affect female fertility and lead to different clinical disorders.

9.4 MUTATION IN P73

The p73 is a transcription factor from the p53 family that inhibits the growth of tumors. The p73 locus is the source of distinct isoform transcriptions. By utilizing two promoters at the N-terminus, it is possible to create an isoform that either fully or partially contains the N-terminal transactivation domain (ΔNp73 or Tap73), with the latter isoform capable of exerting a dominant-negative influence over the former. Furthermore, the C-terminus of both N-terminal variants exhibits alternative splicing. As a true tumor suppressor, Tap73 can cause cell death and cell cycle arrest; ΔNp73, conversely, demonstrates oncogenic properties by impeding the functions of p53 and Tap73. Here, we go over the most recent research connecting p73 to cancer. Determining the relative contributions of TA and ΔNp73 isoforms has been made easier by generating mice that lack specific isoforms [101].

A mutation in the p73 gene can result in different impacts on cell functions and processes. The p73 gene belongs to the p53 gene family, which is vital in controlling cell growth, division, and apoptosis (cell death). When a mutation occurs in the p73 gene, it can disrupt the normal function of the gene. This problem can make you more likely to get cancer because the p73 gene helps manage how cells grow and die when there's DNA damage. Depending on the specific nature of the mutation, it can either result in the gene becoming inactive or acquiring new functions that promote uncontrolled cell growth. These alterations can play a role in the creation and advancement of tumors. In general, mutations in the p73 gene can profoundly impact cellular balance and may potentially result in cancer development. Further research and understanding of these mutations are essential to develop targeted therapies and treatments for individuals affected by such genetic alterations [101].

9.5 THE DOMINANT-NEGATIVE INTERPLAY BETWEEN P73, P63, AND p53 GENES

The function of the p53 gene in preventing tumors is frequently compromised in cancer, even when a normal gene copy is around. This suggests that certain mutations and variations of p53 can have a dominant-negative effect, affecting not just p53 but also its family members, p63 and p73. Research indicates that there might be an intricate interplay where these genes interfere with each other's tumor-suppressing abilities. Yet, the complete scope of particular mutations in p53, along with variations in p53, p63, and p73, is not fully understood and can affect the tumor suppression activity of these genes, along with the underlying mechanisms. Through experiments conducted using yeast, scientists have demonstrated that the dominant-negative effect is common within the p53/p63/p73 family. Many mutations in p53 that lead to loss of function, as well as certain isoforms of p53 and p73, and can produce a dominant-negative effect. The research findings have shed light on the fact that this effect on wild-type p53 occurs through tetramer poisoning, where inactive heterotetramers are formed, rather than through a prion-like mechanism as previously hypothesized. Furthermore, studies have revealed that the mutant p53-R175H can block the function of p63 and p73, although the mechanism for this inhibition is only partially related to tetramerization. The complex connection among p53, p63, and p73 concerning preventing tumor growth presents a complex web of interactions that researchers are actively exploring. The discovery that various mutations and isoforms within these gene families can exert dominant-negative effects provides a valuable understanding of the molecular processes involved in the development and advancement of cancer.

The p53 gene, known as the "guardian of the genome," is essential for protecting cells from DNA damage and stopping tumor formation. In its normal state, p53 works as a tumor suppressor by repairing DNA damage or initiating cell death if the damage is severe. However, in many cancer cases, the tumor suppression activity of p53 is compromised, leading to uncontrolled cell growth and proliferation. One intriguing aspect of p53 dysfunction in cancer is the phenomenon of dominant-negative effects exhibited by certain mutations and isoforms of the gene. A dominant-negative effect occurs when a mutated gene not only loses its normal function but also interferes [41].

The proteins known as p53, p63, and p73 can attach to and trigger the activation of specific genes that contain p53-response elements. Among these proteins, p63 has a unique function as it can also bind to distinct p63-response elements. By doing so, p63 is vital in controlling the activation of specific genes necessary for skin, limb, and facial and skull structure development. In essence, these proteins, especially p63, have the important task of interacting with specific genetic elements to regulate the function of genes related to the intricate processes of skin formation, limb development, and the shaping of facial and cranial features. This intricate mechanism highlights the specialized functions of these proteins in orchestrating the complex processes that underlie the growth and differentiation of various tissues in the body. Certainly recognizing the individual functions of p53, p63, and p73 in gene control is necessary for comprehending their specific contributions to regulating genetic activity. Scientists gain valuable insights into the intricate molecular pathways that govern crucial aspects of embryonic development and tissue differentiation. The ability of p63 to target unique genetic elements underscores its significance in shaping the intricate patterns of gene expression that are necessary for the proper emergence and development of tissues critical for overall development and health [102].

The intricate interplay between family members and their different forms is a fundamental aspect of cancer research. One particularly intriguing area of study involves the interaction among members of the p53 family, such as p53, p73, and p63. These proteins play critical roles in regulating cell growth, apoptosis, and DNA repair, and their dysregulation is associated with various cancers. Central to this interaction is the tumor suppressor p53, famous for stopping damaged cells from multiplying and starting cell death, thereby preventing the accumulation of potentially harmful mutations. However, mutations in the TP53 gene, which encodes p53, are prevalent in human cancers. These mutations can result in the production of dysfunctional p53 variants that not only lose their tumor-suppressing abilities but also gain new functions that promote tumor growth and metastasis. Researchers are increasingly exploring the relationship between mutant p53 and other members of the p53 family, particularly p73 and p63. While p73 and p63 share similarities with p53 in structure and function, they also have distinct roles in various cellular processes. Apart from inducing apoptosis and regulating the cell cycle, p53, p73, and p63 are involved in developmental processes and differentiation. Studies have unveiled a complex network of interactions among these proteins, which have significant implications for cancer progression. Notably, mutant p53 has been observed to interact with and inhibit specific isoforms of p73 and p63, impacting the cell's ability to undergo apoptosis in response to DNA damage or cellular stresses, particularly in the context of carcinogenesis [10, 102].

Mutant p53 suppresses p73 and p63 by a specific mechanism through direct protein–protein interactions. Mutant p53 blocks the DNA-binding regions of p73 and p63, stopping them from binding to specific genes and disrupting their ability to regulate gene expression. Additionally, mutant p53 may sequester p73 and p63 in non-functional protein complexes, further impairing their ability to initiate apoptosis or regulate gene expression. The consequences of these interactions extend beyond the individual proteins involved, influencing broader cellular processes and tumor behavior. For example, when mutant p53 stops p73, it can help cancer cells escape apoptosis, enabling them to grow and spread without control. Moreover, the loss of p73-mediated apoptotic signaling may confer resistance to conventional cancer therapies, complicating treatment strategies for patients with altered p53 tumors. Interestingly, the effects of altered p53 on p73 and p63 isoforms are not uniform and can vary depending on the specific isoform and cellular context. For instance, certain isoforms of p73, such as the Tap73 variants, possess tumor-suppressive functions and can counteract the oncogenic effects of mutant p53. However, other isoforms, such as ΔNp73, may promote cancerous growth and cancer spread, particularly in the presence of mutant p53. Grasping the subtleties of these interactions is crucial for creating precise cancer treatments that focus on rebalancing the signaling of the p53 family within tumors. Strategies to reactivate p73 or p63 function, either by directly targeting mutant p53 or by modulating downstream signaling pathways, hold promise for overcoming therapeutic resistance and improving patient outcomes. In addition to its implications for cancer biology, the way mutant p53 interacts with different forms of p73 and p63 highlights the broader significance of protein families and isoform diversity in cellular regulation. By elucidating the molecular mechanisms underlying these interactions, researchers can gain insights into fundamental biological processes and identify new therapeutic targets for a range of diseases beyond cancer. In summary, the way mutant p53 and p73 and p63 isoforms interact with each other represents a fascinating and clinically relevant aspect of cancer research. Through a combination of biochemical, genetic, and functional studies, researchers are unraveling the complexities of this interaction and exploring its implications for cancer development, progression, and therapy [103–105].

9.5.1 The Dominant-Negative Impact of the p53-R175H Mutant and Various Isoforms of p53, p63, and p73

So, to check how specific mutated versions of p53 and its different forms could influence the functions of p53/p63 and p73, R175H, Δ133-p53α, or Δ160-p53α were introduced alongside the active versions of p53, p63, and p73. By comparing the changes in appearance caused by these altered versions to a standard sample, we could assess their suppressive effect. The results, detailed in Table 9.1, show that these inactive altered forms of p53 can indeed hinder the functions of active p63 and p73.

9.5.2 The Dominant-Negative Influence of ΔN-p73α and ΔN-p73β on the Transactive Isoforms of p53, p63, and p73

To investigate how the inactive forms ΔN-p73α and ΔN-p73β could impact the functions of p53, p63, and p73. The findings are summarized in (Table 9.2), showing that these nonfunctional versions of

TABLE 9.1
The Dominant-Negative Influence Exerted by the Mutant p53-R175H and the Δ133-p53α and Δ160-p53α Isoforms on All Transactive Isoforms within the p53 Family

	p53-R175H	Δ133-p53α	Δ160-p53α
FL-p53α	+++	+	+++
Δ40-p53α	++	+	+
TA-p63α	+	–	–
TA-p63β	+	–	–
TA-p63γ	+	–	–
ΔN-p63α	+	–	–
ΔN-p63β	++	–	++
ΔN-p63γ	+++	++	+++
TA-p73α	++	+	+
TA-p73β	++	–	+
TA-p73γ	+++	++	+++
ΔN-p73γ	+	–	–

TABLE 9.2
The Dominant-Negative Impact of ΔN-p73α and ΔN-p73β on All Transactive Isoforms within the p53 Family

	ΔN-p73α	ΔN-p73β
FL-p53α	+	++
Δ40-p53α	+	++
TA-p63α	–	–
TA-p63β	–	–
TA- p63γ	+	+
ΔN-p63α	–	–
ΔN-p63β	–	++
ΔN-p63γ	–	+++
TA-p73α	–	–
TA-p73β	–	–
TA-p73γ	++	+
ΔN-p73γ	–	+

p73 can disrupt the activities of active p53, p63, and p73. Additionally, the inhibitory effect of ΔN-p73β on FL-p53α-WT wasn't due to a mechanism resembling that of prions in yeast, as it couldn't propagate on its own in the FASAY-RGC and FASAY-p21 systems utilizing the identical glucose-repressed shutdown system as employed in prior experiments conducted. This indicates that the suppressive impact extends broadly throughout the gene family comprising p53, p63, and p73.

9.6 INTERACTION WITH PROMOTERS OF p53, p63, AND p73

Members of the p53 family not only activate similar target genes but also control each other's expression. For instance, p53 and Tap73 can boost DNp73 transcription by binding to its promoter. DNp73, in return, inhibits p53 and Tap73 activity by competing for promoter sites or directly interacting with the proteins. This creates a negative feedback loop similar to the p53/Mdm2 loop. Investigating whether p53/p63/p73 can also bind to and regulate the internal promoter of p63 or p53, potentially forming another feedback loop, would be fascinating. Moreover, understanding the conditions under which these feedback loops favor the expression of one isoform over another would be valuable.

With this knowledge, we might be able to adjust how the p53/p63/p73 isoforms function. For instance, we could potentially alter the p53 reaction from halting the cell cycle to inducing apoptosis. The p53, p63, and p73 family constitutes a group of proteins renowned for their multifaceted functions in terms of maintaining cell balance and reacting to different stress factors. Their intricate interactions, both among themselves and with other cellular components, orchestrate a complex network crucial for maintaining cellular integrity and regulating key biological processes. This paraphrase aims to delve into the nuanced functionalities of these proteins, shedding light on their significance in normal cellular physiology and pathological conditions such as tumor formation. At the core of their functionality lies the capacity of p53/p63/ p73 to combine through direct or indirect protein–protein interactions. These interactions are pivotal for coordinating diverse cellular reactions, encompassing repair of DNA damage, cessation of the cell cycle, and initiation of apoptosis. Moreover, they have a vital role in controlling the expression of target genes by binding to specific promoters, thereby influencing various cellular pathways essential for maintaining genomic stability and preventing aberrant cell proliferation. Despite their shared structural homology and overlapping functions, every member within the p53 family exhibits distinct properties and regulatory mechanisms. This diversity is further accentuated by the existence of various isoforms produced by alternative splicing and post-translational modifications. The differential expression of these isoforms across different tissues and developmental stages underscores their specialized roles in orchestrating tissue-specific responses to various stimuli.

Interestingly, the abundance of a particular isoform does not necessarily correlate with its functional significance. Even isoforms expressed at low levels can exert profound effects on cellular processes by their unique regulatory properties. This underscores the significance of understanding the complex interactions among isoforms when interpreting the functional consequences of the p53 family members in both health and disease contexts. Central to our understanding of the p53 family dynamics is the emerging concept of isoform-specific regulation of target gene promoters. While the canonical roles of p53 in DNA damage response and tumor suppression are well-established, recent studies have unveiled the distinct transcriptional profiles associated with different isoforms. This suggests that the ratio between isoforms may serve as a key factor in determining cell destiny, dictating the outcome of cellular responses to various stress stimuli. Furthermore, the intricate balance between p53 isoforms is not static but subject to dynamic modulation in response to environmental cues and cellular signaling pathways. Perturbations in this delicate equilibrium can have far-reaching consequences, tipping the scales toward either cellular survival or programmed cell death, contingent upon the current cellular environment. Understanding the cellular mechanisms underlying these dynamic changes is vital for elucidating the role of p53 family members in orchestrating cellular decisions in health and disease. In the context of tumor formation, dysfunction in the p53 pathway is a prominent characteristic seen in various types of cancers. Mutations in the TP53 gene, responsible for encoding the p53 protein, are commonly found in genetic changes in human cancers, highlighting its essential role as a protector of the genetic material. However, it is increasingly recognized that alterations in the expression and activity of additional members of the family, p63 and p73, also contribute to tumor development through diverse mechanisms. Moreover, recent studies have implicated isoform-specific dysregulation of the involvement of p53 family members in promoting tumorigenesis and conferring resistance to conventional cancer therapies. For instance, certain p53 isoforms have been shown to exhibit oncogenic properties, promoting cell proliferation and survival in a manner distinct from the standard tumor-inhibiting roles of normal p53. Conversely, other isoforms may act as tumor suppressors, antagonizing the pro-survival effects of their oncogenic counterparts and promoting apoptotic cell death. The significance of isoform-specific regulation in tumor development is further underscored by the intricate crosstalk between the p53 family members and key signaling pathways dysregulated in cancer. For instance, aberrant activation of oncogenic signaling pathways such as the PI3K/AKT/mTOR pathway can influence the expression and function of p53 family members, thereby influencing their contribution to tumor progression and therapeutic response. Furthermore, the emerging involvement of non-coding RNAs, including microRNAs and long non-coding RNAs, in controlling the expression and function of p53 family members adds another layer of complexity to their regulatory network in cancer. These regulatory RNAs can influence the expression of p53 isoforms by directly targeting their mRNA transcripts or by influencing upstream signaling pathways involved in their post-transcriptional regulation. In summary, the p53/p63/p73 proteins represent a paradigmatic example of the intricate interplay between isoform diversity, regulatory complexity, and functional versatility in cellular physiology and disease. Their dynamic regulation and multifaceted roles in orchestrating cellular responses to stress stimuli underscore their significance as central players in maintaining genomic integrity, regulating cell fate decisions, and modulating tumor development. Ongoing investigation into the molecular mechanisms governing the interaction among p53 family members offers the potential for creating new therapeutic approaches aimed at addressing disrupted pathways in cancer and various ailments [13, 106].

9.7 CONCLUSION

In the last five years, research on the newly discovered p53 family members, p63 and p73, has shown that they share many structural and functional traits. The parts of p53 responsible for activating genes, binding to DNA, and forming groups are similar in p63 and p73. Like p53, p63 and p73 can group, attach to DNA, activate genes that p53 usually controls, and start cell death. Moreover, certain proteins in cells and viruses that affect how p53 works can also influence p63 and p73. While p63 and p73 can copy some of p53's jobs in labs, recent studies have shown important differences within the family. Unlike p53, p63 and p73 create various unique protein versions due to how their genes are read and spliced. Some versions, like dominant-negative isoforms, can block certain activities of the full-length proteins. The differences in their abilities to activate genes and cause cell death may come from changes in their gene endings. Also, the α versions have a special SAM part that might be important for new protein interactions. The ways each family member gets activated by signals are also different. Some things that activate p53 may not activate p73. Many parts in cells and viruses can tell the difference between p53 and the newer family members. p63 and p73 don't exactly fit the typical tumor suppressor gene pattern. Mutations in p63 and p73 genes are uncommon in tumors, and congenital mutations in these genes do not induce tumor growth in mice. Instead, mice lacking p63 and p73 exhibit noticeable developmental abnormalities. Consequently, the recently identified members of the p53 family, p63 and p73, possess both shared and distinct biological functions. Despite substantial advancements in discerning the unique roles of each family member, numerous questions remain unanswered. One pivotal query pertains to the expression patterns of different p63 and p73 isoforms during regular development and tumor initiation.

Investigation into isoform-specific expression in tumors could be enhanced by employing antibodies tailored to each isoform. Research utilizing knockout mice devoid of specific isoforms like DNp73 and DNp63 could provide insights into the individual functions of each isoform. Another critical aspect involves defining the roles of the three p53 family members in cellular differentiation and apoptosis across various physiological conditions. For instance, existing evidence links p63 to the maintenance and differentiation of epithelial stem cells and p73 to neuronal cell death. Lastly, interactions among the three family members, both analogous and disparate, may impact tumorigenesis. Understanding the complexities of these interactions could facilitate the development of anti-cancer therapies that activate "p53-responsive" genes in cells lacking functional p53.

The interactions among mutant p53, p63, and p73 proteins have big effects on cell processes. Mutant p53, which is common in cancer, can mess up the normal functions of p63 and p73, causing problems with gene expression and cell activities. This disruption can lead to cells growing out of control, problems with fixing DNA, and changes in how cells respond to stress. Mutant p53 can stop p63 and p73 from working well, which might help tumors grow and cause other cell problems. This complicated relationship shows how important it is to understand how mutant p53 affects p63 and p73 to keep cells healthy and stop them from behaving strangely. Also, the problems caused by mutant p53 together with p63 and p73 can affect lots of cell processes, like controlling cell growth, causing cell death, and responding to DNA damage. This shows why we need more research to figure out how these proteins talk to each other and find treatments that focus on fixing these problems, especially in diseases linked to mutant p53.

In summary, the complex interplay between mutant p53, p63, and p73 proteins significantly influences cellular processes, particularly in the context of oncology development and progression. Understanding the intricate relationships and functional consequences of these interactions is crucial for advancing our knowledge of cancer biology and identifying novel therapeutic approaches to target these pathways effectively.

REFERENCES

1. Yang, A., et al., p63 is essential for regenerative proliferation in limb, craniofacial and epithelial development. *Nature*, 1999. **398**(6729): p. 714–718.
2. De Laurenzi, V., et al., Additional complexity in p73: induction by mitogens in lymphoid cells and identification of two new splicing variants e and z. *Cell Death & Differentiation*, 1999. **6**: p. 389–390.
3. Mills, A.A., et al., p63 is a p53 homologue required for limb and epidermal morphogenesis. *Nature*, 1999. **398**(6729): p. 708–713.
4. Haq, B.U., et al., Targeting p53 misfolding conundrum by stabilizing agents and their analogs in breast cancer therapy: a comprehensive computational analysis. *Frontiers in Pharmacology*, 2024. **14**: p. 1333447.
5. Mir, M.A., M. Bashir, and N. Jan, The Role of Interleukin (IL)-6/IL-6 Receptor Axis in Cancer, in *Cytokine and Chemokine Networks in Cancer*. 2023, Springer. p. 137–164.
6. Yang, A., et al., p73-deficient mice have neurological, pheromonal and inflammatory defects but lack spontaneous tumours. *Nature*, 2000. **404**(6773): p. 99–103.
7. Pozniak, C.D., et al., p73 is required for survival and maintenance of CNS neurons. *Journal of Neuroscience*, 2002. **22**(22): p. 9800–9809.
8. Jan, N., et al., Exploring the role of trifarotene against RAR-α: an investigation of expression pattern and clinicopathological significance of RAR-α in breast cancer. *Frontiers in Pharmacology*, 2024. **15**: p. 1361679.
9. Lane, D.P., p53, guardian of the genome. *Nature*, 1992. **358**(6381): p. 15–16.
10. Mir, M.A., Sumaya, N. Jan, Implications of Chemokine Heterogenicity in Cancer Metastasis, in *Cytokine and Chemokine Networks in Cancer*. 2023, Springer. p. 115–136.
11. Pflaum, J., S. Schlosser, and M. Müller, p53 family and cellular stress responses in cancer. *Frontiers in Oncology*, 2014. **4**: p. 285.
12. Levine, A.J. and M. Oren, The first 30 years of p53: growing ever more complex. *Nature Reviews Cancer*, 2009. **9**(10): p. 749–758.

13. Jan, N., et al., Targeting breast cancer stem cells through retinoids: a new hope for treatment. *Critical Reviews in Oncology/Hematology*, 2023: p. 104156.
14. Vousden, K.H. and C. Prives, Blinded by the light: the growing complexity of p53. *Cell*, 2009. **137**(3): p. 413–431.
15. Hollstein, M., et al., p53 mutations in human cancers. *Science*, 1991. **253**(5015): p. 49–53.
16. Yang, A., et al., p63, a p53 homolog at 3q27–29, encodes multiple products with transactivating, death-inducing, and dominant-negative activities. *Molecular Cell*, 1998. **2**(3): p. 305–316.
17. Kaghad, M., et al., Monoallelically expressed gene related to p53 at 1p36, a region frequently deleted in neuroblastoma and other human cancers. *Cell*, 1997. **90**(4): p. 809–819.
18. Belyi, V.A., et al., The origins and evolution of the p53 family of genes. *Cold Spring Harbor Perspectives in Biology*, 2010. **2**(6): p. a001198.
19. Jan, N., et al., Metronomic chemotherapy and drug repurposing: a paradigm shift in oncology. *Heliyon*, 2024. https://doi.org/10.1016/j.heliyon.2024.e24670
20. Dötsch, V., et al., p63 and p73, the ancestors of p53. *Cold Spring Harbor Perspectives in Biology*, 2010. **2**(9): p. a004887.
21. Deyoung, M. and L. Ellisen, p63 and p73 in human cancer: defining the network. *Oncogene*, 2007. **26**(36): p. 5169–5183.
22. Khoury, M.P. and J.-C. Bourdon, p53 isoforms: an intracellular microprocessor? *Genes & Cancer*, 2011. **2**(4): p. 453–465.
23. Logotheti, S., et al., Functions, divergence and clinical value of TAp73 isoforms in cancer. *Cancer and Metastasis Reviews*, 2013. **32**: p. 511–534.
24. Costanzo, A., et al., TP63 and TP73 in cancer, an unresolved "family" puzzle of complexity, redundancy and hierarchy. *FEBS Letters*, 2014. **588**(16): p. 2590–2599.
25. Conforti, F., et al., Relative expression of TAp73 and ΔNp73 isoforms. *Aging (Albany NY)*, 2012. **4**(3): p. 202.
26. Petitjean, A., et al., Impact of mutant p53 functional properties on TP53 mutation patterns and tumor phenotype: lessons from recent developments in the IARC TP53 database. *Human Mutation*, 2007. **28**(6): p. 622–629.
27. Sofi, S., et al., A comprehensive analysis of notch signaling genes in breast cancer: expression pattern and prognostic significance. *Advances in Cancer Biology-Metastasis*, 2023. **7**: p. 100104.
28. Lehmann, B.D., et al., Evaluation of public cancer datasets and signatures identifies TP53 mutant signatures with robust prognostic and predictive value. *BMC Cancer*, 2015. **15**: p. 1–18.
29. Brachmann, R.K., M. Vidal, and J.D. Boeke, Dominant-negative p53 mutations selected in yeast hit cancer hot spots. *Proceedings of the National Academy of Sciences*, 1996. **93**(9): p. 4091–4095.
30. Mir, M.A., M. Rashid, and N. Jan, Cytokines and Chemokines in Tumor Growth and Progression, in *Cytokine and Chemokine Networks in Cancer*. 2023, Springer. p. 33–77.
31. Di Como, C.J., C. Gaiddon, and C. Prives, p73 function is inhibited by tumor-derived p53 mutants in mammalian cells. *Molecular and Cellular Biology*, 1999. **19**(2): p. 1438–1449.
32. Blagosklonny, M.V., p53 from complexity to simplicity: mutant p53 stabilization, gain-of-function, and dominant-negative effect. *The FASEB Journal*, 2000. **14**(13): p. 1901–1907.
33. Forget, K.J., G. Tremblay, and X. Roucou, p53 aggregates penetrate cells and induce the co-aggregation of intracellular p53. *PLoS One*, 2013. **8**(7): p. e69242.
34. Nomoto, S., et al., Search for mutations and examination of allelic expression imbalance of the p73 gene at 1p36. 33 in human lung cancers. *Cancer Research*, 1998. **58**(7): p. 1380–1383.
35. Moll, U.M., S. Erster, and A. Zaika, p53, p63 and p73–solos, alliances and feuds among family members. *Biochimica et Biophysica Acta (BBA)-Reviews on Cancer*, 2001. **1552**(2): p. 47–59.
36. Dohn, M., S. Zhang, and X. Chen, p63α and ΔNp63α can induce cell cycle arrest and apoptosis and differentially regulate p53 target genes. *Oncogene*, 2001. **20**(25): p. 3193–3205.
37. Courtois, S., C.C.d. Fromentel, and P. Hainaut, p53 protein variants: structural and functional similarities with p63 and p73 isoforms. *Oncogene*, 2004. **23**(3): p. 631–638.
38. Iggo, R. and E. Schärer, Mammalian p53 can function as a transcription factor in yeast. *Cancer Genetics and Cytogenetics*, 1992. **63**(2): p. 113.
39. Flaman, J., et al., A simple p53 functional assay for screening cell lines, blood, and tumors. *Proceedings of the National Academy of Sciences*, 1995. **92**(9): p. 3963–3967.
40. Monti, P., et al., ΔN-P63α and TA-P63α exhibit intrinsic differences in transactivation specificities that depend on distinct features of DNA target sites. *Oncotarget*, 2014. **5**(8): p. 2116.
41. Voisset, C. and M. Blondel, Chemobiology at happy hour: yeast as a model for pharmacological screening. *Medecine Sciences: M/S*, 2014. **30**(12): p. 1161–1168.

42. Hanahan, D. and R.A. Weinberg, The hallmarks of cancer. *Cell*, 2000. **100**(1): p. 57–70.
43. Berenblum, I. and P. Shubik, A new, quantitative, approach to the study of the stages of chemical carcinogenesis in the mouse's skin. *British Journal of Cancer*, 1947. **1**(4): p. 383.
44. Mir, M.A., A. Shabir, and N. Jan, Metronomic Chemotherapy in Breast Cancer, in *Novel Approaches in Metronomic Chemotherapy for Breast Cancer Treatment*. CRC Press. p. 72–86.
45. Knudson Jr, A.G., Mutation and cancer: statistical study of retinoblastoma. *Proceedings of the National Academy of Sciences*, 1971. **68**(4): p. 820–823.
46. Mir, M.A., et al., Metronomics: toward personalized chemotherapy. *Novel Approaches in Metronomic Chemotherapy for Breast Cancer Treatment*, 2024. p. 99–119. https://doi.org/10.1201/9781032632674-8
47. Aylon, Y. and M. Oren, New plays in the p53 theater. *Current Opinion in Genetics & Development*, 2011. **21**(1): p. 86–92.
48. Ahmed, A.A., et al., Driver mutations in TP53 are ubiquitous in high grade serous carcinoma of the ovary. *The Journal of Pathology*, 2010. **221**(1): p. 49–56.
49. Malkin, D., et al., Germ line p53 mutations in a familial syndrome of breast cancer, sarcomas, and other neoplasms. *Science*, 1990. **250**(4985): p. 1233–1238.
50. Mir, M.A., et al., Imaging Techniques, Biomarkers, and Methods for Metronomic Chemotherapy, in *Novel Approaches in Metronomic Chemotherapy for Breast Cancer Treatment*. CRC Press. p. 58–71.
51. Hainaut, P. and M. Hollstein, p53 and human cancer: the first ten thousand mutations. *Advances in Cancer Research*, 1999. **77**: p. 81–137.
52. Sofi, S., et al., Clinicopathological and prognostic significance of Bcl2 in breast cancer: a comprehensive in silico and in vitro study. *Saudi Journal of Biological Sciences*, 2023. **31**(2): p. 103916.
53. Bullock, A.N. and A.R. Fersht, Rescuing the function of mutant p53. *Nature Reviews Cancer*, 2001. **1**(1): p. 68–76.
54. Cho, Y., et al., Crystal structure of a p53 tumor suppressor-DNA complex: understanding tumorigenic mutations. *Science*, 1994. **265**(5170): p. 346–355.
55. Milner, J., E.A. Medcalf, and A.C. Cook, Tumor suppressor p53: analysis of wild-type and mutant p53 complexes. *Molecular and Cellular Biology*, 1991. **11**: p. 12–19.
56. Sigal, A. and V. Rotter, Oncogenic mutations of the p53 tumor suppressor: the demons of the guardian of the genome. *Cancer Research*, 2000. **60**(24): p. 6788–6793.
57. Miller, C., et al., Human p53 gene localized to short arm of chromosome 17. *Nature*, 1986. **319**(6056): p. 783–784.
58. Brosh, R. and V. Rotter, When mutants gain new powers: news from the mutant p53 field. *Nature Reviews Cancer*, 2009. **9**(10): p. 701–713.
59. Oren, M. and V. Rotter, Mutant p53 gain-of-function in cancer. *Cold Spring Harbor Perspectives in Biology*, 2010. **2**(2): p. a001107.
60. Mir, M.A., N. Jan, and S. Sofi, Introduction to Metronomic Chemotherapy, in *Novel Approaches in Metronomic Chemotherapy for Breast Cancer Treatment*. 2024, CRC Press. p. 1–14.
61. Levine, A.J., p53: 800 million years of evolution and 40 years of discovery. *Nature Reviews Cancer*, 2020. **20**(8): p. 471–480.
62. Mir, M.A., et al., Proteomics: Application of Next-Generation Proteomics in Cancer Research, in *Proteomics*. 2023, Elsevier. p. 55–76.
63. Haupt, Y., et al., Mdm2 promotes the rapid degradation of p53. *Nature*, 1997. **387**(6630): p. 296–299.
64. Kubbutat, M.H., S.N. Jones, and K.H. Vousden, Regulation of p53 stability by Mdm2. *Nature*, 1997. **387**(6630): p. 299–303.
65. Kussie, P.H., et al., Structure of the MDM2 oncoprotein bound to the p53 tumor suppressor transactivation domain. *Science*, 1996. **274**(5289): p. 948–953.
66. Kh, V., Live or let die: the cell's response to p53. *Nature Reviews Cancer*, 2002. **2**: p. 594–604.
67. Bieging, K.T. and L.D. Attardi, Deconstructing p53 transcriptional networks in tumor suppression. *Trends in Cell Biology*, 2012. **22**(2): p. 97–106.
68. Vogelstein, B., D. Lane, and A.J. Levine, Surfing the p53 network. *Nature*, 2000. **408**(6810): p. 307–310.
69. Riley, T., et al., Transcriptional control of human p53-regulated genes. *Nature Reviews Molecular Cell Biology*, 2008. **9**(5): p. 402–412.
70. Broz, D.K., et al., Global genomic profiling reveals an extensive p53-regulated autophagy program contributing to key p53 responses. *Genes & Development*, 2013. **27**(9): p. 1016–1031.
71. Freed-Pastor, W.A. and C. Prives, Mutant p53: one name, many proteins. *Genes & Development*, 2012. **26**(12): p. 1268–1286.
72. Armstrong, J.F., et al., High-frequency developmental abnormalities in p53-deficient mice. *Current Biology*, 1995. **5**(8): p. 931–936.

73. Donehower, L.A., et al., Mice deficient for p53 are developmentally normal but susceptible to spontaneous tumours. *Nature*, 1992. **356**(6366): p. 215–221.
74. Holembowski, L., et al., TAp73 is essential for germ cell adhesion and maturation in testis. *Journal of Cell Biology*, 2014. **204**(7): p. 1173–1190.
75. Inoue, S., et al., TAp73 is required for spermatogenesis and the maintenance of male fertility. *Proceedings of the National Academy of Sciences*, 2014. **111**(5): p. 1843–1848.
76. Marshall, C.B., et al., p73 is required for multiciliogenesis and regulates the Foxj1-associated gene network. *Cell Reports*, 2016. **14**(10): p. 2289–2300.
77. Senoo, M., et al., p63 Is essential for the proliferative potential of stem cells in stratified epithelia. *Cell*, 2007. **129**(3): p. 523–536.
78. Suh, E.-K., et al., p63 protects the female germ line during meiotic arrest. *Nature*, 2006. **444**(7119): p. 624–628.
79. Livera, G., et al., p63 null mutation protects mouse oocytes from radio-induced apoptosis. *Reproduction*, 2008. **135**(1): p. 3.
80. Schumacher, B., et al., The C. elegans homolog of the p53 tumor suppressor is required for DNA damage-induced apoptosis. *Current Biology*, 2001. **11**(21): p. 1722–1727.
81. Derry, W.B., A.P. Putzke, and J.H. Rothman, Caenorhabditis elegans p53: role in apoptosis, meiosis, and stress resistance. *Science*, 2001. **294**(5542): p. 591–595.
82. Ollmann, M., et al., Drosophila p53 is a structural and functional homolog of the tumor suppressor p53. *Cell*, 2000. **101**(1): p. 91–101.
83. Ou, H.D., et al., Structural evolution of C-terminal domains in the p53 family. *The EMBO Journal*, 2007. **26**(14): p. 3463–3473.
84. Gebel, J., et al., DNA damaged induced cell death in oocytes. *Molecules*, 2020. **25**(23): p. 5714.
85. Keeney, S., C.N. Giroux, and N. Kleckner, Meiosis-specific DNA double-strand breaks are catalyzed by Spo11, a member of a widely conserved protein family. *Cell*, 1997. **88**(3): p. 375–384.
86. Romanienko, P.J. and R.D. Camerini-Otero, The mouse Spo11 gene is required for meiotic chromosome synapsis. *Molecular Cell*, 2000. **6**(5): p. 975–987.
87. Kerr, J.B., et al., DNA damage-induced primordial follicle oocyte apoptosis and loss of fertility require TAp63-mediated induction of Puma and Noxa. *Molecular Cell*, 2012. **48**(3): p. 343–352.
88. Deutsch, G.B., et al., DNA damage in oocytes induces a switch of the quality control factor TAp63α from dimer to tetramer. *Cell*, 2011. **144**(4): p. 566–576.
89. Coutandin, D., et al., Quality control in oocytes by p63 is based on a spring-loaded activation mechanism on the molecular and cellular level. *Elife*, 2016. **5**: p. e13909.
90. Bolcun-Filas, E., et al., Reversal of female infertility by Chk2 ablation reveals the oocyte DNA damage checkpoint pathway. *Science*, 2014. **343**(6170): p. 533–536.
91. Tuppi, M., et al., Oocyte DNA damage quality control requires consecutive interplay of CHK2 and CK1 to activate p63. *Nature Structural & Molecular Biology*, 2018. **25**(3): p. 261–269.
92. Woodard, T.L. and E. Bolcun-Filas, Prolonging reproductive life after cancer: the need for fertoprotective therapies. *Trends in Cancer*, 2016. **2**(5): p. 222–233.
93. Lena, A.M., et al., The p63 C-terminus is essential for murine oocyte integrity. *Nature Communications*, 2021. **12**(1): p. 383.
94. Serber, Z., et al., A C-terminal inhibitory domain controls the activity of p63 by an intramolecular mechanism. *Molecular and Cellular Biology*, 2002. **22**(24): p. 8601–8611.
95. Romano, R.-A., et al., Δ Np63 knockout mice reveal its indispensable role as a master regulator of epithelial development and differentiation. *Development*, 2012. **139**(4): p. 772–782.
96. Candi, E., et al., Differential roles of p63 isoforms in epidermal development: selective genetic complementation in p63 null mice. *Cell Death & Differentiation*, 2006. **13**(6): p. 1037–1047.
97. Krauskopf, K., et al., Regulation of the activity in the p53 family depends on the organization of the transactivation domain. *Structure*, 2018. **26**(8): p. 1091–1100.e4.
98. Burge, S., et al., Molecular basis of the interactions between the p73 N terminus and p300: effects on transactivation and modulation by phosphorylation. *Proceedings of the National Academy of Sciences*, 2009. **106**(9): p. 3142–3147.
99. Yang, A., et al., Genome-wide mapping indicates that p73 and p63 co-occupy target sites and have similar dna-binding profiles in vivo. *PLoS One*, 2010. **5**(7): p. e11572.
100. Soares, E. and H. Zhou, Master regulatory role of p63 in epidermal development and disease. *Cellular and Molecular Life Sciences*, 2018. **75**(7): p. 1179–1190.
101. Rufini, A., et al., p73 in Cancer. *Genes & Cancer*, 2011. **2**(4): p. 491–502.

102. Inoue, K. and E.A. Fry, Alterations of p63 and p73 in human cancers. *Subcellular Biochemistry*, 2014. **85**: p. 17–40.
103. Lang, G.A., et al., Gain of function of a p53 hot spot mutation in a mouse model of Li-Fraumeni syndrome. *Cell*, 2004. **119**(6): p. 861–872.
104. Olive, K.P., et al., Mutant p53 gain of function in two mouse models of Li-Fraumeni syndrome. *Cell*, 2004. **119**(6): p. 847–860.
105. Strano, S., et al., Physical and functional interaction between p53 mutants and different isoforms of p73. *Journal of Biological Chemistry*, 2000. **275**(38): p. 29503–29512.
106. Grob, T., et al., Human ΔNp73 regulates a dominant negative feedback loop for TAp73 and p53. *Cell Death & Differentiation*, 2001. **8**(12): p. 1213–1223.

10 Role of Post-Translational Modifications in the Regulation of Mutant p53

*Gowhar Masoodi, Nusrat Jan, Asma Jan, and Manzoor Ahmad Mir**

Department of Bioresources, School of Biological Sciences, University of Kashmir, Srinagar, J&K, India
*drmanzoor@kashmiruniversity.ac.in

10.1 INTRODUCTION

In the late 20th century, DNA cancer viruses were intensively explored as a tumorigenic factor and the molecular basis of virus-induced cellular transformations was explored extensively. In such attempts to find proteins interacting with the viral SV40 T antigen, p53 was originally identified as a co-immunoprecipitating protein [1–3]. p53 protein encoded from the *TP53* gene acts as a tumor suppressor helping in the prevention of the transformation of cells [4–6]. Our present understanding of p53's functions has been enriched by the work of numerous laboratories worldwide. These laboratories have explored the protein's roles as a tetramer, which regulates target genes crucial for tumor suppression, and as a labile transcription factor that is heavily mutated in a wide range of cancer types [7–9]. Considerable information has recently been discovered on mutant p53. Mutant p53 can acquire novel gain-of-functions (GOFs) to actively drive tumorigenesis as an oncogenic protein and it is not only a long-lived inactive protein but can also negatively affect the remaining wild-type (WT) p53 protein in an effect known as the dominant-negative (DN) effect [10–13].

The p53 gene is mapped on the short arm of chromosome 17 at position 17p13.1. It is a 16–20 kb cellular DNA fragment that codes for 375 amino acid nuclear phosphoprotein involved in controlling cell proliferation [14, 15]. The p53 gene is a tumor suppressor gene (TSG), meaning that when it is active, tumors cannot grow. If a person receives only one functioning copy of the p53 gene from their parents, they are more likely to develop cancer and often experience many separate tumors in various organs in their early adult years. It is referred to as Li–Fraumeni syndrome and is an uncommon disorder. On the other hand, the majority of tumor types have p53 mutations, which add to the intricate web of molecular processes that cause tumor growth. In the cell, the p53 protein binds DNA, which activates a different gene to generate the protein p21, which interacts with CDK2 (cyclin dependent kinase 2), a protein that drives cell division. The p21–CDK2 complex prevents the cell from proceeding to the subsequent phase of cell division.

In a wide range of human malignancies, the p53 gene is the most often mutated, and in many cancer types, the functions of the wild-type p53 protein are frequently disrupted [16]. Similar to several other transcription factors, the p53 protein possesses a modular structure that is distinguished by the existence of functional domains (Figure 10.1). The DNA binding domain of p53 (between 102 and 109 AA residues) is the site where most mutations occur in cancerous cells. Missense mutations that result in a defective protein make up 90% of these mutations, whereas loss-of-function mutations, which cause no protein through a variety of causes (nonsense or frameshift mutations, deletions),

DOI: 10.1201/9781003520771-10

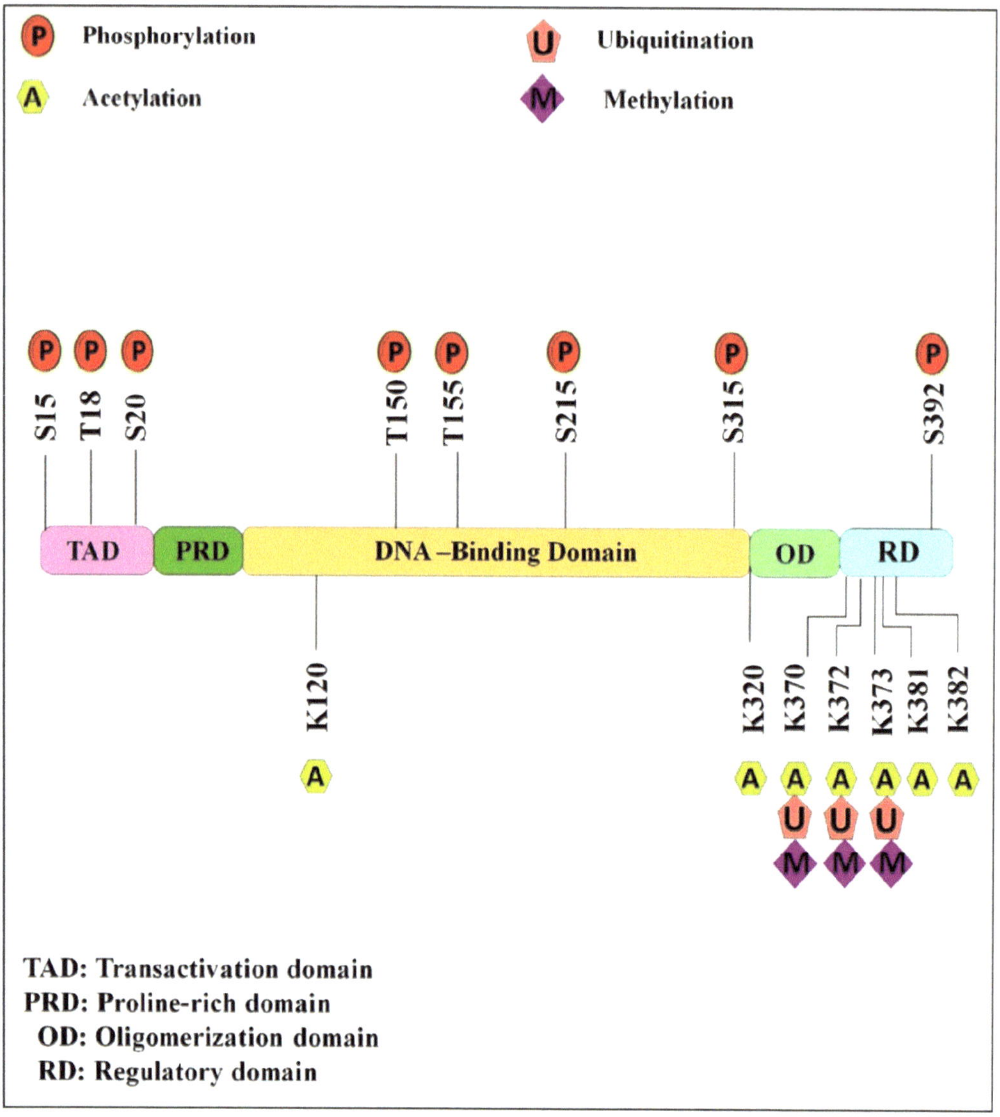

FIGURE 10.1 Domain organization and post-translational modifications of p53 protein.

account for around 10% of these mutations. Loss-of-function mutations impair the protein's capacity to bind selectively to DNA sequence motifs (20 base pairs long) that mediate the transcription of p53-regulated genes. These missense mutations were previously characterized, based on the structure of the p53 DNA binding domain, as mutations that disrupt amino acids that interact with DNA, which contribute specificity to DNA binding, and mutations that affect the conformation of the DNA binding domain [17].

10.2 POST-TRANSLATIONAL MODIFICATIONS (PTMS)

Post-translational modifications (PTMs) are covalent processing events that change the properties of a protein by proteolytic cleavage and adding a modifying group, such as acetyl, phosphoryl, glycosyl, and methyl, to one or more amino acids [18]. In general, post-translational modifications can be either reversible or irreversible. Covalent modifications are found in processes that can be reversed by using specific enzymes that break the covalent bond between the native protein and a chemical group that has been added to it post-translationally. In the irreversible type of modifications, proteolytic modification occurs [19, 20]. PTMs are typically found in proteins that have significant structures/functions, such as secretory proteins, membrane proteins, and histones. These changes influence a variety of protein behaviors and characteristics, such as enzyme function and assembly [21], protein lifespan, protein–protein interactions [22], cell–cell and cell–matrix interactions, molecular trafficking, receptor activation, protein solubility, protein folding, and protein localization [23, 24].

As a result, these changes play an important role in a variety of biological processes, including signal transmission, gene expression regulation, gene activation, DNA repair, and cell cycle control [25, 26]. PTMs appear in different cellular organelles, including the nucleus, cytoplasm, endoplasmic reticulum, and Golgi apparatus [20]. There are about 400 distinct kinds of PTMs [27] that influence several areas of protein function. The dbPTM, one of the most extensive PTM databases, lists 24 significant PTMs and more than 80 experimentally validated reported changed sites [28]. According to the dbPTM database, phosphorylation, acetylation, and ubiquitination account for over 90% of all documented PTMs (about 827,000 sites out of ~908,000). As a result, each amino acid experiences at least three distinct PTMs, with Lys having almost 15 PTM types. Furthermore, based on the entire dbPTM dataset, Cys and Ser are modified with at least 10 PTM types. Finally, phosphorylation on Ser is the most commonly observed PTM type.

10.3 TYPES OF PTMS AFFECTING MUTANT p53

Post-translational modifications occur at more than 60 of the 393 residues of the human p53 (TP53) tumor suppressor in its wild-type form. By controlling protein–protein and protein–DNA interactions, these modifications partially account for alterations in TP53 stability and transcription factor activity in response to a broad range of internal and external stressors. Oncogene activation, DNA damage, oxidative stress, hypoxia, hyperoxia, and nutritional deprivation are among the physical and metabolic stressors linked to cancer. In contrast to most other tumor suppressors, the TP53 gene is commonly mutated in cancers (Figure 10.2). These mutations are primarily missense, which frequently leads to the accumulation of mutant protein, which may have new or altered activities [29–31].

Normal unstressed cells have low levels of p53 due to ubiquitylation caused by MDM2 and MDM4 (MDMX), two of its primary negative regulators that target p53 for proteasomal destruction. Additionally, MDM2/MDM4 binds to transactivation domain 1 (TAD1), inhibiting transcription by blocking TP53 from interacting with transcriptional components. p53 PTMs alter its stability and its interactions with chromatin and several other cofactors that affect target gene transcription or repression mediated by p53. p53 directly stimulates the transcription activation or repression of several genes by binding to response elements in enhancers or close to promoters [32, 33]. p53 also indirectly represses a large number of genes by inducing microRNAs or long non-coding RNAs [34].

Most of the p53 PTMs occur in unstructured regions: (i) the amino (N-) terminal transactivation domains (TAD1 and TAD2); (ii) the linker after the sequence-specific DNA binding domain (DBD); and (iii) the carboxyl (C-) terminal regulatory domain that also serves as a DNA binding domain that is not sequence specific. The majority of the interactions with the numerous proteins (>300) that interact with p53 take place in these regions. PTMs therefore mostly regulate p53 activity by modifying a number of these interactions rather than altering the structure of p53 [29, 35].

Structural changes in the p53 gene itself or alterations in its signaling pathways are the most frequent events in the development of cancer [36] and can be considered hallmarks of cancer cells [13, 37]. Tumor suppressor genes, such as CDKN2A (ARF), RB1, or BRCA1, typically exhibit cancer-associated changes due to gene silencing or deletion. However, p53 mutations arise due to single nucleotide substitution and missense mutation, which frequently lead to the production of a stable mutant protein [38].

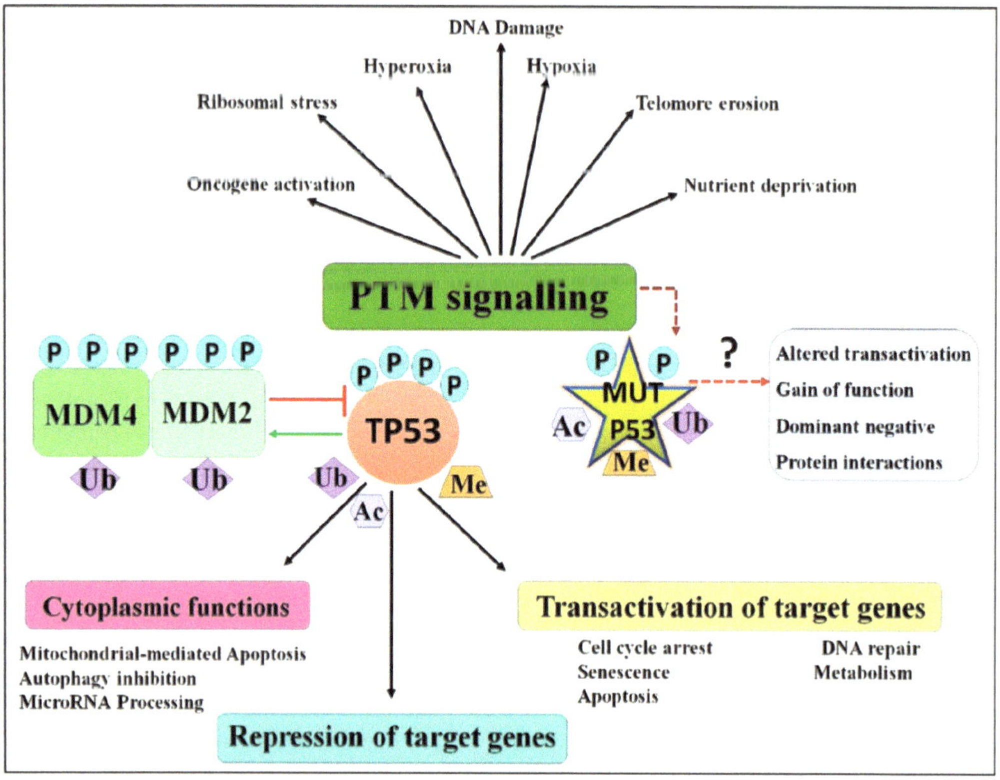

FIGURE 10.2 Cancer-related signaling to WT and MUT TP53.

10.4 PHOSPHORYLATION OF MUT p53

To stabilize p53 and increase p53 transactivating activities at its target genes, phosphorylation of p53 is typically thought to be the initial step. There are almost 30 residues that can be phosphorylated, mostly located in the N- and C-termini. However, the residues that are commonly critical for antiproliferative and antiapoptotic activity p53, such as Ser15, Thr18, Ser20, Ser46, and Ser392, are rarely changed in cancer [29]. The patterns of phosphorylation on MUT p53 can differ from WT patterns. In one of the pioneering studies on PTMs of MUT p53, it was observed that in the absence of stress, phosphorylation of specific residues in MUT p53 was altered compared to WT p53 [39]. Tumor missense mutations of p53 at sites subject to phosphorylation are extremely rare, however, there are certain exceptions for example Thr155 and Ser215 residues located in the DBD. Phosphorylation at Thr155 promotes p53 degradation.

The COP9 signalosome (CSN)-associated kinase complex phosphorylates Thr155, promoting p53 ubiquitylation by both MDM2 and the papillomavirus E6-AP ligases and subsequent proteasomal degradation [36, 40, 41]. One of the few PTM to p53 residues that affects MUT p53 activity and tumor development is Ser392. A protein complex including CK2, hSpt16, and SSRP1 phosphorylates Ser392 in response to UV light, stabilizing the p53 tetramer and triggering the sequence-specific DNA binding activity of p53 [42–44]. In the absence of stress, Ser392 is often reported to be hyperphosphorylated in tumor-derived cell lines that carry the Arg248Trp or Arg273His hotspot mutations [39, 45]. About 60% of the samples with TP53 missense mutations in human transitional cell carcinomas had constitutive phosphorylation of Ser392 [46]. It is unknown how MUT p53 Ser392 phosphorylation aids in tumor development. Certain GOF MUT p53 have been suggested to form tetramers more frequently when they are phosphorylated at Ser392, making them more effective oncoproteins. The Ser392Ala mutation also lowers the half-life of Arg175His misfolded protein, while the Arg248Trp mutant has a longer half-life, which has a native conformation [47].

Ser15 is a crucial residue for p53 activation. The role of Ser15 phosphorylation in MUT p53 function is controversial. During the initial investigations of DNA binding mutants, a deficiency in Ser15 phosphorylation was observed [39, 48]. However, no clear relationship between the Ser15 modification and the abundance, localization, or DNA binding affinity of MUT p53 was found in other studies involving a larger number of MUT p53 cancer cell lines from various tissue origins, indicating that other factors may affect how this modification affects MUT p53 functions under stressed or unstressed conditions [45, 49, 50]. However, constitutive Ser15 phosphorylation is observed in human breast and pancreatic cancer cell lines carrying Arg280Lys, Leu194Phe, and Arg273His mutants, as well as in UV-induced skin tumors in mice. The amount of constitutively phosphorylated MUT TP53 is unaffected by MDM2 overexpression, indicating that phosphorylation of MUT p53 at Ser15 may be involved in stabilization and carcinogenic activity [51]. Ser15 phosphorylation can be crucial in controlling MUT p53 carcinogenic potential and cell survival through the NF-κB signaling pathway. By increasing JNK kinase phosphorylation at Ser15, inhibition of NF-κB signaling stabilizes MUT p53 (Pro223Leu/Val274Phe) [52, 53]. Also, in osteosarcoma SaOs2 cells transfected with p53 proteins altered at residues Ala143 and His175, it was observed that suppression of Ser15 or Ser315 phosphorylation partly restored WT function [54, 55].

10.5 ACETYLATION OF MUT p53

Numerous cancer cell lines have shown evidence of acetylation on several MUT p53 sites. Acetylation and signaling for WT and MUT p53 proteins are not well understood in connection to one another, as is the case with other PTMs. This is primarily because the majority of lysine residues that are targets of acetylation can also be altered by neddylation, ubiquitylation, and methylation, all of which have different inhibitory effects in p53 functioning [56, 57]. p53 has 11 lysine residues that are sites of acetylation. Among these, nine are found at the C-terminus and only two—Lys120 and Lys163—are in the DBD. Histone acetyltransferases include TIP60, hMOF, hMOZ, p300/CBP-associated factor (PCAF), and the physically related p300 and CREB-binding protein (CBP) acetylate p53 [13, 36]. Under stressful conditions, p53 acetylation levels are enhanced and have a strong correlation with TP53 activation, which facilitates the recruitment of cofactors for promoter-specific TP53 transcriptional activity [56, 58]. Acetylation also promotes p53 stabilization by the inhibition of the ubiquitylation process triggered by MDM2/MDM4 repressive complexes [59, 60]. When compared to non-tumorigenic cell lines, the Arg248Trp and Arg273His MUT p53 proteins were hyperacetylated at Lys320, Lys373, or Lys382 in the absence of stress [45, 61]. In a study carried out by Warnock et al. (2011) [62], they discovered a similar finding with Lys382 acetylation in colon cancer cells carrying Arg273 mutations. These strong acetylation patterns may encourage MUT p53 to accumulate in the nucleus [63, 64]. MUT TP53 acetylation significantly affects the metabolic and survival processes in cancer cells. By using the C-terminal acetylation-mimicking variant of TP53 (Gly245Ala-K6Q), autophagic degradation of TP53 is seen, which is dependent on the protein's acetylation state. Therefore, in response to fasting, tumor cells lose control over the autophagic process, which leads to an increase in autophagy and cell death [65, 66].

10.6 UBIQUITYLATION OF MUT p53

The primary contributor of p53 ubiquitylation is the E3 ubiquitin ligase MDM2, although reports have indicated that several other proteins with comparable functions, such as Pirh2, Cop1, TOPORS, and CHIP, can also encourage p53 breakdown on their own in an MDM2-independent manner [67, 68]. Polyubiquitylation is generally responsible for inactivating p53 functions by promoting the degradation of p53 protein. p53 transcriptional target MDM2 creates a negative feedback loop for p53 activity [69]. Furthermore, several tumor forms exhibit overexpression of MDM2, which causes abnormal p53 inactivation. Tumors containing MUT p53 lose the tight regulation that normally occurs between MDM2 and TP53, leading to hyperstability, which is correlated with MUT p53 oncogenic activity. The loss of p53-mediated MDM2 transactivation is linked to hyperstability [70]. Endogenous MUT p53 cell lines produced from tumors demonstrate a striking constitutive p53 stabilization (10–20 times more than WT p53 cancer cell lines) and a total absence of ubiquitylation [71]. The ubiquitylation of MUT p53 by MDM2 is less effective than that of WT p53, even though MDM2 can interact with p53-DBD mutant proteins which are structurally altered [67]. Inhibition of MDM2 and the chaperone CHIP E3 ligases by the HSP90 chaperone machinery can lead to MUT p53 in cancer cells [71, 72]. HSP70 and MDM2 work cooperatively to increase p53Arg175His aggregation and change its subcellular distribution, which stabilizes this MUT p53 [73]. All of these findings point to a more intricate connection between MDM2 and p53 as well as a potential selective impairment of MUT p53 degradation in tumor cells.

Other modifications that p53 can experience include methylation, neddylation, sumoylation, ADP-ribosylation, nitration, and O-linked β-N-acetylglucosamine (O-GlcNAcylation). However, it is unknown how important these alterations are for MUT p53 functions and tumor development.

10.7 THERAPEUTIC IMPLICATIONS

Since more than half of all human malignancies have p53 mutations, MUT p53 has gained attention as a promising target for cancer treatment. MUT p53 typically accumulates at high levels in cancer cells to perform its GOF actions. MUT p53 typically exhibits GOF activities via regulating many downstream signaling pathways in cancer cells. For example, MUT p53 upregulates PDGFRβ and EGFR/integrin recycling to promote tumor metastasis [74, 75]. Various therapeutic strategies target mutp53 for cancer therapy. The first strategy involves directly targeting MUT p53 and either restoring wild-type tumor-suppressive activity or depriving MUT p53 by causing its breakdown. The second strategy is to suppress mutp53 GOF activities by targeting certain mutp53-binding proteins or important downstream signaling pathways of MUT p53 [76, 77]. Small compounds (such as CP-31398, PRIMA-1, and MIRA-1) that selectively target p53 mutants have been developed to restore p53 transcriptional activity and cause tumor cells to undergo cell cycle arrest or apoptosis [78, 79]. MUT p53 stabilization depends on its interaction with the HDAC6/HSP90 chaperone complex. As the first HSP90 inhibitor, geldanamycin is utilized to target MUT p53 and cause its degradation [71, 80, 81]. An analogue of geldanamycin called 7-AAG uses MDM2 and CHIP-mediated ubiquitination to cause the proteasomal destruction of MUT p53 [71]. Moreover, lysosomal and autophagic degradation can also be used for MUT p53 degradation. For example, MCB-613, a small-molecule stimulator of steroid receptor coactivators, causes ubiquitination, nuclear export, and destruction of R175H mutp53 via a lysosome-mediated mechanism by depleting USP15 in ovarian cancer cells [82].

10.8 CONCLUSION

Knowing how PTMs affect MUT p53 stability and function may aid in predicting how tumors containing MUT p53 would react to chemotherapy. The multifaceted landscape of post-translational modifications (PTMs) significantly influences the function and stability of both wild-type (WT) and mutant (MUT) p53 proteins. While PTMs such as phosphorylation, acetylation, and ubiquitylation play crucial roles in regulating WT p53 activity in response to various stressors, they also impact the behavior of MUT p53, often associated with oncogenic activities. Phosphorylation of specific residues in MUT p53 can alter its stability and DNA binding activity, while acetylation patterns contribute to its accumulation in the nucleus and affect cellular processes such as autophagy and cell death. Additionally, the dysregulation of ubiquitylation pathways in tumors containing MUT p53 leads to hyperstability and aberrant oncogenic activity. However, the significance of other PTMs on MUT p53 function and tumor development remains to be fully elucidated. Understanding the intricate interplay between PTMs and mutant p53 may pave the way for targeted therapeutic strategies aimed at restoring normal p53 function and combating cancer progression. Targeting MUT p53 holds great promise for cancer therapy, given its prevalence in malignancies and its pivotal role in promoting tumor progression through gain-of-function activities. Various therapeutic strategies have emerged, including direct targeting of MUT p53 to restore wild-type tumor-suppressive functions or induce its breakdown, as well as suppressing MUT p53 gain-of-function activities by targeting associated proteins or downstream signaling pathways. Small compounds and inhibitors like CP-31398, PRIMA-1, and geldanamycin derivatives have shown efficacy in restoring p53 transcriptional activity or promoting MUT p53 degradation through various mechanisms. Further research and development in this field offer hope for more effective and targeted treatments against p53-mutant cancers.

REFERENCES

1. Kress, M., et al., Simian virus 40-transformed cells express new species of proteins precipitable by anti-simian virus 40 tumor serum. *Journal of Virology*, 1979. **31**(2): p. 472–483.
2. Lane, D.P. and L.V. Crawford, T antigen is bound to a host protein in SY40-transformed cells. *Nature*, 1979. **278**(5701): p. 261–263.
3. Linzer, D.I.H. and A.J. Levine, Characterization of a 54K dalton cellular SV40 tumor antigen present in SV40-transformed cells and uninfected embryonal carcinoma cells. *Cell*, 1979. **17**(1): p. 43–52.
4. Eliyahu, D., et al., Participation of p53 cellular tumour antigen in transformation of normal embryonic cells. *Nature*, 1984. **312**(5995): p. 646–649.
5. Jenkins, J.R., K. Rudge, and G.A. Currie, Cellular immortalization by a cDNA clone encoding the transformation-associated phosphoprotein p53. *Nature*, 1984. **312**(5995): p. 651–654.
6. Parada, L.F., et al., Cooperation between gene encoding p53 tumour antigen and ras in cellular transformation. *Nature*, 1984. **312**(5995): p. 649–651.
7. Menendez, D., A. Inga, and M.A. Resnick, The expanding universe of p53 targets. *Nature Reviews Cancer*, 2009. **9**(10): p. 724–737.
8. Kruiswijk, F., C.F. Labuschagne, and K.H. Vousden, p53 in survival, death and metabolic health: a lifeguard with a licence to kill. *Nature Reviews Molecular Cell Biology*, 2015. **16**(7): p. 393–405.
9. Mir, M.A., Sumaya, N. Jan, Implications of Chemokine Heterogenicity in Cancer Metastasis, in *Cytokine and Chemokine Networks in Cancer*. 2023, Springer. p. 115–136.
10. Sabapathy, K. and D.P. Lane, Therapeutic targeting of p53: all mutants are equal, but some mutants are more equal than others. *Nature Reviews Clinical Oncology*, 2018. **15**(1): p. 13–30.
11. Sabapathy, K., The contrived mutant p53 oncogene–beyond loss of functions. *Frontiers in Oncology*, 2015. **5**: p. 276.
12. Muller, P.A.J. and K.H. Vousden, Mutant p53 in cancer: new functions and therapeutic opportunities. *Cancer Cell*, 2014. **25**(3): p. 304–317.
13. Mir, M.A., M. Rashid, and N. Jan, *Cytokines and Chemokines in Tumor Growth and Progression, in Cytokine and Chemokine Networks in Cancer*. 2023, Springer. p. 33–77.
14. Chang, F., S. Syrjänen, K. Kurvinen, and K. Syrjänen, The p53 tumor suppressor gene as a common cellular target in human carcinogenesis. *The American Journal of Gastroenterology*, 1993. **88**(2): 174–186.
15. Mir, M.A., M. Bashir, and N. Jan, The Role of Interleukin (IL)-6/IL-6 Receptor Axis in Cancer, in *Cytokine and Chemokine Networks in Cancer*. 2023, Springer. p. 137–164.
16. Lozano, G. and A.J. Levine, *The p53 Protein: From Cell Regulation to Cancer*. 2016. Cold Spring Harbor Laboratory Press.
17. Baugh, E.H., et al., Why are there hotspot mutations in the TP53 gene in human cancers? *Cell Death & Differentiation*, 2018. **25**(1): p. 154–160.
18. Ramazi, S., A. Allahverdi, and J. Zahiri, Evaluation of post-translational modifications in histone proteins: a review on histone modification defects in developmental and neurological disorders. *Journal of Biosciences*, 2020. **45**(1): p. 135.
19. Wang, Y.-C., S.E. Peterson, and J.F. Loring, Protein post-translational modifications and regulation of pluripotency in human stem cells. *Cell research*, 2014. **24**(2): p. 143–160.

20. Blom, N., et al., Prediction of post-translational glycosylation and phosphorylation of proteins from the amino acid sequence. *Proteomics*, 2004. **4**(6): p. 1633–1649.
21. Ryšlavá, H., et al., Effect of posttranslational modifications on enzyme function and assembly. *Journal of Proteomics*, 2013. **92**: p. 80–109.
22. Marshall, C.J., Protein prenylation: a mediator of protein-protcin interactions. *Science*, 1993. **259**(5103): p. 1865–1866.
23. Caragea, C., et al., Glycosylation site prediction using ensembles of support vector machine classifiers. *BMC Bioinformatics*, 2007. **8**: p. 1–13.
24. Audagnotto, M. and M. Dal Peraro, Protein post-translational modifications: In silico prediction tools and molecular modeling. *Computational and Structural Biotechnology Journal*, 2017. **15**: p. 307–319.
25. Wang, M., Y. Jiang, and X. Xu, A novel method for predicting post-translational modifications on serine and threonine sites by using site-modification network profiles. *Molecular BioSystems*, 2015. **11**(11): p. 3092–3100.
26. Wei, L., et al., Fast prediction of protein methylation sites using a sequence-based feature selection technique. *IEEE/ACM Transactions on Computational Biology and Bioinformatics*, 2017. **16**(4): p. 1264–1273.
27. Khoury, G.A., R.C. Baliban, and C.A. Floudas, Proteome-wide post-translational modification statistics: frequency analysis and curation of the swiss-prot database. *Scientific Reports*, 2011. **1**(1): p. 90.
28. Huang, K.-Y., et al., dbPTM in 2019: exploring disease association and cross-talk of post-translational modifications. *Nucleic Acids Research*, 2019. **47**(D1): p. D298-D308.
29. Nguyen, T.A., et al., Mutant TP 53 posttranslational modifications: challenges and opportunities. *Human Mutation*, 2014. **35**(6): p. 738–755.
30. Haq, B.U., et al., Targeting p53 misfolding conundrum by stabilizing agents and their analogs in breast cancer therapy: a comprehensive computational analysis. *Frontiers in Pharmacology*, 2024. **14**: p. 1333447.
31. Sofi, S., et al., A comprehensive analysis of notch signaling genes in breast cancer: expression pattern and prognostic significance. *Advances in Cancer Biology-Metastasis*, 2023. **7**: p. 100104.
32. Riley, T., et al., Transcriptional control of human p53-regulated genes. *Nature Reviews Molecular Cell Biology*, 2008. **9**(5): p. 402–412.
33. Sofi, S., et al., Clinicopathological and prognostic significance of Bcl2 in breast cancer: a comprehensive in silico and in vitro study. *Saudi Journal of Biological Sciences*, 2023. **31**(2): p. 103916.
34. Rinn, J.L. and M. Huarte, To repress or not to repress: this is the guardian's question. *Trends in Cell Biology*, 2011. **21**(6): p. 344–353.
35. Sofi, S., et al., Elucidation of interleukin-19 as a therapeutic target for breast cancer by computational analysis and experimental validation. *Saudi Journal of Biological Sciences*, 2023. **30**(9): p. 103774–103774.
36. Petitjean, A., et al., Impact of mutant p53 functional properties on TP53 mutation patterns and tumor phenotype: lessons from recent developments in the IARC TP53 database. *Human Mutation*, 2007. **28**(6): p. 622–629.
37. Pfeifer, G.P. and P. Hainaut, Next-generation sequencing: emerging lessons on the origins of human cancer. *Current Opinion in Oncology*, 2011. **23**(1): p. 62–68.
38. Jan, N., et al., Metronomic chemotherapy and drug repurposing: a paradigm shift in oncology. *Heliyon*, 2024. https://doi.org/10.1016/j.heliyon.2024.e24670
39. Ullrich, S.J., et al., Phosphorylation at Ser-15 and Ser-392 in mutant p53 molecules from human tumors is altered compared to wild-type p53. *Proceedings of the National Academy of Sciences*, 1993. **90**(13): p. 5954–5958.
40. Bech-Otschir, D., et al., COP9 signalosome-specific phosphorylation targets p53 to degradation by the ubiquitin system. *The EMBO Journal*, 2001. **20**(7): p. 1630–1639.
41. Jan, N., et al., Exploring the role of trifarotene against RAR-α: an investigation of expression pattern and clinicopathological significance of RAR-α in breast cancer. *Frontiers in Pharmacology*, 2024. **15**: p. 1361679.
42. Keller, D.M., et al., A DNA damage–induced p53 serine 392 kinase complex contains CK2, hSpt16, and SSRP1. *Molecular Cell*, 2001. **7**(2): p. 283–292.
43. Sakaguchi, K., et al., Phosphorylation of serine 392 stabilizes the tetramer formation of tumor suppressor protein p53. *Biochemistry*, 1997. **36**(33): p. 10117–10124.
44. Hupp, T.R. and D.P. Lane, Two distinct signaling pathways activate the latent DNA binding function of p53 in a casein kinase II-independent manner. *Journal of Biological Chemistry*, 1995. **270**(30): p. 18165–18174.

45. Minamoto, T., et al., Distinct pattern of p53 phosphorylation in human tumors. *Oncogene*, 2001. **20**(26): p. 3341–3347.
46. Furihata, M., et al., Frequent phosphorylation at serine 392 in overexpressed p53 protein due to missense mutation in carcinoma of the urinary tract. *The Journal of Pathology*, 2002. **197**(1): p. 82–88.
47. Gillotin, S., D. Yap, and X. Lu, Mutation at Ser392 specifically sensitizes mutant p53H175 to mdm2-mediated degradation. *Cell Cycle*, 2010. **9**(7): p. 1390–1398.
48. Nagata, Y., et al., The stabilization mechanism of mutant-type p53 by impaired ubiquitination: the loss of wild-type p53 function and the hsp90 association. *Oncogene*, 1999. **18**(44): p. 6037–49.
49. Liu, C., et al., Functional p53 determines docetaxel sensitivity in prostate cancer cells. *Prostate*, 2013. **73**(4): p. 418–27.
50. Ray, D., K.R. Murphy, and S. Gal, The DNA binding and accumulation of p53 from breast cancer cell lines and the link with serine 15 phosphorylation. *Cancer Biology & Therapy*, 2012. **13**(10): p. 848–57.
51. Melnikova, V.O., et al., Mutant p53 is constitutively phosphorylated at Serine 15 in UV-induced mouse skin tumors: involvement of ERK1/2 MAP kinase. *Oncogene*, 2003. **22**(38): p. 5958–66.
52. Zerbini, L.F., et al., Blockage of NF-kappaB induces serine 15 phosphorylation of mutant p53 by JNK kinase in prostate cancer cells. *Cell Cycle*, 2005. **4**(9): p. 1247–53.
53. Mir, M.A., A. Manzoor, and N. Jan, *CCL5/CCR5 Axis in Cancer, in Cytokine and Chemokine Networks in Cancer.* 2023, Springer. p. 219–240.
54. Sugikawa, E., et al., Inhibition of mutant p53 phosphorylation at serine 15 or serine 315 partially restores the function of wild-type p53. *Biochemical and Biophysical Research Communications*, 1999. **261**(2): p. 256–63.
55. Mir, M.A., A. Shabir, and N. Jan, Metronomic Chemotherapy in Breast Cancer, in *Novel Approaches in Metronomic Chemotherapy for Breast Cancer Treatment.* CRC Press. p. 72–86.
56. Carter, S. and K.H. Vousden, Modifications of p53: competing for the lysines. *Current Opinion in Genetics & Development*, 2009. **19**(1): p. 18–24.
57. Kruse, J.P. and W. Gu, Modes of p53 regulation. *Cell*, 2009. **137**(4): p. 609–622.
58. Brooks, C.L. and W. Gu, Ubiquitination, phosphorylation and acetylation: the molecular basis for p53 regulation. *Current Opinion in Cell Biology*, 2003. **15**(2): p. 164–171.
59. Dai, C. and W. Gu, p53 post-translational modification: deregulated in tumorigenesis. *Trends in Molecular Medicine*, 2010. **16**(11): p. 528–536.
60. Mir, M.A., et al., Metronomics: toward personalized chemotherapy. *Novel Approaches in Metronomic Chemotherapy for Breast Cancer Treatment*, 2024. p. 99–119. https://doi.org/10.1201/9781032632674-8
61. Mir, M.A., et al., Proteomics: A Groundbreaking Development in Cancer Biology, in *Proteomics.* 2023, Elsevier. p. 31–53.
62. Warnock, L.J., S.A. Raines, and J. Milner, Aurora A mediates cross-talk between N- and C-terminal post-translational modifications of p53. *Cancer Biology & Therapy*, 2011. **12**(12): p. 1059–1068.
63. Bode, A.M. and Z. Dong, Post-translational modification of p53 in tumorigenesis. *Nature Reviews Cancer*, 2004. **4**(10): p. 793–805.
64. Mir, M.A., et al., Proteomics: Application of Next-Generation Proteomics in Cancer Research, in *Proteomics.* 2023, Elsevier. p. 55–76.
65. Rodriguez, O.C., et al., Dietary downregulation of mutant p53 levels via glucose restriction: mechanisms and implications for tumor therapy. *Cell Cycle*, 2012. **11**(23): p. 4436–4446.
66. Mir, M.A., N. Jan, and S. Sofi, Introduction to Metronomic Chemotherapy, in *Novel Approaches in Metronomic Chemotherapy for Breast Cancer Treatment.* 2024, CRC Press. p. 1–14.
67. Lukashchuk, N. and K.H. Vousden, Ubiquitination and degradation of mutant p53. *Molecular and Cellular Biology*, 2007. **27**(23): p. 8284–8295.
68. *Mir, M.A., M. Rashid, and N. Jan, The Interleukin-8 Pathway in Cancer, in Cytokine and Chemokine Networks in Cancer.* 2023, Springer. p. 165–190.
69. Lee, J.T. and W. Gu, The multiple levels of regulation by p53 ubiquitination. *Cell Death & Differentiation*, 2010. **17**(1): p. 86–92.
70. Midgley, C.A. and D.P. Lane, p53 protein stability in tumour cells is not determined by mutation but is dependent on Mdm2 binding. *Oncogene*, 1997. **15**(10): p. 1179–1189.
71. Galluzzi, L., et al., Mitochondrial liaisons of p53. *Antioxidants & Redox Signaling*, 2011. **15**(6): p. 1691–1714.
72. Mir, M.A., N. Jan, and I. Noor, Therapeutic Implications of Cytokines and Chemokines Network in Cancer, in *Cytokine and Chemokine Networks in Cancer.* 2023, Springer. p. 385–414.
73. Wiech, M., et al., Molecular mechanism of mutant p53 stabilization: the role of HSP70 and MDM2. *PLoS One*, 2012. **7**(12): p. e51426.

74. Muller, P.A., et al., Mutant p53 drives invasion by promoting integrin recycling. *Cell*, 2009. **139**(7): p. 1327–1341.
75. Weissmueller, S., et al., Mutant p53 drives pancreatic cancer metastasis through cell-autonomous PDGF receptor β signaling. *Cell*, 2014. **157**(2): p. 382–394.
76. Blandino, G. and S. Di Agostino, New therapeutic strategies to treat human cancers expressing mutant p53 proteins. *Journal of Experimental & Clinical Cancer Research*, 2018. **37**: p. 1–13.
77. Zhou, X., Q. Hao, and H. Lu, Mutant p53 in cancer therapy-the barrier or the path. *Journal of Molecular and Cellular Biology*, 2019. **11**(4): p. 293–305.
78. Bykov, V.J., et al., Restoration of the tumor suppressor function to mutant p53 by a low-molecular-weight compound. *Nature Medicine*, 2002. **8**(3): p. 282–288.
79. Foster, B.A., et al., Pharmacological rescue of mutant p53 conformation and function. *Science*, 1999. **286**(5449): p. 2507–2510.
80. Peng, Y., et al., Inhibition of MDM2 by hsp90 contributes to mutant p53 stabilization. *Journal of Biological Chemistry*, 2001. **276**(44): p. 40583–4090.
81. Blagosklonny, table M.V., J. Toretsky, and L. Neckers, Geldanamycin selectively destabilizes and conformationally alters mutated p53. *Oncogene*, 1995. **11**(5): p. 933–939.
82. Padmanabhan, A., et al., USP15-dependent lysosomal pathway controls p53-R175H turnover in ovarian cancer cells. *Nature Communications*, 2018. **9**(1): p. 1270.

11 Genetic Alterations Affecting p53 and Emerging Perspectives on Epigenetic Control of p53 in Breast Cancer

*Alia Jabar, Nusrat Jan, Iqra Jan, and Manzoor Ahmad Mir**
Department of Bioresources, School of Biological Sciences, University of Kashmir, Srinagar, J&K, India
*drmanzoor@kashmiruniversity.ac.in

11.1 INTRODUCTION

Breast carcinoma typically begins in the cells of the breast and can arise in various parts, such as the ducts, lobules, or the tissue between them. Its occurrence varies globally, yet it ranks among the most prevalent cancers globally, with millions of new diagnoses each year [1, 2]. The p53 protein acts as a protector of genetic integrity, suppressing tumor development. It plays a crucial role in regulating the equilibrium between cell growth and cell cycle arrest when confronted with genetic stress. Fundamentally, p53 functions as a sentinel, preserving cellular balance by regulating growth and division to prevent tumor formation [3–6]. In its capacity as a transcription factor, the p53 gene possesses essential structural elements, including a central DNA-binding region, a domain responsible for activating transcriptional processes, and a section facilitating the formation of tetramers. Together, these elements facilitate the regulation of genetic activation by the p53 gene through its binding to a particular gene, initiating the transcription of the targeted genetic sequence, and assembling functional protein complexes essential for its regulatory roles [7–9]. Typically, the level of p53 expression remains modest, but it experiences stabilization and amplification when the genome and cellular integrity face various stressors. These stress signals include DNA damage, oxygen deprivation (hypoxia), activation of oncogenes, and deficiencies in critical nutrients. When confronted with such stressors, the expression of p53 is heightened, allowing it to fulfill its role as a sentinel of cellular health by initiating appropriate responses to maintain genomic stability and counteract potential threats to the cell's well-being [10]. When faced with stressors, p53 is stimulated to bind to specific DNA sequences, initiating either the activation or suppression of a group of genes further down the line. These genes are crucial in determining whether the cellular division halts programmed cell death or repairs damaged DNA. Consequently, if p53 malfunctions, it disrupts the delicate equilibrium between cellular expansion and cessation of growth, permitting aberrant cells to multiply unchecked, potentially progressing into cancer. Contrary to classical anti-oncogenes, which are frequently diminished or eliminated in cancerous conditions in human cancers, p53 undergoes mutations more frequently across various types of human malignancies [11, 12]. Analysis of genomic sequencing data from diverse human cancer types demonstrates that the p53 gene stands out as the utmost prevalent and often altered tumor suppressor gene. These mutations are identified in the majority of cancer occurrences, indicating a widespread occurrence of somatic p53 mutations across various cancer types [13–15]. Therefore, targeting mutated p53 aims to restore

DOI: 10.1201/9781003520771-11

its tumor-suppressive function or induce cell death in cancer cells harboring these mutations. This approach could potentially improve treatment outcomes and overcome resistance to conventional therapies in breast cancer patients with p53 mutations. Mutation frequencies rise notably in specific cancer variations, including ovarian serous adenocarcinoma, squamous cell carcinoma of the lung, and triple-negative breast cancer (TNBC) [16–19]. Targeted therapies for mutated p53 in breast cancer are an area of active research. While direct targeting of p53 mutations has been challenging, various strategies aim to indirectly impact p53 function or exploit vulnerabilities caused by p53 mutations. These include approaches such as targeting downstream pathways affected by p53 mutations, utilizing synthetic lethal interactions, and developing drugs that stabilize or restore p53 function. Immunotherapies and combination treatments also hold promise in managing breast cancer with mutated p53. It is now possible to take drugs that either cause the mutant p53 to degrade or bring it back to its normal function. Furthermore, mounting evidence indicates that mutated p53 develops supplementary cancer-promoting capabilities referred to as function-boosting mutations or gain-of-function (GOF) mutations, which aid in malignant spread, dissemination, and insensitivity to medications [20–24]. While there are many systemic treatments for metastatic breast cancer (MBC), most cancers eventually develop resistance to systemic therapy. The outcomes for individuals with solid tumors have seen enhancements due to the introduction of various targeted medications in recent times. Trastuzumab, known as Herceptin and produced by Genentech in South San Francisco, California, is a monoclonal antibody designed to target the human epidermal growth factor receptor 2 (HER2) specifically. It has demonstrated effectiveness in treating breast cancer among women who test positive for the HER2 protein [25–28]. p53 has a significant impact in inhibiting tumor growth by directly controlling the activity of many genes that are critical for regulating cellular division, regulated cell demise, cellular aging (senescence), cell specialization (differentiation), and metabolism in healthy cells [29]. Because of the wide-ranging nature and potent function of p53 mutations in promoting cancer development, they have emerged as a primary focus for treatment in the quest for effective treatments for human cancers. While advancements in conventional cancer treatments like medical treatment, radiation treatment, and surgery procedures have contributed to a decline in cancer-related deaths in recent years, significant challenges persist, often leading to tumor recurrence and fatalities. The investigation of mutation-targeted cancer therapeutics is a result of these difficulties. Standard chemotherapy acts on aberrant proteins encoded by altered genes, while tailored medicines act on malignant and normal cells that divide quickly. Malignant and nonmalignant cells frequently respond to targeted therapies differently because normal cells do not have the tumorigenic mutations that are used to target certain drugs. Because of this, tailored therapy typically results in swift and significant tumor shrinkage while lowering the possibility of the characteristic off-target effects [30, 31]. The progress in targeted therapies has been closely tied to the advancements in sequencing technology over the past 20 years, notably with the transformative emergence of next-generation sequencing (NGS) [32].

11.2 MUTANT p53 AND ITS MECHANISM OF ACTION

Mutant p53 denotes a modified version of the gene responsible for cancer inhibition, p53, which is crucial for preventing cancer formation. Mutations in the p53 gene can result in the creation of a malfunctioning amino acid that loses its ability to regulate cell growth and repair DNA damage effectively. This can play a role in the onset and advancement of different types of cancers. The transition from a non-cancerous cell to a malignant one involves an intricate procedure encompassing numerous stages of changes in DNA and gene expression regulation. These changes offer beneficial traits to the transforming cells. Throughout cancer development, these modifications are thought to empower the developing cancer to generate its growth signals, become resistant to growth-inhibiting signals, evade programmed cell death, acquire the ability to replicate continuously, sustain the continuous formation of new blood vessels, and ultimately develop the capability to infiltrate neighboring tissues and metastasize to distant sites in the body [33]. While many genes contribute to the progression of cancer development, the cancer suppressor p53, produced by the TP53 gene in humans, is notably significant as a crucial anti-cancer agent. It serves as a key regulator of various signaling pathways essential for the tumorigenesis process [34, 35]. p53 serves numerous roles as a tumor suppressor, including prompting cell cycle halt, enhancing DNA mending, instigating cellular aging, and initiating programmed cell death, alongside various other functions [36]. The TP53 gene acts as both a cancer-inhibiting factor and guardian of the genetic material, implying that cells with intact p53 activity are less likely to undergo the conversion from normal to cancerous states [37, 38]. Mutations in the p53 create a conducive environment for the development of carcinoma [39, 40]. Mutations in the TP53 gene are a hallmark of Li–Fraumeni syndrome, a hereditary condition associated with increased cancer susceptibility [41, 42]. The elevated occurrence of mutations in the TP53 gene within tumor cells might be clarified by the selective forces that support the survival of these cells, allowing them to evade immune surveillance and resist programmed cell death [43, 44]. Numerous mutant p53 proteins demonstrate enhanced stability in contrast to wild-type p53 proteins, resulting in their buildup within cells. Additionally, some mutant p53 proteins may possess entirely different functions from those of the wild-type versions [45] and this phenomenon may be caused by changes in the patterns of target genes, the collection of secreted proteins related to mutant p53, or improper interactions between mutant p53 and other proteins [46] (Figure 11.1). Mutated p53 can assist cancer cells in acquiring resistance to treatments. MDR1, also known as P-glycoprotein and encoded by the ATP-binding cassette subfamily B member 1 gene, has been acknowledged as a contributor to shielding cells from the harmful effects of cytotoxic agents and medication therapy [47].

Mutant p53 can disrupt the normal activity of wild-type (WT) p53, suppress the activity of WT p53 through dominant-negative effects, and acquire new oncogenic functions. This mutant p53 influences several cellular processes, including causing genomic instability, altering cellular metabolism, and modifying the tumor microenvironment. These changes lead to enhanced cancer cell growth, increased ability to invade and spread (metastasize), and greater resistance to drugs. As per Figure 12.1, mutations in p53 can acquire cancer-driving features through GOF methods. In these

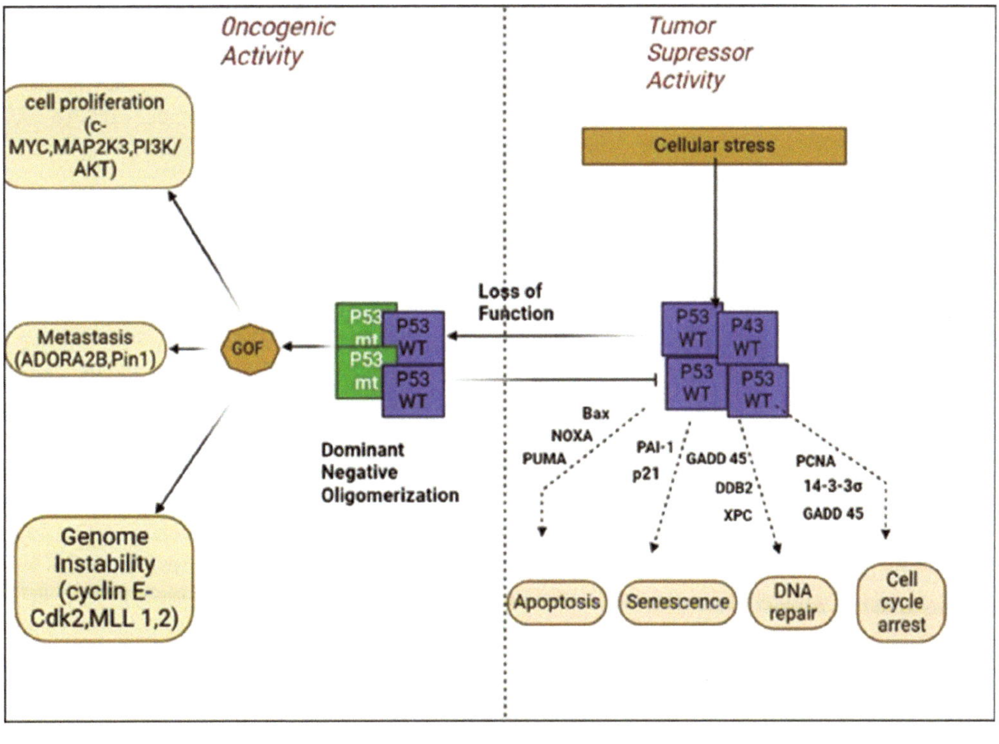

FIGURE 11.1 The mechanisms by which GOF activities and wild-type p53's anticancer function are inactivated in breast cancers harboring altered p53.

instances, the altered protein engages with new transcription factors or cofactors to regulate gene transcription and expression, thereby fostering cancer progression. Additionally, the altered protein exhibits dominant-negative activity, which inhibits the functions of normal p53. Several key mechanisms contribute to the cancer-promoting traits of mtp53, as described in the following sections.

11.2.1 Genome Instability

Genome instability is the core attribute of various malignancies in humans. The gain-of-function activity of altered p53 has been shown to worsen these fluctuations. In samples of breast carcinoma, abnormal copy numbers are associated with mutated p53 [48]. The mutation of the p53 protein where the arginine at position 172 is replaced by histidine (H) or the p53 arginine 172 to histidine (R172H) mutation, which is equivalent to the arginine 175 to histidine (R175H) mutation in mice, leads to abnormalities in centrosomes by modifying the activity of cyclinE-cdk2 at the centrosome, increasing in centrosome numbers [49]. Another investigation found that altered forms of p53 can attach to chromatin and elevate the levels of genes that regulate chromatin, including the enzymes MLL1 and MLL2 (mixed lineage leukemia 1, mixed lineage leukemia 2) responsible for methylation. These enzymes boost the histone modifications (methylation and acetylation), ultimately fostering genetic chaos and promoting the advancement of cancer [50].

11.2.2 Evading Apoptosis

The altered version of the p53 protein prevents programmed cell death by engaging with other members of the p53 family, specifically p63 and p73, to weaken their inherent ability to inhibit tumor growth [51]. Various genetic changes in the p53 gene, including R273H and R175H, have been identified as hindering the programmed cell death process and apoptosis. These mutations achieve this by reducing the levels of BCL2-modifying factor expression through heightened AKT signaling. This alteration in signaling pathways ultimately disrupts the normal apoptotic response, contributing to cell survival and potentially fueling tumor growth [2, 52]. Additionally, these mutations decrease the ability of p73 to regulate transcription on the Bax promoter, which is responsible for regulating the expression of Bax, a protein involved in apoptosis. This reduction in p73's ability to activate Bax expression further disrupts the apoptotic pathway, enabling cancer cells to escape apoptosis and promoting their survival and proliferation [53].

11.2.3 Proliferation

Mutant versions of the p53 protein can stimulate the activation of many genes linked to cell growth, unlike the function of the normal p53 protein. This abnormal transcriptional behavior fuels the unrestrained multiplication of cells, a characteristic trait of cancer. Essentially, the altered p53 protein adopts a new role that enhances cell division, thereby worsening the advancement of cancerous growth [54, 55]. Included in these are genes such as the cellular myelocytomatosis oncogene (c-MYC), mitogen-activated protein kinase 3 (MAP2K3), C-X-C motif chemokine ligand 1 (CXCL1), and cyclin E2 (CCNE2), which mutant p53 can trigger. Moreover, it has been noted that mutant p53 collaborates with various proteins or transcription factors involved in breast cancer progression, including sterol regulatory element-binding proteins (SREBPs), thereby activating the mevalonate pathway [56, 57], poly(ADP-ribose) polymerases (PARPs) [58], nuclear factor Y (NF-Y) [59], and disabled homolog 2-interacting protein (DAB2IP) [60, 61].

11.2.4 Metastasis

Mutant versions of p53 have been documented to increase the aggressiveness of tumors and their propensity to metastasize through various pathways. One such process is the durability or endurance of the mtp53 protein, which is made possible with the secretion of heat shock protein 90 (Hsp90) regulated by the Rab coupling protein. This stabilizing process accelerates cancer cell invasion and metastasis, which advances the disease overall [62, 63]. Mutant forms of the p53 protein also engage with the adenosine A2b receptor (ADORA2B), a member of the G-protein coupled receptor (GPCR) family [64], and Pin [65]. These two interactions correlate with unfavorable clinical results and in cases of cancer affecting the breast and increased invasion and metastasis. This indicates that the development of breast cancer toward highly active and metastatic forms is mostly driven by these molecular interactions mediated by mutant p53, which ultimately has a negative effect on the prognosis of patients.

11.3 CONTRIBUTION OF p53 IN BREAST CANCER

In nearly 30% of instances of breast carcinoma, mutations are found in the p53, making it the gene with the highest frequency of mutations in this type of cancer. Altered TP53 can be found in tumors across all types of breast cancer at the molecular level [66, 67]. A multitude of preclinical and clinical studies have endeavored to understand the contribution of p53 in breast carcinoma. Despite these efforts, the clinical significance of p53 alteration status remains unclear, as different studies have yielded conflicting results, with some indicating that TP53 mutations are linked to negative outcomes, others suggesting neutral effects, and still others showing positive associations [55, 68–71].

11.3.1 TP53 Mutation Analysis and Prognostic Significance in Breast Cancer

Breast malignancy comprises various biological subtypes, each with unique characteristics and responses to treatment [72]. Mutations in the TP53 gene frequently occur in breast carcinoma, impacting about 30% of all instances of the condition [73]. Most p53 mutations occur within the DNA-binding domain, primarily due to missense point mutations that hinder its capacity to control gene transcription. These mutations are closely linked with particular tumor subcategories [64] and correlate with unfavorable outcomes in breast cancer patients [74]. Breast tumors are primarily classified into four molecular subtypes based on gene expression patterns: luminal-like (either luminal-A or luminal-B), basal-like, normal-like, and HER2-positive [75]. The luminal-like subtype has the least frequency of p53 mutations, with 26% occurrence overall. Within this subtype, luminal-A displays a reduced mutation rate of 17% compared to luminal-B, which has a higher rate of 41%. On the other hand, approximately half of the HER2-amplified tumors (53%) and the majority of basal-like cancers (88%) carry p53 mutations. Unlike other subtypes, having a p53 mutation along with HER2 overexpression indicates a notably poorer prognosis [67]. Furthermore, research indicates that mutations of p53 occur more repeatedly in inflammatory breast cancer with a prevalence of 50%, compared to a prevalence of 20–30% in non-inflammatory breast cancer [76]. Additionally, it was discovered that patients with high-grade and advanced-stage cancers had a higher frequency of p53 mutations. Furthermore, these alterations have been linked to aggressive subtypes such as HER2-amplified breast cancer and TNBC [77].

11.3.2 p53 Managing Apoptosis in Breast Carcinoma

In breast malignancy, p53 can have a notable impact in regulating apoptosis, which is a key mechanism for eliminating cancerous cells. Numerous research studies have indicated that the protein p53 is crucial in initiating apoptosis (the process of programmed cell death) [78, 79]. p53 is involved in regulating both primary signaling mechanisms that lead to cell death: the extracellular pathway, triggered by external signals, and the intracellular pathway, activated by internal cellular stress. This protein acts as a mediator in both pathways, ensuring the proper execution of programmed cell death [80]. p53 initiates the extrinsic apoptotic pathway and is enhanced by upregulating the activation of different cell death receptors such as Fas, death receptor 5 (DR5), and the death domain-containing receptor for TRAIL. These receptors are involved in assembling the death-inducing signaling complex (DISC), which initiates a series of events leading to caspase activation, starting with caspase-8 and then caspase-3, ultimately resulting in cell death [81]. p53 additionally triggers the intrinsic apoptotic pathway by enhancing the expression of proapoptotic genes from the Bcl-2 family, including BAX (Bcl 2 associated X protein), Noxa, PUMA (p53 upregulated modulator of apoptosis), and BID (BCL-2-interacting domain death agonist). These genes cooperate to facilitate the assembly and activation of BAX, a crucial step that initiates the release of cytochrome C from the mitochondria. This release subsequently triggers caspase-9, a crucial enzyme in the advancement of apoptosis [82].

11.4 THERAPIES AGAINST MUTANT p53-BEARING BREAST CANCER

Tumor formation, advancement, and spread are mediated by mutant p53, which is commonly observed in HER2-positive and TNBC subtypes [1, 83]. This renders it a compelling focus for breast carcinoma therapy. In TNBC, p53 mutations are also most commonly clonal [84]. Breast carcinoma is recognized for its diverse nature, but targeting mutant p53 offers an uncommon consistency in the treatment approach. The therapeutic potential of targeting mutant p53 is highlighted by the fact that TNBC tumors, which are particularly severe and lack many targeted treatment options, could significantly benefit from this strategy. Therapies targeting tumors with mutant p53 primarily aim to (1) restore mutant p53 to its normal function, (2) promote its degradation, (3) induce synthetic lethality, (4) inhibit interactions or pathways associated with its harmful functions, (5) leverage immunotherapies, and (6) use gene therapies to deliver the normal p53 gene into tumor cells.

11.4.1 Restoring Mutant p53 to Its Normal Function

Most TP53 mutations predominantly manifest as missense mutations indicating that one amino acid change occurs in the p53 protein, disrupting its ability to bind to DNA [85, 86]. Numerous compounds, including quinuclidines, pyrazoles 2-sulfonyl pyrimidines, and thiosemicarbazones, have been created to help mutant p53 regain functions similar to those of wtp53.

(i) **Quinuclidines**: Prodrugs founded on quinuclidines, such as PRIMA-1 and its methylated derivative APR-246 (also known as PRIMA-1MET), undergo in vivo metabolism to provide 2-methylene-3-quinuclidinone (MQ), which is the active metabolite. By focusing on exposed cysteine residues located in the central domain of the altered p53 protein, MQ, acting as a nucleophile acceptor, rectifies the protein's folding and reinstates its DNA-binding capacity. This is achieved by modifying thiol groups through a chemical reaction known as Michael addition. MQ is recognized for its ability to specifically target Cys-124 and Cys-277, critical residues responsible for enhancing the stability of the mutant p53 R175H [87]. In addition to reinstating the function of altered p53, PRIMA-1 also mitigates the dominant-negative effect by inhibiting the aggregation of the mutant p53 protein [88]. Moreover, it increases the expression of downstream genes regulated by p53, including p21, BAX, PUMA, and NOXA. Additionally, it triggers the activation of caspase-2, caspase-3, and caspase-9 to initiate apoptosis in various cancers, including breast carcinoma [1, 89].
   1. PRIMA-1 as well as APR-246 have been observed to specifically block altered p53 in breast carcinoma cell lines and mouse tumor grafts, demonstrating a preference for altered p53 over wild-type p53 [88]. Curiously, heightened levels of naturally occurring p53 expression are linked to enhanced responsiveness to APR-246 among different breast cancer cell lines [90, 91].

(ii) **2-sulfonyl pyrimidines**: In mutant p53 Y220C and V143A, the 2-sulfonyl pyrimidine chemical PK11007 preferentially alkylates cysteine residues to improve the thermal integrity of the DNA-interacting region [82]. This leads to the restoration of mutant p53 [92]. Additionally, PK11007 selectively triggers apoptosis and suppresses proliferation in p53 mutant breast cancer cells at a lower dosage than in wtp53 cells. Gene ontology and RNA sequencing data demonstrate that PK11007 upregulates gene activation related to the induction of apoptosis following p53 reactivation, intracellular communication, protein refolding, and cell migration [93].

(iii) **Thiosemicarbazones**: Another category of compounds capable of reactivating mutant p53 are thiosemicarbazones. Zinc ions serve as essential cofactors for the wild-type p53, allowing it to interact with DNA. Mutations within the residues that coordinate zinc interfere with p53's zinc-binding ability, thereby hindering its DNA binding [94]. Thiosemicarbazones function as agents that bind zinc, facilitating its attachment to mutant p53. COTI-2, among these compounds, can boost the ability to bind DNA, prompting the induction of p53 target genes such as NOXA, PUMA, and p21. Experimental analyses have demonstrated that breast carcinoma cells containing mutant p53 demonstrate notably lower IC50 values in vitro compared to those with wild-type p53 [95].

(iv) **Natural p53 reactivators**: Numerous naturally derived compounds were discovered to rejuvenate the function of altered p53. Among them are KSS-9 [96], R-goniothalamin (GON) [97], phenethyl isothiocyanate [98], HO-3867 [99], chetomin [100], and 2-[(4-hydroxybenzyl) amino] phenol (HBAP) [101]. Such compounds have the potential to reinstate the p53 protein's capacity to regulate gene expression by rejuvenating its transcriptional activity. Additionally, they exhibit a greater propensity to stimulate mutated variations of p53 in contrast to cells harboring the standard or wild-type iteration of the p53 gene. This preference is observed across different models of breast cancer, whether studied within laboratory settings (in vitro) or in living organisms (in vivo).

11.4.2 Inducing Altered p53 Degradation

Inducing altered p53 breakdown in breast carcinoma involves targeting and breaking down the abnormal, mutated forms associated with p53 detected in malignancies. By promoting the degradation of altered p53, this approach aims to reduce the harmful effects of the mutated protein and potentially inhibit cancer growth. This strategy often involves the use of various compounds or therapies designed to specifically target and degrade mutant p53 proteins, offering a promising avenue for cancer treatment. Various inhibitors were developed to enhance the breakdown of altered p53 including Hsp90 inhibitors and histone deacetylase inhibitors.

(i) **Hsp90 inhibitors**: In cancer cells, chaperones like Hsp90 stabilize the mutant p53 molecule, unlike normal cells. Targeting Hsp90 could therefore be a strategy against tumors with mutant p53 [102]. Geldanamycin along with its derivative 17-allylamino-17-demethoxygeldanamycin (17-AAG), was the pioneering inhibitor of heat shock protein 90 (Hsp90) to be developed. They were found to destabilize different mutant forms of the p53 protein, causing them to be broken down by E3 ligases such as murine double minute 2 (MDM2) or carboxyl terminus of Hsc70-interacting protein (CHIP) [103]. Ganetespib, a more powerful version, was subsequently created and shown to trigger the breakdown of mutant p53 in mouse models of breast carcinoma with multiple p53 genetic alterations [104].

(ii) **HDAC inhibitors**: Histone deacetylase (HDAC) inhibitors, recognized for their involvement in regulating epigenetics, have been discovered to affect mutant p53 through both transcriptional and post-transcriptional processes. Examples include vorinostat (suberoylanilide hydroxamic acid, SAHA) and sodium butyrate (NaB), which belong to the class I histone deacetylase inhibitors. They impede the transcription process of altered p53 by targeting HDAC8 and the Yin Yang-1 complex specifically in triple-negative breast cancer [105]. Additionally, vorinostat can promote the breakdown of p53 by reducing its stability via the inhibition of HDAC6, which is pivotal in controlling Hsp90. Other histone deacetylase inhibitors such as Trichostatin A, sodium butyrate, and FR901228 have been observed to decrease the extent of various altered forms of p53 proteins, including R175H, P223L, V274F, R249S, and R280K [106]. Although clinical trials have evaluated how effective Hsp90 and HDAC inhibitors are in treating breast cancer sufferers, there hasn't been a thorough investigation into their correlation with the mutational status of p53.

(iii) **Other inducers of mutant p53 degradation**: In addition to Hsp90 and histone deacetylase inhibitors, there are other natural or synthetic compounds identified for inducing mutant p53 degradation in breast carcinoma studies. Among them is arsenic trioxide [107], gambogic acid [108], Spautin-1 [109], YK-3-237 [110], triptolide, *Origanum majorana* extract (OSE) [111, 112], THZ1 [113], BEZ235 [114], CBISC [115], capsaicin [116], and disulfiram [117].

11.4.3 Induce Synthetic Lethality

The G1/S checkpoint is vital for controlling the progression of the cellular division to ensure accurate DNA duplication [118]. When DNA injury occurs, normal p53 triggers a halt at the G1/S checkpoint to facilitate DNA repair before entering the S phase [119]. Even when DNA damage is present, cancer cells containing mutated p53 can circumvent this checkpoint. As a result, their means of maintaining genomic stability hinges solely on the G2/M checkpoint [120]. Disabling the G2-M phase transition checkpoint can result in the early commencement of mitosis despite significant DNA damage, triggering mitotic disaster or failure. Targeting this vulnerability might indicate a hopeful remedial approach for tumors with altered p53.

11.4.4 Targeting the G2 Checkpoint

Synthetic lethality targeting the G2 checkpoint in breast cancer involves exploiting vulnerabilities in carcinoma cells, particularly those with mtp53, to enhance therapeutic outcomes. Many combination therapy approaches for breast cancer treatments are governed by the vulnerability of mtp53 during the G2 checkpoint. For example, it has been shown that giving roscovitine, a pan-CDK inhibitor, before doxorubicin causes synthetic lethality only in mtp53 TNBC cells. When doxorubicin is added, roscovitine stops these cellular entities in the G2/M transition phase and increases dsDNA breaks while blocking genetic maintenance by lowering genetic recombination-related proteins. When roscovitine and doxorubicin are administered sequentially instead of simultaneously or with a single drug, the general survival rate of mutant p53 TNBC xenografts is improved and the tumor volume is significantly reduced [121]. DNA damage is also increased by a different combination therapy that uses PARP inhibitors and deoxyuridine analogs. Mutant p53-carrying cells, on the other hand, cannot activate the p53–p21 signaling pathway, which would otherwise cause the cell to stop at G1 to repair DNA. As a result, these cells with accumulated DNA damage are stopped at G2. As expected, this combination therapy works best in cases of mutant p53 breast cancer, markedly suppressing progression and enhancing overall life expectancy in the transplant of altered p53 in triple-negative breast cancer [122].

Synthetic lethality related to mtp53 is not limited to G2 phase dependence. Computational analysis of gene expression profiles with mutant p53 has uncovered several potential gene targets linked to synthetic lethality. These potential genes include aurora kinase A (AURKA), polo-like kinase 1 (PLK1), and polo-like kinase 4 (PLK4), for which inhibitors are available in the market [123]. When contrasted with luminal cell lines with a prevalent wild-type p53, treatment with the PLK1 inhibitor onvansertib in TNBC cell lines with prevalent mutant p53 demonstrated a more pronounced effect. Furthermore, the combination of paclitaxel and onvansertib has shown notable efficacy in xenograft models and breast cancer cell lines carrying mtp53 [124]. Phosphatidylinositol 5-phosphate 4-kinase (PI5P4K) is recognized as another significant synthetic target. Research has shown that PI5P4K levels are raised in a subset of breast carcinoma, and this elevation is linked to deletions or mutations in the p53 gene [125]. Apart from the known targets, additional undiscovered synthetic lethal targets related to mutant p53 might exist. These discoveries could emerge new treatment possibilities for addressing tumors harboring mtp53.

11.4.5 Inhibiting Mutant p53 Gain-of-Function Interactors or Pathways

Based on the understanding of proteins that interact with mutant p53, another therapeutic approach involves creating inhibitors that target pathways or interactions connected to the GOF tasks exhibited by altered p53.

(i) **Mutant p53-Nrf2**: In breast cancer models, the complex formed by altered p53 and Nrf2 stimulates the transcriptional activation of genes encoding proteasome subunits, leading to heightened protein turnover [126]. Combining the proteasome inhibitor carfilzomib with APR-246 was shown to diminish the growth and spread of primary tumors in breast carcinoma xenografts carrying mutant p53 [127].

(ii) **Mutant p53-SREBPs**: The partnership between SREBP and mutated p53 triggers the start of SREBP target gene activation, resulting in heightened sterol production through the mevalonate pathway. This, in turn, triggers the activation of Yes-associated protein (YAP) and transcriptional coactivator with PDZ-binding motif (TAZ) cofactors, which promotes cell proliferation [56]. In breast cancer cells containing mutated p53, researchers found that cholesterol-lowering medications like statins caused the relocation of YAP/TAZ to the cytoplasm [128]. Furthermore, they were seen to break down altered p53 and halt its activities associated with GOF.

(iii) **Mtp53-Pin1**: An additional protein involved in the increased functionality of mutant p53 in mammary carcinoma is peptidyl-prolyl cis-trans isomerase NIMA-interacting 1 (Pin1). Pin1 induces changes in the structure of mutant p53, affecting its interactions and gene expression pattern. Additionally, Pin1 collaborates with mutated p53 to boost the expression of genes like DEPDC1, thereby amplifying the ability of breast cancer cells to migrate and invade [65]. Suppressors directed at Pin1, including all-trans retinoic acid (ATRA) and KPT-6566, have shown a decrease in Pin1-induced cancer-promoting activities and tumor growth in living organisms, along with a suppression of the ability of breast carcinoma stem cells to regenerate themselves. The effectiveness of KPT-6566 in breast carcinoma cells also corresponds with the levels of Pin1 expression [129].

(iv) **Mutant p53-PARP**: PARP1 binds to the domain at the carboxy-terminal (CTD) of mtp53, particularly the R273H variant, during DNA replication, inhibiting DNA repair processes [130]. The pairing of the PARP inhibitor talazoparib with the alkylating agent temozolomide demonstrates synergistic cytotoxic effects in MDA-MB-468 cells harboring the R273H mutation. Overexpression of R273H further enhances this synergistic effect [58]. Moreover, removing the CTD of the R273H mutant disrupts its interaction with PARP1, leading to hindered cell advancement through the G2/M checkpoint, slower cell growth, and reduced responsiveness to the combination of talazoparib and temozolomide [131]. Such discoveries highlight the possible practical use of PARP inhibitors, especially in breast cancers carrying the R273H p53 mutation. Overall, although these inhibitors display a level of specificity toward mutant p53 models, this method represents an indirect means for addressing altered p53.

11.4.6 Genetic Approaches

Transporting the normal p53 gene into cancer cells using viral or plasmid vectors can cause these cells to undergo senescence or die [132]. A notable example is Gendicine (also known as Ad-p53) incorporates an adenovirus serotype-5 vector carrying the normal human p53 gene. When used alongside the EGFR inhibitor gefitinib, Gendicine demonstrated improved suppression of cellular proliferation in laboratory conditions and reduced the size of tumors in MDA-MB-468 xenograft models [133]. Gendicine has undergone testing as a treatment for TNBC in a clinical trial where one group received Gendicine combined with capecitabine, and the other group received capecitabine alone. The pairing of Gendicine and capecitabine yielded elevated response rates of 84.4% compared to 71.8% with capecitabine alone, indicating that Gendicine shows clinical potential for treating TNBC with prevalent mutant p53 [134].

Apart from viral vectors, plasmid vectors can be transported into carcinoma cells via nanoparticles for p53 gene therapies. One instance is transferrin-SiNPs-p53, a nanoparticle loaded with transferrin carrying the wild-type p53 plasmid. Treatment of MCF-7 cells with transferrin-SiNPs-p53 enhances wild-type p53 activation, resulting in suppression of cell growth and induction of programmed cell death both in laboratory settings (in vitro) and within living organisms (in vivo) [135].

11.4.7 Mutant p53 Immunotherapies and Immune Checkpoint Inhibitors

Mutant p53 can avoid being broken down by E3 ligases, yet it remains susceptible to breakdown via proteasome-dependent mechanisms not mediated by MDM2. Its peptides are presented on the surface of tumor cells through major histocompatibility complex (MHC) class I molecules, rendering them susceptible to targeting by immunotherapies. By identifying the antigen expression levels of altered p53-expressing cells, including breast carcinoma cells, the designed T cell receptor-like antibody P1C1TM, tailored for a particular wild-type p53 peptide associated with the wild-type p53 protein, induces targeted cell death and restrains growth when attached to the HLA-A24 class I MHC allele [136]. The capacity to discern minute variations in antigen expression between cells harboring wild-type p53 and those containing mutant p53 is critical for the future development of analogous antibodies or chimeric antigen receptor (CAR) T cells. This will lessen off-target impacts and improve target specificity. Immunotherapy against mutant p53 also includes administering a vaccine using a modified Ankara virus to cancer patients that expresses human p53 in its wild-type form (p53MVA). This strategy makes use of the oncogenic mutant p53's high expression to activate the body's immune system to generate a targeted cytotoxic T-lymphocyte reaction against mutant p53. According to phase I trials, the p53MVA vaccine induces a potent CD8+ T cell reaction targeting p53 in the bloodstream while also being well-tolerated and not associated with any serious side effects [137]. When patients with advanced solid tumors, such as breast cancer, were treated with both the p53MVA vaccine and the anti-PD-1 drug pembrolizumab, three out of eleven patients experienced disease control. Additionally, two patients exhibited elevated and sustained levels of CD8+ T cells that responded to p53 [138]. In another case, detailed examination of a patient diagnosed with TNBC, the combination therapy resulted in the complete disappearance of metastasis. This was associated with the stimulation of T cells targeting p53 and activation of genes associated with immune response in the bloodstream [139]. These results suggest that utilizing a vaccine to target mutant p53 could offer a hopeful avenue for treating breast cancer.

Recent studies suggest a link between p53 and immune checkpoint regulation in cancer, suggesting that the effectiveness of immune checkpoint inhibitors (ICIs) may be influenced by the status of p53 [140]. ICIs might offer a solution to resistance against endocrine therapy in luminal-B breast cancer instances with elevated levels of immunologic gene expression [141]. However, ICIs alone have limited effectiveness in treating breast carcinoma, especially in subtypes with common altered p53, such as TNBC. Therefore, new strategies are needed to improve the therapeutic benefits of ICIs [142]. Research indicates that employing p53 gene therapies leads to heightened inflammation markers and interferon signaling within tumors. This correlates with an increase in the CD8+ T cell marker, which is correlated with better responses to ICIs in clinical scenarios [143, 144]. Consequently, ICIs are now being extensively studied in combination with various targeted therapies that specifically target p53. The p53-modified vaccinia Ankara (p53MVA) [145], SGT-53 [146], and Adenovirus-delivered p53 (Ad-p53) [147] in combination with CD122/132, APR-246 along with anti-programmed cell death protein 1 (anti-PD-1) in various cancer models and OBP-702 (an oncolytic adenovirus expressing normal p53), alongside CXCR4-targeted p53 messenger RNA (mRNA) nanoparticles [148] are a few examples. Yet, most of these combinations have not been studied concerning breast carcinoma.

11.5 INNOVATIVE THERAPIES/DRUGS IN CLINICAL TRIALS TARGETING MUTANT p53 RESTORATION

Some drugs are undergoing clinical trials to restore the normal activity of dysfunctional p53 proteins. The objective is to create treatments that can effectively counteract or reverse the damaging effects of p53 mutations, potentially improving outcomes for patients with cancers driven by these mutations. Several drugs aimed at restoring function to mutated p53 are currently undergoing clinical trials. Some of these are explained in the following sections.

11.5.1 Eprenetapopt (APR246)

In 2002, Bykov and his team discovered APR-246 through cell-based screening [149]. After being converted, this prodrug targets p53 mutants with altered conformations and restores them to their original structure [150]. This restoration reactivates their transcriptional functions, allowing them to regulate the expression of target genes such as p53 upregulated modulator of apoptosis, phorbol-12-myristate-13-acetate-induced protein 1, and Bcl-2-associated X protein, thus promoting apoptosis [149, 151]. Eprenetapopt, previously known as APR-246, is the most extensively studied drug for reactivating mutant p53 [152]. Eprenetapopt initially transforms into MQ, which subsequently binds to specific thiol groups within the p53 DNA-binding domain, thereby enhancing the drug's anti-tumor efficacy. Whether or if p53 binds to DNA determines the altered thiol residues of MQ. The altered p53 structurally reconfigures to take on the wild-type conformation after MQ binding. It can now perform wild-type tasks again, including triggering programmed cell death and inhibiting the proliferation of cells, thanks to this transformation [153]. In short, eprenetapopt has been shown to increase levels of reactive oxygen species in malignant cells, which may contribute to its anti-cancer effects by promoting cell death and potentially facilitating the degradation of altered p53. This double mode of operation makes eprenetapopt a promising candidate for reinstating the activity of altered p53 and combating breast cancer driven by p53 mutations.

11.5.2 COTI-2

COTI-2, also known as cancer targeting compound 2, aims to reinstate the function of altered p53 in breast cancer by targeting and reactivating mutant p53 proteins. The third-generation thiosemicarbazone drug COTI-2 is claimed to possess a broad spectrum of anti-cancer characteristics [154]. COTI-2 blocks mTOR signaling and stimulates AMP-activated protein kinase (AMPK). As wild-type p53 is recognized for its ability to activate AMPK and suppress mTOR, these actions hint that COTI-2 could be restoring p53 to its original, wild-type state [155]. These actions of COTI-2 may further amplify its anticancer potential. The inhibition of mTOR using drugs like everolimus is a well-established approach for treating certain types of cancers [156].

11.5.3 Arsenic Trioxide (ATO)

Arsenic trioxide (ATO) shows potential as a treatment option for attacking the p53 gene in breast cancer. Although ATO has traditionally been employed in the treatment of acute promyelocytic leukemia, it has demonstrated the capacity to reactivate structurally altered mutant forms of p53. This reactivation can successfully hinder tumor cell growth and restore normal function in both living organisms and laboratory experiments [157]. In contrast to eprenetapopt, ATO has a unique mechanism of action. Studying the ability of ATO to revive mutated p53 in breast carcinoma is in line with the overall objective of targeting the p53 gene, as it doesn't trigger the activation of mutant p53 with contact mutations or stimulate the transcription of target genes harboring such mutations [158]. Arsenic trioxide works by targeting and destabilizing proteins that degrade p53, allowing the mutated p53 to accumulate and potentially restore some of its tumor-suppressing functions. This can lead to apoptosis (cell death) in cancer cells, including those in breast cancer, where mutated p53 is often found.

11.5.4 PC14586

When examining new methods to focus on the p53 gene in breast cancer, scientists are especially looking into the Y220C mutation. This mutation provides a particular method for evaluating putative low-molecular-weight p53 mutant inhibitors. In cells bearing the p53 Y220C mutation, the chemical PC14586 has demonstrated promise by stabilizing and reactivating the mutant protein. Cell cycle arrest results from this and crucial genes regulated by the normal (wild-type) p53 are stimulated [159].

11.5.5 MDM2 Inhibitors

MDM2 inhibitors aim to reinstate the function of altered p53 in breast carcinoma by blocking the interplay or relationship between MDM2 and p53. Normally, MDM2 binds to p53 and targets it for degradation, which diminishes p53's tumor suppressor functions. By inhibiting MDM2, these drugs prevent the breakdown of p53, thereby stabilizing and activating p53's tumor-suppressing activities, potentially resulting in the inhibition of cancer cell proliferation. Inulanolide A, leariifolianoid A, and JapA 71 [160] are among the substances that can directly bind to MDM2 and cause its downregulation or destruction. These substances not only cause the MDM2 protein to degrade and suppress its transcription, but the latter two also prevent the expression of MDM2 transactivator NFAT1, which is often overexpressed in breast cancer [161, 162].

11.5.6 PRIMA- 1

The first p53 reactivator chemical to be identified was PRIMA-1 (stands for p53 reactivation with induction of massive apoptosis-1) [149]. Numerous unfolded p53 alterations are brought back to a WT-like conformation by PRIMA-1, which promotes cell death and activates several p53 target genes [150, 163, 164]. PRIMA-1 seeks to revive the activity of mutated p53 in breast cancer by transforming it into a structure that mirrors the functional, wild-type p53. It does this by binding to the mutant p53 protein and promoting its refolding, thereby restoring its ability to function as a cancer-inhibiting agent, inducing apoptosis, and halting cancer cell proliferation.

11.6 TARGETED THERAPIES AGAINST THE ALTERED p53 IN BREAST CANCER

Alterations in the p53 gene, responsible for producing the tumor suppressor protein p53, are frequently found in various cancers, including breast carcinoma. Targeted therapies for mutated p53 in breast cancer aim to reinstate the normal function of p53 or exploit the vulnerabilities of cancer cells harboring these mutations. Following are some of the targeted therapies being investigated or used.

11.6.1 Small-Molecule Inhibitors

Small molecules are a class of compounds that have shown promise in targeting mutant p53 proteins in cancer cells, including those found in breast cancer. One notable small molecule is PRIMA-1. PRIMA-1 was initially discovered through screening a library of low-molecular-weight compounds known as the NCI Diversity Set for their capability to reinstate the normal functions of mutant p53

[149]. After screening approximately 2000 compounds, scientists discovered a compound named PRIMA-1 (short for p53 reactivation and induction of massive apoptosis 1), which was found to reinstate normal activities to the mutated p53 protein, such as targeted DNA binding and the initiation of cell death. Later, by adding a methyl group, the pro-apoptotic effects and membrane permeability of PRIMA-1 were boosted, resulting in the creation of PRIMA-1MET or APR-246 [163]. Liang et al. [165] in the early stages of research, demonstrated that PRIMA-1 hindered the growth of breast cancer cells carrying mutated p53. Their initial investigation showed that PRIMA-1 influenced the survival of mutated p53 cell lines BT-474, HCC-1428, and T47-D, while it had no effect on the viability of cells expressing normal p53, such as endothelial cells, normal breast cells, or MCF-7 cells. Additionally, PRIMA-1 prompted a conversion of mutated p53 into its normal conformation, as confirmed by fluorescent labeling using p53 antibodies specific to distinct conformations [89, 166]. Just like PRIMA-1, APR-246 has shown its capability to halt the growth of breast carcinoma cells in preclinical studies. Synnott and colleagues conducted experiments using various breast cancer cell lines in laboratory settings, uncovering APR-246's effectiveness with IC50 values ranging from 0.9 to 31.1 μM across the panel. They noted a strong association between the response to APR-246 and the existence of altered p53 or elevated levels of native p53 protein, indicating that these factors could act as predictive markers for its effectiveness. However, the response to APR-246 remained unaffected by the estrogen receptor (ER) status, HER2 status, or molecular subtype of the investigated cell lines. Additionally, APR-246 not only hindered cell proliferation but also triggered cell death and diminished migration in the mutp53 breast carcinoma cell lines under investigation [90]. As APR-246 is improbable to be used as a standalone treatment for breast carcinoma, scientists have investigated its anticancer properties when paired with different chemotherapy drugs. Notably, a considerable synergistic effect in suppressing cell growth was noted when APR-246 was used in conjunction with eribulin across six distinct breast cancer cell lines harboring mutated p53 [167].

Another compound under investigation for its potential to inhibit cancer in breast carcinoma cells is PK11007. Similar to APR-246, PK11007 stabilizes and restores functionality to altered p53. Another common feature shared with APR-246 is the capacity to enhance the creation of ROS [92]. PK11007 has demonstrated its ability to specifically induce programmed cell death and decrease both the growth and mobility of breast carcinoma cells carrying mutant p53, in contrast to breast cancer cell lines with wild-type p53. This aligns with its ability to reactivate mutant p53 [93, 168]. Among the breast carcinoma cell lines studied, it was observed that triple-negative (TN) cell lines were more prone to growth inhibition by PK11007 compared to non-TN cell lines [92]. COTI-2, as mentioned earlier in this chapter, is another example.

11.6.2 MDM2 Inhibitors

MDM2 inhibitors represent another class of targeted therapies aimed at addressing altered p53 in breast carcinoma. The detailed crystal structure of the interplay between MDM2 and p53 has revealed a hydrophobic surface pocket composed of phenylalanine 19 (Phe 19), tryptophan 23 (Trp 23), and leucine 26 (Leu 26) [169]. This finding aids in the creation of small molecules engineered to disrupt the MDM2–p53 interaction, thereby restoring p53 functions in cancer cells. More than 20 different chemical classes have been proposed to inhibit this interaction [170], Research mainly targets three types of compounds: nutlins, spirooxindoles, and benzodiazepinediones. Nutlin-based and spirooxindole compounds are the most commonly used inhibitors of the MDM2–p53 interaction in breast cancer research, valued for their drug-like properties.

Nutlins are small molecules designed to imitate the p53 protein's binding site, enabling them to competitively bind to MDM2. By physically blocking MDM2 at its binding site on p53 through steric hindrance, nutlins stabilize p53. This stabilization prompts the activation of p53, leading to the halting of the cell cycle and induction of cell death in cancerous cells with elevated MDM2 levels [171].

Spirooxindoles, commonly referred to as the MI-series, are chemical compounds that share a structural resemblance with nutlins. These derivatives mimic the hydrophobic pocket residues present in the MDM2–p53 interaction that are crucial for binding. By inhibiting this interaction, spirooxindoles prevent the breakdown of the p53 protein. This preservation of p53 allows it to regain its function in regulating cell growth and inducing apoptosis in cancerous cells. Besides nutlins and spirooxindoles, many other small molecule inhibitors targeting the MDM2–p53 interaction have been tested in breast cancer studies. However, all of these inhibitors remain in the preclinical phase of development [172–178].

11.6.3 Immunotherapy

Immunotherapy directed at mutated p53 in breast cancer aims to utilize the body's natural immune system to identify and eliminate cancerous cells containing altered p53 proteins. Despite the gathering of mutp53 and its capacity to avoid degradation mediated by MDM2, it can still undergo breakdown via an MDM2-independent, proteasome-dependent pathway. This results in the production of peptides that are presented on the exterior of cancer cells through class I molecules of the MHC. As a result, both mutp53 and the mutant peptide–MHC complexes derived from p53 could be considered potential targets for immunotherapies [179, 136]. While peptides containing mutp53 sequences are seldom found because of MHC interaction limitations, a T cell receptor-like (TCRL) antibody called P1C1TM has been custom-engineered. This antibody is designed to specifically target mutp53 [180]. The peptide, displayed by the HLA-A24:02 (HLA-24) MHC allele can differentiate between cells expressing altered and normal p53 based on the levels of antigen expression. The complex interaction between mutated p53 within cells and the peptide–MHC complex on the cell surface that can be targeted allows for effective antibody-dependent cellular cytotoxicity (ADDC) of cells exhibiting mutp53 in both experimental conditions and biological systems [136]. In a nutshell, immunotherapy aimed at mutant p53 in breast cancer presents promising opportunities to enhance treatment effectiveness and surmount resistance to conventional therapies. Continuing research and clinical trials are assessing the effectiveness and safety of these approaches, with the aspiration of introducing novel therapeutic alternatives for individuals afflicted with breast cancer.

11.6.4 Gene Therapy

Gene therapy designed to address mutated p53 in breast cancer aims to reinstate the typical function of the p53 tumor suppressor gene, which is commonly altered in cases of breast cancer. Gene therapy, when used alongside traditional treatments, employs genetic methods to boost the immune system's ability to combat tumors and transport cytotoxic substances or therapeutic genes directly to cancer cells. This approach is being studied in multiple clinical trials [181]. The mechanisms used include gene addition or gene replacement, gene suppression, gene inactivation, and gene insertion. Each of these treatments is applied using carriers or vectors for delivery [182]. Gene therapy utilizes both viral and non-viral delivery methods to administer therapeutic drugs or genes, selected depending on the desired specificity. Targeted gene therapy is often favored over the use of recombinant peptides, as peptides typically suffer from low bioavailability, instability, high toxicity, and high costs [183]. In breast cancer, gene therapy targets mutated p53 by delivering a functional p53 gene or corrective genetic material into cancer cells. This can restore the tumor-inhibiting role of p53, inhibit tumor growth, and promote cancer cell death.

In addition to these targeted therapies, chemotherapy and radiotherapy are typically used as part of a multimodal treatment approach, often in combination with other therapies to achieve the best possible outcomes.

11.7 EMERGING PERSPECTIVES ON EPIGENETIC CONTROL OF p53 IN BREAST CANCER

Emerging perspectives on the epigenetic control of p53 in breast cancer focus on how epigenetic mechanisms regulate the function and p53 tumor suppressor activity. Heritable DNA alterations that impact gene expression but do not alter DNA sequence are referred to as epigenetics. Numerous regular biological functions, such as cell division and development, are influenced by epigenetic control [184]. The three main epigenetic alterations are the production of non-coding RNA, alterations of histone after translation, and changes in the addition of methyl groups to DNA. These changes play a part in the early stages of breast cancer carcinogenesis and act as an indicator for early identification, prognostic assessment, and therapy response [185].

11.7.1 DNA Methylation

The chemical modification referred to as DNA methylation happens when a methyl group is added to cytosine in CpG dinucleotides, forming 5-methyl-cytosine (5mC). Three enzymes, DNMT1, DNMT3A, and DNMT3B, transfer methyl groups from S-adenosyl-L-methionine. DNMT3A and DNMT3B initiate new methylation, while DNMT1 maintains existing methylation patterns during DNA replication [186]. DNA methylation in promoter regions inhibits gene expression by either binding to proteins with a methyl-binding domain (MBD) that are more likely to bind to promoters or by preventing the attachment of the transcriptional machinery to their recognition sequences [187]. MBD proteins recruit histone deacetylase complexes and chromatin remodeling factors, leading to the condensation of chromatin and consequently link epigenetic alterations involving DNA methylation and histone modifications [188].

In breast cancer, DNA methylation controls how the p53 gene works and how much of it is produced, mainly by overmethylating its promoter region. Aberrant methylation of the p53 promoter region can silence its expression, contributing to tumorigenesis. Hypomethylation strategies are being explored to reactivate p53. Targeting these methylation changes holds the potential for reactivating p53 and restoring its tumor-suppressive functions in breast cancer therapy. Additionally, there is a clear pattern in DNA methylation that is seen in several breast cancer subtypes. For instance, ER-positive/luminal breast cancer has been demonstrated to exhibit a greater occurrence of DNA methylation compared to ER-negative/basal-like tumors [189, 190]. In addition, well-differentiated breast cancers exhibit lower levels of cytosine–phosphate–guanine (CpG) island methylation compared to poorly differentiated tumors, which display a higher degree of methylation in these regions [191]. Similarly, increased methylation of the promoter region of the progesterone receptor gene is elevated in breast cancers that do not express the progesterone receptor (PR-negative) [192]. Distinct methylation patterns in the ER, PR, or HER2 genes can impact the expression of these receptors within breast tumors, potentially altering the tumors' response to endocrine or hormonal therapies. The DNA methylation profiles of luminal-A, luminal-B, and basal-like breast cancer subtypes were examined by analyzing 807 genes associated with cancer. The research unveiled unique methylation patterns for each subtype, indicating substantial differences among them [190].

Changes in methylated DNA detected in healthy breast tissue or adjacent tissues close to cancer can provide important insights into the likelihood of developing breast cancer. Specifically, variations in the methylation state of certain genes associated with cancer in normal breast tissue may occur before the onset of breast cancer [193]. Furthermore, the specific categories of breast cancer can be linked to particular precursor cell groups based on their methylation patterns. This helps resolve questions regarding their originating cell or biological diversity [194]. Recent research comparing breast cancer with normal breast tissue has pinpointed seven methylation biomarkers specific to breast cancer and six CpG sites that could potentially forecast patient survival [195]. An extensive examination of DNA methylation and gene expression patterns throughout the genome in breast cancer and normal breast tissue has identified PRAC2, TDR10, and TMEM132C as novel markers associating DNA methylation with genes, providing diagnostic and prognostic significance in breast cancer [196].

11.7.2 Histone Modification

Chromatin is a flexible arrangement consisting of nucleosomes, with histones serving as the fundamental constituents of these units. These foundational proteins assemble to form an octamer, composed of two identical sets of four histones: histone 2A (H2A), histone 2B (H2B), histone 3 (H3), and histone 4 (H4). Within each nucleosome core particle, approximately 147 base pairs of DNA are wrapped around the histone octamer in nearly two helical turns [197]. Histones are proteins that are preserved across species and can experience post-translational modifications at specific amino acid residues located on both their C-terminal and N-terminal tails [198]. Non-sequential alterations to the DNA sequence and histone alterations after translation (PTMs) can influence gene expression by altering chromatin structure. These modifications shift histones from an open, transcriptionally active configuration known as euchromatin to a dense, inactive form called heterochromatin. Various covalent post-translational modifications (PTMs) such as the addition of methyl groups (methylation), acetyl groups (acetylation), phosphate groups (phosphorylation), SUMO (small ubiquitin-like modifier) proteins (sumoylation), sugar moieties (glycosylation), ubiquitin proteins (ubiquitination), ADP-ribose groups (ADP-ribosylation), and carboxyl groups (carboxylation) can occur on the residues located on histone tails [199, 200]. As an illustration, the addition of acetyl groups to histone H3 and the presence of di- or tri-methyl groups on histone H3 at lysine 4 (H3K4me2, H3K4me3) within the promoter region can activate the expression of genes. Conversely, gene repression typically involves the removal of acetyl groups from histones and the presence of tri-methyl groups on histone H3 at lysine 27 (H3K27me3) and lysine 9 (H3K9me3) [201, 202]. It's not surprising that numerous cancer cases display abnormal changes in histone modifications because of their essential functions in DNA-related cellular activities. Specifically, a common decrease in acetylation at lysine K16 and tri-methylation at lysine K20 on histone H4 is a characteristic marker of numerous cancers [203]. Post-translational modifications of histones, such as the addition of acetyl groups (acetylation), methyl groups (methylation), and phosphate groups (phosphorylation), can alter the chromatin organization around the tumor protein (TP53 gene), hence modulating its activity. Specific histone modifications can either enhance or suppress p53 transcription in breast cancer cells. In breast cancer, tumors with poor prognosis frequently show reduced levels of lysine acetylation (H3K9ac, H3K18ac, and H4K12ac), lysine methylation (H3K4me2, H4K20me3), and arginine methylation (H4R3me2). Additionally, a decrease in H4K16ac and its associated enzyme, histone acetyltransferase (HAT) hMOF, is an early marker in most primary breast tumors [204, 205].

Changes at the molecular level influencing the activity of enzymes that alter histones can contribute to the initiation and progression of cancer. In breast cancer, various modifications have been identified, such as heightened levels of p300, HBO1, histone deacetylase 1 (HDAC1), histone deacetylase 2 (HDAC2), histone deacetylase 3 (HDAC3), and histone deacetylase 6 (HDAC6) [206]; enhanced expression of enhancer of zeste homolog 2 (EZH2) [207], Jumonji domain-containing protein 2B (JMJD2B) [208], and a decrease in lysine-specific demethylase 1 (LSD1) [209].

11.7.3 Non-Coding RNAs

Non-coding RNAs, which are functional RNA molecules that do not encode proteins, exert important regulative activities and influence the performance of specific genes implicated in breast cancer. This category encompasses long non-coding RNAs (lncRNAs) and microRNAs (miRNAs). MiRNAs, in particular, have been extensively researched for their role in epigenetic regulation, where they can activate or inhibit key biological pathways and mechanisms essential for breast cancer development. Notably, the let-7 family of miRNAs is highly significant in breast cancer, and its suppression is linked to the formation of metastases and aggressive hormone-negative breast

TABLE 11.1
Clinical Trials Conducted on Epigenetic Targets and Other Combination Inhibitors as Breast Cancer Treatments

Target	Epigenetic Agent	Clinical Trial Identifier	Phase
HDAC	Entinostat*	NCT03538171	III
HDAC	Romidepsin*	NCT00098397 (metastatic BC)	II
DNMT plus HDAC	Azacitidine Entinostat	NCT01349959	II
HDAC plus chemotherapy	Etinostat* Capecitabine	NCT03473639	I
HDAC plus anti-PD-L1 antibody, anti-VEGF antibody, aromatase inhibitor, estrogen receptor inhibitor	Etinostst* Atezolizumab* Bevacizumab, Exemestane, Fulvestrant, Tamoxifen Ipatasertib	NCT03280563	I/ II
HDAC plus HER1/HER2 kinase inhibitor, anti-HER antibody	Etinostst* Lepatinib, Trastuzumab	NCT01434303	I
HDAC plus anti-PD-L1 antibody	Entinostat* Atezolizumab	NCT02708680 (for TNBC	I/ II
HDAC plus anti-PD-1 antibody, chemotherapy	Romidepsin,* Nivolumab Cisplatin	NCT02393794	I/ II
BET inhibitor plus estrogen receptor inhibitor	Molibresib* Fulvestrant	NCT02964507	II

* Particular epigenetic agent.

tumors [210–212]. Several microRNAs, including microRNA-663, microRNA-148, microRNA-9-1, microRNA-152, and microRNA-124a3, have been documented to exhibit abnormal hypermethylation in primary breast tumors [213]. These small ncRNAs can bind to the mRNA of p53, leading to its degradation or inhibition of translation. For instance, miR-125b targets p53 mRNA, reducing its expression and impairing its tumor-suppressive functions. Scientists have observed an unusual increase in the methylation of H19, a lncRNA, in invasive breast cancer compared to normal breast tissue, suggesting that H19 may possess tumor-suppressive functions [214]. Another lncRNA, HOTAIR (HOX transcript antisense RNA), has been implicated in the progression of breast cancer. Studies have revealed that several writer proteins, including MLL1, MLL3, and P300/CBP, are attracted to the promoter region of HOTAIR. This process results in greater histone acetylation and elevated H3K4me3 levels, which support breast cancer progression by preventing cell death (apoptosis) [215].

Therefore, epigenetic processes offer various avenues for treating breast cancer. Because the changes brought about by DNMTs and HDACs can be undone and are not permanent. Numerous ongoing investigations seek to identify the optimal doses and treatment regimens for different epigenetic drugs used in breast cancer therapy (Table 11.1) [216].

11.8 ADVANCED METHODS IN BREAST CANCER THERAPY

Breast cancer is a multifaceted and intricate illness, offering numerous treatment options. These can include different combinations of surgeries, chemotherapy plans, and hormone replacement therapies (HRTs). Additionally, there are treatments aimed at the HER2. In certain situations, choosing not to undergo treatment is also an option [86, 217]. Within each of these treatment categories, there are numerous specific options available [218]. In breast cancer clinics, chemotherapies using anthracyclines and non-anthracyclines that cause DNA damage are commonly employed. Doxorubicin and epirubicin are two anthracycline-based drugs that trigger cell death by intercalating between DNA strands bound by topoisomerase II, thereby disrupting DNA replication [219, 220]. The mechanism of action of non-anthracycline based DNA-damaging treatments is broader and includes DNA-alkylating drugs like cyclophosphamide [57, 221] and antimetabolites that obstruct DNA synthesis, such as 5-fluorouracil [222]. In a similar vein, radiation therapy damages DNA by producing strand breaks [223]. Non-DNA damaging taxanes that alter microtubule activity to impede mitotic cell division are also used to treat breast cancer [224]. Chemotherapy can be administered before surgery to reduce tumor size (neoadjuvant therapy) or following surgery to destroy any remaining cancer cells and lower the chance of recurrence (adjuvant therapy) [225]. Adjuvant therapies are treatments given following the main treatment, such as the surgical removal of a tumor. In contrast, neoadjuvant therapies are administered before the main therapy. This approach enables pathologists to assess the effectiveness of the treatment in reducing the tumor by examining the residual disease, classified into (i) complete response (CR), (ii) partial response, (iii) stable disease, and (iv) progressive disease (PD) [226, 227].

HRTs are frequently employed to control HR-positive breast cancers by disrupting the hormone receptor signaling pathways responsible for driving these cancer types. HRTs encompass a range of medications, including selective estrogen receptor modulators, selective estrogen receptor degraders, and aromatase inhibitors [228–231].

Besides biological factors, breast cancer treatment can differ among patients based on individual and physician preferences, institutional protocols, healthcare accessibility, insurance coverage [218], and financial reimbursement incentives [232–234]. Put plainly, breast cancer is a complicated illness that demands various treatment methods, influenced by many biological and non-biological factors.

11.9 CONCLUSION

The advancement of targeted therapies for mutated 53 in breast cancer marks a crucial step toward personalized medicine and better patient outcomes. Through extensive research and clinical trials, several promising therapeutic strategies have been developed to specifically target the defective p53 pathway. A key approach involves using small molecule inhibitors to reactivate mutant p53, thereby restoring its tumor-suppressive functions and making cancer cells more susceptible to conventional treatments. Additionally, immunotherapy techniques, including cancer vaccines and adoptive cell therapies, hold promise in leveraging the immune system to detect and eliminate cells with mutant p53. Moreover, advances in molecular profiling techniques have allowed for the identification of patient subgroups that are most likely to benefit from targeted therapies, enabling treatment plans to be customized based on individual genetic profiles. This precision medicine approach not only enhances therapeutic effectiveness but also reduces unnecessary side effects. Despite these advancements, challenges remain, such as the development of resistance to targeted treatments and the need for better delivery methods to ensure optimal drug distribution within tumors. Additionally, further research is needed to understand the complex interactions between mutant p53 and other signaling pathways, which could lead to the creation of combination therapies with synergistic effects. Furthermore, the chapter likely concludes key findings and implications of research on how epigenetic modifications regulate the p53 gene in breast cancer, emphasizing the importance of understanding these mechanisms for the development of targeted therapies and improved patient outcomes. In summary, targeted therapies for mutated p53 in breast cancer present promising opportunities for enhancing patient outcomes and signify a major shift toward personalized, precision medicine. Sustained interdisciplinary research, along with ongoing clinical trials, is crucial for unlocking the full potential of these therapeutic approaches and ultimately revolutionizing breast cancer treatment.

REFERENCES

1. Jan, N., et al., Targeting breast cancer stem cells through retinoids: a new hope for treatment. *Critical Reviews in Oncology/Hematology*, 2023: p. 104156.
2. Jan, N., et al., Metronomic chemotherapy and drug repurposing: a paradigm shift in oncology. *Heliyon*, 2024. https://doi.org/10.1016/j.heliyon.2024.e24670
3. Brown, C.J., et al., Awakening guardian angels: drugging the p53 pathway. *Nature Reviews Cancer*, 2009. **9**(12): p. 862–873.
4. Mandinova, A. and S.W. Lee, The p53 pathway as a target in cancer therapeutics: obstacles and promise. *Science Translational Medicine*, 2011. **3**(64): p. 64rv1–64rv1.
5. Reinhardt, H.C. and B. Schumacher, The p53 network: cellular and systemic DNA damage responses in aging and cancer. *Trends in Genetics*, 2012. **28**(3): p. 128–136.
6. Pellegata, N.S., et al., DNA damage and p53-mediated cell cycle arrest: a reevaluation. *Proceedings of the National Academy of Sciences*, 1996. **93**(26): p. 15209–15214.
7. Hainaut, P. and K.G. Wiman, 30 years and a long way into p53 research. *The Lancet Oncology*, 2009. **10**(9): p. 913–919.
8. Jan, N., et al., Exploring the role of trifarotene against RAR-α: an investigation of expression pattern and clinicopathological significance of RAR-α in breast cancer. *Frontiers in Pharmacology*, 2024. **15**: p. 1361679.
9. Vousden, K.H. and X. Lu, Live or let die: the cell's response to p53. *Nature Reviews Cancer*, 2002. **2**(8): p. 594–604.
10. Vazquez, A., et al., The genetics of the p53 pathway, apoptosis and cancer therapy. *Nature Reviews Drug Discovery*, 2008. **7**(12): p. 979–987.
11. Muller, P.A. and K.H. Vousden, p53 mutations in cancer. *Nature Cell Biology*, 2013. **15**(1): p. 2–8.
12. Kandoth, C., et al., Mutational landscape and significance across 12 major cancer types. *Nature*, 2013. **502**(7471): p. 333–339.
13. Muller, P.A. and K.H. Vousden, Mutant p53 in cancer: new functions and therapeutic opportunities. *Cancer Cell*, 2014. **25**(3): p. 304–317.
14. Gurpinar, E. and K.H. Vousden, Hitting cancers' weak spots: vulnerabilities imposed by p53 mutation. *Trends in Cell Biology*, 2015. **25**(8): p. 486–495.
15. Kruiswijk, F., C.F. Labuschagne, and K.H. Vousden, p53 in survival, death and metabolic health: a lifeguard with a licence to kill. *Nature Reviews Molecular Cell Biology*, 2015. **16**(7): p. 393–405.
16. Gibbons, D.L., L.A. Byers, and J.M. Kurie, Smoking, p53 mutation, and lung cancer. *Molecular Cancer Research*, 2014. **12**(1): p. 3–13.
17. Haq, B.U., et al., Targeting p53 misfolding conundrum by stabilizing agents and their analogs in breast cancer therapy: a comprehensive computational analysis. *Frontiers in Pharmacology*, 2024. **14**: p. 1333447.
18. Duffy, M.J., et al., p53 as a target for the treatment of cancer. *Cancer Treatment Reviews*, 2014. **40**(10): p. 1153–1160.
19. Corney, D.C., et al., Role of p53 and Rb in ovarian cancer. *Ovarian Cancer: State of the Art and Future Directions in Translational Research*, 2008: p. 99–117.
20. Oren, M. and V. Rotter, Mutant p53 gain-of-function in cancer. *Cold Spring Harbor Perspectives in Biology*, 2010. **2**(2): p. a001107.
21. Zhou, G., et al., Gain-of-function mutant p53 promotes cell growth and cancer cell metabolism via inhibition of AMPK activation. *Molecular Cell*, 2014. **54**(6): p. 960–974.
22. Lu, X., D. Liu, and Y. Xu, The gain of function of p53 cancer mutant in promoting mammary tumorigenesis. *Oncogene*, 2013. **32**(23): p. 2900–2906.
23. Sturm, I., et al., Mutation of p53 and consecutive selective drug resistance in B-CLL occurs as a consequence of prior DNA-damaging chemotherapy. *Cell Death & Differentiation*, 2003. **10**(4): p. 477–484.
24. Powell, E., D. Piwnica-Worms, and H. Piwnica-Worms, Contribution of p53 to metastasis. *Cancer Discovery*, 2014. **4**(4): p. 405–414.
25. Slamon, D.J., et al., Use of chemotherapy plus a monoclonal antibody against HER2 for metastatic breast cancer that overexpresses HER2. *New England Journal of Medicine*, 2001. **344**(11). p. 783–792.
26. Andreopoulou, E., et al., Feasibility and cardiac safety of pegylated liposomal doxorubicin plus trastuzumab in heavily pretreated patients with recurrent HER2-overexpressing metastatic breast cancer. *Clinical Breast Cancer*, 2007. **7**(9): p. 690–696.

27. Cobleigh, M.A., et al., Multinational study of the efficacy and safety of humanized anti-HER2 monoclonal antibody in women who have HER2-overexpressing metastatic breast cancer that has progressed after chemotherapy for metastatic disease. *Journal of Clinical Oncology*, 1999. **17**(9): p. 2639–2639.
28. Romond, E.H., et al., Trastuzumab plus adjuvant chemotherapy for operable HER2-positive breast cancer. *New England Journal of Medicine*, 2005. **353**(16): p. 1673–1684.
29. Kastenhuber, E.R. and S.W. Lowe, Putting p53 in context. *Cell*, 2017. **170**(6): p. 1062–1078.
30. Yang, Y., Cancer Immunotherapy: harnessing the immune system to battle cancer. *The Journal of Clinical Investigation*, 2015. **125**(9): p. 3335–3337.
31. Sofi, S., et al., A comprehensive analysis of notch signaling genes in breast cancer: expression pattern and prognostic significance. *Advances in Cancer Biology-Metastasis*, 2023. 7: p. 100104.
32. Levy, S.E. and R.M. Myers, Advancements in next-generation sequencing. *Annual Review of Genomics and Human Genetics*, 2016. **17**: p. 95–115.
33. Hanahan, D. and R.A. Weinberg, The hallmarks of cancer. *Cell*, 2000. **100**(1): p. 57–70.
34. Levine, A.J. and M. Oren, The first 30 years of p53: growing ever more complex. *Nature Reviews Cancer*, 2009. **9**(10): p. 749–758.
35. Lane, D.P., p53, guardian of the genome. *Nature*, 1992. **358**(6381): p. 15–16.
36. Aylon, Y. and M. Oren, New plays in the p53 theater. *Current Opinion in Genetics & Development*, 2011. **21**(1): p. 86–92.
37. Matozaki, T., et al., p53 gene mutations in human gastric cancer: wild-type p53 but not mutant p53 suppresses growth of human gastric cancer cells. *Cancer Research*, 1992. **52**(16): p. 4335–4341.
38. Wb, I., Wild-Type p53 suppresses growth of human prostate cancer cells containing mutant p53 alleles. *Cancer Research*, 1991. **51**: p. 4716–4720.
39. Menon, A., et al., Chromosome 17p deletions and p53 gene mutations associated with the formation of malignant neurofibrosarcomas in von Recklinghausen neurofibromatosis. *Proceedings of the National Academy of Sciences*, 1990. **87**(14): p. 5435–5439.
40. Maxwell, K.N., et al., Inherited TP53 variants and risk of prostate cancer. *European Urology*, 2022. **81**(3): p. 243–250.
41. Malkin, D., et al., Germ line p53 mutations in a familial syndrome of breast cancer, sarcomas, and other neoplasms. *Science*, 1990. **250**(4985): p. 1233–1238.
42. McBride, K.A., et al., Li-Fraumeni syndrome: cancer risk assessment and clinical management. *Nature Reviews Clinical Oncology*, 2014. **11**(5): p. 260–271.
43. Cooper, M.J., et al., p53 mutations in bladder carcinoma cell lines. *Oncology Research*, 1994. **6**(12): p. 569–579.
44. Goh, A.M., C.R. Coffill, and D.P. Lane, The role of mutant p53 in human cancer. *The Journal of Pathology*, 2011. **223**(2): p. 116–126.
45. Dittmer, D., et al., Gain of function mutations in p53. *Nature Genetics*, 1993. **4**(1): p. 42–46.
46. Ghosh, M., et al., Mutant p53 suppresses innate immune signaling to promote tumorigenesis. *Cancer Cell*, 2021. **39**(4): p. 494–508.e5.
47. Robey, R.W., et al., Revisiting the role of ABC transporters in multidrug-resistant cancer. *Nature Reviews Cancer*, 2018. **18**(7): p. 452–464.
48. Jain, A.N., et al., Quantitative analysis of chromosomal CGH in human breast tumors associates copy number abnormalities with p53 status and patient survival. *Proceedings of the National Academy of Sciences*, 2001. **98**(14): p. 7952–7957.
49. Murphy, K.L., A.P. Dennis, and J.M. Rosen, A gain of function p53 mutant promotes both genomic instability and cell survival in a novel p53-null mammary epithelial cell mode. *The FASEB Journal*, 2000. **14**(14): p. 2291–2302.
50. Zhu, J., et al., Gain-of-function p53 mutants co-opt chromatin pathways to drive cancer growth. *Nature*, 2015. **525**(7568): p. 206–211.
51. Lim, L., et al., Mutant p53 mediates survival of breast cancer cells. *British Journal of Cancer*, 2009. **101**(9): p. 1606–1612.
52. Mir, M.A., et al., Proteomics: Application of Next-Generation Proteomics in Cancer Research, in *Proteomics*. 2023, Elsevier. p. 55–76.
53. Di Como, C.J., C. Gaiddon, and C. Prives, p73 function is inhibited by tumor-derived p53 mutants in mammalian cells. *Molecular and Cellular Biology*, 1999. **19**(2): p. 1438–1449.
54. Kim, E. and W. Deppert, Transcriptional activities of mutant p53: when mutations are more than a loss. *Journal of Cellular Biochemistry*, 2004. **93**(5): p. 878–886.
55. Mir, M.A., et al., Metronomics: toward personalized chemotherapy. *Novel Approaches in Metronomic Chemotherapy for Breast Cancer Treatment*, 2024. p. 99–119. https://doi.org/10.1201/9781032632674-8

56. Freed-Pastor, W.A., et al., Mutant p53 disrupts mammary tissue architecture via the mevalonate pathway. *Cell*, 2012. **148**(1): p. 244–258.
57. Mir, M.A., M. Bashir, and N. Jan, The Role of Interleukin (IL)-6/IL-6 Receptor Axis in Cancer, in *Cytokine and Chemokine Networks in Cancer.* 2023, Springer. p. 137–164.
58. Xiao, G., et al., Gain-of-function mutant p53 R273H interacts with replicating DNA and PARP1 in breast cancer. *Cancer Research*, 2020. **80**(3): p. 394–405.
59. Di Agostino, S., et al., Gain of function of mutant p53: the mutant p53/NF-Y protein complex reveals an aberrant transcriptional mechanism of cell cycle regulation. *Cancer Cell*, 2006. **10**(3): p. 191–202.
60. Valentino, E., et al., Mutant p53 potentiates the oncogenic effects of insulin by inhibiting the tumor suppressor DAB2IP. *Proceedings of the National Academy of Sciences*, 2017. **114**(29): p. 7623–7628.
61. Sofi, S., et al., Clinicopathological and prognostic significance of Bcl2 in breast cancer: a comprehensive in silico and in vitro study. *Saudi Journal of Biological Sciences*, 2023. **31**(2): p. 103916.
62. Zhang, S., et al., Mutant p53 drives cancer metastasis via RCP-mediated Hsp90α secretion. *Cell Reports*, 2020. **32**(1): p. 107879.
63. Mir, M.A., et al., Imaging Techniques, Biomarkers, and Methods for Metronomic Chemotherapy, in *Novel Approaches in Metronomic Chemotherapy for Breast Cancer Treatment.* CRC Press. p. 58–71.
64. Horigome, E., et al., Mutant TP53 modulates metastasis of triple negative breast cancer through adenosine A2b receptor signaling. *Oncotarget*, 2018. **9**(77): p. 34554.
65. Girardini, J.E., et al., A Pin1/mutant p53 axis promotes aggressiveness in breast cancer. *Cancer Cell*, 2011. **20**(1): p. 79–91.
66. Shang, J., et al., Identification of lung adenocarcinoma specific dysregulated genes with diagnostic and prognostic value across 27 TCGA cancer types. *Oncotarget*, 2017. **8**(50): p. 87292.
67. Mir, M.A., N. Jan, and S. Sofi, Introduction to Metronomic Chemotherapy, in *Novel Approaches in Metronomic Chemotherapy for Breast Cancer Treatment.* 2024, CRC Press. p. 1–14.
68. Berns, E.M., et al., Complete sequencing of TP53 predicts poor response to systemic therapy of advanced breast cancer. *Cancer Research*, 2000. **60**(8): p. 2155–2162.
69. Bertheau, P., et al., TP53 status and response to chemotherapy in breast cancer. *Pathobiology*, 2008. **75**(2): p. 132–139.
70. Silwal-Pandit, L., et al., TP53 mutation spectrum in breast cancer is subtype specific and has distinct prognostic relevance. *Clinical Cancer Research*, 2014. **20**(13): p. 3569–3580.
71. Chen, M.-B., et al., Value of TP53 status for predicting response to neoadjuvant chemotherapy in breast cancer: a meta-analysis. *PloS One*, 2012. **7**(6): p. e39655.
72. Yersal, O. and S. Barutca, Biological subtypes of breast cancer: Prognostic and therapeutic implications. *World Journal of Clinical Oncology*, 2014. **5**(3): p. 412.
73. Ungerleider, N.A., et al., Breast cancer survival predicted by TP53 mutation status differs markedly depending on treatment. *Breast Cancer Research*, 2018. **20**: p. 1–8.
74. Lai, H., et al., Spectrum of p53 tumor suppressor gene mutations and breast cancer survival. *Breast Cancer Research and Treatment*, 2004. **83**: p. 57–66.
75. Sørlie, T., et al., Repeated observation of breast tumor subtypes in independent gene expression data sets. *Proceedings of the National Academy of Sciences*, 2003. **100**(14): p. 8418–8423.
76. Matsuda, N., et al., Identification of frequent somatic mutations in inflammatory breast cancer. *Breast Cancer Research and Treatment*, 2017. **163**: p. 263–272.
77. Curtis, C., et al., The genomic and transcriptomic architecture of 2,000 breast tumours reveals novel subgroups. *Nature*, 2012. **486**(7403): p. 346–352.
78. Clarke, A., et al., Thymocyte apoptosis induced by p53-dependent and independent pathways. *Nature*, 1993. **362**(6423): p. 849–852.
79. Lowe, S.W. and H.E. Ruley, Stabilization of the p53 tumor suppressor is induced by adenovirus 5 E1A and accompanies apoptosis. *Genes & Development*, 1993. **7**(4): p. 535–545.
80. Riley, T., et al., Transcriptional control of human p53-regulated genes. *Nature Reviews Molecular Cell Biology*, 2008. **9**(5): p. 402–412.
81. Tait, S.W. and D.R. Green, Mitochondria and cell death: outer membrane permeabilization and beyond. *Nature Reviews Molecular Cell Biology*, 2010. **11**(9): p. 621–632.
82. Chen, J., The cell-cycle arrest and apoptotic functions of p53 in tumor initiation and progression. *Cold Spring Harbor Perspectives in Medicine*, 2016. **6**(3): p. a026104.
83. Silwal-Pandit, L., A. Langerød, and A.-L. Børresen-Dale, TP53 mutations in breast and ovarian cancer. *Cold Spring Harbor Perspectives in Medicine*, 2017. **7**(1): p. a026252.
84. Berke, T.P., S.H. Slight, and S.M. Hyder, Role of reactivating mutant p53 protein in suppressing growth and metastasis of triple-negative breast cancer. *OncoTargets and Therapy*, 2022: p. 23–30.

85. Rivlin, N., et al., Mutations in the p53 tumor suppressor gene: important milestones at the various steps of tumorigenesis. *Genes & Cancer*, 2011. **2**(4): p. 466–474.
86. Mir, M.A., Sumaya, N, Jan, Implications of Chemokine Heterogenicity in Cancer Metastasis, in *Cytokine and Chemokine Networks in Cancer*. 2023, Springer. p. 115–136.
87. Zhang, Q., et al., APR-246 reactivates mutant p53 by targeting cysteines 124 and 277. *Cell Death & Disease*, 2018. **9**(5): p. 439.
88. Rangel, L.P., et al., p53 reactivation with induction of massive apoptosis-1 (PRIMA-1) inhibits amyloid aggregation of mutant p53 in cancer cells. *Journal of Biological Chemistry*, 2019. **294**(10): p. 3670–3682.
89. Liang, Y., C. Besch-Williford, and S.M. Hyder, PRIMA-1 inhibits growth of breast cancer cells by re-activating mutant p53 protein. *International Journal of Oncology*, 2009. **35**(5): p. 1015–1023.
90. Synnott, N., et al., Mutant p53: a novel target for the treatment of patients with triple-negative breast cancer? *International Journal of Cancer*, 2017. **140**(1): p. 234–246.
91. Mir, M.A., A. Shabir, and N. Jan, Metronomic Chemotherapy in Breast Cancer, in *Novel Approaches in Metronomic Chemotherapy for Breast Cancer Treatment*. CRC Press. p. 72–86.
92. Bauer, M.R., A.C. Joerger, and A.R. Fersht, 2-Sulfonylpyrimidines: Mild alkylating agents with anti-cancer activity toward p53-compromised cells. *Proceedings of the National Academy of Sciences*, 2016. **113**(36): p. E5271–E5280.
93. Synnott, N.C., et al., Mutant p53 as a therapeutic target for the treatment of triple-negative breast cancer: Preclinical investigation with the anti-p53 drug, PK11007. *Cancer Letters*, 2018. **414**: p. 99–106.
94. Kogan, S. and D.R. Carpizo, Zinc metallochaperones as mutant p53 reactivators: a new paradigm in cancer therapeutics. *Cancers*, 2018. **10**(6): p. 166.
95. Synnott, N.C., et al., COTI-2 reactivates mutant p53 and inhibits growth of triple-negative breast cancer cells. *Breast Cancer Research and Treatment*, 2020. **179**: p. 47–56.
96. Punganuru, S.R., et al., Design and synthesis of a C7-aryl piperlongumine derivative with potent anti-microtubule and mutant p53-reactivating properties. *European Journal of Medicinal Chemistry*, 2016. **107**: p. 233–244.
97. Punganuru, S.R., et al., Selective killing of human breast cancer cells by the styryl lactone (R)-goniothalamin is mediated by glutathione conjugation, induction of oxidative stress and marked reactivation of the R175H mutant p53 protein. *Carcinogenesis*, 2018. **39**(11): p. 1399–1410.
98. Aggarwal, M., et al., Reactivation of mutant p53 by a dietary-related compound phenethyl isothiocyanate inhibits tumor growth. *Cell Death & Differentiation*, 2016. **23**(10): p. 1615–1627.
99. Madan, E., et al., The curcumin analog HO-3867 selectively kills cancer cells by converting mutant p53 protein to transcriptionally active wildtype p53. *Journal of Biological Chemistry*, 2018. **293**(12): p. 4262–4276.
100. Hiraki, M., et al., Small-molecule reactivation of mutant p53 to wild-type-like p53 through the p53-Hsp40 regulatory axis. *Chemistry & Biology*, 2015. **22**(9): p. 1206–1216.
101. Xu, C., J. Zhuang, and X. Zhang, 2-[(4-Hydroxybenzyl) amino] phenol (HBAP) restores the mutated p53 to the level similar to that of wild-type p53 protein and inhibits breast cancer growth in vivo to by inducing tumor cells apoptosis. *Frontiers in Cell and Developmental Biology*, 2020. **8**: p. 574799.
102. Mahalingam, D., et al., Targeting HSP90 for cancer therapy. *British Journal of Cancer*, 2009. **100**(10): p. 1523–1529.
103. Hao, Q., Y. Chen, and X. Zhou, The janus face of p53-targeting ubiquitin ligases. *Cells*, 2020. **9**(7): p. 1656.
104. Alexandrova, E.M., et al., Improving survival by exploiting tumour dependence on stabilized mutant p53 for treatment. *Nature*, 2015. **523**(7560): p. 352–356.
105. Wang, Z.-T., et al., Histone deacetylase inhibitors suppress mutant p53 transcription via HDAC8/YY1 signals in triple negative breast cancer cells. *Cellular Signalling*, 2016. **28**(5): p. 506–515.
106. Gomes, A.S., et al., Structural and drug targeting insights on mutant p53. *Cancers*, 2021. **13**(13): p. 3344.
107. Yan, W., et al., Arsenic trioxide reactivates proteasome-dependent degradation of mutant p53 protein in cancer cells in part via enhanced expression of Pirh2 E3 ligase. *PLoS One*, 2014. **9**(8): p. e103497.
108. Wang, J., et al., Gambogic acid-induced degradation of mutant p53 is mediated by proteasome and related to CHIP. *Journal of Cellular Biochemistry*, 2011. **112**(2): p. 509–519.
109. Vakifahmetoglu-Norberg, H., et al., Chaperone-mediated autophagy degrades mutant p53. *Genes & Development*, 2013. **27**(15): p. 1718–1730.
110. Yi, Y.W., et al., Targeting mutant p53 by a SIRT1 activator YK-3-237 inhibits the proliferation of triple-negative breast cancer cells. *Oncotarget*, 2013. **4**(7): p. 984.
111. Liu, J., et al., Effects of triptolide from Tripterygium wilfordii on ERα and p53 expression in two human breast cancer cell lines. *Phytomedicine*, 2009. **16**(11): p. 1006–1013.

112. Al Dhaheri, Y., et al., Mitotic arrest and apoptosis in breast cancer cells induced by Origanum majorana extract: upregulation of TNF-α and downregulation of survivin and mutant p53. *PLoS One*, 2013. **8**(2): p. e56649.
113. Peng, J., et al., Targeting mutated p53 dependency in triple-negative breast cancer cells through CDK7 inhibition. *Frontiers in Oncology*, 2021. **11**: p. 664848.
114. Cai, J., et al., The PI3K/mTOR dual inhibitor NVP-BEZ235 stimulates mutant p53 degradation to exert anti-tumor effects on triple-negative breast cancer cells. *FEBS Open Bio*, 2020. **10**(4): p. 535–545.
115. Ronayne, C.T., et al., Synthesis and biological evaluation of a novel anticancer agent CBISC that induces DNA damage response and diminishes levels of mutant-p53. *Biochemical and Biophysical Research Communications*, 2021. **562**: p. 127–132.
116. Zhao, D., et al., Molecularly targeted therapies for p53-mutant cancers. *Cellular and Molecular Life Sciences*, 2017. **74**: p. 4171–4187.
117. Paranjpe, A. and K.S. Srivenugopal, Degradation of NF-κB, p53 and other regulatory redox-sensitive proteins by thiol-conjugating and-nitrosylating drugs in human tumor cells. *Carcinogenesis*, 2013. **34**(5): p. 990–1000.
118. Barnum, K.J. and M.J. O'Connell, Cell cycle regulation by checkpoints. *Cell Cycle Control: Mechanisms and Protocols*, 2014: p. 29–40.
119. Williams, A.B. and B. Schumacher, p53 in the DNA-damage-repair process. *Cold Spring Harbor Perspectives in Medicine*, 2016. **6**(5): p. a026070.
120. Visconti, R., R. Della Monica, and D. Grieco, Cell cycle checkpoint in cancer: a therapeutically targetable double-edged sword. *Journal of Experimental & Clinical Cancer Research*, 2016. **35**: p. 1–8.
121. Jabbour-Leung, N.A., et al., Sequential combination therapy of CDK inhibition and doxorubicin is synthetically lethal in p53-mutant triple-negative breast cancer. *Molecular Cancer Therapeutics*, 2016. **15**(4): p. 593–607.
122. Zonneville, J., et al., Selective therapeutic strategy for p53-deficient cancer by targeting dysregulation in DNA repair. *Communications Biology*, 2021. **4**(1): p. 862.
123. Jung, Y., et al., Crosstalk between Plk1, p53, cell cycle, and G2/M DNA damage checkpoint regulation in cancer: computational modeling and analysis. *NPJ Systems Biology and Applications*, 2021. **7**(1): p. 46.
124. Giordano, A., et al., Polo-like kinase 1 inhibitor onvansertib synergizes with paclitaxel in breast cancer carrying p53 mutation. *Annals of Oncology*, 2019. **30**: p. v125–v126.
125. Emerling, B.M., et al., Depletion of a putatively druggable class of phosphatidylinositol kinases inhibits growth of p53-null tumors. *Cell*, 2013. **155**(4): p. 844–857.
126. Lisek, K., D. Walerych, and G. Del Sal, Mutant p53–Nrf2 axis regulates the proteasome machinery in cancer. *Molecular & Cellular Oncology*, 2017. **4**(1): p. e1217967.
127. Walerych, D., et al., Proteasome machinery is instrumental in a common gain-of-function program of the p53 missense mutants in cancer. *Nature Cell Biology*, 2016. **18**(8): p. 897–909.
128. Di Agostino, S., et al., YAP enhances the pro-proliferative transcriptional activity of mutant p53 proteins. *EMBO Reports*, 2016. **17**(2): p. 188–201.
129. Campaner, E., et al., A covalent PIN1 inhibitor selectively targets cancer cells by a dual mechanism of action. *Nature Communications*, 2017. **8**(1): p. 15772.
130. Polotskaia, A., et al., Proteome-wide analysis of mutant p53 targets in breast cancer identifies new levels of gain-of-function that influence PARP, PCNA, and MCM4. *Proceedings of the National Academy of Sciences*, 2015. **112**(11): p. E1220–E1229.
131. Lundine, D., et al., The C-terminus of gain-of-function mutant p53 R273H is required for association with PARP1 and Poly-ADP-Ribose. *Molecular Cancer Research*, 2022. **20**(12): p. 1799–1810.
132. Valente, J.F., J.A. Queiroz, and F. Sousa, p53 as the focus of gene therapy: past, present and future. *Current Drug Targets*, 2018. **19**(15): p. 1801–1817.
133. Wang, X., et al., Ad-p53 enhances the sensitivity of triple-negative breast cancer MDA-MB-468 cells to the EGFR inhibitor gefitinib. *Oncology Reports*, 2015. **33**(2): p. 526–532.
134. Zhang, W.-W., et al., The first approved gene therapy product for cancer Ad-p53 (Gendicine): 12 years in the clinic. *Human Gene Therapy*, 2018. **29**(2): p. 160–179.
135. Rejeeth, C. and S. Kannan, p53 gene therapy of human breast carcinoma: using a transferrin-modified silica nanoparticles. *Breast Cancer*, 2016. **23**: p. 101–110.
136. Low, L., et al., Targeting mutant p53-expressing tumours with a T cell receptor-like antibody specific for a wild-type antigen. *Nature Communications*, 2019. **10**(1): p. 5382.
137. Hardwick, N.R., et al., p53MVA therapy in patients with refractory gastrointestinal malignancies elevates p53-specific CD8+ T-cell responses. *Clinical Cancer Research*, 2014. **20**(17): p. 4459–4470.

138. Chung, V., et al., Evaluation of safety and efficacy of p53MVA vaccine combined with pembrolizumab in patients with advanced solid cancers. *Clinical and Translational Oncology*, 2019. **21**: p. 363–372.
139. Yuan, Y., et al., Complete regression of cutaneous metastases with systemic immune response in a patient with triple negative breast cancer receiving p53MVA vaccine with pembrolizumab. *Oncoimmunology*, 2017. **6**(12): p. e1363138.
140. Daneste, H., et al., Immunoexpression of p53 mutant-type in Iranian patients with primary and recurrence oral squamous cell carcinoma. *European Journal of Translational Myology*, 2023. **33**(1). https://doi.org/10.4081/ejtm.2022.10847
141. Halim, F., et al., p53 mutation as plausible predictor for endocrine resistance therapy in luminal breast cancer. *F1000Research*, 2022. **11**. https://doi.org/10.12688/f1000research.108628.1
142. Zeng, W., et al., Advances in Doxorubicin-based nano-drug delivery system in triple negative breast cancer. *Frontiers in Bioengineering and Biotechnology*, 2023. **11**. https://doi.org/10.3389/fbioe.2023.1271420
143. Sobol, R.E., et al., Analysis of adenoviral p53 gene therapy clinical trials in recurrent head and neck squamous cell carcinoma. *Frontiers in Oncology*, 2021. **11**: p. 645745.
144. Chada, S., et al., Tumor suppressor immune gene therapy to reverse immunotherapy resistance. *Cancer Gene Therapy*, 2022. **29**(6): p. 825–834.
145. Johnson, R.L., et al., Barriers to immunotherapy in ovarian cancer: metabolic, genomic, and immune perturbations in the tumour microenvironment. *Cancers*, 2021. **13**(24): p. 6231.
146. Kim, S.-S., et al., A novel P53 nanomedicine reduces immunosuppression and augments anti-PD-1 therapy for non-small cell lung cancer in syngeneic mouse models. *Cells*, 2022. **11**(21): p. 3434.
147. Kunimura, N., et al., Combination of rAd-p53 in situ gene therapy and anti-PD-1 antibody immunotherapy induced anti-tumor activity in mouse syngeneic urogenital cancer models. *Scientific Reports*, 2020. **10**(1): p. 17464.
148. Xiao, Y., et al., Combining p53 mRNA nanotherapy with immune checkpoint blockade reprograms the immune microenvironment for effective cancer therapy. *Nature Communications*, 2022. **13**(1): p. 758.
149. Bykov, V.J., et al., Restoration of the tumor suppressor function to mutant p53 by a low-molecular-weight compound. *Nature Medicine*, 2002. **8**(3): p. 282–288.
150. Bykov, V.J., et al., Reactivation of mutant p53 and induction of apoptosis in human tumor cells by maleimide analogs. *Journal of Biological Chemistry*, 2005. **280**(34): p. 30384–30391.
151. Mohell, N., et al., APR-246 overcomes resistance to cisplatin and doxorubicin in ovarian cancer cells. *Cell Death & Disease*, 2015. **6**(6): p. e1794–e1794.
152. Duffy, M.J., et al., Targeting mutant p53 for cancer treatment: moving closer to clinical use? *Cancers*, 2022. **14**(18): p. 4499.
153. Sallman, D.A., et al., Eprenetapopt (APR-246) and azacitidine in TP53-mutant myelodysplastic syndromes. *Journal of Clinical Oncology*, 2021. **39**(14): p. 1584.
154. Lindemann, A., et al., COTI-2, a novel thiosemicarbazone derivative, exhibits antitumor activity in HNSCC through p53-dependent and-independent mechanisms. *Clinical Cancer Research*, 2019. **25**(18): p. 5650–5662.
155. Tang, M., J. Crown, and M.J. Duffy, Degradation of MYC by the mutant p53 reactivator drug, COTI-2 in breast cancer cells. *Investigational New Drugs*, 2023. **41**(4): p. 541–550.
156. Nagourney, A.J., et al., Therapeutic targeting of P53: a comparative analysis of APR-246 and COTI-2 in human tumor primary culture 3-D explants. *Genes*, 2023. **14**(3): p. 747.
157. Chen, S., et al., Arsenic trioxide rescues structural p53 mutations through a cryptic allosteric site. *Cancer Cell*, 2021. **39**(2): p. 225–239.
158. Hu, X., et al., Arsenic trioxide targets Hsp60, triggering degradation of p53 and survivin. *Chemical Science*, 2021. **12**(32): p. 10893–10900.
159. Dumble, M., et al., PC14586: The first orally bioavailable small molecule reactivator of Y220C mutant p53 in clinical development. *Cancer Research*, 2021. **81**. https://doi.org/10.1158/1538-7445.am2021-lb006
160. Qin, J.-J., et al., Identification of a new class of natural product MDM2 inhibitor: In vitro and in vivo anti-breast cancer activities and target validation. *Oncotarget*, 2015. **6**(5): p. 2623.
161. Qin, J.-J., et al., Inulanolide A as a new dual inhibitor of NFAT1-MDM2 pathway for breast cancer therapy. *Oncotarget*, 2016. **7**(22): p. 32566.
162. Qin, J.-J., et al., Identification of lineariifolianoid A as a novel dual NFAT1 and MDM2 inhibitor for human cancer therapy. *Journal of Biomedical Research*, 2016. **30**(4): p. 322.
163. Bykov, V.J., et al., PRIMA-1MET synergizes with cisplatin to induce tumor cell apoptosis. *Oncogene*, 2005. **24**(21): p. 3484–3491.

164. Lambert, J., et al., Mutant p53 reactivation by PRIMA-1MET induces multiple signaling pathways converging on apoptosis. *Oncogene*, 2010. **29**(9): p. 1329–1338.
165. Liang, Y., et al., Re-activation of the p53 pathway inhibits in vivo and in vitro growth of hormone-dependent human breast cancer cells. *International Journal of Oncology*, 2007. **31**(4): p. 777–784.
166. Liang, Y., et al., Targeting mutant p53 protein and the tumor vasculature: an effective combination therapy for advanced breast tumors. *Breast Cancer Research and Treatment*, 2011. **125**: p. 407–420.
167. Synnott, N.C., et al., *Combined Treatment Using the Anti-p53 Drug, APR-246 and Eribulin: Synergistic Growth Inhibition in p53-Mutated Breast Cancer Cells.* 2017, American Society of Clinical Oncology.
168. Synnott, N.C., et al., *Targeting Mutant p53 with PK11007: A New Approach for the Treatment of Patients with Triple-Negative Breast Cancer?* 2017, American Society of Clinical Oncology.
169. Baek, S., et al., Structure of the stapled p53 peptide bound to Mdm2. *Journal of the American Chemical Society*, 2012. **134**(1): p. 103–106.
170. Nag, S., et al., Targeting MDM2-p53 interaction for cancer therapy: are we there yet? *Current Medicinal Chemistry*, 2014. **21**(5): p. 553–574.
171. Vassilev, L.T., et al., In vivo activation of the p53 pathway by small-molecule antagonists of MDM2. *Science*, 2004. **303**(5659): p. 844–848.
172. Ding, K., et al., Structure-based design of spiro-oxindoles as potent, specific small-molecule inhibitors of the MDM2– p53 interaction. *Journal of Medicinal Chemistry*, 2006. **49**(12): p. 3432–3435.
173. Islam, M.S., et al., Synthesis, anticancer activity, and molecular modeling of new halogenated spiro [pyrrolidine-thiazolo-oxindoles] derivatives. *Applied Sciences*, 2020. **10**(6): p. 2170.
174. Wang, S., et al., SAR405838: an optimized inhibitor of MDM2–p53 interaction that induces complete and durable tumor regression. *Cancer Research*, 2014. **74**(20): p. 5855–5865.
175. Lu, J., et al., Reactivation of p53 by MDM2 inhibitor MI-77301 for the treatment of endocrine-resistant breast cancer. *Molecular Cancer Therapeutics*, 2016. **15**(12): p. 2887–2893.
176. Saxena, R., et al., Spiro-oxindole derivative 5-chloro-4′, 5′-diphenyl-3′-(4-(2-(piperidin-1-yl) ethoxy) benzoyl) spiro [indoline-3, 2′-pyrrolidin]-2-one triggers apoptosis in breast cancer cells via restoration of p53 function. *The International Journal of Biochemistry & Cell Biology*, 2016. **70**: p. 105–117.
177. Mu, J., et al., Discovery of spirooxindole–ferrocene hybrids as novel MDM2 inhibitors. *Chinese Chemical Letters*, 2021. **32**(6): p. 1897–1901.
178. Liu, S.-J., et al., Design, synthesis, and biological evaluation of nitroisoxazole-containing spiro [pyrrolidin-oxindole] derivatives as novel glutathione peroxidase 4/mouse double minute 2 dual inhibitors that inhibit breast adenocarcinoma cell proliferation. *European Journal of Medicinal Chemistry*, 2021. **217**: p. 113359.
179. Sobhani, N., et al., Mutant p53 as an antigen in cancer immunotherapy. *International Journal of Molecular Sciences*, 2020. **21**(11): p. 4087.
180. Zhang, Y., et al., Therapeutic potential of ReACp53 targeting mutant p53 protein in CRPC. *Prostate Cancer and Prostatic Diseases*, 2020. **23**(1): p. 160–171.
181. Chung-Faye, G.A., et al., Gene therapy strategies for colon cancer. *Molecular Medicine Today*, 2000. **6**(2): p. 82–87.
182. Steele, F.R., A moving target gene therapy: therapeutic mechanisms and strategies. *Molecular Therapy*, 2001. **3**(4): p. 429–430.
183. Sharma, A.R., et al., Next generation delivery system for proteins and genes of therapeutic purpose: why and how? *BioMed Research International*, 2014. **2014**. https://doi.org/10.1155/2014/327950
184. Sharma, S., T.K. Kelly, and P.A. Jones, Epigenetics in cancer. *Carcinogenesis*, 2010. **31**(1): p. 27–36.
185. Kanwal, R. and S. Gupta, Epigenetic modifications in cancer. *Clinical Genetics*, 2012. **81**(4): p. 303–311.
186. Veeck, J. and M. Esteller, Breast cancer epigenetics: from DNA methylation to microRNAs. *Journal of Mammary Gland Biology and Neoplasia*, 2010. **15**: p. 5–17.
187. Moore, L.D., T. Le, and G. Fan, DNA methylation and its basic function. *Neuropsychopharmacology*, 2013. **38**(1): p. 23–38.
188. Esteller, M., Epigenetic gene silencing in cancer: the DNA hypermethylome. *Human Molecular Genetics*, 2007. **16**(R1): p. R50–R59.
189. Győrffy, B., et al., Aberrant DNA methylation impacts gene expression and prognosis in breast cancer subtypes. *International Journal of Cancer*, 2016. **138**(1): p. 87–97.
190. Holm, K., et al., Molecular subtypes of breast cancer are associated with characteristic DNA methylation patterns. *Breast Cancer Research*, 2010. **12**: p. 1–16.
191. Yan, P.S., et al., CpG island arrays: an application toward deciphering epigenetic signatures of breast cancer. *Clinical Cancer Research*, 2000. **6**(4): p. 1432–1438.

192. Lapidus, R.G., et al., Methylation of estrogen and progesterone receptor gene 5′ CpG islands correlates with lack of estrogen and progesterone receptor gene expression in breast tumors. *Clinical Cancer Research: An Official Journal of the American Association for Cancer Research*, 1996. **2**(5): p. 805–810.
193. Ennour-Idrissi, K., et al., DNA methylation and breast cancer risk: an epigenome-wide study of normal breast tissue and blood. *Cancers*, 2020. **12**(11): p. 3088.
194. Dedeurwaerder, S., et al., DNA methylation profiling reveals a predominant immune component in breast cancers. *EMBO Molecular Medicine*, 2011. **3**(12): p. 726–741.
195. Zhang, M., et al., Integrative analysis of DNA methylation and gene expression to determine specific diagnostic biomarkers and prognostic biomarkers of breast cancer. *Frontiers in Cell and Developmental Biology*, 2020. **8**: p. 529386.
196. de Almeida, B.P., et al., Roadmap of DNA methylation in breast cancer identifies novel prognostic biomarkers. *BMC Cancer*, 2019. **19**: p. 1–12.
197. Audia, J.E. and R.M. Campbell, Histone modifications and cancer. *Cold Spring Harbor Perspectives in Biology*, 2016. **8**(4): p. a019521.
198. Chervona, Y. and M. Costa, Histone modifications and cancer: biomarkers of prognosis? *American Journal of Cancer Research*, 2012. **2**(5): p. 589.
199. Kurdistani, S., Histone modifications as markers of cancer prognosis: a cellular view. *British Journal of Cancer*, 2007. **97**(1): p. 1–5.
200. Stoccoro, A., et al., Epigenetic effects of nano-sized materials. *Toxicology*, 2013. **313**(1): p. 3–14.
201. Horn, P.J. and C.L. Peterson, Heterochromatin assembly: a new twist on an old model. *Chromosome Research*, 2006. **14**: p. 83–94.
202. Yan, W., J.G. Herman, and M. Guo, Epigenome-based personalized medicine in human cancer. *Epigenomics*, 2016. **8**(1): p. 119–133.
203. Fraga, M.F., et al., Loss of acetylation at Lys16 and trimethylation at Lys20 of histone H4 is a common hallmark of human cancer. *Nature Genetics*, 2005. **37**(4): p. 391–400.
204. Elsheikh, S.E., et al., Global histone modifications in breast cancer correlate with tumor phenotypes, prognostic factors, and patient outcome. *Cancer Research*, 2009. **69**(9): p. 3802–3809.
205. Kapoor-Vazirani, P., et al., Role of hMOF-dependent histone H4 lysine 16 acetylation in the maintenance of TMS1/ASC gene activity. *Cancer Research*, 2008. **68**(16): p. 6810–6821.
206. Buocikova, V., et al., Epigenetics in breast cancer therapy—New strategies and future nanomedicine perspectives. *Cancers*, 2020. **12**(12): p. 3622.
207. Yang, X., et al., CDKN1C (p57KIP2) is a direct target of EZH2 and suppressed by multiple epigenetic mechanisms in breast cancer cells. *PLoS One*, 2009. **4**(4): p. e5011.
208. Shi, L., et al., Histone demethylase JMJD2B coordinates H3K4/H3K9 methylation and promotes hormonally responsive breast carcinogenesis. *Proceedings of the National Academy of Sciences*, 2011. **108**(18): p. 7541–7546.
209. Wang, Y., et al., LSD1 is a subunit of the NuRD complex and targets the metastasis programs in breast cancer. *Cell*, 2009. **138**(4): p. 660–672.
210. Lu, L., et al., Let-7a regulation of insulin-like growth factors in breast cancer. *Breast Cancer Research and Treatment*, 2011. **126**: p. 687–694.
211. Yun, J., et al., Signalling pathway for RKIP and Let-7 regulates and predicts metastatic breast cancer. *The EMBO Journal*, 2011. **30**(21): p. 4500–4514.
212. Aure, M.R., et al., Individual and combined effects of DNA methylation and copy number alterations on miRNA expression in breast tumors. *Genome Biology*, 2013. **14**: p. 1–20.
213. Lehmann, U., et al., Epigenetic inactivation of microRNA gene hsa-mir-9-1 in human breast cancer. *The Journal of Pathology: A Journal of the Pathological Society of Great Britain and Ireland*, 2008. **214**(1): p. 17–24.
214. Barrow, T.M., et al., Aberrant methylation of imprinted genes is associated with negative hormone receptor status in invasive breast cancer. *International Journal of Cancer*, 2015. **137**(3): p. 537–547.
215. Bhan, A., et al., Antisense transcript long noncoding RNA (lncRNA) HOTAIR is transcriptionally induced by estradiol. *Journal of Molecular Biology*, 2013. **425**(19): p. 3707–3722.
216. Feng, S. and D.D. De Carvalho, Clinical advances in targeting epigenetics for cancer therapy. *The FEBS Journal*, 2022. **289**(5): p. 1214–1239.
217. Gonzalez-Angulo, A.M., F. Morales-Vasquez, and G.N. Hortobagyi, Overview of resistance to systemic therapy in patients with breast cancer. *Breast Cancer Chemosensitivity*, 2007: p. 1–22. https://doi.org/10.1093/annonc/mdq612
218. Waks, A.G. and E.P. Winer, Breast cancer treatment: a review. *Jama*, 2019. **321**(3): p. 288–300.

219. Roninson, I.B., E.V. Broude, and B.-D. Chang, If not apoptosis, then what? Treatment-induced senescence and mitotic catastrophe in tumor cells. *Drug Resistance Updates*, 2001. **4**(5): p. 303–313.
220. Gianni, L., et al., Role of anthracyclines in the treatment of early breast cancer. *Journal of Clinical Oncology*, 2009. **27**(28): p. 4798–4808.
221. Fu, D., J.A. Calvo, and L.D. Samson, Balancing repair and tolerance of DNA damage caused by alkylating agents. *Nature Reviews Cancer*, 2012. **12**(2): p. 104–120.
222. Longley, D.B., D.P. Harkin, and P.G. Johnston, 5-fluorouracil: mechanisms of action and clinical strategies. *Nature Reviews Cancer*, 2003. **3**(5): p. 330–338.
223. Vignard, J., G. Mirey, and B. Salles, Ionizing-radiation induced DNA double-strand breaks: a direct and indirect lighting up. *Radiotherapy and Oncology*, 2013. **108**(3): p. 362–369.
224. Sparreboom, A., et al., Preclinical pharmacokinetics of paclitaxel and docetaxel. *Anti-Cancer Drugs*, 1998. **9**(1): p. 1–17.
225. Buchholz, T.A., et al., Neoadjuvant chemotherapy for breast carcinoma: multidisciplinary considerations of benefits and risks. *Cancer: Interdisciplinary International Journal of the American Cancer Society*, 2003. **98**(6): p. 1150–1160.
226. Eisenhauer, E., et al., 32 INVITED New response evaluation criteria in solid tumors: revised RECIST guideline version 1.1. *European Journal of Cancer Supplements*, 2008. **6**(12): p. 13.
227. Mir, M.A., M. Rashid, and N. Jan, Cytokines and Chemokines in Tumor Growth and Progression, in *Cytokine and Chemokine Networks in Cancer*. 2023, Springer. p. 33–77.
228. Osborne, C.K., H. Zhao, and S.A. Fuqua, Selective estrogen receptor modulators: structure, function, and clinical use. *Journal of Clinical Oncology*, 2000. **18**(17): p. 3172–3186.
229. Osborne, C.K. and R. Schiff, Aromatase inhibitors: future directions. *The Journal of Steroid Biochemistry and Molecular Biology*, 2005. **95**(1–5): p. 183–187.
230. Nasrazadani, A., et al., Precision medicine in hormone receptor-positive breast cancer. *Frontiers in Oncology*, 2018. **8**: p. 144.
231. Fabian, C.J., The what, why and how of aromatase inhibitors: hormonal agents for treatment and prevention of breast cancer. *International Journal of Clinical Practice*, 2007. **61**(12): p. 2051–2063.
232. Mitchell, A.P., et al., Association between reimbursement incentives and physician practice in oncology: a systematic review. *JAMA Oncology*, 2019. **5**(6): p. 893–899.
233. Epstein, A.J. and S.J. Johnson, Physician response to financial incentives when choosing drugs to treat breast cancer. *International Journal of Health Care Finance and Economics*, 2012. **12**: p. 285–302.
234. Hadley, J., et al., Medicare breast surgery fees and treatment received by older women with localized breast cancer. *Health Services Research*, 2003. **38**(2): p. 553–573.

12 Targeted Therapies against Mutated p53 in Breast Cancer

Samridhi Kaul[1], Kirti Hooda[2], Mary Chatterjee[1], Asma Jan[3], and Manzoor Ahmad Mir[,3]*

[1]Department of Biotechnology Engineering, University Institute of Engineering & Technology, Panjab University, Chandigarh, India
[2]Centre for Nanoscience and Nanotechnology, Panjab University, Chandigarh, India
[3]Department of Bioresources, School of Biological Sciences, University of Kashmir, Srinagar, J&K, India
*drmanzoor@kashmiruniversity.ac.in

12.1 INTRODUCTION

About 30% of instances of breast cancer are caused by mutations in the p53 gene, which is the most often altered gene in breast cancer [1]. Missense point mutations that block p53's transcriptional activity are the primary cause of most p53 alterations, which are found inside the DNA-binding domain. These mutations are linked to lower overall survival and more severe illness. While the frequency of p53 mutations in breast cancer is lower than in other solid tumors, there are higher frequencies in some kinds of the disease, such as those that develop in carriers of germ-line BRCA1 and BRCA2 mutations [2, 3]. A p53 mutation has been connected to reduce overall survival, breast cancer-corrected survival, and relapse-free survival in breast cancer, all of which are associated with a worse prognosis [4, 5]. One important tumor suppressor route that helps stop breast cancer from developing is the p53 pathway. The p53 protein, which controls cell growth and division, is normally disrupted by mutations in the p53 gene, which can result in the development of breast cancer [6]. Triple-negative breast cancer (TNBC) is a compelling therapeutic target due to the high frequency of tumor protein 53 (TP53) mutations, which also serve as a marker to predict chemotherapy response. Nonetheless, there is still much to learn about how TP53 mutations affect therapy response and consequences [7–9]. The four most frequent p53 mutation types seen in breast cancer are missense, truncating, in-frame, and splice mutations. Single amino-acid alterations brought about by missense mutations have the potential to exhibit gain-of-function activity during the tumorigenic process. Proteins with truncations caused by truncating mutations have the potential to encourage the growth of tumors. Nucleotide insertions or deletions result in in-frame mutations. They may result in the formation of novel domains that may aid in carcinogenesis or the loss of functioning domains. Splice mutations that take place at the splice site may result in the loss of functional domains or the production of abnormal transcripts [10, 11]. p53 mutations largely cause targeted therapy resistance in breast cancer. Through the formation of a more aggressive and therapy-resistant phenotype, p53 mutations can contribute to chemotherapy resistance. Furthermore, resistance to radiation and chemotherapy can be predicted by the existence of p53 mutations. A p53 mutation may increase a tumor cell's capacity to repair DNA damage brought on by drugs, making the cell resistant to chemotherapy. DNA repair processes including nucleotide excision repair and mismatch repair are activated to do this. Additionally, mutant p53 can encourage cancer-causing processes like invasion, migration, angiogenesis, and proliferation, all of which can increase a patient's resistance to targeted treatment [12, 13]. In TNBC, where p53 mutations are present in

 DOI: 10.1201/9781003520771-12

70–80% of cases, targeting p53 mutations is a potentially effective treatment strategy for breast cancer. Among the tactics are genetically based methods employing vectors and designed antibodies, stapled peptides, PROTACs, small molecule pharmacologic inhibitors, and the use of circular RNA circ-Ccnbl to block the activity of mutant p53 [6]. The most promising molecularly targeted therapies for breast cancer include the standard of care for adjuvant treatment of breast tumors overexpressing HER2 trastuzumab, which is directed against the human epidermal growth factor receptor 2 (HER2) [14, 15]. Another authorized targeted drug for the treatment of breast cancer is lapatinib, which is directed against HER2. Bevacizumab is used in conjunction with chemotherapy that targets vascular endothelial growth factor (VEGF) in the treatment of breast cancer [16, 17]. Neratinib is a HER2-targeting small molecule tyrosine kinase inhibitor (TKI) that has demonstrated efficacy in treating HER2-positive breast cancer [18, 19]. The goal of developing targeted therapeutics against mutated p53 is to either stop the carcinogenic consequences of mutant p53 or restore the functions of wild-type p53. These tactics include immunotherapies, gene therapies, causing synthetic lethality, encouraging degradation, blocking gain-of-function-associated interactors or pathways, and reactivating or restoring mutant p53 to wild-type p53 capabilities [13, 20, 21].

TP53 is an essential modulator of cellular mechanisms that avert the development of cancer. It is engaged in several cellular processes, such as ensuring that damaged DNA is not copied and transferred to daughter cells, which is a major function of p53 in controlling the cell cycle. In reaction to cellular stressors such as DNA damage, p53 can trigger cellular senescence, which is an irreversible stoppage of the cell cycle. By activating genes involved in DNA repair pathways, p53 contributes to the repair of DNA damage (Table 12.1). When cells experience cellular stress or damage to their

TABLE 12.1
Functions of p53

Function of p53	Description	References
Induction of cellular senescence	A permanent stop to the cell cycle known as cellular senescence can be brought on by p53 in response to cellular stress. One way that cellular senescence suppresses cancer is by halting the proliferation of damaged cells.	[22–24]
DNA damage repair	Through the activation of genes involved in DNA repair mechanisms, p53 plays a critical role in DNA damage repair pathways. It makes it easier for DNA damage to be repaired, preserving genomic stability and averting the buildup of mutations that might eventually cause cancer.	[25–27]
Induction of apoptosis	When cells are under cellular stress or have damage to their DNA, p53 can cause programmed cell death, often known as apoptosis. p53 prevents damaged DNA-containing cells from multiplying and perhaps developing into cancer by inducing apoptosis.	[28–30]
Regulation of autophagy	The autophagic process, which includes the breakdown and recycling of harmed or dysfunctional cellular components, is regulated by p53. Through the regulation of autophagy, p53 aids in the preservation of cellular homeostasis and hinders the buildup of detrimental cellular debris, which may be a factor in the development of cancer.	[31, 32]
Control of cell cycle	By preventing damaged DNA from being copied and passed on to daughter cells, p53 controls the cell cycle. In reaction to biological stressors such as DNA damage, it causes cell cycle arrest, which stops damaged cells from multiplying and possibly developing into cancer.	[27, 33]
Regulation of cellular metabolism	The regulation of cellular metabolism by p53 impacts a cell's capacity for environmental adaptation. To meet the energy and nutritional needs of cells, it controls metabolic pathways, which affect cellular survival, proliferation, and stress response.	[34–36]

DNA, p53 can trigger programmed cell death, or apoptosis, which stops the cells with damaged DNA from proliferating [9, 37]. It has been demonstrated that p53 controls autophagy, a physiological process that recycles harmed or malfunctioning cellular components to preserve cellular homeostasis. The regulation of cellular metabolism by p53 affects a cell's capacity to adjust to its surroundings. Ferroptosis, a type of planned cell death marked by the buildup of lipid peroxides, has been linked to the control of p53 [38]. Mutations in p53 can have a variety of implications on the protein's actions in breast cancer cells, including tumor-suppressive and carcinogenic effects. The most prevalent kind of p53 mutation is the missense mutation, which results in a full-length mutant p53 protein (mutp53) that differs from the wild-type p53 protein by just one amino acid. The bulk of these mutations affect the DNA-binding domain of the p53 gene, which affects the protein's capacity to bind to target genes and, consequently, its transcriptional activity. These mutations can occur in any location of the p53 gene. It is well known that when DNA damage occurs, wild-type p53 can cause senescence, apoptosis, and cell cycle arrest. These capabilities may be lost due to p53 gene mutations, which could allow damaged cells to continue proliferating and eventually result in cancer. Nonetheless, it has been demonstrated that certain mutp53 proteins can develop novel carcinogenic properties separate from wild-type p53, potentially accelerating the development of cancer. These carcinogenic effects may involve influencing the capacity of cancer cells to divide, evade apoptosis, invade, and spread [39, 40]. Because of the high incidence of p53 gene mutations and the carcinogenic properties of mutp53 in cancer, targeting p53 for cancer therapy is a viable strategy. Reactivating the mutant p53 protein into its functional wild-type conformation has been demonstrated to inhibit triple-negative breast cancer spread and growth. Furthermore, p53 targeting has been investigated in cancer treatment, with an emphasis on the reactivation of mutant p53 protein [1, 6].

12.2 TARGETING MUTATED p53: RATIONALE AND STRATEGIES

Since TP53 mutations are common in human malignancies, targeting mutp53 for cancer therapy is an appealing approach. These mutations not only reduce TP53's antitumor efficacy but also give the mutant protein carcinogenic qualities. Because the medicine must selectively target mutp53 in cancer cells while not affecting normal cells retaining wild-type p53 (wtp53), the development of p53-targeted therapies is difficult. In addition, different mutp53 protein structures that are challenging to target are produced by numerous p53 mutations (Figure 12.1) [41].

Targeting mutp53 directly entails using tiny compounds that can either shield p53 from its negative regulators or make mutant p53 proteins functional again. One tactic used in indirect methods is

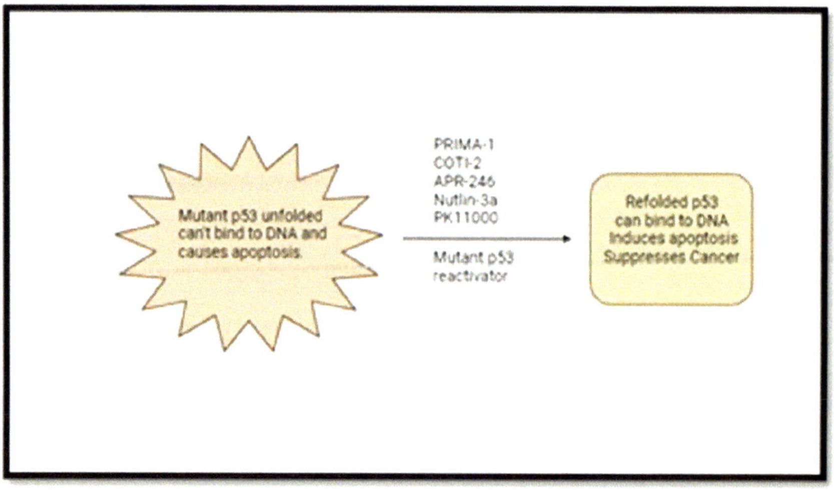

FIGURE 12.1 Various p53 reactivators of p53. (Image created using Biorender.com).

to take advantage of synthetic lethal interactions with mutp53, in which cell death can result from the disruption of p53-interacting genes. Targeting noncoding RNAs may have potential synthetic fatal effects in tumors with p53 mutations, as evidenced by research on noncoding RNAs and the ability to disrupt noncoding RNA networks to have a beneficial antitumor effect [19, 42, 43]. Targeting the stability of mutant p53, which is strongly associated with treatment resistance and a bad prognosis, is a further strategy. The characteristics of mutant p53's protein structure, the control of E3 ubiquitin ligase, and the action of molecular chaperones are the primary mechanisms of mutant p53 stabilization. Reducing the amount of mutant p53, increasing its ubiquitination, preventing the formation of aggregates, and interfering with mutant p53's ability to form other protein complexes are some methods for modifying these interrelated mechanisms in cancer treatment [44]. For several reasons, targeting mutp53 for cancer therapy is a difficult undertaking. Among these difficulties are the diverse architectures and functions exhibited by mtp53 proteins that pose a challenge in the development of a single therapeutic strategy capable of efficiently addressing all types of mutations. The majority of mutp53 variants do not have an appropriate pocket for the high-affinity binding of low-molecular-weight drugs, which are frequently employed in cancer treatments. Because of its position in tumor cells, mutp53 is essentially inaccessible to certain types of medications, such as those that need the protein to bind in a particular shape [13, 20]. It is difficult to reactivate mutp53 into a wtp53-like condition since this necessitates the restoration of the protein's original structure and functionality. Mutp53 degradation is a multistep process involving the control of several different pathways and interactions with different proteins. Mutp53's oncogenic effects must be disrupted while retaining its tumor-suppressive functions, making the challenge of disrupting its function and reactivating wild-type function difficult. It is difficult to target mutp53 stability, binding partners, and downstream pathways since doing so necessitates a thorough comprehension of the molecular mechanisms underlying the protein and the creation of potent treatment approaches [45]. A potential strategy is immunological targeting of p53, which entails stimulating the immune system to identify and destroy cancer cells that express mutant p53. It is difficult to restore the function of downstream effector genes that control tumor suppression since doing so necessitates the creation of potent treatment plans that can get past the difficulties associated with mutp53-mediated malignancy. It is past time for a national p53 program to be implemented, as it would offer a structure for tackling the difficulties in mutp53 targeting and creating potent treatment plans. To overcome the difficulties in targeting mutp53, persistence, and naivete are crucial since they might result in creative solutions and the creation of successful treatment plans [46]. Targeting mutp53 for cancer therapy involves numerous techniques, including small drugs, gene therapy, and immunotherapy, each with its advantages and drawbacks. Small molecules that can either protect p53 from its negative regulators or restore the functionality of mutant p53 proteins are gaining interest. These compounds seek to restore the tumor-suppressive properties of p53, which are deactivated in cancerous cells as a result of mutations. Because these compounds may specifically target cancer cells while preserving normal cells, their development is essential for cancer therapy [44]. Gene therapy techniques, such as the use of clustered regularly interspaced short palindromic repeats (CRISPR)/Cas9, are being examined to restore the TP53 414delC mutation to the wild-type TP53 genotype and stop the cell. This approach involves the genetic editing of p53 to restore its wild-type function, which can lead to the suppression of tumor growth. Immunotherapy targeting mutant p53 to suppress tumor growth is becoming a promising approach in cancer therapy. This entails using vaccinations, which have been studied in numerous phase I/II clinical trials involving various cancer types, to boost T cell responses against tumors that contain mutant p53 [47].

12.3 SMALL MOLECULE INHIBITORS OF MUTANT p53

Targeting mutp53 with small molecule inhibitors is a promising strategy for cancer treatment because it aims to restore the tumor-suppressive functions of p53 that are lost in cancer cells as a result of mutations.

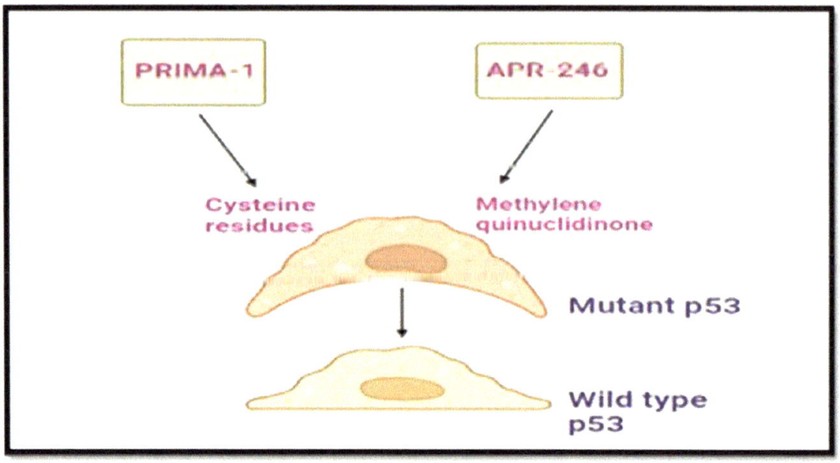

FIGURE 12.2 Small molecule inhibitors PRIMA-1 and APR-246 restoration of p53. (Image created using Biorender.com).

These inhibitors fall into two general categories: MDM2 inhibitors and p53 corrector mutations [48]. By attaching to the MDM2 protein, a negative regulator of p53, MDM2 antagonists stop the degradation of the p53 protein. By inhibiting MDM2, these drugs allow p53 to concentrate and perform its tumor-suppressive effects. Clinical trials for MDM2 inhibitors have been completed, suggesting that they may have therapeutic uses. By focusing on particular mutations that render p53 inactive, these substances can restore the tumor-suppressive properties of p53. The ability of mutant p53 correctors to specifically target cancer cells while preserving normal cells makes them essential for use in cancer therapy (Figure 12.2) [49].

Targeting mutp53, small molecule inhibitors seek to restore the tumor-suppressive properties of p53 that are lost in cancer cells as a result of mutations. These inhibitors fall into two general categories: mutant p53 correctors and MDM2 antagonists. By attaching to the MDM2 protein, a negative regulator of p53, MDM2 antagonists stop the degradation of the p53 protein [50]. Mutant p53 correctors seek to rectify the structure or function of mutant p53 proteins to restore their functionality [51]. Increasing mutant p53 ubiquitination, preventing aggregation formation, and interfering with mutant p53's interaction with other protein complexes are some methods for addressing the stabilization of mutant p53. One of the most sought-after goals in developing treatments has been the creation of small molecule inhibitors targeting mutant p53; several different drugs are being researched to restore wild-type p53 function to these mutants [52]. Some of these compounds, which were developed by inhibiting MDM2, have advanced to clinical testing. Dual inhibitors of MDM2 and MDMX, as well as a restricted number of small compounds, are nevertheless able to revive the function of mutant p53 [53]. These inhibitors work in different ways, but, generally speaking, they work by focusing on a subset of p53 missense mutations, giving the mutant proteins their original structure and function, boosting p53-mediated gene expression, and causing tumor regression [52]. The bulk of the nine most frequent p53 mutations are DNA contact mutants, which are the most often targeted p53 mutations by small molecule inhibitors. Unlike "conformational" mutations, which reduce DNA binding by destabilizing the protein structure, these changes take place in locations that come into direct contact with target DNA sequences [54]. The MDM2–p53 association is the target of the majority of small chemical inhibitors that target mutant p53, including nutlins, benzodiazepinediones, and spirooxindoles. The mutant protein, which is overexpressed in cancer cells, is the specific target of small molecule inhibitors targeting mutant p53. This selectivity minimizes damage to normal cells and lowers the possibility of off-target effects. Because these inhibitors can be made reversible, p53 function may be restored without the protein being permanently altered. This selectivity minimizes damage to normal cells and lowers the possibility of off-target effects. Because these inhibitors can be made reversible, p53 function may be restored without the protein being permanently altered. Because of its reversibility, there may be a lower chance of long-term negative effects when treating cancer. In certain cancers, stages, populations, subpopulations, genetic mutations, comorbidities, cancer stem cells, tumor microenvironment, and immune system, small molecule inhibitors can be engineered to prevent both cancer-associated morbidity and mortality. One example of this would be early-stage breast cancer in elderly patients with particular genetic mutations and comorbidities. Immunotherapy and small molecule inhibitors can be combined to strengthen the immune system's defenses against cancer cells. This strategy can be especially useful in tumors where the immune system is unable to identify and eradicate cancer cells due to a p53 mutation. To increase the efficacy of treatment, small molecule inhibitors can be used in conjunction with targeted medicines or radiation therapy [55].

The process of creating small molecule inhibitors that specifically target mutant p53 in breast cancer is difficult because of the variety of p53 mutations and the requirement for targeted and efficient treatments. Because mutant p53 proteins have different conformations and activities, it is challenging to create tiny compounds with the same potency as wild-type p53 proteins. The creation of targeted therapeutics that can specifically restart the activity of particular mutant proteins is required due to the large degree of structural and conformational heterogeneity across mutant p53 proteins. Despite these obstacles, scientists have made strides in discovering tiny compounds like PRIMA-1, which has demonstrated promise in preclinical research that can restore the function of mutant p53 proteins [43]. Moreover, the development of effective treatments is hampered by the unclear mechanisms by which mutant p53 proteins contribute to carcinogenesis and the lack of a therapeutic approach that works for all mutant p53 malignancies. A thorough grasp of the molecular pathways generating p53 mutations is necessary for the development of small molecule inhibitors targeting mutant p53 for breast cancer, as is the creation of tailored therapeutics that can successfully restart the function of particular mutant proteins [50].

12.4 GENE THERAPY APPROACHES FOR MUTANT p53

Research on developing gene therapies that specifically target mutant p53 in breast cancer is ongoing to find efficient cures that can restart the activity of particular mutant p53 proteins. Since it enables the creation of substances that can disrupt contact and activate p53 functions in cancer cells, the MDM2–p53 interaction is a crucial target for small molecule inhibitors. By reactivating mutant p53 and preventing the proliferation of cancer cells, compounds including PRIMA-1, APR-246, PK11007, and COTI-2 have been found as possible treatments for breast cancer, especially triple-negative breast cancer. These substances are being researched as possible breast cancer treatment approaches because preclinical research on them has demonstrated promise (Figure 12.3) [42, 56]. By reactivating the mutant p53 protein, which is frequently present in breast cancer, PRIMA-1 prevents the proliferation of breast cancer cells [57]. It has been demonstrated that PRIMA-1 can cause apoptosis in breast cancer cells that have lost the p53 gene and can stop breast cancer cells from growing by reactivating the mutant p53 protein. Compared to other small molecules, PRIMA-1 is more successful in halting the growth of tumors and triggering apoptosis in tumor cells in mouse models. PRIMA-1 has been linked to the induction of apoptosis through the promotion of Bax activation while blocking JNK signaling. The Epstein–Barr virus-encoded EBNA-5 protein has been reported to undergo nucleolar translocation upon exposure to PRIMA-1. It has been demonstrated that PRIMA-1 triggers several signaling cascades that culminate in apoptosis. PRIMA-1 has been discovered to target mutant versions of p63 and p73, members of the p53 family [58]. Treatment for p53-mutated breast tumors, including the subset with triple-negative disease, may now be possible with PRIMA-1 [59]. It has been discovered that PRIMA-1 is a prodrug that covalently interacts with cysteine residue thiol groups in the mutp53 core domain to restore wtp53 conformation. It has been discovered that PRIMA-1 induces the release of cytochrome c from the mitochondria in a manner that is dependent on BAX, which in turn triggers the activation of caspase. By directly binding to

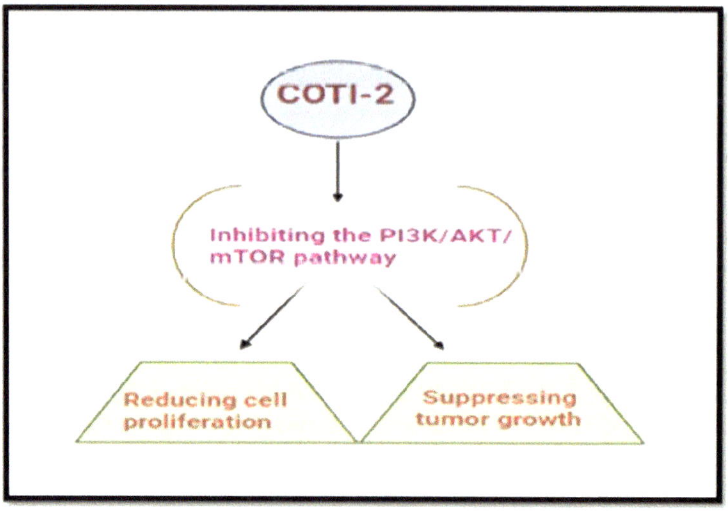

FIGURE 12.3 COTI-2 mechanism of action.

cysteine in glutathione and blocking thioredoxin reductase, PRIMA-1 has been shown to alter the cellular redox balance. This disruption of a critical homeostatic mechanism that is necessary to preserve cell viability leads to the promotion of cancer cell death. It has been discovered that PRIMA-1 is a potentially effective treatment for breast cancer [3, 43].

PRIMA-1 may cause resistance in breast cancer cells, which could reduce its efficacy as a therapeutic agent. PRIMA-1 may be harmful to healthy breast cells or other tissues, which could cause unfavorable patient reactions. It's possible that PRIMA-1 isn't selective enough to target solely mutant p53 proteins, which could have harmful or off-target consequences. The therapeutic potential of PRIMA-1 may be limited if it is unable to successfully pass the blood-brain barrier or reach the tumor location [60]. These difficulties point to the necessity of additional study and advancement to get over PRIMA-1's drawbacks and enhance its therapeutic potential for individuals with breast cancer. One gene therapy strategy called APR-246 has been studied for its ability to restore wild-type p53 function in breast cancer. One effective medication-targeted approach to treating breast cancer with mtp53 expression is the restoration of p53 function [63]. APR-246 can reactivate mutant p53 and stop the growth of cancer cells because it has been demonstrated to cause cell cycle arrest, enhance apoptosis, and upregulate many p53 target genes [62, 63]. Reactivating mutant p53 and modifying reactive oxygen species (ROS) are two distinct processes by which APR-246 can impede the development of cancer cells and induce their demise. APR-246 was reported to cause changes in the expression of 162 genes in BT549 cells, however, only 26 genes in MDA-MB-468 and MCF7 cells treated with APR-246 displayed altered expression. In all three of the cell lines that were studied, APR-246 was shown to upregulate the expression of six genes: TRIM16, SLC7A11, TXNRD1, SRXN1, LOC344887, and SLC7A11-AS1. It has been established that APR-246 upregulates the expression of TRIM16, SLC7A11, and SRXN1 in both new breast cancer cell lines and wild-type TP53-carrying MCF7 cells [13, 64]. APR-246's potential for therapeutic use is demonstrated by the fact that it is presently being investigated in a phase II clinical trial for high-grade serous ovarian cancer. APR-246 is a potentially effective treatment for breast cancer since it has been demonstrated to reinstate the transcriptional activity of unfolded wild-type or mutant p53 [65]. APR-246 might not be selective enough to target just mutant p53 proteins, which could have harmful or off-target consequences. Because breast cancer is a genetically diverse illness, APR-246 might not be effective against every mutation or subtype. To improve treatment outcomes and overcome resistance to APR-246, it is imperative to comprehend the processes underlying resistance. To optimize the dosage and administration of APR-246, a thorough understanding of its pharmacokinetics and pharmacodynamics is necessary. These difficulties show how much more study and development are required to get over APR-246's drawbacks and maximize its therapeutic potential for breast cancer patients [66].

The possibility of using COTI-2, a gene therapy technique, to restore wild-type p53 function in breast cancer has been studied. Through at least two distinct mechanisms, the reactivation of mutant p53 and the regulation of reactive oxygen species COTI-2 can impede the development of cancer cells and induce cell death. It has been discovered that COTI-2 induces changes in the expression of 162 genes in BT549 cells, however, only 26 genes in COTI-2-treated MDA-MB-468 and MCF7 cells exhibited altered expression. In all three of the cell lines examined, COTI-2 has been shown to upregulate the expression of six genes: TRIM16, SLC7A11, TXNRD1, SRXN1, LOC344887, and SLC7A11-AS1. It has been demonstrated that COTI-2 upregulates the expression of TRIM16, SLC7A11, and SRXN1 in both new breast cancer cell lines and wild-type TP53-carrying MCF7 cells [67]. A phase II clinical trial including high-grade serous ovarian cancer is presently testing COTI-2, suggesting that the drug may find use in therapeutic settings. COTI-2 is a potentially effective treatment for breast cancer since it has been demonstrated to reinstate the transcriptional activity of unfolded wild-type or mutant p53 [68]. It has been demonstrated that COTI-2 inhibits the development of triple-negative breast cancer cells and reactivates mutant p53. Patients with breast cancer may benefit from better treatment outcomes if it is combined with other targeted medicines that focus on distinct processes. It has been demonstrated that COTI-2 inhibits the development of triple-negative breast cancer cells and reactivates mutant p53. Its combination with targeted medications that address several processes may help patients with breast cancer receive better treatment outcomes [69].

12.5 IMMUNOTHERAPY TARGETING MUTATED p53

Immunotherapy is a tool used in immunotherapeutic techniques to target breast cancer cells that contain mutant p53 proteins by stimulating the immune system to identify and fight these cells. Among these strategies is immunotherapy, which targets mutant p53 to inhibit tumor growth and is quickly emerging as a promising cancer treatment modality [70]. Additionally, effective methods for treating mutp53-expressing cancers include gene editing, immunotherapy, siRNA silencing, and synthetic lethality. These tactics seek to produce synthetic lethality, target mutp53 for degradation, and restore mutp53's transcriptional activity and wild-type conformation. To accomplish these therapeutic objectives, a variety of strategies have been investigated, including synthetic tiny peptides, CRISPR/Cas9-mediated genome editing, small interference RNAs (RNAi), small chemical drugs, and immunotherapies. Targeting mutant p53 with immunotherapy may strengthen the immune system's defenses against breast cancer cells, improving the prognosis of breast cancer patients undergoing treatment [71]. The various forms of immunotherapy directed against p53-mutant breast cancer cells include immunotherapy directed against p53 mutants to inhibit tumor growth. Using immunotherapy, this strategy aims to inhibit the growth of tumors by specifically targeting mutant p53-expressing breast cancer cells [70]. T cell receptor-like (TCLR) antibodies can bind to particular mutant p53 proteins and trigger the body's defense mechanism against cancerous cells. By exposing the immune system to p53 antigens, p53-based vaccinations can elicit an immunological response against cancer cells [72]. Immunotherapy directed toward p53 degradation makes use of immunotherapy directed at p53 mutants for degradation, which has the potential to eradicate cancer cells. Immunotherapy is used in synthetic lethality-based therapy to cause cancer cells that depend on mutant p53 for survival to become fatal. Genetic mutations that lead to the onset and spread of breast cancer, such as those in the TP53 gene, can be corrected by the use of gene editing technologies like CRISPR/Cas9. RNAi can be used to mute the mRNA for mutp53, which can kill cancer cells [73]. Immunotherapy directed toward mutant p53 for apoptosis makes use of immunotherapy directed toward mutant p53 for apoptosis, which has the potential to eradicate cancer cells [74]. p53 plays a complicated role in the development of breast cancer, acting to both stimulate and inhibit tumor growth. Immunotherapy can target p53 mutations that result in the development of immunogenic activity in breast cancer. Nonetheless, TNBCs, which are notorious for their poor prognosis because of their aggressive behavior and lack of viable treatment choices, account for the bulk of breast cancers with mutant p53. Immunotherapy directed against breast cancer cells that carry mutant p53 proteins entails triggering the immune system to identify and assault certain types of breast cancer cells. This strategy makes use of the fact that mutant p53 proteins can trigger an immune response against cancer cells and are frequently immunogenic. There are several ways to target mutant p53 with immunotherapy, including blocking the MDM2–p53 connection, bringing back p53 function, or causing synthetic lethality [73]. Research on the practical application of p53 activation to elicit an immunological response is ongoing, with multiple clinical trials examining the combination of immunotherapy and p53-restoring drugs or vaccines. Although the outcomes of these clinical trials have been inconsistent, they indicate that certain patients may experience an immunological response when p53 is activated [74]. Because altered p53 proteins are frequently immunogenic and can trigger an immune response against cancer cells, immunotherapy directed against p53-mutant breast cancer cells is a promising strategy. Because p53 mutations are the basis of tumors, p53 is a prime candidate for cancer therapy. Treatment approaches that target p53 can be broadly classified into three groups: restoring p53's wild-type conformation and transcriptional activity; targeting p53 for degradation; and inducing synthetic lethality. To accomplish these therapeutic objectives, researchers have looked into small chemical drugs, synthetic small peptides, CRISPR/Cas9-mediated genome editing, small interference RNAs (RNAi), and immunotherapies [71]. Furthermore, immunotherapies are made feasible by the mutant peptides generated by the degradation of altered p53 [75].

12.6 FUTURE DIRECTIONS AND CONCLUSIONS

Future options for targeted therapy against p53 mutations in breast cancer include several approaches designed to minimize damage to normal cells while effectively targeting the altered protein. Some of these approaches include reactivation or restoration of wild-type functions in mutant p53, which entails finding substances that can make mutant p53 function again. By doing so, it may be possible to counteract several pro-cancer driving factors, such as reactivating host immunity against the cancer that is being treated. Another strategy is to create medications that can encourage the p53 mutation to break down, perhaps reducing the oncogenic consequences of the altered protein called promoting degradation. Blocking gain-of-function-associated interactors or pathways entails concentrating on the proteins or pathways that a mutant p53 activates, as these can aid in the initiation and spread of cancer. The goal of immunotherapies is to strengthen the immune system's defense against cancer cells that carry p53 mutations. This can entail focusing on the tumor microenvironment to encourage the body to fight cancer through immunological response [76].

The idea of synthetic lethality states that although it is fine to disrupt one gene on its own, doing so completely disrupts both genes and causes cell death. This technique entails locating genes that interact with synthetically lethal mutant p53 in a way that permits targeted therapy without endangering healthy cells [42]. Using CRISPR-Cas9 technology for gene editing, a therapeutic strategy to fix mutated p53 genes in cancer cells has been investigated [41].

In conclusion, missense point mutations in the DNA-binding domain of the p53 gene, in particular, are linked to more aggressive types of illness and decreased overall survival rates. As a potential treatment approach, targeting these mutations shows promise, particularly in triple-negative breast cancer where p53 mutations are common. The goal of several strategies, including gene therapy, immunotherapy, and small molecule inhibitors, is to either cause synthetic lethality in cancer cells that possess mutant p53 or restore the tumor-suppressive effects of p53. Small chemical inhibitors have the potential to restore p53 activity and stop tumor growth. In particular, those that target the MDM2–p53 interaction show promise. It has been shown that gene therapy methods such as APR-246 and COTI-2 can reactivate mutant p53 and cause cancer cells to die. Furthermore, immunotherapy directed against mutant p53 seeks to activate the immune system to recognize and eliminate breast cancer cells that harbor mutant p53 proteins. There is promise for better outcomes in breast cancer therapy due to continuing research targeting mutant p53, despite obstacles such as treatment resistance and the heterogeneous nature of p53 mutations.

REFERENCES

1. Haq, B.U., et al., Targeting p53 misfolding conundrum by stabilizing agents and their analogs in breast cancer therapy: a comprehensive computational analysis. *Frontiers in Pharmacology*, 2024. **14**: p. 1333447.
2. Gasco, M., S. Shami, and T. Crook, The p53 pathway in breast cancer. *Breast Cancer Research*, 2002. **4**(2): p. 70–76.
3. Sofi, S., et al., Clinicopathological and prognostic significance of Bcl2 in breast cancer: a comprehensive in silico and in vitro study. *Saudi Journal of Biological Sciences*, 2023. **31**(2): p. 103916.
4. Sjögren, S., et al., The p53 gene in breast cancer: prognostic value of complementary DNA sequencing versus immunohistochemistry. *JNCI: Journal of the National Cancer Institute*, 1996. **88**(3–4): p. 173–182.
5. Mir, M.A., et al., Proteomics: A Groundbreaking Development in Cancer Biology, in *Proteomics*. 2023, Elsevier. p. 31–53.
6. Berke, T.P., S.H. Slight, and S.M. Hyder, Role of reactivating mutant p53 protein in suppressing growth and metastasis of triple-negative breast cancer. *OncoTargets and Therapy*, 2022: p. 23–30.
7. Mitri, Z.I., et al., Impact of TP53 mutations in triple negative breast cancer. *NPJ Precision Oncology*, 2022. **6**(1): p. 64.
8. Jan, N., et al., Metronomic chemotherapy and drug repurposing: a paradigm shift in oncology. *Heliyon*, 2024. https://doi.org/10.1016/j.heliyon.2024.e24670
9. Jan, N., et al., Exploring the role of trifarotene against RAR-α: an investigation of expression pattern and clinicopathological significance of RAR-α in breast cancer. *Frontiers in Pharmacology*, 2024. **15**: p. 1361679.
10. Chen, X., et al., Mutant p53 in cancer: from molecular mechanism to therapeutic modulation. *Cell Death & Disease*, 2022. **13**(11): p. 974.
11. Sofi, S., et al., Elucidation of interleukin-19 as a therapeutic target for breast cancer by computational analysis and experimental validation. *Saudi Journal of Biological Sciences*, 2023. **30**(9): p. 103774–103774.
12. Hientz, K., et al., The role of p53 in cancer drug resistance and targeted chemotherapy. *Oncotarget*, 2017. **8**(5): p. 8921–8946.
13. Sofi, S., et al., A comprehensive analysis of notch signaling genes in breast cancer: expression pattern and prognostic significance. *Advances in Cancer Biology-Metastasis*, 2023. **7**: p. 100104.
14. Schlotter, C.M., et al., Molecular targeted therapies for breast cancer treatment. *Breast Cancer Research*, 2008. **10**(4): p. 211.
15. Mir, M.A., M. Bashir, and N. Jan, The Role of Interleukin (IL)-6/IL-6 Receptor Axis in Cancer, in *Cytokine and Chemokine Networks in Cancer*. 2023, Springer. p. 137–164.
16. Munagala, R., F. Aqil, and R.C. Gupta, Promising molecular targeted therapies in breast cancer. *Indian J Pharmacol*, 2011. **43**(3): p. 236–245.
17. Mir, M.A., Sumaya, N. Jan, Implications of Chemokine Heterogenicity in Cancer Metastasis, in *Cytokine and Chemokine Networks in Cancer*. 2023, Springer. p. 115–136.
18. Ke, X. and L. Shen, Molecular targeted therapy of cancer: The progress and future prospect. *Frontiers in Laboratory Medicine*, 2017. **1**(2): p. 69–75.
19. Mir, M.A., M. Rashid, and N. Jan, Cytokines and Chemokines in Tumor Growth and Progression, in *Cytokine and Chemokine Networks in Cancer*. 2023, Springer. p. 33–77.
20. Duffy, M.J., et al., Targeting mutant p53 for cancer treatment: moving closer to clinical use? *Cancers*, 2022. **14**(18): p. 4499.
21. Mir, M.A., A. Manzoor, and N. Jan, CCL5/CCR5 Axis in Cancer, in *Cytokine and Chemokine Networks in Cancer*. 2023, Springer. p. 219–240.
22. Zingoni, A., et al., The senescence journey in cancer immunoediting. *Molecular Cancer*, 2024. **23**(1): p. 68.

23. Shreeya, T., et al., Senescence: A DNA damage response and its role in aging and Neurodegenerative Diseases. *Frontiers in Aging*, 2024. **4**: p. 1292053.
24. Chandrakar, L., R. Ambatwar, and G.L. Khatik, Cellulur senescence and senolytic agents: recent updates on their role and applications. *Current Topics in Medicinal Chemistry*, 2024. **24**(2): p. 157–178.
25. Shi, T. and T.B. Dansen, Reactive oxygen species induced p53 activation: DNA damage, redox signaling, or both? *Antioxidants & Redox Signaling*, 2020. **33**(12): p. 839–859.
26. Stead, E.R. and I. Bjedov, Balancing DNA repair to prevent ageing and cancer. *Experimental Cell Research*, 2021. **405**(2): p. 112679.
27. Patil, M.R. and A. Bihari, A comprehensive study of p53 protein. *Journal of Cellular Biochemistry*, 2022. **123**(12): p. 1891–1937.
28. Capuozzo, M., et al., p53: from fundamental biology to clinical applications in cancer. *Biology*, 2022. **11**(9): p. 1325.
29. Rather, R.A., M. Bhagat, and S.K. Singh, Oncogenic BRAF, endoplasmic reticulum stress, and autophagy: Crosstalk and therapeutic targets in cutaneous melanoma. *Mutation Research/Reviews in Mutation Research*, 2020. **785**: p. 108321.
30. Ceder, S., *Mechanisms of Cancer Cell Death by Mutant p53-Reactivating Compound APR-246*. 2021, Karolinska Institutet (Sweden).
31. Wu, Q. and D. Sharma, Autophagy and breast cancer: connected in growth, progression, and therapy. *Cells*, 2023. **12**(8): p. 1156.
32. Gerada, C. and K.M. Ryan, Autophagy, the innate immune response and cancer. *Molecular Oncology*, 2020. **14**(9): p. 1913–1929.
33. Malumbres, M., Control of the Cell Cycle, in *Abeloff's Clinical Oncology*. 2020, Elsevier. p. 56–73.e5.
34. Voskarides, K. and N. Giannopoulou, The role of TP53 in adaptation and evolution. *Cells*, 2023. **12**(3): p. 512.
35. Martínez-Reyes, I. and N.S. Chandel, Cancer metabolism: looking forward. *Nature Reviews Cancer*, 2021. **21**(10): p. 669–680.
36. Zhang, J., S. Zou, and L. Fang, Metabolic reprogramming in colorectal cancer: regulatory networks and therapy. *Cell & Bioscience*, 2023. **13**(1): p. 25.
37. Hernández Borrero, L.J. and W.S. El-Deiry, Tumor suppressor p53: Biology, signaling pathways, and therapeutic targeting. *Biochimica et Biophysica Acta - Reviews on Cancer*, 2021. **1876**(1): p. 188556.
38. Capuozzo, M., et al., p53: from fundamental biology to clinical applications in cancer. *Biology*, 2022. **11**(9): p. 1325.
39. Zhang, C., et al., Gain-of-function mutant p53 in cancer progression and therapy. *Journal of Molecular Cell Biology*, 2020. **12**(9): p. 674–687.
40. Marei, H.E., et al., p53 signaling in cancer progression and therapy. *Cancer Cell International*, 2021. **21**(1): p. 703.
41. Wang, H., et al., Targeting p53 pathways: mechanisms, structures, and advances in therapy. *Signal Transduction and Targeted Therapy*, 2023. **8**(1): p. 92.
42. Hu, J., et al., Targeting mutant p53 for cancer therapy: direct and indirect strategies. *Journal of Hematology & Oncology*, 2021. **14**(1): p. 157.
43. Hassin, O. and M. Oren, Drugging p53 in cancer: one protein, many targets. *Nature Reviews Drug Discovery*, 2023. **22**(2): p. 127–144.
44. Wang, J., et al., Targeting mutant p53 stabilization for cancer therapy. *Frontiers in Pharmacology*, 2023. **14**: p. 1215995.
45. Dolma, L. and P.A.J. Muller, GOF mutant p53 in cancers: a therapeutic challenge. *Cancers (Basel)*, 2022. **14**(20). https://doi.org/10.3390/cancers14205091
46. El-Deiry, W.S., Targeting mutated p53: naivete and enthusiasm to attempt the impossible. *Cancer Research*, 2023. **83**(7): p. 979–982.
47. Zhang, S., et al., Advanced strategies for therapeutic targeting of wild-type and mutant p53 in cancer. *Biomolecules*, 2022. **12**(4). https://doi.org/10.3390/biom12040548
48. Fallatah, M.M., et al., Small-molecule correctors and stabilizers to target p53. *Trends in Pharmacological Sciences*, 2023. https://doi.org/10.1016/j.tips.2023.02.007
49. Fallatah, M.M.J., et al., Small-molecule correctors and stabilizers to target p53. *Trends in Pharmacological Sciences*, 2023. **44**(5): p. 274–289.
50. Yu, X., et al., Small molecule compounds targeting the p53 pathway: are we finally making progress? *Apoptosis*, 2014. **19**(7): p. 1055–1068.
51. Vassilev, L.T., p53 Activation by small molecules: application in oncology. *Journal of Medicinal Chemistry*, 2005. **48**(14): p. 4491–4499.

52. Kogan, S. and D. Carpizo, Pharmacological targeting of mutant p53. *Translational Cancer Research*, 2016. **5**(6): p. 698–706.
53. Aguilar, A. and S. Wang, Therapeutic strategies to activate p53. *Pharmaceuticals*, 2022. **16**(1): p. 24.
54. Chasov, V., et al., Key players in the mutant p53 team: Small molecules, gene editing, immunotherapy. *Frontiers in Oncology*, 2020. **10**: p. 1460.
55. Lopes, E.A., et al., Small molecules targeting mutant p53: a promising approach for cancer treatment. *Current Medicinal Chemistry*, 2019. **26**(41): p. 7323–7336.
56. Duffy, M.J., N.C. Synnott, and J. Crown, Mutant p53 in breast cancer: potential as a therapeutic target and biomarker. *Breast Cancer Research and Treatment*, 2018. **170**(2): p. 213–219.
57. Lima, Z.S., et al., Recent advances of therapeutic targets based on the molecular signature in breast cancer: genetic mutations and implications for current treatment paradigms. *Journal of Hematology & Oncology*, 2019. **12**(1): p. 38.
58. Perdrix, A., et al., PRIMA-1 and PRIMA-1Met (APR-246): from mutant/wild type p53 reactivation to unexpected mechanisms underlying their potent anti-tumor effect in combinatorial therapies. *Cancers*, 2017. **9**(12): p. 172.
59. Synnott, N.C., et al., PRIMA-1MET (APR-246): A novel targeted therapy for triple negative breast cancer? *Journal of Clinical Oncology*, 2015. **33**(15_suppl): p. e12072–e12072.
60. Liang, Y., C. Besch-Williford, and S.M. Hyder, PRIMA-1 inhibits growth of breast cancer cells by re-activating mutant p53 protein. *International Journal of Oncology*, 2009. **35**(5): p. 1015–1023.
61. Liang, Y., et al., A combination of p53-activating APR-246 and phosphatidylserine-targeting antibody potently inhibits tumor development in hormone-dependent mutant p53-expressing breast cancer xenografts. *Breast Cancer: Targets and Therapy*, 2018: p. 53–67.
62. Duffy, M.J., et al., Targeting p53 for the treatment of cancer. *Seminars in Cancer Biology*, 2022. **79**: p. 58–67.
63. Mir, M.A., et al., Proteomics: Application of Next-Generation Proteomics in Cancer Research, in *Proteomics*. 2023, Elsevier. p. 55–76.
64. Synnott, N.C., et al., The mutant p53-targeting compound APR-246 induces ROS-modulating genes in breast cancer cells. *Translational Oncology*, 2018. **11**(6): p. 1343–1349.
65. Lehmann, S., et al., Targeting p53 in vivo: a first-in-human study with p53-targeting compound APR-246 in refractory hematologic malignancies and prostate cancer. *Journal of Clinical Oncology*, 2012. **30**(29): p. 3633–3639.
66. McCubrey, J.A., et al., APR-246-the mutant TP53 reactivator-increases the effectiveness of berberine and modified berberines to inhibit the proliferation of pancreatic cancer cells. *Biomolecules*, 2022. **12**(2). https://doi.org/10.3390/biom12020276
67. Tyagi, A., et al., Nicotine promotes breast cancer metastasis by stimulating N2 neutrophils and generating pre-metastatic niche in lung. *Nature Communications*, 2021. **12**(1): p. 474.
68. Murayama, M.A., et al., Nicotine treatment regulates PD-L1 and PD-L2 expression via inhibition of Akt pathway in HER2-type breast cancer cells. *PLoS One*, 2022. **17**(1): p. e0260838.
69. Synnott, N., et al., COTI-2 reactivates mutant p53 and inhibits growth of triple-negative breast cancer cells. *Breast Cancer Research and Treatment*, 2020. **179**. https://doi.org/10.1007/s10549-019-05435-1
70. Zhang, S., et al., Advanced strategies for therapeutic targeting of wild-type and mutant p53 in cancer. *Biomolecules*, 2022. **12**(4): p. 548.
71. Zhu, G., et al., Mutant p53 in cancer progression and targeted therapies. *Frontiers in Oncology*, 2020. **10**: p. 595187.
72. Sobhani, N., et al., Mutant p53 as an antigen in cancer immunotherapy. *International Journal of Molecular Sciences*, 2020. **21**(11): p. 4087.
73. Liu, Z., et al., TP53 mutations promote immunogenic activity in breast cancer. *Journal of Clinical Oncology*, 2019. **2019**: p. 5952836.
74. Carlsen, L., et al., The role of p53 in anti-tumor immunity and response to immunotherapy. *Frontiers in Molecular Biosciences*, 2023. **10**. https://doi.org/10.3389/fmolb.2023.1148389
75. Zhu, G., et al., Mutant p53 in cancer progression and targeted therapies. *Front Oncol*, 2020. **10**: p. 595187.
76. Duffy, M.J., et al., Targeting mutant p53 for cancer treatment: moving closer to clinical use? *Cancers*, 2022. **14**(18): p. 4499.

13 The Role of the Mevalonate Pathway in Cancer Progression with Mutant p53

*Janifar Yasin, Nusrat Jan, Mehvish Feroz, and Manzoor Ahmad Mir**

Department of Bioresources, School of Biological Sciences, University of Kashmir, Srinagar, J&K, India

*drmanzoor@kashmiruniversity.ac.in

13.1 INTRODUCTION

Uncontrolled cell growth and proliferation are characteristic features of the complex condition referred to as cancer. A primary factor contributing to the initiation and advancement of cancer constitutes the mutation associated with tumor suppression genes, including TP53. Altered p53 no longer can suppress cancers. However, it can also develop oncogenic characteristics, which can lead to changes in metabolic pathways and other elements of cancer biology. One such metabolic system that has been linked to cancer is the mevalonic acid pathway, particularly when p53 is mutated. A vital metabolic route found in the majority of eukaryotic cells is the mevalonate pathway, accountable for the biosynthesis of numerous essential biomolecules, including the production of cholesterol, steroid hormones, bile acids, and isoprene-derived compounds [1]. Isoprene-derived compounds serve as precursors for a diverse range of molecules engaged in various biological processes, including the formation of cell membranes, the attachment of prenyl groups to proteins, and signaling molecule synthesis. Mutant p53 proteins have the potential to actively contribute to the development of cancer, as p53 is a frequently targeted mutation in human malignancies. A study conducted utilized a three-dimensional growing setup wherein cells related to breast cancer also have a highly disordered appearance, while breast epithelial cells that are not cancerous mature into spheroids that mimic in vivo acinar structures. It has been noted that depleting mutant p53 is the only way to induce phenotypic alterations in breast cancer cells to resemble alveolar cells. The mutant p53 significantly increased the mevalonic acid pathway, according to a genome-wide expression investigation. Statins and intermediates in the production of sterols have demonstrated that this pathway is deemed essential and satisfactory for the phenotypic impacts of mutant p53 on breast tissue structure. The connection between mutant p53 and sterol gene promoters is mediated, at least in part, by sterol regulatory element-binding protein (SREBP) transcription factors [2, 3]. Mutations in the tumor suppressor gene p53 are responsible for over 50% of all human malignancies, making them the most prevalent genetic abnormalities in tumors [4]. Missense mutations constitute the majority of p53 genetic alterations, which cause tumors to accumulate dysfunctional p53 protein. Often exhibiting oncogenic gain-of-function activities, these mutations intensify the malignant characteristics of cancer cells, including drug resistance and metastasis. There is growing evidence that p53 mutation stability affects the cancer-causing activities of the protein in tumors, and that p53 depletion reduces the malignant properties of cancer cells. Thus, a preferable pharmacological target for cancer treatment is mutant p53. Various strategies have been employed to create

 DOI: 10.1201/9781003520771-13

small-molecule drugs that selectively target p53 mutants. Among these are substances that reinstate transcriptional activity and wild-type conformation [5]. The study provides further evidence suggesting that mutated p53 proteins, traditionally associated with tumor suppression, can acquire new functions akin to oncogenes. Specifically, it proposes that certain mutations in the p53 gene enable the resulting proteins to hinder the MRN–ATM signaling pathway. This discovery clarifies the intricate functions that p53 mutations play in the initiation and spread of cancer [6, 7]. The mevalonic acid pathway is crucial for creating compounds derived from the isoprene unit and is essential for various cellular functions from cholesterol production to regulating disease progression. Feedback mechanisms regulate two important enzymes and receptors for low-density lipoproteins in this pathway, ensuring adequate mevalonic acid production for various end-products. Modifying this regulatory system could be beneficial in targeting particular cancer types and the heart [8–10].

13.2 OVERVIEW OF THE KEY STEPS IN THE MEVALONIC ACID PATHWAY

(i) **Acetyl-CoA conversion**: Acetyl-CoA acetyltransferase, commonly known as thiolase, facilitates the merging of two acetyl-CoA molecules to produce acetoacetyl-CoA, initiating the pathway.

(ii) **Generation of HMG-CoA**: Next, acetoacetyl-CoA reacts with another molecule of acetyl-CoA via the enzyme HMG-CoA synthase, resulting in the formation of 3-hydroxy-3-methylglutaryl-CoA (HMG-CoA).

(iii) **Mevalonate phosphorylation**: Mevalonate kinase catalyzes the phosphorylation of mevalonate, leading to the formation of 5-phosphomevalonate, a process that requires ATP.

(iv) **Formation of isopentenyl pyrophosphate (IPP)**: The generation of isopentenyl pyrophosphate (IPP) and dimethylallyl pyrophosphate (DMAPP), essential for the formation of building blocks for synthesizing isoprenoid compounds, occurs after the decarboxylation of 5-phosphomevalonate as shown in Figure 13.1.

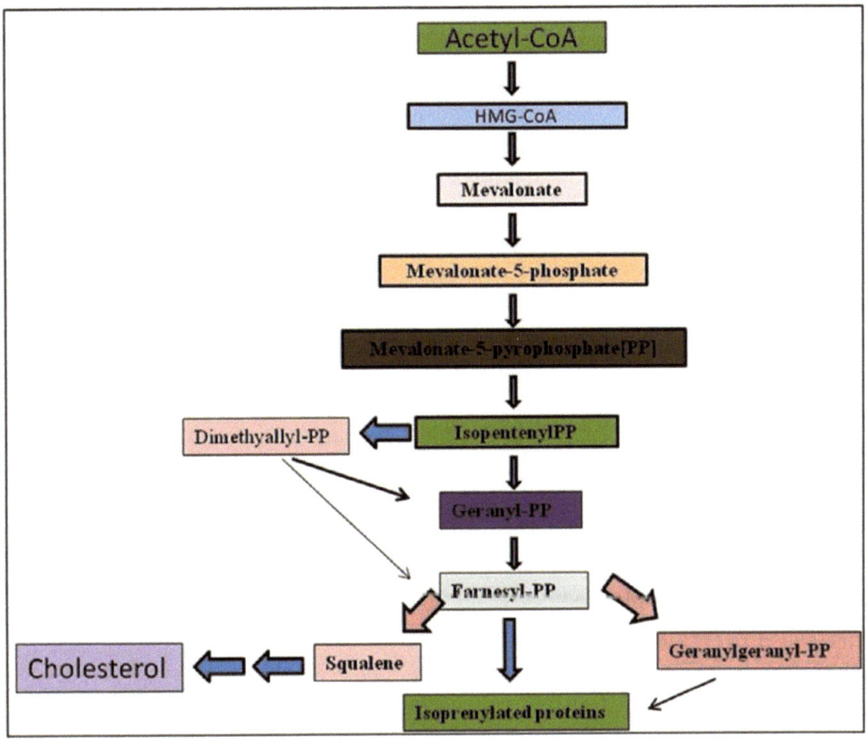

FIGURE 13.1 Mevalonic acid pathway.

(v) **Isoprenoid synthesis**: Several isoprenoids, such as farnesyl pyrophosphate (FPP), geranylgeranyl pyrophosphate (GGPP), and geranyl pyrophosphate (GPP), are produced utilizing IPP and DMAPP as starting materials. The modification of proteins after translation (prenylation), which is crucial for various cellular processes including cell signaling, membrane trafficking, and cytoskeletal organization, relies on these isoprenoid compounds (Figure 13.1).

(vi) **Cholesterol synthesis**: Mevalonic acid is also a precursor to the production of cholesterol, crucial for cell membrane integrity, and serves as a precursor for bile acids and steroid hormones. Several enzymatic steps are involved in cholesterol biosynthesis, including the conversion of mevalonic acid to squalene, which undergoes cyclization and modification to form lanosterol, the first cyclic transitional stage in cholesterol synthesis. Overall, the mevalonic acid pathway is indispensable for the production of essential biomolecules required for cellular structure, signaling, and metabolism. This pathway's imbalance has been associated with various human conditions, including cancer, heart disease, and metabolic disorders, making it an important target for therapeutic intervention. Previously, it was believed that the main therapeutic effect was the lowering of blood levels of low-density lipoprotein (LDL) cholesterol, which led to the first rationale for treating cardiovascular disease [1, 11]. Nonetheless, it is becoming clearer that statins' advantageous effects in cardiovascular medicine are not only due to their ability to decrease cholesterol [12] [13]. Thus, it became clear that statins alter the immune response at the same time that it was discovered that coronary disease has a significant inflammatory component [14–16] as shown in (Figure 13.1).

Tumor hypoxia and the activation of the progression are linked with hypoxia-inducible factor 1 (HIF-1) of cancer. Here, we show that non-transcriptional suppression of HIF-1 function by the transcription factor TAp73 affects tumor angiogenesis. Larger vascularization in both spontaneously occurring and chemically induced tumors is more common in mice missing TAp73. TAp73's mechanistic interaction with the HIF-1 regulatory subunit (α) brings the mouse double minute 2 homolog into the protein complex. This promotes the polyubiquitination of HIF-1α leading to the subsequent, oxygen-independent degradation of the protein by the proteasome. The expression of TAp73 is linked to reduced HIF-1 activation and angiogenesis, and it is a robust predictor of a favorable patient prognosis in human lung cancer datasets. Our results, which have important implications for personalized treatment, reveal a mechanism for regulating HIF-1 that is not dependent on oxygen levels based on in vivo and clinical evidence [3, 9, 17]. There is increasing awareness that the metabolic profile of cells within tumors differs from that of their normal counterparts and is heterogeneous. The breakdown of glucose, lactate, pyruvate, hydroxybutyrate, acetate, glutamine, and fatty acids in metabolism is generally significantly higher in tumor cells compared to non-tumor cells. Yet, the metabolic dynamics of tumors are intricate due to the presence of numerous metabolic compartments connected through the exchange of these breakdown products. Tumor cells' flexibility along with variable metabolism allows them to generate ATP as a source of energy, which also allows for the viability, proliferation, and expansion of the cells, i.e., for them to allocate resources to biosynthesis that also maintains the redox equilibrium. Crucially, based on experimental evidence, it appears that cell populations with different but complementary metabolic properties might metabolically couple to promote the formation of cancer. Thus, concentrating on the metabolic variations between cancer and healthy cells has potential as a novel anticancer tactic [18–21].

13.3 THERAPEUTIC IMPLICATIONS

One possible therapeutic approach in tumors with p53 mutations is to target the mevalonic acid pathway. Researchers have looked into inhibitors of HMG-CoA reductase, such as statins for their ability to inhibit tumor proliferation and enhance cancer cell sensitivity to chemotherapy. Additionally, inhibitors of downstream targets in the mevalonate pathway, such as farnesyltransferase inhibitors (FTIs) and geranylgeranyltransferase I (GGTI) inhibitors, have shown promise in preclinical studies and clinical trials [18, 22].

13.4 MEVALONIC ACID PATHWAY AND CANCER

The extremely conserved mevalonate system provides the enzymatic building blocks needed to produce essential cellular components such as cholesterol and prenyl pyrophosphates, which act as substrates for the post-translational prenylation of various proteins. Proteins with attached prenyl groups of the Ras superfamily are thought to represent a prominent target in the treatment of cancer because they are essential in controlling the proliferation, viability, invasion, and spread of cancerous cells. The route is also thought to be overactive in cancer cells. Cells of the immune system and cancer cells respond differently to amino-containing bisphosphonates, for example, in terms of the buildup of intermediates earlier in the mevalonic acid pathway and the decrease of intermediates farther down the pathway. Therefore, by encouraging cancer immune surveillance, mevalonic acid pathway modification can influence tumor biology, whether through direct or indirect means [23, 24]. The mevalonic acid pathway for the attachment of prenyl groups to proteins and cholesterol synthesis is connected to multiple facets of tumor growth and progression. Some medication groups, such as bisphosphonates and statins, have also been investigated as anticancer agents because they block the metabolism of mevalonic acid. The finding that p53 mutations, which account for more than half of human cancer cases, could significantly increase protein prenylation and mevalonic metabolism in carcinoma cells provides compelling evidence for this hypothesis. Mevalonic acid pathway inhibitors have already shown the first indication that they could be able to change the cancerous phenotype. Furthermore, statins and bisphosphonates recently identified immunomodulatory qualities may be a factor in their established anti-tumor advantages. The suppression of protein prenylation by drugs can result in a series of different cellular stress reactions, such as the unfolded protein response and autophagy, leading to the eventual initiation of innate immunity that is both caspase 1 and inflammasome-dependent [25, 26]. It is well recognized that higher concentrations and the effectiveness of 3-hydroxy-3-methylglutaryl-CoA reductase result in elevated rates of mevalonic acid synthesis in cancerous cells. It is unknown if mevalonic acid stimulates the growth of tumor cells or if this increased synthesis of mevalonic acid results from a higher demand for a metabolite generated from mevalonic acid in response to rapid growth. To explore this topic, the MDA-MB-435 human cancer cells were injected and transformed into nude mice via micro-osmotic pumps, which then administered mevalonic acid in the mice. Following 13 weeks of growth, tumors within mice treated with mevalonic acid showed a notable increase in size compared to those in animals administered with saline (1.52 ± 0.26 grams compared to 0.81 ± 0.27 grams, respectively, with a significance level of less than 0.05). Higher rates of proliferation were also observed in the mevalonic acid-exposed cancer cells in culture, which were associated with a quicker cell progression into the S phase. These cells increased the triggering phosphorylation of CDK-2, reduced the inhibitory interaction between CDK-2 and p21Cip1, and increased the overall activity of CDK-dependent kinase-2 (CDK-2), both in total and in its cyclin A-bound form [27]. Moreover, the prognosis is poorer for breast cancer patients whose mevalonate pathway-associated protein expression is higher [28, 29]. The increased expression of HMGCoAR in the human hepatocellular carcinoma cell line HepG2 and the non-tumorigenic breast epithelial cell line MCF10A stimulates the formation of HepG2 tumors in xenograft models and their anchorage-independent cell proliferation as shown in Figure 13.2.

13.5 FUNCTIONS OF MUTANT p53 IN HUMAN CANCER

Mutations in the TP53 (p53) gene occur in a considerable proportion of human malignancies, and these tumors often exhibit high but diverse levels of mutant p53 proteins. The therapeutic significance of this level of proteins is still unclear. Mutant p53 proteins have been demonstrated

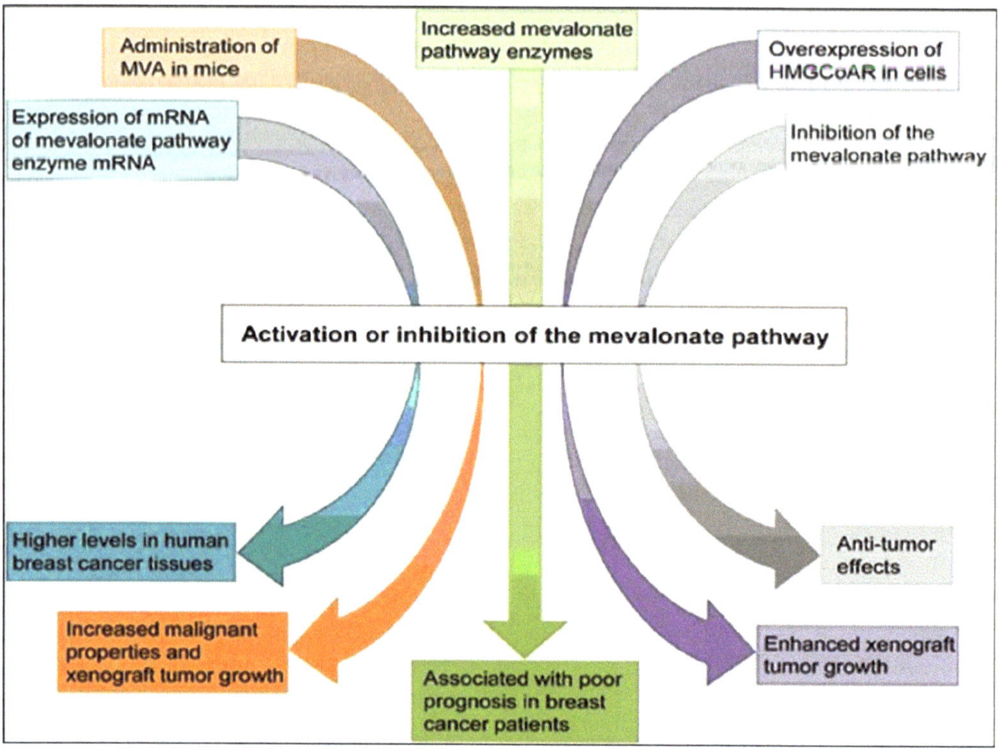

FIGURE 13.2 The consequences of activating or inhibiting the mevalonate pathway. Activation, shown by increased enzyme expression and administration of mevalonate (MVA) in mice, leads to higher levels in human breast cancer tissues, increased malignancy, and poor prognosis. Inhibition, via HMG-CoAR suppression, results in anti-tumor effects and reduced xenograft tumor growth.

to promote tumor initiation, aggression, and metastatic spread in mouse models with p53 knock-in mutations by inhibiting wild-type p53 through a dominant negative mechanism and gaining function or "neomorphic" actions that can suppress or enhance the activity of other proteins. Moreover, these models illustrate that stability is not solely conferred by mutation alone. Thus, the diverse staining patterns of mutant proteins seen in human malignancies suggest the activation of tumor-specific mechanisms that stabilize p53. Thus, inhibiting the production and function of mutant p53 proteins might offer new avenues for oncological treatment and diagnosis. Yet, the activation of these proteins by chemotherapy may paradoxically reduce the efficacy of these interventions [30].

13.6 THE ROLE OF STATINS IN REDUCING THE RISK OF CANCER AND THEIR APPLICATION IN CANCER TREATMENT

Statins, initially formulated as medications to lower lipid levels in individuals with hypercholesterolemia, inhibit HMG-CoA reductase, the enzyme responsible for the initial step in the mevalonic acid pathway [31]. Statins not only halt cholesterol synthesis but also inhibit the prenylation branch of proteins. Statins inhibit HMG-CoA reductase, resulting in a downstream reduction of farnesyl phosphate (FPP) and geranylgeranyl phosphate (GGPP). This keeps the cell from completing post-translational protein prenylation. Statins have been suggested as a potential cancer treatment due to their capacity to inhibit HMG-CoA reductase, which selectively and sensitively promotes programmed cell death in various types of tumor cells [31]. Due to their pleiotropic properties, statins may also have an effect on cancer. HMG-CoA reductase serves as the main enzyme regulating the rate at which HMG-CoA undergoes conversion to mevalonic acid; statins competitively inhibit this enzyme. The molecules responsible for attaching lipids to small G proteins like Ras, Rho, and Rac are called non-steroidal isoprenoids, and mevalonic acid is one of their precursors. It has been demonstrated that statins block the activity of HMG-CoA reductase, thus halting the production of mevalonic acid. Consequently, statins may prevent the production of isoprenoids and can decrease the activation of small G proteins. Moreover, statins have immunoregulatory, anti-angiogenic, and pro-apoptotic properties that may stop the spread of cancer. Statins can impede the proliferation of multiple types of cancer cells, including neuroblastoma, melanoma, mesothelioma, gastric, pancreatic, breast carcinoma, and myeloid leukemia. They exhibit inducing apoptosis in various cancer cell lines, even though different cancer cell types are not all equally susceptible to statin-induced cell death. Several effects of statins on the formation of blood vessels have been proposed in relation to their anti-angiogenic properties. These effects include the inhibition of endothelial cell proliferation, suppression by decreasing the activity of pro-angiogenic factors, and inhibition of angiogenesis. Inhibiting vascular endothelial growth factor (VEGF) can prevent cells from adhering to the extracellular matrix by blocking intercellular adhesion molecules. One common route connected to the molecular processes of statin immunomodulation involves controlling the expression of genes that encode immune system components and significant molecules engaged in presenting antigens and thereafter regulating the immune response. A further technique is the reductions in the activity of nuclear factor-kappa-B (NFκ-B), a regulator of numerous genes involved in immunologic pathways, such as cyclooxygenase-2, monocyte chemoattractant protein 1, and interferon-inducible protein-10. Numerous observational studies have associated statins with a significantly decreased incidence of lymphoma, lung, pancreatic, ovarian, breast, and colorectal cancers [32, 33].

13.7 INTERPLAY BETWEEN MUTANT p53 AND MEVALONIC ACID PATHWAY

The manner that the mevalonic acid pathway and mutp53 interact with several biochemical processes, including mutp53 stability, the production of cholesterol, and the process of attaching prenyl or lipid groups to proteins (such as Ras farnesylation or Rho geranylgeranylation), and the mevalonic acid pathway can accelerate the spread of cancer. The interaction between mutp53 and DNAJA1 is facilitated by the metabolic process involving mevalonate-5-phosphate (MVP) in the mevalonic acid pathway. This interaction maintains the stability of mutp53 by inhibiting its degradation via the proteasome and preventing its ubiquitination catalyzed by the CHIP ubiquitin ligase. Research has demonstrated that mutp53 interacts with SREBP2, increasing the levels of mevalonate-5-phosphate (MVP) and the synthesis of enzymes that are part of the mevalonic acid pathway. This creates a self-amplifying cycle by stabilizing mutp53. Therefore, inhibition of the mevalonate pathway with statins, zoledronic acid, or GGTI inhibitors (GGTI-2133, GGTI-298) may represent a novel therapeutic strategy of targeting cancers with mutp53 by inhibiting mutp53 GOF activities, prenylation of oncogenes, and cholesterol synthesis, as well as inducing mutp53 degradation.

The coenzymes HMG-CoA synthase and HMG-CoA reductase are responsible for hydroxylmethylglutaryl coenzyme A synthase and reductase, respectively, and MVK, PMVK, and MVD mevalonate diphosphate decarboxylase, pyrophosphate, GGTI, and FDPS (farnesyl diphosphate synthase). Alterations caused by missense mutations in the TP53 gene cause oncogenic gain-of-function (GOF) activity in tumors with defective TP53 proteins. The GOF requires the stabilizing mutated TP53, or mutp53. However, it is unclear how exactly mutp53 promotes the growth of cancer and how its stability is controlled. Recent research conducted has shown that statins, which are mevalonic acid pathway inhibitors, degrade conformational mutp53. By blocking the interaction between mutant TP53 and DNAJA1, a member of the Hsp40 family, the misfolded TP53 protein undergoes degradation mediated by the CHIP ubiquitin ligase when the metabolic step mevalonate-5-phosphate (MVP) is specifically reduced, either by statins or knockdown of mevalonate kinase (MVK). This implies that the stability of mutant TP53 is reliant on the mevalonate pathway. The connection between mutant TP53 and the mevalonate pathway is strengthened as it has been observed to accelerate cancer development by boosting the mRNA expression of enzymes in the pathway through binding to SREBP2, consequently enhancing the activities of oncogenic proteins associated with the mevalonic acid pathway such as Ras, Rho, and YAP/TAZ (Figure 13.3).

13.8 RHO ACTIVITY REGULATION VIA mutp53 AND THE MEVALONIC ACID PATHWAY

Cell signal transducers that regulate cellular processes include cytoskeleton regulation, vesicle transportation, cell polarity, and cell cycle progression belong to the Ras homolog family (Rho) of GTPases [21, 34]. Similar to Ras and Rho, to perform their intended functions GTPases need to bind to the cell membrane in a prenylation-dependent way [35]. A subset of the Ras superfamily of GTP hydrolases is the Rho/Rac proteins. Despite being first linked to the regulation of cytoskeletal events, these GTPases are presently recognized to control several biological processes, including the cell cycle, vesicular trafficking, transcriptomic dynamics, and cell polarity [35]. GGPP, which is produced by the mevalonic pathway, is necessary for Rho geranylgeranyl modification [9, 36]. Rho prenylation increases with activation of the mevalonic acid pathway, which in turn accelerates the growth of cancer. Ginestier et al. demonstrate that statins prevent spheroid formation along with a reduction in the stem cell population and demonstrated breast cancer cells grown in non-adherent, serum-free spheroid conditions express more enzymes involved in the mevalonate pathway [37]. Since GGPP supplementation restores the attributes or properties characteristic of stem cells that statins impair, the noted decline in the attributes or characteristics of stem cells caused by statins is dependent on Rho geranylgeranylation rather than cholesterol synthesis or Ras farnesylation. Furthermore, pharmacological blocking of GGTI, an enzyme necessary for geranylgeranylation of Rho, diminishes the stem cell pool within breast cancer cells and suppresses tumor growth and development of a mouse model of xenografts derived from breast cancer patients [37].

Moreover, pancreatic cancer cells that have had their mevalonic acid pathway blocked through the use of statins or zoledronic acid exhibit reduced viable cell proliferation and death, which can be reversed by supplementing with GGPP [38]. Consequently, geranylgeranylation of Rho is essential for the development of cancer. Mutp53 may be crucial for the prenyl attachment and activation of Rho because it increases the enzymes involved in the mevalonic acid pathway. Moreover, Mizuarai et al.'s research [34] shows that p53 mutants (p53V157F, p53R175H, and p53R248Q) may be expressed inducibly in U2OS cells, which dramatically increases RhoA is subsequently activated by the outcome of GEF-H1, a guanine nucleotide exchange factor for RhoA. Furthermore, mutp53 knockdown prevents some malignant cells with decreased GEF-H1 expression from proliferating viable [34]. Additionally, compared to cells expressing wtp53 or null for p53, those expressing mutp53 typically had higher levels of GEF-H1 mRNA expression [34]. Thus, GEF-H1 and the mevalonic acid pathway allow mutp53 to indirectly modulate Rho activity. Cancers that express mutp53 might be treated by targeting the mutp53–RhoA axis.

13.9 MEVALONATE PATHWAY AND mutp53 CONTROL RAS ACTIVITY

Prenylation of proteins is crucial for various biological processes, such as cellular division, migration, and survival [39]. In particular, the mevalonate pathway-regulated farnesylation of Ras GTPase is essential for both tumor development and Ras activation [36, 40]. The establishment of foci formed by primary mouse embryonic fibroblasts (MEFs) is increased by co-overexpressing Ras and HMGCoAR [41], indicating that the modification of normal cells is mediated via the mevalonic acid pathway in conjunction with Ras. Additionally, when HMGCoAR and FDPS, two factors that

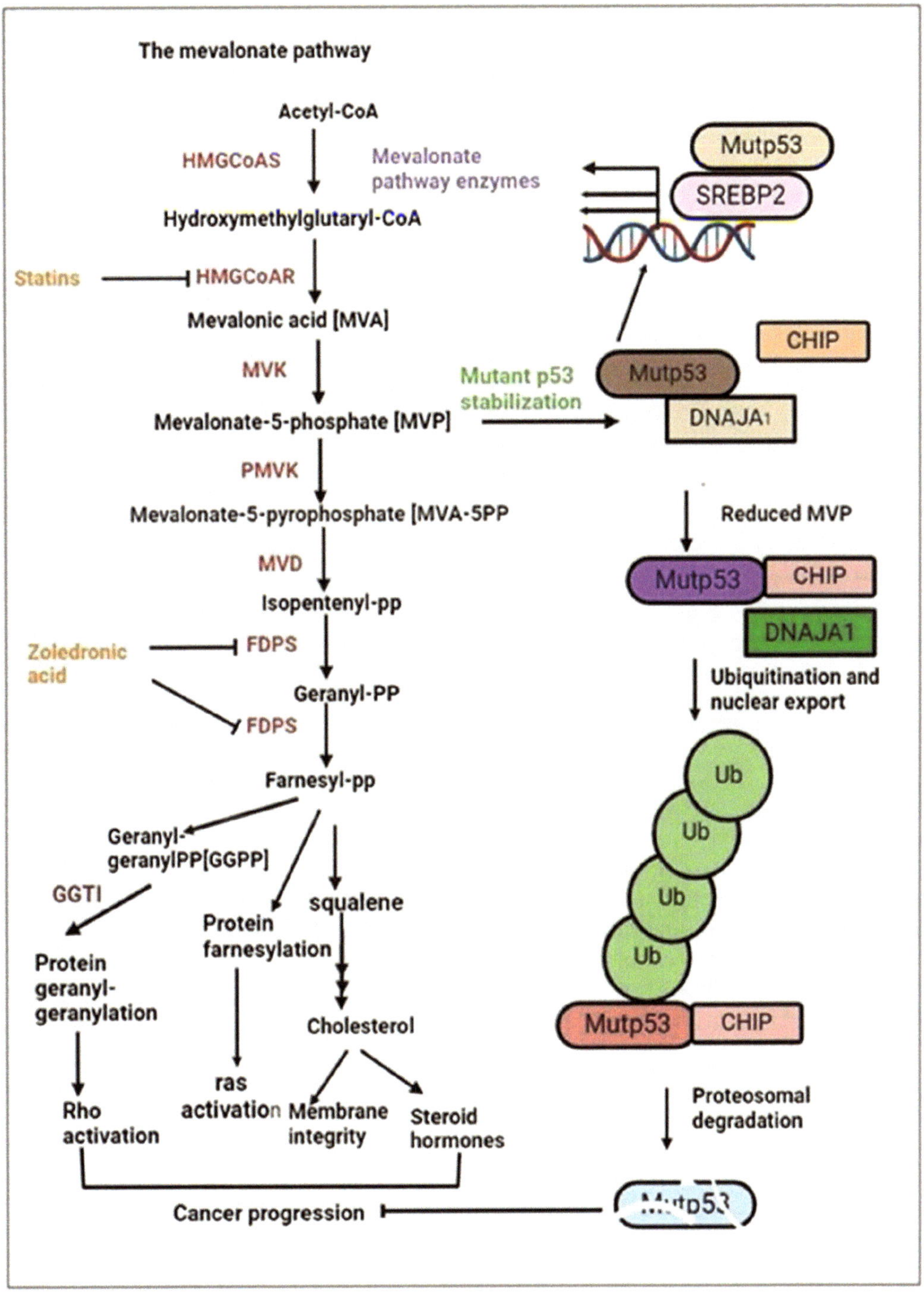

FIGURE 13.3 This figure depicts the mevalonate pathway, showing how statins and zoledronic acid inhibit various steps, reducing mutant p53 (Mutp53) stabilization. Key enzymes and intermediates are outlined, demonstrating their roles in protein prenylation, cholesterol synthesis, and cancer progression. DNAJA1 and CHIP proteins facilitate Mutp53 ubiquitination and degradation.

contribute to the formation of FPP, are blocked, pancreatic and breast cancer cells demonstrate suppressed viable cell proliferation with lower Ras farnesylation [42]. Supplementing with FPP partially alleviates the observed reduction of cell growth [38, 43]. These findings indicate a role for the Ras farnesylation pathway facilitated by the mevalonic acid pathway in the advancement of cancer patients. Accordingly, the discovery that mutp53 increases the activity of the mevalonate pathway by upregulating the manifestation of its enzymes [44] raises the possibility that mutp53, as one of its oncogenic GOF, may indirectly raise Ras activity. Furthermore, it has been demonstrated that conformational p53R175H and p53H179R interact along with the B-cell translocation gene 2 (BTG2), which acts as a suppressor of H-RasV12, to increase oncogenic H-RasV12 activity [45]. Oncogenic Ras activates the Ras–MEK1/2/–ERK1/2 pathway, which is controlled by extracellular signal-regulated kinase 1/2 (ERK1/2) [44]. When membrane tyrosine kinase receptors (RTKs) are activated, it leads to Ras-mediated movement of ERK1/2 into the cell nucleus and triggers the activation of numerous transcription factors implicated in cell proliferation, migration, and cancer advancement [46]. Furthermore, in cancer cells derived from the breast (MDA-MB-231) and lung (H1299), it has been shown that mutp53 (p53R273H) decreases the expression of miR-27a. This leads to an increase in EGFR expression and activates the Ras–ERK1/2 pathway [47]. Additionally, the expression of EGFR, the activity of ERK1/2, cell proliferation, and tumor growth, are all reduced in MDA-MB-231 cells with downregulated mutp53 [47]. All of these findings point to the possibility that mutp53 may raise Ras activity via both independent and dependent pathways on the mevalonic acid pathway.

13.10 MEVALONATE PATHWAY AND mutp53 CONTROL YAP/TAZ ACTIVITY

Two targets of the Hippo signaling pathway, which governs stem cell characteristics, tissue renewal, and organ growth, are the yes-associated protein (YAP) and transcriptional coactivator with PDZ-binding motif (TAZ) [42]. Moreover, it is commonly acknowledged that YAP and TAZ contribute to the proliferation of cancer [48]. A recent high-throughput drug screening investigation employing fluorescence microscopy shows that statins prevent YAP/TAZ from being nuclearly localized in MDA-MB-231 cells [49]. Additionally, in various cancer cell lines, transcription of genes targeted by YAP/TAZ is inhibited by blocking the mevalonate pathway by GGTI-298 (a GGTI inhibitor), zoledronic acid, or statins [49]. Moreover, zoledronic acid and statins suppress the proliferation and multiplication of breast cancer cells into tumors, which is linked to a decrease in YAP/TAZ activity [49]. Accordingly, Wang et al. [50] also show that staining and Rho knockdown decrease YAP activity by lowering the mRNA levels of RHAMM (the receptor for hyaluronan-mediated motility). This, in turn, prevents MDA-MB-231 breast cancer cells from migrating or invading, and phosphorylating ERK1/2. These findings imply that Rho activity and the mevalonic acid pathway control the nuclear localization and activity of YAP/TAZ. Since Rho prevents phosphorylation of YAP via LATS1/2 [51]. Thus, the Rho-YAP/TAZ axis and the mevalonic acid pathway impact the growth and spread of breast cancer. In addition to its indirect impact on YAP/TAZ activation via the Rho axis-mediated mevalonate pathway, to boost the transcription of genes that encourage cell proliferation, mutant p53 can physically interact with YAP in breast cancer cells [52]. The target genes downstream, including cyclin A, cyclin B, and cyclin-dependent kinase 1 (CDK1) genes, require binding to the NF-Y response sites in these genes, and mutp53 mechanistically creates a complex comprising YAP and NF-Y [52]. This increases the transcription of these genes. Mutp53 or YAP knockdown reduces the expression of genes targeted by NF-Y in SK-Br-3 and CAL27 breast cancer cells and stops viable cell growth [52]. In human breast tumors, elevated mutp53 levels are associated with exhibiting elevated YAP activity profiles and heightened expression of YAP target genes, including CDK1, cyclin A, and cyclin B [52].

In cells from glioblastoma and breast cancer, mutp53 has also been demonstrated to enhance YAP/TAZ nuclear translocation and stabilization. The process is aided by the enhanced capability of mutant p53 to recycle EGFR and integrins, leading to increased activity of Akt2-WIP (WASP interacting protein) signaling and promoting the nuclear translocation of YAP/TAZ. In terms of biology, mutp53 overexpression results in astrocyte cells with higher YAP/TAZ activity and stem cell-like characteristics, whereas knockdown of mutp53 or WIP results in the emergence of stem cell markers to express less frequently tumor development, and proliferation in cells derived from glioblastoma and breast cancer that express mutp53 [53]. These results indicate the presence of a unique mutp53 GOF that activates the signaling pathway involving Akt2, WIP, YAP, and TAZ, promotes the process of recycling integrin/EGFR, and confers malignant features similar to stem cells on cancer cells.

13.11 THE mutp53 AXIS–MEVALONATE PATHWAY

The transcription factors called basic helix-loop-helix leucine zipper and SREBPs predominantly regulate the expression of lipogenic enzymes, including those participating in the mevalonic acid pathway. As demonstrated by SREBP2's binding to oncogenic mutp53, more mevalonate pathway enzymes, including FDPS, MVK, and HMGCoAR, are expressed [2]. When statins, a GGTI inhibitor, or other drugs block this pathway, breast cancer cells expressing mutant p53 in three-dimensional (3D) culture regain their disrupted mammary architecture. In 3D culture, the disruption of the mammary architecture in breast cancer cells is also eradicated by mutp53 knockdown [2]. Notably, p53 mutations in human breast cancer tissue and elevated production of enzymes in the mevalonate pathway are linked to a bad prognosis for those associated with breast cancer [2]. These findings imply that oncogenic GOF mutp53 promotes the development of breast cancer based on the mevalonic acid pathway.

13.12 MUTANT p53 DISTURBS BREAST TISSUE THROUGH THE MEVALONATE PATHWAY

Breast cancer is believed to originate from structures formed by mammary epithelial cells termed acini, which combine to create in each acinus of the terminal ductal lobular units; a singular layer of polarized luminal epithelial cells surrounds an empty lumen. Although traditional two-dimensional (2D) cell culture has provided insights into the process of breast carcinogenesis, the in vivo microenvironment experienced by cells differs from the conditions observed in such in vitro culture settings. Conversely, when normal mammary epithelial cells are embedded in an extracellular matrix rich in laminin, they can create 3D formations that resemble acinar structures present in the body. Given that an aspect of breast carcinogenesis involves the disruption of the architecture of mammary tissue, it is easy to discriminate The distinction between normal and tumorigenic tissue is based on morphological characteristics under 3D culture settings. Furthermore, Bissell et al. (2005) discovered that blocking significant oncogenic signaling pathways is all that is needed to induce phenotypic reversion in breast cancer cells cultured in three dimensions. Here, we show that the damage caused by mutant p53 to acinar morphology is both necessary and sufficient when utilizing the mevalonate pathway. Additionally, we identify a possible mechanism through which mutant p53 enhances the expression of genes involved in the mevalonic acid pathway [2].

13.13 MEVALONIC ACID METABOLISM CONTROLS STEM CELLS FROM BASAL BREAST CARCINOMA AND MAY BE A TARGET FOR TREATMENT

An increasing body of research indicates that breast cancers are hierarchical in structure, with cancer stem cells (CSCs), a subset of cancer cells with tumorigenic properties being in charge of sustaining tumor growth. It is critical to characterize the protein networks that control CSC behavior to create innovative therapy approaches that specifically target this cell subpopulation. Using CSCs derived from 13 specific breast cancer cell lines classified as either luminal or basal/mesenchymal subtype, we have attempted to pinpoint certain molecular pathways. The gene expression profiles of corresponding tumorsphere cultures and cancer cells grown under adherent conditions were compared. No particular pathway was identified to be regularly controlled in luminal tumorspheres despite a slight CSC enrichment in tumorspheres derived from luminal cell lines. Conversely, basal/mesenchymal tumorspheres exhibited overexpression of enzymes in the mevalonate metabolic pathway but cognate adherent cells did not exhibit this. The amount of breast CSC declined when inhibitors of hydroxy-3-methylglutaryl CoA reductase were used to block this pathway, regardless of the inhibition of protein farnesylation and cholesterol biosynthesis. Additional adjustment of this metabolic pathway revealed the geranylgeranylation of proteins, or geranylgeranylation, is essential for the survival of breast CSCs. A compound that inhibits the enzyme GGTI decreased the subpopulation of breast cancer stem cells in vitro and primary breast cancer xenografts. We observed that increased P27kip1 nucleus accumulation and the protein Ras homolog family member A (RhoA) inactivation mediates the GGTI action on the CSC subpopulation [37].

In addition to being a major medical challenge, breast cancer represents a significant risk to public health. To create novel therapeutic approaches capable of overcoming resistance to established treatments and metastatic spread, the CSC idea offers an appealing oncogenesis model [54].

13.14 INCREASED ACTIVITY IN MUTANT p53

The mutation of the tumor suppressor gene is the most commonly observed genetic change in human malignancies. The majority of alterations in tp53 are due to missense point mutations, which typically aggregate within the DNA binding domain. An increasing body of evidence indicates that numerous mutations result in altered p53 proteins with altered biological and biochemical characteristics. Mutant p53 is assumed to participate in this gain-of-function activity, which in turn increases tumor aggressiveness. Our goal was to investigate the possibility of using mutant p53 as a target for innovative anticancer therapies. Via three distinct lines of cancer cells that naturally produce altered p53 proteins, the production of the p53 mutant is suppressed via RNA interference and the impact on the molecular mechanisms required for the p53 mutant to become functional. It has been demonstrated that mutant p53 depletion decreases cell proliferation, tumorigenicity both in laboratory settings and in living organisms, and sensitivity to anticancer medications. Our findings improve our knowledge of the processes behind the increased functional activity of mutant p53 in human cancers and demonstrate that p53 mutation lowers the pathogenicity of human cancer cells [55].

13.15 DEGRADATION OF MUTANT p53

When cells are stimulated, the protein that the p53 tumor suppressor gene makes accumulates, which sets off a cascade of events that includes DNA repair, apoptosis, and cell cycle arrest. In its role as a transcriptional regulator, p53 stimulates the expression of multiple target genes that are responsible for mediating the p53 responses [56]. The proline-rich regulatory domain, the central domain for sequence-specific DNA binding (DBD), the N-terminal transactivation domains, and a C-terminal are the structural components of the p53 regulatory region that houses the oligomerization domain and sequences for nuclear import and export as shown in Figure 13.4.

The activity of the oncoprotein murine double minute 2 (Mdm2), a crucial p53 negative regulator, is one of the many mechanisms that keep p53 inactive in normal cells [57]. Under conditions of cellular stress, the short-lived p53 tumor suppressor protein is stabilized. A carcinogenic E3 ligase called Mdm2 is primarily responsible for causing p53 to become tagged with ubiquitin and degrade. Stress signals induce covalent changes in Mdm2 and p53 or alter interactions between proteins, which both result in the stability of p53. The post-ubiquitination activity of Mdm2 helps target p53 tagged with ubiquitin to the proteasome. p53 gets tagged with ubiquitin as it leaves the nucleus and enters the cytoplasm. However, the precise point to which p53 declined is still up for debate. Ubiquitination of p53 is linked to its transport from the nucleus to the cytoplasm. However, there is no conflict over the

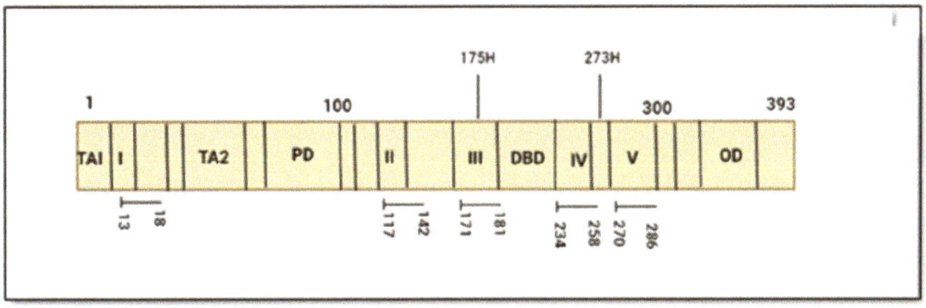

FIGURE 13.4 The figure illustrates the configuration of the p53 protein. The locations of conserved boxes I through V and the accompanying deletions (ΔI to ΔV), as well as the primary domains of p53 and point mutations 175H and 273H, are shown. TA1 and TA2 stand for transactivation domains 1 and 2, OD for oligomerization domain, and PD for proline-rich domain. The numerical positions of amino acids are shown.

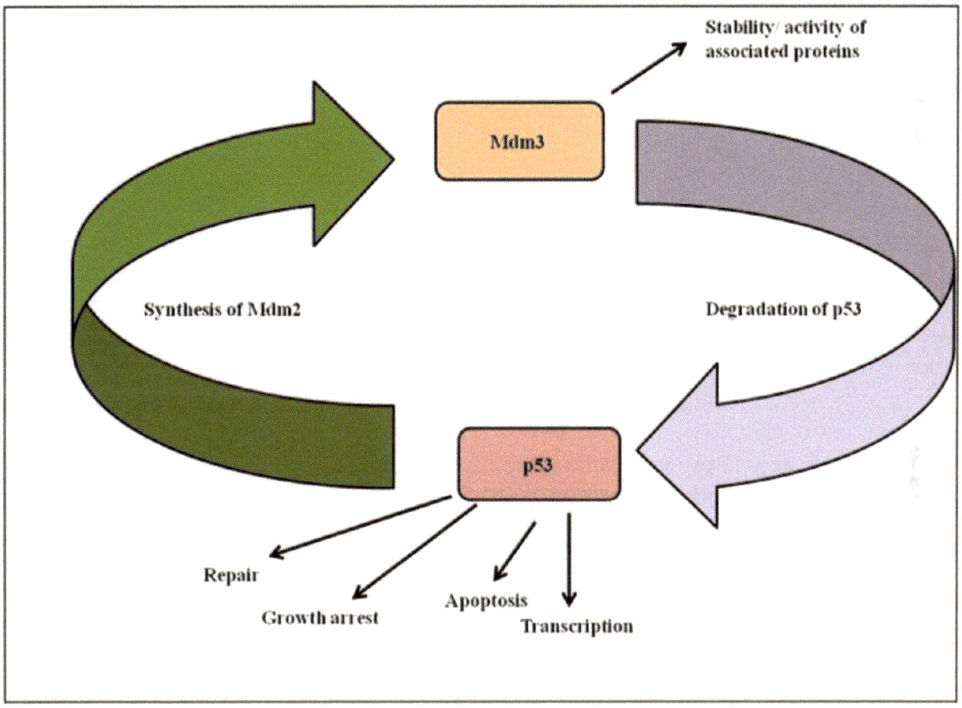

FIGURE 13.5 Major activation implicated for p53 and Mdm2.

precise location of p53 degradation. Other E3 ligases besides Mdm2 and non-proteasomal pathways may also target p53. There is still much to learn about p53 degradation, as evidenced by the abundance of unanswered questions (Figure 13.5) [58].

13.16 DRUGS INFLUENCING THE MEVALONIC ACID PATHWAY

13.16.1 Statins

Originally found in fungi, statins are a class of medications, many of which are now manufactured. Numerous species, including oysters, mushrooms, Aspergillus, and Monascus fungus, naturally contain statins [59]. Currently, lovastatin, simvastatin, pravastatin, fluvastatin, atorvastatin, rosuvastatin, and pitavastatin are the seven medications that make up the statin medicine group [60]. Cerivastatin was taken off the market in 2001 because of a higher risk of myopathy, which includes muscle breakdown syndrome. The original approved use of statins was to treat hypercholesterolemia. However, because of their multifaceted antiatherogenic effects, they are also utilized in preventing further cardiovascular diseases after an initial occurrence. Research is being conducted on their wider applications, which include treating cancer, osteoporosis, and Alzheimer's disease [61]. Statins competitively inhibit HMGR by preventing HMG-CoA from being converted to mevalonate [28]. De novo cholesterol production is disrupted, mostly in the liver, when statins, which are the main drug target for treating and preventing cardiovascular disease, inhibit HMGR. As a result, LDL receptors on the surface of hepatocyte cells and microsomal HMGR synthesis are activated. This subsequently causes circulatory LDL to be absorbed into cells, where it is digested and changed into bile salts, causing the blood's LDL levels to significantly drop. In addition to their main function in reducing cholesterol, it is believed that statins play a significant role in preventing tumor growth and differentiation. However, there is a lot of disagreement among oncologists regarding its application. Statins cause angiogenesis, apoptosis, and cell growth halt. They also prevent metastasis.

13.16.2 Bisphosphonates

Bisphosphonates (BPs) are divided into two classes based on variations in their chemical arrangements and modes of action. The nitrogen-containing compounds in the second group are alendronate, ibandronate, olpadronate, pamidronate, risedronate, and zoledronate. Nitrogen-free compounds in the initial group include etidronate, clodronate, and tiludronate. BP is utilized in skeletal-associated diseases because it causes osteoclasts to undergo apoptosis, which means it can also promote pro-apoptosis. Nitrogenous BP is crucial to the mevalonic acid pathway because it inhibits FPP synthase, an enzyme that is necessary to limit the generation of FPP and GGPP. As FPP synthase is further inhibited, IPP accumulates and changes into the ATP analog ApppI, which is cytotoxic. It causes mitochondrial apoptosis directly, which could have detrimental undesirable effects. As such, these properties of BPs may inhibit the development of tumors or the transformation of malignant cells. The mevalonic acid pathway, which possesses antiproliferative and anticancer characteristics, can be blocked by BPs comprising nitrogen. The addition of prenyl groups to small GTPases inhibits the attachment of tumor cells facilitated by integrin to the bone accumulation of unprenylated Rap1, which in turn inhibits the growth of mesothelioma cells blocking geranylgeranylation leading to the deactivation of Rho proteins, which obstructs cancer cells' ability to migrate [62].

13.16.3 Farnesyltransferase Inhibitors

FTIs are a novel class of signal transduction inhibitors that specifically target the crucial post-translational modification of Ras. Compounds with both actions and those competing with farnesyl pyrophosphate or the CAAX domain in FTs are classified as FTIs. Any of these compounds that are active cause cell growth arrest and block Ras farnesylation. FTIs can function in a way that is independent of Ras because FTIs nonspecifically inhibit farnesylation, which impairs the functioning of numerous distinct cellular proteins [63]. For example, it is doubtful that inhibiting RhoB farnesylation will result in RhoB with reduced prenylation because, as mentioned earlier, RhoB can also undergo geranylgeranylation. Nevertheless, RhoB-GG may have an additional antiproliferative impact, which could increase the effectiveness of FTIs. It has been proposed that FTIs may one day be used to treat cancer. Following numerous others, lonafarnib was the inaugural FTI to undergo clinical trials. The phase III trial demonstrated no notable impact on survival rates in solid tumors. None of the FTIs were able to pass it. Most phase I and II clinical studies were effective in establishing a significant anticancer activity with a tolerable toxicity profile [63]. According to specific studies, when farnesylation is prevented, some Ras proteins can go through alternative geranylgeranylation by GGTI. This has been shown in an animal model dependent on K-Ras, suggesting that farnesylation is not necessary for cancer.

13.17 THE CLINICAL SIGNIFICANCE OF STATINS IN THE ADVANCEMENT OF CANCER

Clinical research showing statins' effectiveness in reducing human cancer is still debatable [64, 65]. In individuals with multiple cancers, such as high-grade malignancies of the uterus [66], colon and rectal cancer [67], renal cancer [67], and plasma cell myeloma [68], there has been a proposal to improve overall survival with statins. The use of statins has also been linked to reduced overall mortality rates among cancer patients, according to statistics [69], and a decreased chance of cancer linked to insulin in diabetic people [70]. Moreover, post-diagnostic statin use is linked to better recurrence-free survival than pre-diagnostic statin use [69]. Nonetheless, certain findings are debatable, such as the following: the usage of the association between statins and the likelihood of breast cancer are unrelated [71], and taking statins raises the likelihood of developing prostate cancer [72]. Therefore, even though multiple clinical studies demonstrate the favorable benefits of the effectiveness of statins in suppressing human cancer or impacting patient prognosis, the efficacy of statins may vary depending on the kind or dosage of statins, the type of cancer, as well as the nature of genetic alterations in tumors. In fact, the in vivo mouse model experiments show tumors containing conformational/misfolded p53 mutants respond more favorably to statins than tumors with wild-type p53, p53 null, and p53 mutants lacking DNA-contact capabilities [73]. Additionally, the research indicates that to limit tumor growth in mice, a larger dose of statins—near the highest amount clinically permitted—is needed [5, 73]. Therefore, the clinical result of the p53 status and statin dosage may have an impact on the tumor suppression properties of statins. To the best of our knowledge, no clinical study has looked at the effects of statins. To our current understanding, no clinical investigation has examined how statin dosage or the p53 status of tumors affects the way that statins reduce tumor growth. Clinical trials have investigated other mevalonic acid pathway inhibitors, with encouraging outcomes. Patients with multiple myeloma have better clinical outcomes while using zoledronic acid [74]. Prostate and metastatic breast cancer, as well as preexisting bone metastases, are the subjects of additional clinical trials involving zoledronic acid [75]. In preclinical models of cancer, GGTI inhibitors and FTIs have also demonstrated encouraging outcomes; yet, their effectiveness in clinical trials does not seem to match expectations [76–78]. It should be observed that the p53 status of the tumors is not taken into account in any of these trials, even though this could be a crucial factor in predicting how well mevalonic acid pathway inhibitors work.

13.18 CONCLUSION

The mevalonic acid pathway, particularly concerning mutant p53, is demonstrated to be significant in cancer progression. A tumor's buildup of defective TP53 proteins, which display carcinogenic gain-of-function characteristics, and mutations in the TP53 gene can lead to this condition. Recent research has shown that statins, which affect the mevalonic acid pathway inhibitors, can degrade mutant p53, which is necessary to stabilize these functions. Through a particular mechanism involving CHIP ubiquitin ligase, statins cause the conformational mutant p53 to be degraded by lowering mevalonate-5-phosphate levels. Disrupting the connection between mutant p53 and DNAJA1 is how this degradation is accomplished. Mutant p53 can speed up the development of cancer by increasing the expression of enzymes in the mevalonate pathway, thereby enhancing the activity of carcinogenic proteins associated with the mevalonate pathway. The mevalonate route is crucial in preserving the stability of mutant p53. The link between mutant p53 and the mevalonate pathway is established through a reinforcing loop of positive feedback emphasizing their shared functions in promoting the spread of cancer. The association between mutant p53 and the mevalonate pathway reveals potential implications for cancer treatment strategies. The importance of targeting the mevalonate pathway in therapeutic interventions is underscored by its involvement in cancer development, especially in the context of p53 mutations. Mutant p53 can disrupt several biological functions, including lipid metabolism, which increases the activity of the mevalonic acid pathway. Because of this dysregulation, there is an increase in the production of subsequent metabolites such as cholesterol and isoprenoids, which support the growth and spread of tumors as well as oncogenic signaling. By concentrating on key enzymes in the mevalonate pathway, cancer may be prevented from spreading, especially when p53 mutations are present. Therefore, understanding the connection between mutant p53 and the mevalonate pathway offers important new insights into potential cancer-fighting therapy approaches.

REFERENCES

1. Mir, M.A., M. Bashir, and N. Jan, The Role of Interleukin (IL)-6/IL-6 Receptor Axis in Cancer, in *Cytokine and Chemokine Networks in Cancer*. 2023, Springer. p. 137–164.
2. Freed-Pastor, W.A., et al., Mutant p53 disrupts mammary tissue architecture via the mevalonate pathway. *Cell*, 2012. **148**(1): p. 244–258.
3. Mir, M.A., et al., Metronomics: toward personalized chemotherapy. *Novel Approaches in Metronomic Chemotherapy for Breast Cancer Treatment*, 2024. p. 99–119. https://doi.org/10.1201/9781032632674-8
4. Sofi, S., et al., A comprehensive analysis of notch signaling genes in breast cancer: expression pattern and prognostic significance. *Advances in Cancer Biology-Metastasis*, 2023. **7**: p. 100104.
5. Parrales, A. and T. Iwakuma, Targeting oncogenic mutant p53 for cancer therapy. *Frontiers in Oncology*, 2015. **5**: p. 288.
6. Kastan, M.B. and E. Berkovich, p53: a two-faced cancer gene. *Nature Cell Biology*, 2007. **9**(5): p. 489–491.
7. Jan, N., et al., Exploring the role of trifarotene against RAR-α: an investigation of expression pattern and clinicopathological significance of RAR-α in breast cancer. *Frontiers in Pharmacology*, 2024. **15**: p. 1361679.
8. Goldstein, J.L. and M.S. Brown, Regulation of the mevalonate pathway. *Nature*, 1990. **343**(6257): p. 425–430.
9. Jan, N., et al., Targeting breast cancer stem cells through retinoids: a new hope for treatment. *Critical Reviews in Oncology/Hematology*, 2023: p. 104156.
10. Mir, M.A., M. Rashid, and N. Jan, Cytokines and Chemokines in Tumor Growth and Progression, in *Cytokine and Chemokine Networks in Cancer*. 2023, Springer. p. 33–77.
11. LaRosa, J.C., J. He, and S. Vupputuri, Effect of statins on risk of coronary disease: a meta-analysis of randomized controlled trials. *Jama*, 1999. **282**(24): p. 2340–2346.
12. Maron, D.J., S. Fazio, and M.F. Linton, Current perspectives on statins. *Circulation*, 2000. **101**(2): p. 207–213.
13. Palinsk, W., New evidence for beneficial effects of statins unrelated to lipid lowering. *Arteriosclerosis, Thrombosis, and Vascular Biology*, 2001. **21**(1): p. 3–5.
14. Wick, G., et al., Is atherosclerosis an immunologically mediated disease? *Immunology Today*, 1995. **16**(1): p. 27–33.
15. Ludewig, B., R.M. Zinkernagel, and H. Hengartner, Arterial inflammation and atherosclerosis. *Trends in Cardiovascular Medicine*, 2002. **12**(4): p. 154–159.
16. Vaughan, C.J., M.B. Murphy, and B.M. Buckley, Statins do more than just lower cholesterol. *The Lancet*, 1996. **348**(9034): p. 1079–1082.
17. Amelio, I., et al., TAp73 opposes tumor angiogenesis by promoting hypoxia-inducible factor 1α degradation. *Proceedings of the National Academy of Sciences*, 2015. **112**(1): p. 226–231.
18. Martinez-Outschoorn, U.E., et al., Cancer metabolism: a therapeutic perspective. *Nature Reviews Clinical Oncology*, 2017. **14**(1): p. 11–31.
19. Jan, N., et al., Metronomic chemotherapy and drug repurposing: a paradigm shift in oncology. *Heliyon*, 2024. https://doi.org/10.1016/j.heliyon.2024.e24670
20. Mir, M.A., N. Jan, and S. Sofi, *Introduction to Metronomic Chemotherapy, in Novel Approaches in Metronomic Chemotherapy for Breast Cancer Treatment*. 2024, CRC Press. p. 1–14.

21. Mir, M.A., Sumaya, N. Jan, *Implications of Chemokine Heterogenicity in Cancer Metastasis, in Cytokine and Chemokine Networks in Cancer.* 2023, Springer. p. 115–136.
22. Haq, B.U., et al., Targeting p53 misfolding conundrum by stabilizing agents and their analogs in breast cancer therapy: a comprehensive computational analysis. *Frontiers in Pharmacology*, 2024. **14**: p. 1333447.
23. Thurnher, M., G. Gruenbacher, and O. Nussbaumer, Regulation of mevalonate metabolism in cancer and immune cells. *Biochimica et Biophysica Acta (BBA)-Molecular and Cell Biology of Lipids*, 2013. **1831**(6): p. 1009–1015.
24. Mir, M.A., et al., Imaging Techniques, Biomarkers, and Methods for Metronomic Chemotherapy, in *Novel Approaches in Metronomic Chemotherapy for Breast Cancer Treatment.* CRC Press. p. 58–71.
25. Thurnher, M., O. Nussbaumer, and G. Gruenbacher, Novel aspects of mevalonate pathway inhibitors as antitumor agents. *Clinical Cancer Research*, 2012. **18**(13): p. 3524–3531.
26. Sofi, S., et al., Clinicopathological and prognostic significance of Bcl2 in breast cancer: a comprehensive in silico and in vitro study. *Saudi Journal of Biological Sciences*, 2023. **31**(2): p. 103916.
27. Duncan, R.E., A. El-Sohemy, and M.C. Archer, Mevalonate promotes the growth of tumors derived from human cancer cells in vivo and stimulates proliferation in vitro with enhanced cyclin-dependent kinase-2 activity. *Journal of Biological Chemistry*, 2004. **279**(32): p. 33079–33084.
28. Istvan, E.S., Structural mechanism for statin inhibition of 3-hydroxy-3-methylglutaryl coenzyme A reductase. *American Heart Journal*, 2002. **144**(6): p. S27–S32.
29. Mir, M.A., A. Shabir, and N. Jan, Metronomic Chemotherapy in Breast Cancer, in *Novel Approaches in Metronomic Chemotherapy for Breast Cancer Treatment.* CRC Press. p. 72–86.
30. Goh, A.M., C.R. Coffill, and D.P. Lane, The role of mutant p53 in human cancer. *The Journal of Pathology*, 2011. **223**(2): p. 116–126.
31. Wong, W.W., et al., HMG-CoA reductase inhibitors and the malignant cell: the statin family of drugs as triggers of tumor-specific apoptosis. *Leukemia*, 2002. **16**(4): p. 508–519.
32. Vallianou, N., et al., Statins and cancer. *Anti-Cancer Agents in Medicinal Chemistry (Formerly Current Medicinal Chemistry-Anti-Cancer Agents)*, 2014. **14**(5): p. 706–712.
33. Mir, M.A., et al., Proteomics: Application of Next-Generation Proteomics in Cancer Research, in *Proteomics.* 2023, Elsevier. p. 55–76.
34. Mizuarai, S., K. Yamanaka, and H. Kotani, Mutant p53 induces the GEF-H1 oncogene, a guanine nucleotide exchange factor-H1 for RhoA, resulting in accelerated cell proliferation in tumor cells. *Cancer Research*, 2006. **66**(12): p. 6319–6326.
35. Bustelo, X.R., V. Sauzeau, and I.M. Berenjeno, GTP-binding proteins of the Rho/Rac family: regulation, effectors and functions in vivo. *Bioessays*, 2007. **29**(4): p. 356–370.
36. Mullen, P.J., et al., The interplay between cell signalling and the mevalonate pathway in cancer. *Nature Reviews Cancer*, 2016. **16**(11): p. 718–731.
37. Ginestier, C., et al., Mevalonate metabolism regulates Basal breast cancer stem cells and is a potential therapeutic target. *Stem Cells*, 2012. **30**(7): p. 1327–1337.
38. Göbel, A., et al., Combined inhibition of the mevalonate pathway with statins and zoledronic acid potentiates their anti-tumor effects in human breast cancer cells. *Cancer Letters*, 2016. **375**(1): p. 162–171.
39. Buhaescu, I. and H. Izzedine, Mevalonate pathway: a review of clinical and therapeutical implications. *Clinical Biochemistry*, 2007. **40**(9–10): p. 575–584.
40. Goldstein, J. L., R. A. DeBose-Boyd, and M. S. Brown, Protein sensors for membrane sterol. *Cell*, 2006. **124**: p. 35–46.
41. Clendening, J.W., et al., Dysregulation of the mevalonate pathway promotes transformation. *Proceedings of the National Academy of Sciences*, 2010. **107**(34): p. 15051–15056.
42. Likus, W., et al., Could drugs inhibiting the mevalonate pathway also target cancer stem cells? *Drug Resistance Updates*, 2016. **25**: p. 13–25.
43. Elsayed, M., et al., Synergistic antiproliferative effects of zoledronic acid and fluvastatin on human pancreatic cancer cell lines: an in vitro study. *Biological and Pharmaceutical Bulletin*, 2016. **39**(8): p. 1238–1246.
44. Buganim, Y., et al., p53 Regulates the Ras circuit to inhibit the expression of a cancer-related gene signature by various molecular pathways. *Cancer Research*, 2010. **70**(6): p. 2274–2284.
45. Peifer, M., et al., Integrative genome analyses identify key somatic driver mutations of small-cell lung cancer. *Nature Genetics*, 2012. **44**(10): p. 1104–1110.
46. Zhang, W. and H.T. Liu, MAPK signal pathways in the regulation of cell proliferation in mammalian cells. *Cell Research*, 2002. **12**(1): p. 9–18.

47. Wang, W., et al., Mutant p53-R273H gains new function in sustained activation of EGFR signaling via suppressing miR-27a expression. *Cell Death & Disease*, 2013. **4**(4): p. e574–e574.
48. Moroishi, T., C.G. Hansen, and K.-L. Guan, The emerging roles of YAP and TAZ in cancer. *Nature Reviews Cancer*, 2015. **15**(2): p. 73–79.
49. Sorrentino, G., et al., Metabolic control of YAP and TAZ by the mevalonate pathway. *Nature Cell Biology*, 2014. **16**(4): p. 357–366.
50. Wang, Z., et al., Interplay of mevalonate and Hippo pathways regulates RHAMM transcription via YAP to modulate breast cancer cell motility. *Proceedings of the National Academy of Sciences*, 2014. **111**(1): p. E89–E98.
51. Mo, J. S., et al., Regulation of the Hippo–YAP pathway by protease-activated receptors (PARs). *Genes & Development*, 2012. **26**(19): p. 2138–2143.
52. Di Agostino, S., et al., YAP enhances the pro-proliferative transcriptional activity of mutant p53 proteins. *EMBO Reports*, 2016. **17**(2): p. 188–201.
53. Escoll, M., et al., Mutant p53 oncogenic functions in cancer stem cells are regulated by WIP through YAP/TAZ. *Oncogene*, 2017. **36**(25): p. 3515–3527.
54. Wicha, M.S., S. Liu, and G. Dontu, Cancer stem cells: an old idea—a paradigm shift. *Cancer Research*, 2006. **66**(4): p. 1883–1890.
55. Bossi, G., et al., Mutant p53 gain of function: reduction of tumor malignancy of human cancer cell lines through abrogation of mutant p53 expression. *Oncogene*, 2006. **25**(2): p. 304–309.
56. Vousden, K.H., Outcomes of p53 activation-spoilt for choice. *Journal of Cell Science*, 2006. **119**(24): p. 5015–5020.
57. Alarcon-Vargas, D. and Z.e. Ronai, p53–Mdm2—the affair that never ends. *Carcinogenesis*, 2002. **23**(4): p. 541–547.
58. Michael, D. and M. Oren. *The p53–Mdm2 Module and the Ubiquitin System in Seminars in Cancer Biology*. 2003. Elsevier.
59. Gunde-Cimerman, N. and A. Cimerman, Pleurotus fruiting bodies contain the inhibitor of 3-hydroxy-3-methylglutaryl-coenzyme A reductase—lovastatin. *Experimental Mycology*, 1995. **19**(1): p. 1–6.
60. Schaefer, E.J., et al., Comparisons of effects of statins (atorvastatin, fluvastatin, lovastatin, pravastatin, and simvastatin) on fasting and postprandial lipoproteins in patients with coronary heart disease versus control subjects. *The American Journal of Cardiology*, 2004. **93**(1): p. 31–39.
61. Graaf, M.R., et al., Effects of statins and farnesyltransferase inhibitors on the development and progression of cancer. *Cancer Treatment Reviews*, 2004. **30**(7): p. 609–641.
62. Wakchoure, S., et al., Bisphosphonates inhibit the growth of mesothelioma cells in vitro and in vivo. *Clinical Cancer Research*, 2006. **12**(9): p. 2862–2868.
63. Crul, M., et al., Ras biochemistry and farnesyl transferase inhibitors: a literature survey. *Anti-Cancer Drugs*, 2001. **12**(3): p. 163–184.
64. Brunner, T.B., et al., Farnesyltransferase inhibitors: an overview of the results of preclinical and clinical investigations. *Cancer Research*, 2003. **63**(18): p. 5656–5668.
65. Alfaqih, M.A., et al., The current evidence on statin use and prostate cancer prevention: are we there yet? *Nature Reviews Urology*, 2017. **14**(2): p. 107–119.
66. Feng, C.H., et al., Statin use significantly improves overall survival in high-grade endometrial cancer. *International Journal of Gynecologic Cancer*, 2016. **26**(9): p. 1642–1649.
67. Nayan, M., et al., Statin use and kidney cancer survival outcomes: a systematic review and meta-analysis. *Cancer Treatment Reviews*, 2017. **52**: p. 105–116.
68. Sanfilippo, K.M., et al., Statins are associated with reduced mortality in multiple myeloma. *Journal of Clinical Oncology*, 2016. **34**(33): p. 4008.
69. Mei, Z., et al., Effects of statins on cancer mortality and progression: a systematic review and meta-analysis of 95 cohorts including 1,111,407 individuals. *International Journal of Cancer*, 2017. **140**(5): p. 1068–1081.
70. Kautzky-Willer, A., S. Thurner, and P. Klimek, Use of statins offsets insulin-related cancer risk. *Journal of Internal Medicine*, 2017. **281**(2): p. 206–216.
71. Undela, K., V. Srikanth, and D. Bansal, Statin use and risk of breast cancer: a meta-analysis of observational studies. *Breast Cancer Research and Treatment*, 2012. **135**(1): p. 261–269.
72. Nordström, T., et al., The risk of prostate cancer for men on aspirin, statin or antidiabetic medications. *European Journal of Cancer*, 2015. **51**(6): p. 725–733.
73. Parrales, A., et al., DNAJA1 controls the fate of misfolded mutant p53 through the mevalonate pathway. *Nature Cell Biology*, 2016. **18**(11): p. 1233–1243.

74. Aviles, A., et al., Randomized clinical trial of zoledronic acid in multiple myeloma patients undergoing high-dose chemotherapy and stem-cell transplantation. *Current Oncology*, 2013. **20**(1): p. 13–20.
75. Coleman, R.E. and J.J. Seaman. *The Role of Zoledronic Acid in Cancer: Clinical Studies in the Treatment and Prevention of Bone Metastases in Seminars in Oncology*. 2001. Elsevier.
76. Lobell, R.B., et al., Preclinical and clinical pharmacodynamic assessment of L-778,123, a dual inhibitor of farnesyl: protein transferase and geranylgeranyl: protein transferase type-I. *Molecular cancer Therapeutics*, 2002. **1**(9): p. 747–758.
77. Dudakovic, A., H. Tong, and R.J. Hohl, Geranylgeranyl diphosphate depletion inhibits breast cancer cell migration. *Investigational New Drugs*, 2011. **29**: p. 912–920.
78. Appels, N.M., J.H. Beijnen, and J.H. Schellens, Development of farnesyl transferase inhibitors: a review. *The Oncologist*, 2005. **10**(8): p. 565–578.

14 Interactions and Implications of p53 in Hormonal Signaling Pathways in Breast Cancer

*Asma Jan, Nusrat Jan, and Manzoor Ahmad Mir**

Department of Bioresources, School of Biological Sciences, University of Kashmir, Srinagar, J&K, India

*drmanzoor@kashmiruniversity.ac.in

14.1 INTRODUCTION

One of the most common cancers diagnosed worldwide and the leading cause of death for women is breast cancer (BC) [1–3]. BC is associated with several risk factors, such as hereditary and genetic susceptibility [4, 5]. A common feature of many malignancies, including BC, is the absence or mutation of the tumor suppressor p53. The p53 tumor suppressor is primarily activated by post-translational changes in response to stress signals such as DNA damage, hypoxia, oncogene activation, and ribosomal stress. Among the important signaling pathways regulated by active p53 are cell cycle regulation, DNA repair, metabolism, senescence, autophagy, and cell death. During cell cycle progression, for example, p53 will efficiently regulate the expression levels of the important kinases CDK and p21, which will inhibit the cyclin E-CDK2 complex and prevent the G1 phase [6–9]. Also when DNA damage is detected, p53 triggers the production of p21. This protein binds to and blocks the activity of complexes cyclinD-CDK4/6 and cyclinE-CDK2, ultimately causing cells to stop in the G1 phase**.** The cell can fix the damaged DNA before moving on to S-phase replication by arresting the cell cycle. To trigger programmed cell death, p53 triggers the activation of apoptotic target genes like Bax and PUMA when the cell is unable to repair DNA damage [10, 11]. Figure 14.1 depicts the arrangement of the p53 protein in humans, along with its distinct regions. It shows that the human p53 protein consists of three primary domains: the NTD (N-terminal domain), the DBD (DNA-binding domain), and the CTD (C-terminal domain). The NTD comprises the transcription activation region at the N-terminus and a region rich in proline. CTD is comprised of a TD (tetramerization domain) and an RD (regulatory domain). Hence, tumor development follows abnormal cell proliferation and cell death caused by p53 depletion. It is worth noting that p53 inactivation is present in nearly all human tumors, with rates ranging from 20% to 80% depending on the specific kind, stage, and cause of cancer [12, 13]. Multiple tumors develop prematurely in p53-knockout mice and people with Li–Fraumeni syndrome when p53 function is lost [14–16]. Nevertheless, estrogen-responsive tumors do not frequently exhibit p53 mutation. This figure is significantly lower in endometrial cancer (18%), cervical cancer (1.5%), and breast cancer (20%) [17–19].

Estrogen has a crucial role in the maturation of the mammary glands and the proper functioning of the reproductive organs. Estrogen controls a wide variety of other physiological processes related to the circulatory, neurological, skeletal systems, and immunological. The actions of estrogen are controlled by ERs (estrogen receptors), which include ERα and ERβ. Intracellular nuclear hormone receptors ERα and ERβ mainly activate target genes through transcription to facilitate estrogen signaling. An integral membrane protein called G-protein coupled receptor 30 (GPR30) may also

 DOI: 10.1201/9781003520771-14

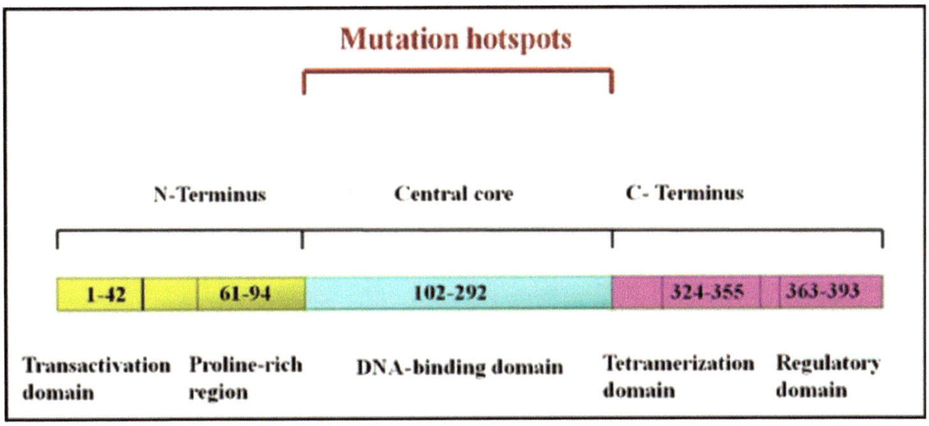

FIGURE 14.1 Structure of p53 shown schematically. Three functional domains—an N terminal activation domain, a DNA-binding domain, and a C-terminal tetramerization domain—make up the 393-amino-acid protein p53.

detect estrogen. When estrogen is present, GPR30 starts non-genomic processes like transporting calcium inside the cell, activating adenylyl cyclase, making nuclear PIP3 (phosphatidylinositol (3,4,5)-trisphosphate), and triggering the MAPK and PI3K signaling pathways [20, 21]. The significance of GPR30 in hormone-dependent cancer is poorly understood because it operates independently of ERα and ERβ. Deregulated expression of ERα and signaling in cell proliferation, survival, and migration can generate tumors in estrogen-regulated tissues such as the colon, endometrial, and breast [22, 23]. For individuals with ER-positive (estrogen receptor positive) breast cancer, anti-estrogen medications like tamoxifen have been developed, as over 70% of these tumors express ERα [24]. Chemotherapy is also the primary or adjuvant treatment for breast cancers that have spread outside the breast or for tumors that are sensitive to estrogen [25]. A better knowledge of the interaction between p53 and ER signaling might enhance the effectiveness of current breast cancer therapy strategies, as p53 is a primary mediator for chemotherapy [26, 27].

14.2 THE SIGNALING PATHWAYS OF THE ER

Although ERα and ERβ are on distinct chromosomes, their DNA-binding domains are 97% identical and their ligand-binding domains are 55% the same. Six functional domains comprise ERα and Erβ. Transcriptional activity requires activation function-1 (AF-1) which is found in the N-terminal A/B domains and interacts with coactivators. Within the C domain is the DNA-binding region. A nuclear localization signal is found in the D domain, sometimes known as the hinge area. A dimerization domain, AF-2, ligand-binding area, and extranuclear localization signal are all found in the E domain. The C-terminal ligand-binding region, or F domain, is strictly controlled by agonists and antagonists [28, 29].

The N-terminal AF-1 is absent from ERα46, the other of the two primary isoforms of human ERα. Full-length ERα may form a heterodimer with ERα46, which suppresses ERα transactivation activity [30, 31]. Transactivation domains AF-1 and AF-2 are absent from ERα36, a third isoform [32]. ERα36 is thought to facilitate non-genomic estrogen signaling in the plasma membrane and cytoplasm, which is different from the functions of full-length ERα and ERα46 [33]. Alternative splicing allows for the expression of more than five isoforms of human Erβ [34]. The whole-length receptor is called ERβ1. Since their AF-2 ligand-binding domain is shortened, ERβ2–5 is unable to bind ligands. Although ERβ2–5 cannot form functional homodimers, they can regulate the function of ERα or ERβ1 by forming heterodimers [35, 36].

ERα and ERβ assemble into homo- and heterodimers that operate as transcription factors when they bind to 17β-estradiol, an estrogen. Activator protein 1 (AP1), NFκB, or Sp1 are examples of additional transcription factors with which these nuclear hormone receptors interact secondary to, or directly to, an estrogen response element (ERE) in the promoters of their target genes [37, 38]. EREs may be a non-consensus sequence [39, 40] or a half-consensus sequence of 5′-GGTCA-3′ (where "n" is any nucleotide). Remarkably, the tissue expression patterns of the two estrogen receptors differ and they control distinct sets of genes as well as common ones [41]. The mammary gland and the uterus are home to the primary estrogen receptor in the female reproductive system, ERα [42]. The main estrogen receptors in the prostate, colon, lungs, cardiovascular system, and central nervous system are ERβ [43]. Seventy percent of BCs are ER-positive, or expressing ERα [44]. Generally speaking, ER-positive BC indicates a favorable prognosis for the patient and response to anti-estrogen therapy, including tamoxifen [45]. But 50% of tamoxifen-responding tumors become resistant to therapy [46, 47]. Patients who acquire resistance to tamoxifen therapy as well as ER-positive BC patients who have de novo resistance to the drug are usually receptive to ICI 182,780 [48]. Following binding to the ER, ICI 182,780 (fulvestrant), a pure ER antagonist, prevents dimerization [49]. Furthermore, by accelerating receptor degradation via the ubiquitin-proteasome pathway, ICI 182,780 lowers ERα levels [50]. Reduction of ERα levels can result in an ER-negative tumor state and treatment resistance. ER-negative tumors are linked to aggressive tumor development, increased invasiveness, poor patient prognosis, and resistance to anti-estrogen therapy.

Although the expression of ERα is linked to tumor growth, that of ERβ may suppress the development of tumors [51]. Low ERβ expression has been demonstrated in breast cancer, and ectopic ERβ expression reduces the proliferation and/or invasion of MCF7, T47D, and MDA-MB-231 cells among other breast cancer cells [52–55]. Reports did, however, also demonstrate that ERβ is expressed by ERα-negative invasive breast tumors and that overexpression of ERβ promoted the proliferation and/or dissemination of MDA-MB-435 and MDA-MB-231 BC cells [56–58]. It follows that ERβ is probably able to either stimulate or prevent breast cancer cells from proliferating and spreading. It would be fascinating to investigate in the future how ERβ functions in breast carcinogenesis and how patient prognosis is related to ERβ expression in clinical samples of breast tumors.

14.3 p53 AND ERα IN BREAST CANCER

Breast cancer is three times more likely to develop in a woman's lifetime if her first full-term pregnancy happens before the age of 18 compared to a woman whose first birth comes after the age of 30 [59]. The risk of cancer in parous mice exposed to chemical carcinogens was also lower than in virgin rodents [60–62]. To add to that, estrogen and progesterone, which are hormones produced by the ovaries, have been shown to boost p53-dependent responses and decrease BC cases in mice and rats when treated for brief periods [63–65]. According to a study conducted on nulliparous mice lacking p53, animals with abnormal ERα expression showed less apoptosis and increased proliferation of mammary epithelial cells [66]. It is worth noting that p53-null animals who were given estrogen had a shorter latency for ERα-positive mammary tumors, compared to those that were not given estrogen, which resulted in ERα-negative tumors [67]. Tumor behavior following anti-estrogen treatment, radiation therapy, or chemotherapy, as well as the emergence of resistance to these treatments, remain largely unexplained, although these findings of p53 and estrogen interaction in human clinical cases and animal models seem to correlate with findings from molecular investigations.

When it comes to ER-positive breast cancer, tamoxifen is the gold standard for both pre- and post-menopausal women. There was a 31% decrease in the death rate for individuals using tamoxifen to treat ER-positive breast cancer as compared to those who did not. Tamoxifen had no discernible effect on ER-negative breast cancer patients, as predicted [68]. Combining cyclophosphamide, doxorubicin, and paclitaxel as chemotherapeutic drugs for ER-negative breast tumors led to a 22.8% increase in disease-free survival after five years. In contrast, for ER-positive patients, adding these chemotherapy drugs to tamoxifen treatment resulted in only a 7% improvement in disease-free survival [69]. Because of its dual role as an estrogen antagonist in breast tissue and an estrogen agonist in heart and bone tissue, tamoxifen is referred to as a selective estrogen receptor modulator (SERM) [70]. To create the active metabolite 4-hydroxytamoxifen (OHT), the liver metabolizes the prodrug tamoxifen. Next, in competition with estrogen, this metabolite binds to the ligand-binding domain of ERα in bovine tissue. When bound, OHT causes a conformational shift that moves helix 12 out of the way of the AF-2 domain's coactivator binding groove. Consequently, corepressors like NCR and SMRT bind to ERα and control a separate group of genes [70–72]. The number of cells in S-phase drops precipitously and the number of cells in the G1 fraction increases when tamoxifen is administered. The exact process by which tamoxifen causes cell cycle arrest is not yet known, although it is believed to be mediated by ERα since ER-negative cells do not respond as strongly to tamoxifen as ER-positive cells [73]. When ER-positive, p53 wild-type cells were treated with tamoxifen, there was a dose-dependent rise in the levels of p53 and p21 proteins, which suggested that a p53-dependent cycle arrest mechanism had been activated [74, 75]. By increasing cyclin D1 protein levels and cyclin D1/CDK4 and cyclin D1/CDK2 kinase activity, estrogen caused tamoxifen-treated G1 arrested cells to enter the S-phase [76–80]. This evidence suggests that the hormone therapy that targets ERα is influenced by the p53 protein's capacity to halt the cell cycle. Regardless of estrogen receptor status, disease-free survival rates are poorer for breast cancer patients with mutant p53 [81]. In ER-positive cells with wild-type p53, tamoxifen raised p53 levels and activated downstream p53 target genes, but in ER-positive cells with mutant p53, this effect was not observed. The effects of tamoxifen would be diminished if alterations in p53 inhibited ERα expression, as p53 controls ERα expression [82]. Whether treatment success is caused by additional pathway connections or by direct interaction between p53 and ERα remains unclear.

14.4 THE INTERACTION OF ERα AND ERβ IN BREAST CANCER

Certain researchers think that variations in ERα and ERβ expression in the healthy breast provide evidence for a direct relationship between the nuclear expression of ERs and the breast's proliferative characteristics [83]. The activity of several signaling pathways involved in cell proliferation and the response to endocrine treatment are correlated with the relative amounts of ERα and ERβ in BC [84, 85]. Wild-type p53 function is enhanced by ERβ1, which also inhibits ERα-dependent regulation of p53 (Figure 14.2). Research reveals that when ERα and ERβ are coexpressed, HER2 expression is often negative while the Ki-67 index is up, suggesting a link between this particular combination of biomarkers and the aggressiveness of BC [86]. Furthermore, via downregulating basal ERα promoter activity, increased ERβ can influence ERα expression at the transcriptional level. The downregulation of ERα in breast cancer cells caused by ERβ requires the presence of the proximal GC-rich motifs at –223 and –214. Histone H4 hypoacetylation, RNA polymerase II displacement, recruitment of a corepressor complex comprising the nuclear receptor corepressor NCoR, and Erβ–Sp1 protein interactions inside the ERα promoter region are the mechanisms responsible for this downregulation of ERα [87]. When an ERβ-specific agonist is used, MCF-7 BC cells' ERα expression and functional activity are markedly reduced. This is accompanied by a reduction in the transcription of BCA2 (breast cancer-associated gene 2), a downstream effector [88].

More data demonstrates that uncoupling protein (UCP), antioxidant enzyme protein levels, oxidative damage, and sirtuin 3 (SIRT3) protein levels are all elevated in tumors with low ERα/ERβ ratios. The ERα/ERβ ratio has a positive correlation with glutathione peroxidase, complex II, complex III, complex IV, complex V, stress-activated protein kinase (SAPK), and protein kinase B (AKT) and ERα. On the other hand, the ratio has a negative correlation with SIRT3, UCP5, Cu-Zn superoxide dismutase, catalase, carbonyl groups, and ERβ [89]. It is plausible to propose that the presence of an imbalance between two ERs might be the cause of BC.

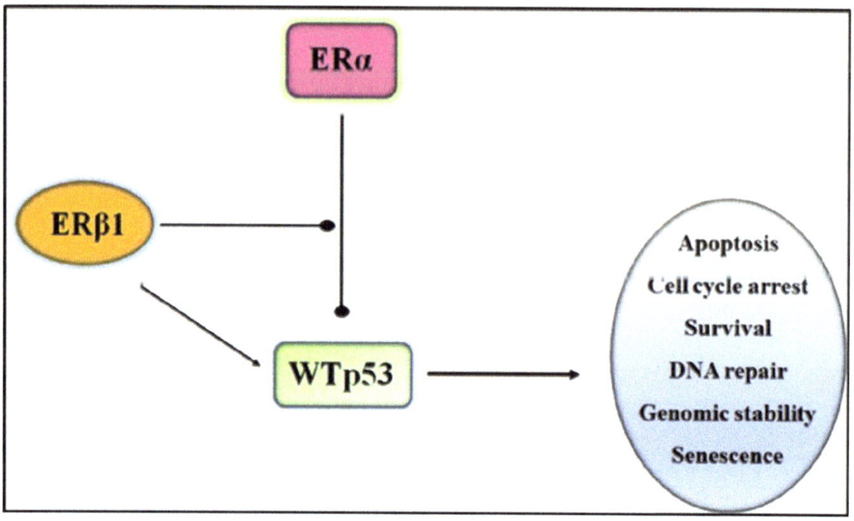

FIGURE 14.2 Wild-type p53 function is enhanced by ERβ1, which also inhibits ERα-dependent regulation of p53.

14.5 INTERACTION OF ERβ AND p53

p53 is believed to interact with ERβ, an activator of wild-type p53-dependent transcription. Nuclear p53 expression is elevated during ERβ overexpression or ERβ agonist activation [90, 91]. One of the key factors in breast cancer incidence and progression is the cooperative action of ERβ and p53 inactivation activities [92]. p53 status and the ESR2 mutant both have antiproliferative effects in triple-negative breast cancer (TNBC) [93]. ERβ1 downregulates prometastatic factors and increases the mutant p53's target genes that are linked to a normal phenotype [94]. Using a mammary tumor model using mice, depletion of p53 and ERβ speeds up the growth of tumors [92]. Following exposure to cisplatin and doxorubicin, ERβ expression results in the G2/M checkpoints mediated by Chk1/Cdc25C and S-phase disruption. It's interesting to note that p53 wild-type mammary cells do not exhibit this impact; only p53-defective breast cancer cells do [95]. Furthermore, the interaction between p53 and ERα contributes to ERβ's proapoptotic and antiproliferative activities in breast cancer cells. By interacting with p53, ERβ decreases ERα-p53 binding, which antagonizes ERα-p53-mediated transcriptional regulation. Furthermore, RNA polymerase II and histone H3 lys4 trimethylation (H3K4me3) on ERα-repressed genes are stimulated by ERβ. This results in the epigenetic activation of H3K4me3-related suppressor gene transcription, which in turn promotes p53-based tumor suppression. ERβ1 forms a connection with mutant p53 in order to regulate the expression of certain genes that are involved in epithelial–mesenchymal transition (EMT), invasion, and metastasis. Thus, ERβ1 may act in opposition to cancer growth, thereby enhancing its function as a tumor suppressor. In general, ERβ1 has the ability to safeguard cells from developing cancer and spreading to other parts of the body. Therefore, it is considered a promising option for enhancing the rate of survival in cancer patients (Figure 14.3). By decreasing SMRT recruitment by ERα and corepressor NCoR, ERβ also lessens the cross-talk between ERα and p53 [96].

14.6 p53 ALTERATIONS AND RESPONSE TO THERAPY

It is believed that a key indicator of cancer's resistance to chemotherapy and radiation therapy in numerous cancers is the lack of functioning p53. Significant support for this theory comes from studies on cell death in mice with p53 knockouts and from correlations found between the p53 status ascertained by immunochemistry or SSCP (single-strand conformational polymorphism) analysis

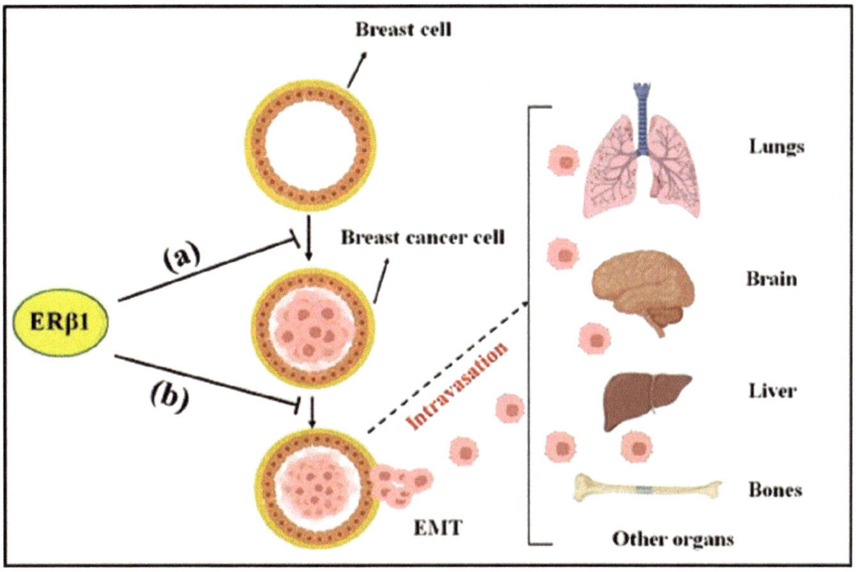

FIGURE 14.3 Tumor suppressive functions of ERβ1 in BC. (a) Tumor development and genetic mutations are inhibited by ERβ1. (b) EMT (epithelial-to-mesenchymal transition), invasion, and metastasis are inhibited by ERβ1.

and the therapeutic response of human tumors in vivo [97]. It is essentially possible that p53, in addition to activating proapoptotic genes such as bax transcriptionally and suppressing genes like bcl-2 that prevent, might boost chemosensitivity by causing apoptosis through mechanisms separate from transcription. p53 may likewise regulate the drug-induced suicide pathway mediated by the CD95/CD95 ligand system [98].

p53, however, may lessen chemosensitivity by promoting differentiation, p21-mediated and p21-independent growth arrest, and DNA repair. It may also do this by increasing the transcription of antiapoptotic genes such as bcl-x. The cellular environment appears to be a key factor in determining how p53 status modification impacts chemosensitivity, according to research conducted on cell cultures [99]. Chemosensitivity may be increased rather than decreased in normally healthy, non-cancerous cells when p53 failure occurs. Targeted p53 gene disruption, however, results in enhanced radiation sensitivity in some cell types produced from p53-knockout mice rather than decreased susceptibility. In most cases, when the p53 function is blocked, altered cells that have retained the p53 function become chemoresistance [98]. Consequently, rather than only p53 activity loss, tumor cells may also acquire chemoresistance from preexisting molecular alterations or a later accumulation of abnormalities in the molecules after loss of p53 [100]. Finally, significant drug- and tumor-cell-specific patterns of p53-mediated regulation of chemosensitivity are beginning to emerge. Although p53 gene transfer into cancer cells can also increase the cell's resistance to the majority of chemotherapy medications, it is often the cause of growth arrest [101].

14.7 CHALLENGES IN DEVELOPING TREATMENT PLANS THAT TARGET p53 AND FUTURE PERSPECTIVES

Finding inhibitors against p53 is a difficult task. This is explained by the fact that it is a transcription factor without an enzyme-active site or receptor-ligand interaction accessibility. Still, the structure of p53 and its interaction partners have made it easier to find and create a wide range of drugs that may be able to restore p53's tumor-suppressing effects. Although most of them are still in the pre-clinical phases of research, several small molecule drugs with different degrees of complexity have been developed to target both wild-type and mutant p53-bearing tumors. Only a small number of potential medications have been studied in early-phase clinical trials including breast cancer patients (Table 14.3) and despite their encouraging pre-clinical results, the outcomes have been mixed with low-effectiveness signals and high-grade toxicities. Even if the precise causes of the variations in patient response to the small molecule inhibitors are yet unclear, it is important to take into account the unexpected effects of blocking a specific p53 target. For instance, the suppression or elimination of MDM2 in tumors with functioning p53 might cause other carcinogenic pathways to become activated [102]. Furthermore, focusing on p53 negative regulators might result in broad p53 activation that could impact both healthy and malignant cells.

14.8 CONCLUSION

In healthy cells, estrogen encourages the division of cells. The increased proliferation in response to estrogen stimulation may be offset by the concomitant rise in p53. Despite increased p53 levels, estrogen-stimulated growth via the ER and p53-mediated growth inhibition are out of balance in cells with dysregulated p53 and ER levels, resulting in unchecked tumor development.

The vast majority of malignancies in the breast, cervical, and endometrial regions are ER-positive, however numerous other variables also play a role in tumor development. Although it is speculated that mutant p53 can suppress ERα transcription, the exact mechanism by which ER-positive tumors with wild-type p53 transform into ER-negative tumors with mutant p53 remains a mystery. Even more puzzling is the fact that treatment resistance develops in 50% of individuals whose ER-positive tumors responded initially to tamoxifen. The formation and progression of hormone-dependent cancer can be better understood by completely comparing the signaling pathways used by normal and malignant cells when it comes to the interplay between p53 and ER. To enhance patient treatment, further clinical and molecular research into the tumor response to anti-estrogen therapy for ER-positive malignancies and DNA damage-induced chemotherapies for ER-negative cancers is required.

REFERENCES

1. Haq, B.U., et al., Targeting p53 misfolding conundrum by stabilizing agents and their analogs in breast cancer therapy: a comprehensive computational analysis. *Frontiers in Pharmacology*, 2024. **14**: p. 1333447.
2. Jan, N., et al., Exploring the role of trifarotene against RAR-α: an investigation of expression pattern and clinicopathological significance of RAR-α in breast cancer. *Frontiers in Pharmacology*, 2024. **15**: p. 1361679.
3. Jan, N., et al., Targeting breast cancer stem cells through retinoids: a new hope for treatment. *Critical Reviews in Oncology/Hematology*, 2023: p. 104156.
4. Jan, N., et al., Metronomic chemotherapy and drug repurposing: a paradigm shift in oncology. *Heliyon*, 2024. https://doi.org/10.1016/j.heliyon.2024.e24670
5. Sofi, S., et al., Clinicopathological and prognostic significance of Bcl2 in breast cancer: a comprehensive in silico and in vitro study. *Saudi Journal of Biological Sciences*, 2023. **31**(2): p. 103916.
6. Mir, M.A. and A. Jan, *Introduction to Cell Cycle and Its Regulators in Therapeutic Potential of Cell Cycle Kinases in Breast Cancer.* 2023, Springer. p. 53–82.
7. Sofi, S., et al., A comprehensive analysis of notch signaling genes in breast cancer: expression pattern and prognostic significance. *Advances in Cancer Biology-Metastasis*, 2023. **7**: p. 100104.
8. Mir, M.A., et al., Proteomics: A Groundbreaking Development in Cancer Biology, in *Proteomics*. 2023, Elsevier. p. 31–53.
9. Sofi, S., et al., Elucidation of interleukin-19 as a therapeutic target for breast cancer by computational analysis and experimental validation. *Saudi Journal of Biological Sciences*, 2023. **30**(9): p. 103774–103774.
10. Takaoka, A., et al., Integration of interferon-α/β signalling to p53 responses in tumour suppression and antiviral defence. *Nature*, 2003. **424**(6948): p. 516–523.

11. Mir, M.A., et al., Proteomics: Application of Next-Generation Proteomics in Cancer Research, in *Proteomics*. 2023, Elsevier. p. 55–76.
12. Petitjean, A., et al., Impact of mutant p53 functional properties on TP53 mutation patterns and tumor phenotype: lessons from recent developments in the IARC TP53 database. *Human Mutation*, 2007. **28**(6): p. 622–629.
13. Olivier, M., M. Hollstein, and P. Hainaut, TP53 mutations in human cancers: origins, consequences, and clinical use. *Cold Spring Harbor Perspectives in Biology*, 2010. **2**(1): p. a001008.
14. Malkin, D., et al., Germ line p53 mutations in a familial syndrome of breast cancer, sarcomas, and other neoplasms. *Science*, 1990. **250**(4985): p. 1233–1238.
15. Lavigueur, A., et al., High incidence of lung, bone, and lymphoid tumors in transgenic mice overexpressing mutant alleles of the p53 oncogene. *Molecular and Cellular Biology*, 1989. https://doi.org/10.1128/mcb.9.9.3982-3991.1989
16. Mir, M.A., M. Bashir, and N. Jan, The Role of Interleukin (IL)-6/IL-6 Receptor Axis in Cancer, in *Cytokine and Chemokine Networks in Cancer*. 2023, Springer. p. 137–164.
17. Pharoah, P., N. Day, and C. Caldas, Somatic mutations in the p53 gene and prognosis in breast cancer: a meta-analysis. *British Journal of Cancer*, 1999. **80**(12): p. 1968–1973.
18. Westhof, G., et al., Comparison of cytosolic p53 protein levels in the female genital tract and breast, and their tumors. *Tumor Biology*, 2000. **21**(3): p. 123–134.
19. Mir, M.A., M. Rashid, and N. Jan, Cytokines and Chemokines in Tumor Growth and Progression, in *Cytokine and Chemokine Networks in Cancer*. 2023, Springer. p. 33–77.
20. Mosselman, S., J. Polman, and R. Dijkema, ERβ: identification and characterization of a novel human estrogen receptor. *FEBS Letters*, 1996. **392**(1): p. 49–53.
21. Mir, M.A., Sumaya, N. Jan, *Implications of Chemokine Heterogenicity in Cancer Metastasis, in Cytokine and Chemokine Networks in Cancer*. 2023, Springer. p. 115–136.
22. Kuiper, G.G., et al., Comparison of the ligand binding specificity and transcript tissue distribution of estrogen receptors α and β. *Endocrinology*, 1997. **138**(3): p. 863–870.
23. Mir, M.A., et al., Metronomics: toward personalized chemotherapy. *Novel Approaches in Metronomic Chemotherapy for Breast Cancer Treatment*, 2024. p. 99–119. https://doi.org/10.1201/9781032632674-8
24. Mir, M.A., et al., Imaging Techniques, Biomarkers, and Methods for Metronomic Chemotherapy, in *Novel Approaches in Metronomic Chemotherapy for Breast Cancer Treatment*. CRC Press. p. 58–71.
25. Mir, M.A., N. Jan, and I. Noor, Therapeutic Implications of Cytokines and Chemokines Network in Cancer, in *Cytokine and Chemokine Networks in Cancer*. 2023, Springer. p. 385–414.
26. Mir, M.A., N. Jan, and S. Sofi, Introduction to Metronomic Chemotherapy, in *Novel Approaches in Metronomic Chemotherapy for Breast Cancer Treatment*. 2024, CRC Press. p. 1–14.
27. Mir, M.A., N. Jan, and H. Qayoom, Conventional Chemotherapy vs. Metronomic Chemotherapy, *in Novel Approaches in Metronomic Chemotherapy for Breast Cancer Treatment*. CRC Press. p. 27–42.
28. Green, S., et al., Human oestrogen receptor cDNA: sequence, expression and homology to v-erb-A. *Nature*, 1986. **320**(6058): p. 134–139.
29. Mir, M.A., A. Manzoor, and N. Jan, CCL5/CCR5 Axis in Cancer, in *Cytokine and Chemokine Networks in Cancer*. 2023, Springer. p. 219–240.
30. Flouriot, G., et al., Identification of a new isoform of the human estrogen receptor-alpha (hER- α) that is encoded by distinct transcripts and that is able to repress hER- α activation function 1. *The EMBO journal*, 2000. **19**(17): p. 4688–700.
31. Mir, M.A., A. Shabir, and N. Jan, Metronomic Chemotherapy in Breast Cancer, in *Novel Approaches in Metronomic Chemotherapy for Breast Cancer Treatment*. CRC Press. p. 72–86.
32. Wang, Z., et al., Identification, cloning, and expression of human estrogen receptor-α36, a novel variant of human estrogen receptor-α66. *Biochemical and Biophysical Research Communications*, 2005. **336**(4): p. 1023–1027.
33. Shi, L., et al., Expression of ER-α36, a novel variant of estrogen receptor α, and resistance to tamoxifen treatment in breast cancer. *Journal of Clinical Oncology*, 2009. **27**(21): p. 3423.
34. Moore, J.T., et al., Cloning and characterization of human estrogen receptor β isoforms. *Biochemical and Biophysical Research Communications*, 1998. **247**(1): p. 75–78.
35. Leung, Y.-K., et al., Estrogen receptor (ER)-β isoforms: a key to understanding ER-β signaling. *Proceedings of the National Academy of Sciences*, 2006. **103**(35): p. 13162–13167.
36. Omoto, Y., et al., Estrogen receptor (ER) β1 and ERβcx/β2 inhibit ERα function differently in breast cancer cell line MCF7. *Oncogene*, 2003. **22**(32): p. 5011–5020.
37. Cerillo, G., et al., The oestrogen receptor regulates NFκB and AP-1 activity in a cell-specific manner. *The Journal of Steroid Biochemistry and Molecular Biology*, 1998. **67**(2): p. 79–88.

38. Krishnan, V., X. Wang, and S. Safe, Estrogen receptor-Sp1 complexes mediate estrogen-induced cathepsin D gene expression in MCF-7 human breast cancer cells. *Journal of Biological Chemistry*, 1994. **269**(22): p. 15912–15917.
39. Walker, P., et al., Sequence homologies in the region preceding the transcription initiation site of the liver estrogen-responsive vitellogenin and apo-VLDLII genes. *Nucleic Acids Research*, 1984. **12**(22): p. 8611–8626.
40. El-Ashry, D., et al., Estrogen induction of TGF-α is mediated by an estrogen response element composed of two imperfect palindromes. *The Journal of Steroid Biochemistry and Molecular Biology*, 1996. **59**(3–4): p. 261–269.
41. Hall, J.M. and D.P. McDonnell, The estrogen receptor β-isoform (ERβ) of the human estrogen receptor modulates ERα transcriptional activity and is a key regulator of the cellular response to estrogens and antiestrogens. *Endocrinology*, 1999. **140**(12): p. 5566–5578.
42. Hanstein, B., et al., p300 is a component of an estrogen receptor coactivator complex. *Proceedings of the National Academy of Sciences*, 1996. **93**(21): p. 11540–11545.
43. Taylor, A. and F. Al-Azzawi, Immunolocalisation of oestrogen receptor beta in human tissues. *Journal of Molecular Endocrinology*, 2000. **24**(1): p. 145.
44. Group, E.B.C.T.C., Tamoxifen for early breast cancer: an overview of the randomised trials. *Lancet (London, England)*, 1998. **351**(9114): p. 1451–1467.
45. Bentzon, N., et al., Prognostic effect of estrogen receptor status across age in primary breast cancer. *International Journal of Cancer*, 2008. **122**(5): p. 1089–1094.
46. Clarke, R., et al., Antiestrogen resistance in breast cancer and the role of estrogen receptor signaling. *Oncogene*, 2003. **22**(47): p. 7316–7339.
47. Hurtado, A., et al., Regulation of ERBB2 by oestrogen receptor–PAX2 determines response to tamoxifen. *Nature*, 2008. **456**(7222): p. 663–666.
48. Howell, A., et al., Response to a specific antioestrogen (ICI 182780) in tamoxifen-resistant breast cancer. *The Lancet*, 1995. **345**(8941): p. 29–30.
49. Dauvois, S., R. White, and M.G. Parker, The antiestrogen ICI 182780 disrupts estrogen receptor nucleocytoplasmic shuttling. *Journal of Cell Science*, 1993. **106**(4): p. 1377–1388.
50. Long, X. and K.P. Nephew, Fulvestrant (ICI 182,780)-dependent interacting proteins mediate immobilization and degradation of estrogen receptor-α. *Journal of Biological Chemistry*, 2006. **281**(14): p. 9607–9615.
51. Thomas, C. and J.-Å. Gustafsson, The different roles of ER subtypes in cancer biology and therapy. *Nature Reviews Cancer*, 2011. **11**(8): p. 597–608.
52. Paruthiyil, S., et al., Estrogen receptor β inhibits human breast cancer cell proliferation and tumor formation by causing a G2 cell cycle arrest. *Cancer Research*, 2004. **64**(1): p. 423–428.
53. Roger, P., et al., Decreased expression of estrogen receptor β protein in proliferative preinvasive mammary tumors. *Cancer Research*, 2001. **61**(6): p. 2537–2541.
54. Ström, A., et al., Estrogen receptor β inhibits 17β-estradiol-stimulated proliferation of the breast cancer cell line T47D. *Proceedings of the National Academy of Sciences*, 2004. **101**(6): p. 1566–1571.
55. Lazennec, G., et al., ERβ inhibits proliferation and invasion of breast cancer cells. *Endocrinology*, 2001. **142**(9): p. 4120–4130.
56. Tonetti, D.A., et al., Stable transfection of an estrogen receptor beta cDNA isoform into MDA-MB-231 breast cancer cells. *The Journal of Steroid Biochemistry and Molecular Biology*, 2003. **87**(1): p. 47–55.
57. Shaaban, A.M., et al., Declining estrogen receptor-beta expression defines malignant progression of human breast neoplasia. *The American Journal of Surgical Pathology*, 2003. **27**(12): p. 1502–1512.
58. Hou, Y.F., et al., ERbeta exerts multiple stimulative effects on human breast carcinoma cells. *Oncogene*, 2004. **23**(34): p. 5799–806.
59. MacMahon, B., et al., Age at first birth and breast cancer risk. *Bulletin of the World Health Organization*, 1970. **43**(2): p. 209.
60. Medina, D. and G.H. Smith, Chemical carcinogen-induced tumorigenesis in parous, involuted mouse mammary glands. *Journal of the National Cancer Institute*, 1999. **91**(11): p. 967–969.
61. Marchant, J., Influence of pregnancy and lactation on the incidence of mammary carcinoma induced with methylcholanthrene in female mice of the "IF" strain. *Journal of Pathology and Bacteriology*, 1955. **70**: p. 415–418.
62. Moon, R.C., Relationship between previous reproductive history and chemically induced mammary cancer in rats. *International Journal of Cancer*, 1969. **4**(3): p. 312–317.
63. Becker, K.A., et al., Estrogen and progesterone regulate radiation-induced p53 activity in mammary epithelium through TGF-β-dependent pathways. *Oncogene*, 2005. **24**(42): p. 6345–6353.

64. Huggins, C., R.C. Moon, and S. Morii, Extinction of experimental mammary cancer, I. Estradiol-17β and progesterone. *Proceedings of the National Academy of Sciences*, 1962. **48**(3): p. 379–386.
65. Sivaraman, L., et al., p53 is a potential mediator of pregnancy and hormone-induced resistance to mammary carcinogenesis. *Proceedings of the National Academy of Sciences*, 2001. **98**(22): p. 12379–12384.
66. Díaz-Cruz, E.S. and P.A. Furth, Deregulated estrogen receptor α and p53 heterozygosity collaborate in the development of mammary hyperplasia. *Cancer Research*, 2010. **70**(10): p. 3965–3974.
67. Shai, A., H.C. Pitot, and P.F. Lambert, p53 Loss synergizes with estrogen and papillomaviral oncogenes to induce cervical and breast cancers. *Cancer Research*, 2008. **68**(8): p. 2622–2631.
68. Love, R.R., et al., Effects of tamoxifen on bone mineral density in postmenopausal women with breast cancer. *New England Journal of Medicine*, 1992. **326**(13): p. 852–856.
69. Shang, Y., et al., Cofactor dynamics and sufficiency in estrogen receptor–regulated transcription. *Cell*, 2000. **103**(6): p. 843–852.
70. Jackson, T.A., et al., The partial agonist activity of antagonist-occupied steroid receptors is controlled by a novel hinge domain-binding coactivator L7/SPA and the corepressors N-CoR or SMRT. *Molecular Endocrinology*, 1997. **11**(6): p. 693–705.
71. Frasor, J., et al., Gene expression preferentially regulated by tamoxifen in breast cancer cells and correlations with clinical outcome. *Cancer Research*, 2006. **66**(14): p. 7334–7340.
72. Love, R.R., Tamoxifen therapy in primary breast cancer: biology, efficacy, and side effects. *Journal of Clinical Oncology*, 1989. **7**(6): p. 803–815.
73. Ichikawa, A., J. Ando, and K. Suda, G1 arrest and expression of cyclin-dependent kinase inhibitors in tamoxifen-treated MCF-7 human breast cancer cells. *Human Cell*, 2008. **21**: p. 28–37.
74. Varma, H. and S.E. Conrad, Reversal of an antiestrogen-mediated cell cycle arrest of MCF-7 cells by viral tumor antigens requires the retinoblastoma protein-binding domain. *Oncogene*, 2000. **19**(41): p. 4746–4753.
75. El-Deiry, W.S., et al., WAF1, a potential mediator of p53 tumor suppression. *Cell*, 1993. **75**(4): p. 817–825.
76. Bergh, J., et al., Complete sequencing of the p53 gene provides prognostic information in breast cancer patients, particularly in relation to adjuvant systemic therapy and radiotherapy. *Nature Medicine*, 1995. **1**(10): p. 1029–1034.
77. Berry, D.A., et al., Estrogen-receptor status and outcomes of modern chemotherapy for patients with node-positive breast cancer. *Jama*, 2006. **295**(14): p. 1658–1667.
78. Planas-Silva, M.D. and R.A. Weinberg, Estrogen-dependent cyclin E-cdk2 activation through p21 redistribution. *Molecular and Cellular Biology*, 1997. https://doi.org/10.1128/mcb.17.7.4059
79. Prall, O.J., et al., Estrogen-induced activation of Cdk4 and Cdk2 during G1-S phase progression is accompanied by increased cyclin D1 expression and decreased cyclin-dependent kinase inhibitor association with cyclin E-Cdk2. *Journal of Biological Chemistry*, 1997. **272**(16): p. 10882–10894.
80. Watts, C., et al., Antiestrogen inhibition of cell cycle progression in breast cancer cells in associated with inhibition of cyclin-dependent kinase activity and decreased retinoblastoma protein phosphorylation. *Molecular Endocrinology*, 1995. **9**(12): p. 1804–1813.
81. Lim, L., et al., Mutant p53 mediates survival of breast cancer cells. *British Journal of Cancer*, 2009. **101**(9): p. 1606–1612.
82. Berger, C., Y. Qian, and X. Chen, The p53-estrogen receptor loop in cancer. *Current Molecular Medicine*, 2013. **13**(8): p. 1229–1240.
83. Dall, G.V., et al., Estrogen receptor subtypes dictate the proliferative nature of the mammary gland. *Journal of Endocrinology*, 2018. **237**(3): p. 323–336.
84. Madeira, M., et al., Estrogen receptor alpha/beta ratio and estrogen receptor beta as predictors of endocrine therapy responsiveness–a randomized neoadjuvant trial comparison between anastrozole and tamoxifen for the treatment of postmenopausal breast cancer. *BMC Cancer*, 2013. **13**: p. 1–12.
85. Chang, E.C., et al., Impact of estrogen receptor β on gene networks regulated by estrogen receptor α in breast cancer cells. *Endocrinology*, 2006. **147**(10): p. 4831–4842.
86. Oueslati, M., et al., ERα and ERβ co-expression: An indicator of aggressive tumors and hormonal sensitivity. *Oncology Letters*, 2017. **14**(2): p. 1675–1682.
87. Bartella, V., et al., Estrogen receptor beta binds Sp1 and recruits a corepressor complex to the estrogen receptor alpha gene promoter. *Breast Cancer Research and Treatment*, 2012. **134**: p. 569–581.
88. Lee, Y.-H., et al., Regulation of DNA damage response by estrogen receptor β-mediated inhibition of Breast Cancer Associated Gene 2. *Biomedicines*, 2015. **3**(2): p. 182–200.
89. Sastre-Serra, J., et al., The oxidative stress in breast tumors of postmenopausal women is ERα/ERβ ratio dependent. *Free Radical Biology and Medicine*, 2013. **61**: p. 11–17.

90. Cotrim, C., et al., Estrogen receptor beta growth-inhibitory effects are repressed through activation of MAPK and PI3K signalling in mammary epithelial and breast cancer cells. *Oncogene*, 2013. **32**(19): p. 2390–2402.
91. Bado, I., et al., ERβ alters the chemosensitivity of luminal breast cancer cells by regulating p53 function. *Oncotarget*, 2018. **9**(32): p. 22509.
92. Bado, I., et al., Somatic loss of estrogen receptor beta and p53 synergize to induce breast tumorigenesis. *Breast Cancer Research*, 2017. **19**: p. 1–10.
93. Mukhopadhyay, U.K., et al., TP53 status as a determinant of pro-vs anti-tumorigenic effects of estrogen receptor-beta in breast cancer. *JNCI: Journal of the National Cancer Institute*, 2019. **111**(11): p. 1202–1215.
94. Bado, I., et al., ERβ decreases the invasiveness of triple-negative breast cancer cells by regulating mutant p53 oncogenic function. *Oncotarget*, 2016. **7**(12): p. 13599.
95. Thomas, C.G., et al., Estrogen receptor beta decreases survival of p53-defective cancer cells after DNA damage by impairing G 2/M checkpoint signaling. *Breast Cancer Research and Treatment*, 2011. **127**: p. 417–427.
96. Lu, W. and B.S. Katzenellenbogen, Estrogen Receptor-β modulation of the ERα-p53 loop regulating gene expression, proliferation, and apoptosis in breast cancer. *Hormones and Cancer*, 2017. **8**: p. 230–242.
97. Marei, H.E., et al., p53 signaling in cancer progression and therapy. *Cancer Cell International*, 2021. **21**(1): p. 703.
98. Alvarado-Ortiz, E., et al., Mutant p53 gain-of-function: role in cancer development, progression, and therapeutic approaches. *Frontiers in Cell and Developmental Biology*, 2021. **8**: p. 607670.
99. Vaddavalli, P.L. and B. Schumacher, The p53 network: cellular and systemic DNA damage responses in cancer and aging. *Trends in Genetics*, 2022. **38**(6): p. 598–612.
100. Hu, J., et al., Targeting mutant p53 for cancer therapy: direct and indirect strategies. *Journal of Hematology & Oncology*, 2021. **14**(1): p. 157.
101. Timofeev, O., et al., Residual apoptotic activity of a tumorigenic p53 mutant improves cancer therapy responses. *The EMBO Journal*, 2019. **38**(20): p. e102096.
102. Shostak, K., et al., MDM2 restrains estrogen-mediated AKT activation by promoting TBK1-dependent HPIP degradation. *Cell Death & Differentiation*, 2014. **21**(5): p. 811–824.

15 p53 as a Diagnostic Biomarker in Breast Cancer

*Asma Jan, Nusrat Jan, and Manzoor Ahmad Mir**

Department of Bioresources, School of Biological Sciences, University of Kashmir, Srinagar, J&K, India
*drmanzoor@kashmiruniversity.ac.in

15.1 INTRODUCTION

The most prevalent form of cancer and the second leading cause of death for women is breast cancer (BC) [1, 2]. It's a complex disorder with several biological subgroups, each with unique characteristics and therapeutic responses [3, 4]. TP53 is the gene that is crucial for preventing genetic alterations in the body and is more likely to undergo mutations, as shown in various malignancies including breast cancer, accounting for almost 30% of all instances of breast cancer [5–7]. The gene consists of 11 exons that cover a distance of 20 kilobases and is located at 17p13. It is part of a family of genes that are quite similar and also include TP63 and TP73, which produce p63 and p73, respectively. The protein is composed of 393 amino acids and contains four primary functional domains. In the context of cancer, p53 suppresses cell proliferation in reaction to many stimuli, such as DNA damage, lack of nutrients, low oxygen levels, and excessive signals for cell growth [8]. This mechanism effectively hinders the development of tumors. Missense point mutations cause most p53 alterations, which are found in the DBD (DNA-binding domain) that hinder its ability to activate transcription (Figure 15.1).

The presence of these mutations is strongly correlated with tumor subtypes [9] and is connected to a worse chance of survival in breast cancer patients [10]. The oncoprotein MDM2 inhibits p53 activity [11]. When cells experience stress, p53 goes through several changes after it is translated into a protein. These changes include phosphorylation, which makes p53 more stable by interrupting its interaction with MDM2. Additionally, p53 binds to specific sequences of DNA and activates or suppresses certain genes that are responsible for regulating the cell cycle, repairing DNA, and triggering senescence and apoptosis (Figure 15.2) [12].

p53 isoforms, present in normal tissues, are involved in several biological processes such as cell cycle arrest, tissue regeneration, apoptosis, and carcinogenesis. Evidence has demonstrated that the p53 isoforms are expressed typically in several types of human malignancies, highlighting the importance of these proteins in the onset and advancement of cancer. To improve cancer treatment and predict clinical outcomes, it is crucial to understand the many p53 isoforms [13].

The p53 isoforms have diverse activities. p53 isoforms can regulate both innate and adaptive immunological responses, as well as influence macrophage activity and the recruitment of immune cells. Imbalances in the expression of different p53 isoforms can lead to a range of health issues, including cancer, premature aging, neurological disorders, inflammation, developmental defects in embryos, and impaired tissue regeneration. In *Drosophila melanogaster*, the shorter p53A isoform is primarily responsible for regulating the transcription of pro-apoptotic genes and initiating apoptosis in response to DNA damage [14]. The p53 isoforms aid the cell in distinguishing between different stresses and initiating the right response. Regulating the expression of p53 isoforms can effectively control the cellular response to treatment [15].

DOI: 10.1201/9781003520771-15

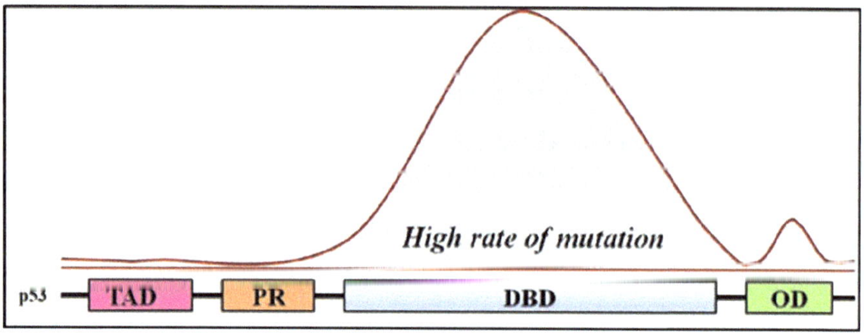

FIGURE 15.1 Sites of p53 mutations: The DBD (DNA-binding domain) of the p53 protein is mostly affected by mutations. There are fewer mutations in the TAD (transactivation domain), proline-rich domain (PR), and oligomerization domain (OD).

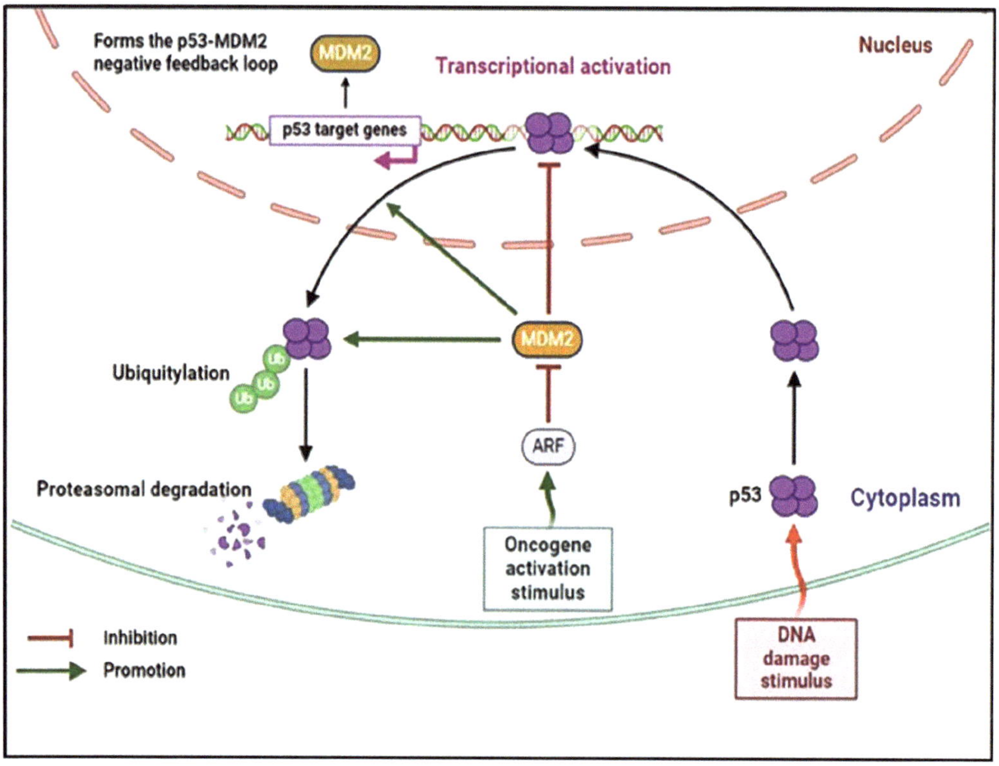

FIGURE 15.2 p53 signaling pathway.

15.2 UNDERSTANDING FUNCTIONALITY OF p53

15.2.1 DNA Repair

p53, acting as a tumor suppressor, is crucial for preserving the integrity of the genome by providing sufficient time for the DNA repair machinery to remove damaged lesions before the proliferation of cells restarts [16]. The p53 protein regulates many DNA repair pathways, including DNA

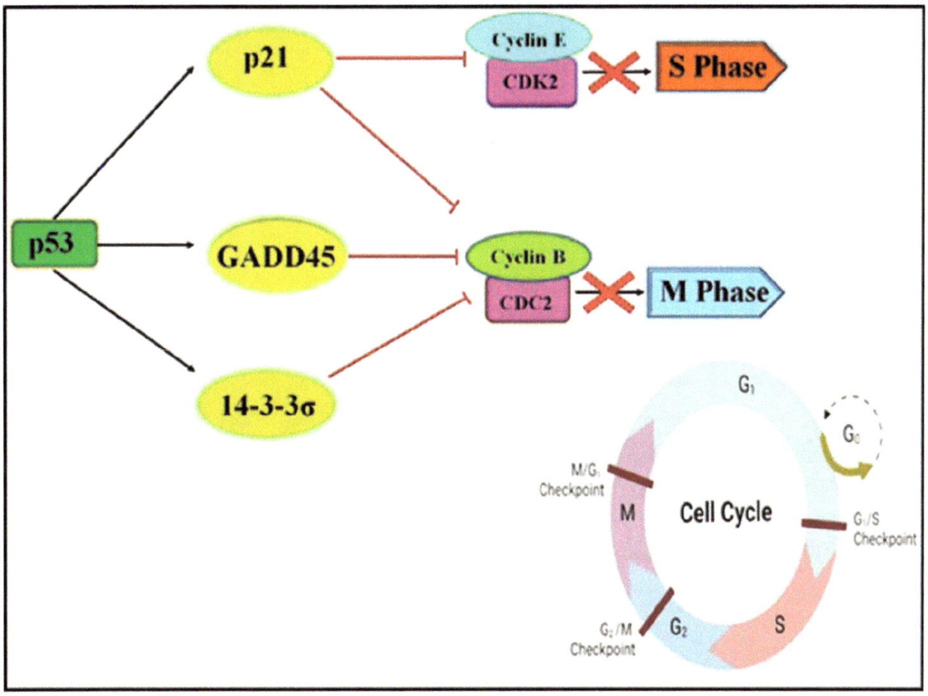

FIGURE 15.3 Significance of p53 in cell cycle arrest.

double-stranded break repair, nucleotide excision repair, base excision repair, and mismatch repair. Homologous recombination and non-homologous end joining are two of these repair pathways [17].

15.2.2 Regulation of Cell Cycle

The essential regulatory pathway that controls the sequence and length of the cell cycle transition is the cell cycle checkpoint and it helps the cell to preserve the chromosomal distribution and DNA replication quality [11]. When DNA damage occurs, p53 becomes active to control the restriction points of the G1-S and G2-M phases. When activated, p53 controls the transcription of GADD45, Cdc25c, 14-3-3σ, and p21 to induce cell cycle halt [18]. According to the findings, p53 predominantly causes G1 arrest by activating p21. p21 suppresses the activity of cyclin E/CDK2, therefore preventing excessive phosphorylation of Rb (retinoblastoma). Therefore, retinoblastoma remains attached to E2F, preventing the E2F-mediated transcription of cell cycle genes that are crucial for the passage from the G1 to the S phase. p53 inhibits the actions of cyclin B1/cdc2 and prevents the G2/M phase of the cell cycle by boosting the production of 14-3-3σ in response to DNA damage [19] (Figure 15.3).

15.2.3 Apoptosis

Numerous investigations have established that p53 plays a crucial role in initiating apoptosis [20, 21]. Both the extrinsic and intrinsic mechanisms that transmit apoptosis are regulated by p53 [22]. p53 initiates the extrinsic apoptotic cascade by stimulating the production of death receptor 5, the cell death receptor Fas, and the death-domain-containing receptor for TRAIL. This leads to the creation of the death-inducing signaling complex, which initiates a series of caspase activation events, including caspase-8 and caspase-3 [23]. p53 activates the intrinsic apoptotic pathway by causing the transcription of pro-apoptotic genes from the Bcl2 family, including BID, PUMA, Noxa, and BAX.

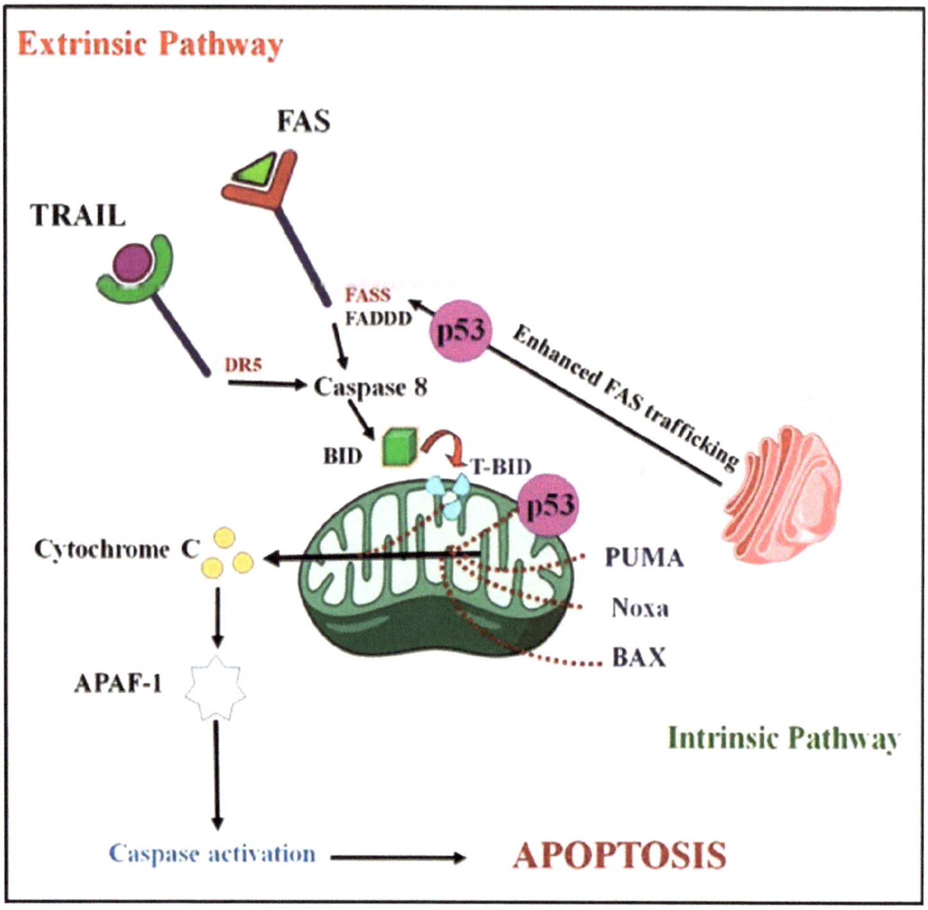

FIGURE 15.4 The role of p53 in both the intrinsic and extrinsic apoptotic pathways.

The interplay between these genes enhances the formation of multiple units and the initiation of functional activity of BAX, which in turn induces the release of cytochrome c. This ultimately leads to the activation of caspase 9 [24, 25] (Figure 15.4).

15.2.4 Senescence

Senescence is the permanent halt in the cell cycle that can be triggered by several forms of cellular stress. When senescence is initiated, p53 is activated by either ATM/ATR or Chk1/2 protein to stimulate the transactivation of p21, which in turn activates the Rb pathway [26, 27]. It is important to mention that the levels, kinetics, and threshold of stressor intensity of p53 can determine whether a cell chooses to undergo apoptosis or senescence [28].

15.3 p53 MUTATION IN BC

A significant number of persons with the Li–Fraumeni cancer susceptibility syndrome have germline mutations in the p53 gene, which leads to a higher likelihood of developing BC [29]. This suggests that the deactivation of p53 is involved in the progression of BC, and there has been much research on the composition and p53 activity concerning BC. Previous research has shown that BC cell lines exhibit the presence of mutated p53 [30, 31]. LOH (loss of heterozygosity) in the p53 gene

TABLE 15.1
Frequency of p53 Mutation in Molecular Subtypes of BC

Molecular Subtypes of Breast Cancer	Frequency of p53 Mutation
Luminal A	17%
Luminal B	41%
Basal-like tumors	88%
HER2+	53%

is frequently observed in primary BCs [32, 33], often followed by mutation of the remaining allele in certain instances. The great majority of colon carcinomas have a mutant residual p53 allele, but in BC, wild-type p53 alleles are still present in at least 60% of LOH patients [32, 34]. However, other investigations have shown coding mutations in the p53 gene in BC. This is now widely acknowledged as a frequent, though not universal, genetic alteration in BC. A thorough meta-analysis has shown that mutant p53 is expressed in only around 20% of all instances [35]. Multiple research has aimed to determine the specific stage of BC development in which mutation in p53 occurs. Thorough examinations of micro-dissected tumor samples reveal that low-grade DCIS (ductal carcinoma in situ) has very few mutations, while high-grade DCIS tends to have a higher frequency of mutations [36].

While approximately 20% of cases of BC had a mutation in p53 [35], some subtypes of the illness exhibit greater rates (Table 15.1). Several studies have found a higher occurrence of p53 mutations in malignancies that develop in individuals with inherited BRCA1 and BRCA2 mutations [37–39]. Furthermore, these carcinomas have a unique range of p53 mutations [40]. Remarkably, the p53 mutation is present in 100% of instances in typical medullary breast carcinomas [41]. This is particularly intriguing because it is now well-acknowledged that medullary breast tumors have clinicopathological characteristics with instances associated with the BRCA1 gene. BRCA1 expression is frequently silenced through methylation-dependent mechanisms in medullary breast tumors [42, 43].

15.4 p53 ANTIBODIES AS DIAGNOSTIC MARKERS FOR CANCER

One interesting direction in the study of the therapeutic potential of p53 gene targeting in BC is the examination of antibodies against p53 as cancer diagnostic markers. These antibodies have become important diagnostic tools in the field of cancer in recent years because of their ability to identify and describe p53 protein expression. The complex relationship between changes in the p53 gene and cancer development emphasizes the need to create accurate diagnostic markers to improve early identification and prognostic evaluation. The use of p53 antibodies in precisely detecting abnormalities in the expression of p53 has been shown in pioneering investigations, which helps to stratify breast cancer patients according to unique clinicopathological features [44]. Furthermore, the sensitivity and specificity of p53 antibodies support their possible use in identifying subtypes of breast cancer and forecasting treatment outcomes. p53 antibody incorporation into diagnostic methods has the potential for enhancing patient outcomes generally, enabling prompt interventions, and refining individualized treatment plans [45]. As scientists learn more about the complex terrain of p53 in BC, using antibodies against p53 as diagnostic markers is an important development in the field. Sophisticated diagnostic methods are required to meet the complex role of the p53 system in cancer development, and p53 antibodies seem to be essential in this regard. The investigation of p53 antibodies as diagnostic markers is evidence of the continuous attempts to use creative approaches to decipher the complexity of breast cancer, paving the way for a day when early detection and focused therapies combine to improve patient care [46, 47].

15.5 p53 AS A PROGNOSTIC BIOMARKER

Mutations in the p53 gene are frequently linked to a negative outcome in BC [48, 49]. The nuclear p53 accumulation or the presence of p53 mutation is linked to a rapid rate of cancer growth, early recurrence of the illness, and early mortality in breast cancers that have not spread to the lymph nodes [50, 51]. Additionally, it is often seen as an indicator of more aggressive malignancy [52]. While several studies have shown that p53 overexpression can be a standalone indicator for delayed recurrence and overall survival in node-negative resectable BC [53]. The prognostic significance of p53 on its own is limited. It is most effective when used in conjunction with other cellular and molecular factors [54]. These indicators, such as estrogen and progesterone receptor expression, are used to assess the response to endocrine therapy [55]. The Bcl-2 proto-oncogene can be used as a reliable indicator for determining the effectiveness of adjuvant hormone therapy [56]. Additionally, the c-erb-2 (Her-2/neu) gene is associated with the tumor's ability to proliferate [57, 58]. The Ki67 antigen can be used as a predictor for both survival and recurrence [59]. Additionally, microvessel density can serve as a prediction for relapse-free survival, while the rate of cancer cell proliferation can indicate the malignant potential of the tumor [60, 61].

Although some markers, such as p53 coexpression and P-glycoprotein, consistently provide reliable results in indicating a worse prognosis than with p53 alone for locally advanced BC, there is considerable variation in findings across different studies [62, 63]. This has been unequivocally shown while examining p53 and c-erb-2. Studies have demonstrated that the overexpression of p53 and c-erb-2 proteins is associated with a more significant indication of a high likelihood of malignancy prediction of overall survival and a prediction of the interval without metastasis in cancers that do not involve the lymph nodes [64, 65]. These findings align with the results of previous studies conducted in patients with positive lymph nodes [66], where individuals who had an overexpression of c-erb-2 had a worse prognosis. On the other hand, some research groups have shown the opposite, which is that overexpression of c-erb-2 is linked to higher survival rates [67]. However, more recent studies have concluded that the coexpression of c-erb-2 and p53 does not have any meaningful impact as prognostic indicators [68, 69]. Based on the available information, p53 has little predictive ability as a standalone biological marker for predicting response to current therapies and illness outcomes.

15.6 p53 AS A PREDICTOR FOR TREATMENT STRATEGY OR DISEASE RESPONSE

Systemic adjuvant therapy, such as hormonal or systemic chemotherapy, has been proven to effectively decrease the recurrence of BC that is operable and extend the lifespan of patients [70–72]. Likewise, using chemotherapy as a neoadjuvant, together with subsequent surgery, radiation, or a combination of both, has the potential to enhance the prognosis of individuals diagnosed with locally advanced BC. Unfortunately, it has been challenging to definitively determine which groups of patients would benefit from further therapy and which groups would not, perhaps rendering such treatment ineffective or unnecessary. Multiple studies have indicated that the state of p53 plays a crucial role in determining how tumors respond to anti-cancer drugs [73–75]. Particular genetic alterations in the p53 gene have been linked to a negative reaction to first systemic treatment or reduced overall survival. The lack of normal p53 activity in breast tumors might lead to a decreased sensitivity to chemotherapeutic medicines. This is because p53 plays a crucial role in causing cell death or apoptosis, which is the main mechanism of action for many anti-cancer drugs [76–78].

The role of p53 as a reliable predictor for treatment response is still uncertain and is now being investigated in ongoing clinical studies. Currently, the presence of p53 mutation alone does not seem to accurately predict the response of BC to systemic treatment in clinical settings [79, 80]. In addition, recent research conducted in laboratory settings (in vitro) [81, 82] and in living organisms (in vivo) [64] have indicated that the activity of p53 may be separate from drug resistance and other cellular variables that are likely to have a significant impact on how the body responds to therapy. Therefore, current research is prioritizing the integration of data on the functionality and condition of p53 in its function of responding to therapy, together with information on other genes and products that are also recognized to play a part in cellular response. p53 regulates apoptosis by controlling the expression of Bcl-2 and Bax, which have opposing effects on apoptosis by inhibiting and promoting it, respectively [83–85]. The cellular response to apoptotic stimuli can be determined by the ratio of Bcl-2 to Bax, which can either promote cell survival or induce cell death [86]. The decrease in Bcl-2 and the increase in Bax expression, which occur in a p53-dependent way after systemic chemotherapy, indicate that evaluating the Bcl-2/Bax ratio and the p53 status can provide more useful information about cancer response to systemic chemotherapy [87]. The reliability of p53 as a standalone indicator for treatment response appears to be mostly influenced by the clinical stage of BC during the first diagnosis. While the nuclear accumulation of p53 is an important prognostic factor in early breast cancer (stage II/III), it does not appear to have the same independent prognostic importance in locally advanced BC (stage IIIA/IIIB) [62].

15.7 CONCLUSION

The occurrence of p53 gene mutations is common among BC patients, and this gene plays a crucial role in regulating cell proliferation and preventing the development of malignancies. Although the promise of a biomarker for mutant p53 in BC has been extensively studied, the therapeutic usefulness of measuring the mutant protein has not been confirmed. Nevertheless, the recent development of mutation-specific antibodies targeting various p53 mutations is expected to revive the investigation into the potential of mutant p53 as a biomarker. Until recently, there has been limited research on using the mutant protein as a therapeutic target for breast cancer, in contrast to its significance as a biomarker. Nevertheless, the discovery of numerous drugs that may restore the folded structure and activity of the mutant p53 protein has led to a probable surge in research focused on targeting mutant p53 in the next years. Restoring the activity of mutant p53 might be particularly crucial for patients with TN breast cancer, as they presently do not have a specific treatment available. While TN breast cancer exhibits significant heterogeneity, p53 mutations are present in as many as 80% of these individuals. Given the significant occurrence rate, it is imperative to prioritize the investigation of mutant p53 as a key focus in the study on TNBC therapy. Future studies should focus on determining the efficacy of the aforementioned medications against other p53 mutations, as well as their ability to bind to proteins other than p53. It is crucial that we promptly determine if the aforementioned chemicals have anti-cancer properties against human tumors.

REFERENCES

1. Jan, N., et al., Exploring the role of trifarotene against RAR-α: an investigation of expression pattern and clinicopathological significance of RAR-α in breast cancer. *Frontiers in Pharmacology*, 2024. **15**: p. 1361679.
2. Jan, N., et al., Targeting breast cancer stem cells through retinoids: a new hope for treatment. *Critical Reviews in Oncology/Hematology*, 2023: p. 104156.
3. Yersal, O. and S. Barutca, Biological subtypes of breast cancer: Prognostic and therapeutic implications. *World Journal of Clinical Oncology*, 2014. **5**(3): p. 412.
4. Jan, N., et al., Elucidation of interleukin-19 as a therapeutic target for breast cancer by computational analysis and experimental validation. *Saudi Journal of Biological Sciences*, 2023. **30**(9): p. 103774.
5. Ungerleider, N.A., et al., Breast cancer survival predicted by TP53 mutation status differs markedly depending on treatment. *Breast Cancer Research*, 2018. **20**: p. 1–8.
6. Haq, B.U., et al., Targeting p53 misfolding conundrum by stabilizing agents and their analogs in breast cancer therapy: a comprehensive computational analysis. *Frontiers in Pharmacology*, 2024. **14**: p. 1333447.

7. Jan, N., et al., Metronomic chemotherapy and drug repurposing: a paradigm shift in oncology. *Heliyon*, 2024. https://doi.org/10.1016/j.heliyon.2024.e24670
8. Pitolli, C., et al., Do mutations turn p53 into an oncogene? *International Journal of Molecular Sciences*, 2019. **20**(24). p. 6241.
9. Desmedt, C., et al., Next-generation sequencing in breast cancer: first take home messages. *Current Opinion in Oncology*, 2012. **24**(6): p. 597–604.
10. Lai, H., et al., Spectrum of p53 tumor suppressor gene mutations and breast cancer survival. *Breast Cancer Research and Treatment*, 2004. **83**: p. 57–66.
11. Mir, M.A. and A. Jan, *Introduction to Cell Cycle and Its Regulators in Therapeutic Potential of Cell Cycle Kinases in Breast Cancer.* 2023, Springer. p. 53–82.
12. Gottifredi, V. and C. Prives, Getting p53 out of the nucleus. *Science*, 2001. **292**(5523): p. 1851–1852.
13. Khoury, M.P. and J.-C. Bourdon, The isoforms of the p53 protein. *Cold Spring Harbor Perspectives in Biology*, 2010. **2**(3): p. a000927.
14. Zhang, B., et al., The function of Drosophila p53 isoforms in apoptosis. *Cell Death & Differentiation*, 2015. **22**(12): p. 2058–2067.
15. Zhao, L. and S. Sanyal, p53 isoforms as cancer biomarkers and therapeutic targets. *Cancers*, 2022. **14**(13): p. 3145.
16. Georgakilas, A.G., O.A. Martin, and W.M. Bonner, p21: a two-faced genome guardian. *Trends in Molecular Medicine*, 2017. **23**(4): p. 310–319.
17. Williams, A.B. and B. Schumacher, p53 in the DNA-damage-repair process. *Cold Spring Harbor Perspectives in Medicine*, 2016. **6**(5): p. a026070.
18. Giono, L.E. and J.J. Manfredi, The p53 tumor suppressor participates in multiple cell cycle checkpoints. *Journal of Cellular Physiology*, 2006. **209**(1): p. 13–20.
19. Helton, E.S. and X. Chen, p53 modulation of the DNA damage response. *Journal of Cellular Biochemistry*, 2007. **100**(4): p. 883–896.
20. Clarke, A., et al., Thymocyte apoptosis induced by p53-dependent and independent pathways. *Nature*, 1993. **362**(6423): p. 849–852.
21. Lowe, S.W. and H.E. Ruley, Stabilization of the p53 tumor suppressor is induced by adenovirus 5 E1A and accompanies apoptosis. *Genes & Development*, 1993. **7**(4): p. 535–545.
22. Riley, T., et al., Transcriptional control of human p53-regulated genes. *Nature Reviews Molecular Cell Biology*, 2008. **9**(5): p. 402–412.
23. Tait, S.W. and D.R. Green, Mitochondria and cell death: outer membrane permeabilization and beyond. *Nature Reviews Molecular Cell Biology*, 2010. **11**(9): p. 621–632.
24. Chen, J., The cell-cycle arrest and apoptotic functions of p53 in tumor initiation and progression. *Cold Spring Harbor Perspectives in Medicine*, 2016. **6**(3): p. a026104.
25. Sofi, S., et al., Clinicopathological and prognostic significance of Bcl2 in breast cancer: a comprehensive in silico and in vitro study. *Saudi Journal of Biological Sciences*, 2023. **31**(2): p. 103916.
26. Dolan, D.W., et al., Integrated stochastic model of DNA damage repair by non-homologous end joining and p53/p21-mediated early senescence signalling. *PLoS Computational Biology*, 2015. **11**(5): p. e1004246.
27. Sofi, S., et al., A comprehensive analysis of notch signaling genes in breast cancer: expression pattern and prognostic significance. *Advances in Cancer Biology-Metastasis*, 2023. **7**: p. 100104.
28. Mijit, M., et al., Role of p53 in the regulation of cellular senescence. *Biomolecules*, 2020. **10**(3): p. 420.
29. Malkin, D., et al., Germ line p53 mutations in a familial syndrome of breast cancer, sarcomas, and other neoplasms. *Science*, 1990. **250**(4985): p. 1233–1238.
30. Bartek, J., et al., Genetic and immunochemical analysis of mutant p53 in human breast cancer cell lines. *Oncogene*, 1990. **5**(6): p. 893–899.
31. Mir, M.A., et al., Metronomics: toward personalized chemotherapy. *Novel Approaches in Metronomic Chemotherapy for Breast Cancer Treatment*, 2024. p. 99–119. https://doi.org/10.1201/9781032632674-8
32. Davidoff, A.M., et al., Genetic basis for p53 overexpression in human breast cancer. *Proceedings of the National Academy of Sciences*, 1991. **88**(11): p. 5006–5010.
33. Mir, M.A., N. Jan, and I. Noor, Therapeutic Implications of Cytokines and Chemokines Network in Cancer, in *Cytokine and Chemokine Networks in Cancer.* 2023, Springer. p. 385–414.
34. Mir, M.A., A. Manzoor, and N. Jan, CCL5/CCR5 Axis in Cancer, in *Cytokine and Chemokine Networks in Cancer.* 2023, Springer. p. 219–240.
35. Pharoah, P., N. Day, and C. Caldas, Somatic mutations in the p53 gene and prognosis in breast cancer: a meta-analysis. *British Journal of Cancer*, 1999. **80**(12): p. 1968–1973.

36. Done, S.J., et al., p53 missense mutations in microdissected high-grade ductal carcinoma in situ of the breast. *Journal of the National Cancer Institute*, 2001. **93**(9): p. 700–704.
37. Smith, P.D., et al., Novel p53 mutants selected in BRCA-associated tumours which dissociate transformation suppression from other wild-type p53 functions. *Oncogene*, 1999. **18**(15): p. 2451–2459.
38. Phillips, K.-A., et al., Frequency of p53 mutations in breast carcinomas from Ashkenazi Jewish carriers of BRCA1 mutations. *Journal of the National Cancer Institute*, 1999. **91**(5): p. 469–473.
39. Mir, M.A., A. Shabir, and N. Jan, Metronomic Chemotherapy in Breast Cancer, in *Novel Approaches in Metronomic Chemotherapy for Breast Cancer Treatment*. CRC Press. p. 72–86.
40. Greenblatt, M.S., et al., TP53 mutations in breast cancer associated with BRCA1 or BRCA2 germline mutations: distinctive spectrum and structural distribution. *Cancer Research*, 2001. **61**(10): p. 4092–4097.
41. de Cremoux, P., et al., p53 mutation as a genetic trait of typical medullary breast carcinoma. *Journal of the National Cancer Institute*, 1999. **91**(7): p. 641–643.
42. Esteller, M., et al., Promoter hypermethylation and BRCA1 inactivation in sporadic breast and ovarian tumors. *JNCI: Journal of the National Cancer Institute*, 2000. **92**(7): p. 564–569.
43. Mir, M.A., N. Jan, and H. Qayoom, Conventional Chemotherapy vs. Metronomic Chemotherapy, in *Novel Approaches in Metronomic Chemotherapy for Breast Cancer Treatment*. CRC Press. p. 27–42.
44. Xiao, Y., et al., Combining p53 mRNA nanotherapy with immune checkpoint blockade reprograms the immune microenvironment for effective cancer therapy. *Nature Communications*, 2022. **13**(1): p. 758.
45. Levine, A.J., P53 and the immune response: 40 years of exploration—a plan for the future. *International Journal of Molecular Sciences*, 2020. **21**(2): p. 541.
46. Li, L., M. Li, and X. Wang, Cancer type-dependent correlations between TP53 mutations and antitumor immunity. *DNA Repair*, 2020. **88**: p. 102785.
47. Mir, M.A., et al., Proteomics: Application of Next-Generation Proteomics in Cancer Research, in *Proteomics*. 2023, Elsevier. p. 55–76.
48. Elledge, R.M. and D.C. Allred, The p53 tumor suppressor gene in breast cancer. *Breast Cancer Research and Treatment*, 1994. **32**: p. 39–47.
49. Sjögren, S., et al., The p53 gene in breast cancer: prognostic value of complementary DNA sequencing versus immunohistochemistry. *JNCI: Journal of the National Cancer Institute*, 1996. **88**(3–4): p. 173–182.
50. Allred, D.C., et al., Association of p53 protein expression with tumor cell proliferation rate and clinical outcome in node-negative breast cancer. *JNCI: Journal of the National Cancer Institute*, 1993. **85**(3): p. 200–206.
51. Mir, M.A., et al., Proteomics: A Groundbreaking Development in Cancer Biology, in *Proteomics*. 2023, Elsevier. p. 31–53.
52. Falette, N., et al., Prognostic value of P53 gene mutations in a large series of node-negative breast cancer patients. *Cancer Research*, 1998. **58**(7): p. 1451–1455.
53. Silvestrini, R., et al., p53 as an independent prognostic marker in lymph node-negative breast cancer patients. *JNCI: Journal of the National Cancer Institute*, 1993. **85**(12): p. 965–970.
54. Ostrowski, J., et al., p53 expression in human breast cancer related to survival and prognostic factors: an immunohistochemical study. *The Journal of Pathology*, 1991. **164**(1): p. 75–81.
55. Allegra, J.C., et al., Estrogen receptor status: an important variable in predicting response to endocrine therapy in metastatic breast cancer. *European Journal of Cancer (1965)*, 1980. **16**(3): p. 323–331.
56. Gasparini, G., et al., Expression of bcl-2 protein predicts efficacy of adjuvant treatments in operable node-positive breast cancer. *Clinical Cancer Research: An Official Journal of the American Association for Cancer Research*, 1995. **1**(2): p. 189–198.
57. Allred, D.C., et al., HER-2/neu in node-negative breast cancer: prognostic significance of overexpression influenced by the presence of in situ carcinoma. *Journal of Clinical Oncology*, 1992. **10**(4): p. 599–605.
58. Gusterson, B., et al., Prognostic importance of c-erbB-2 expression in breast cancer. International (Ludwig) Breast Cancer Study Group. *Journal of Clinical Oncology*, 1992. **10**(7): p. 1049–1056.
59. Clark, G.M., et al., Prediction of relapse or survival in patients with node-negative breast cancer by DNA flow cytometry. *New England Journal of Medicine*, 1989. **320**(10): p. 627–633.
60. Isola, J., et al., Association of overexpression of tumor suppressor protein p53 with rapid cell proliferation and poor prognosis in node-negative breast cancer patients. *JNCI: Journal of the National Cancer Institute*, 1992. **84**(14): p. 1109–1114.
61. Mir, M.A., N. Jan, and S. Sofi, Introduction to Metronomic Chemotherapy, in *Novel Approaches in Metronomic Chemotherapy for Breast Cancer Treatment*. 2024, CRC Press. p. 1–14.

62. Honkoop, A., et al., Prognostic role of clinical, pathological and biological characteristics in patients with locally advanced breast cancer. *British Journal of Cancer*, 1998. **77**(4): p. 621–626.
63. Linn, S., et al., p53 and P-glycoprotein are often co-expressed and are associated with poor prognosis in breast cancer. *British Journal of Cancer*, 1996. **74**(1): p. 63–68.
64. MacGrogan, G., et al., Primary chemotherapy in breast invasive carcinoma: predictive value of the immunohistochemical detection of hormonal receptors, p53, c-erbB-2, MiB1, pS2 and GST pi. *British Journal of Cancer*, 1996. **74**(9): p. 1458–1465.
65. Mir, M.A., et al., Imaging Techniques, Biomarkers, and Methods for Metronomic Chemotherapy, in *Novel Approaches in Metronomic Chemotherapy for Breast Cancer Treatment*. CRC Press. p. 58–71.
66. Gasparini, G., et al., Human breast cancer: prognostic significance of the c-erbB-2 oncoprotein compared with epidermal growth factor receptor, DNA ploidy, and conventional pathologic features. *Journal of Clinical Oncology*, 1992. **10**(5): p. 686–695.
67. Muss, H.B., et al., c-erbB-2 expression and response to adjuvant therapy in women with node-positive early breast cancer. *New England Journal of Medicine*, 1994. **330**(18): p. 1260–1266.
68. Rozan, S., et al., No significant predictive value of c-erbB-2 or p53 expression regarding sensitivity to primary chemotherapy or radiotherapy in breast cancer. *International Journal of Cancer*, 1998. **79**(1): p. 27–33.
69. Mir, M.A., M. Bashir, and N. Jan, The Role of Interleukin (IL)-6/IL-6 Receptor Axis in Cancer, in *Cytokine and Chemokine Networks in Cancer*. 2023, Springer. p. 137–164.
70. Group, E.B.C.T.C., Tamoxifen for early breast cancer: an overview of the randomised trials. *Lancet (London, England)*, 1998. **351**(9114): p. 1451–1467.
71. Goldhirsch, A., et al., Meeting highlights: international consensus panel on the treatment of primary breast cancer. *Journal of the National Cancer Institute*, 1998. **90**(21): p. 1601–1608.
72. Mir, M.A., Sumaya, N. Jan, Implications of Chemokine Heterogenicity in Cancer Metastasis, in *Cytokine and Chemokine Networks in Cancer*. 2023, Springer. p. 115–136.
73. Lowe, S.W., et al., p53 status and the efficacy of cancer therapy in vivo. *Science*, 1994. **266**(5186): p. 807–810.
74. Clahsen, P.C., et al., p53 protein accumulation and response to adjuvant chemotherapy in premenopausal women with node-negative early breast cancer. *Journal of Clinical Oncology*, 1998. **16**(2): p. 470–479.
75. Mir, M.A., M. Rashid, and N. Jan, Cytokines and Chemokines in Tumor Growth and Progression, in *Cytokine and Chemokine Networks in Cancer*. 2023, Springer. p. 33–77.
76. Carson, D.A. and J.M. Ribeiro, Apoptosis and disease. *The Lancet*, 1993. **341**(8855): p. 1251–1254.
77. Fisher, D.E., Apoptosis in cancer therapy: crossing the threshold. *Cell*, 1994. **78**(4): p. 539–542.
78. Thompson, C.B., Apoptosis in the pathogenesis and treatment of disease. *Science*, 1995. **267**(5203): p. 1456–1462.
79. Hazar, B., et al., p53 protein expression in gastrointestinal lymphomas. *Oncology*, 1997. **54**(1): p. 84–87.
80. Paradiso, A., et al., p53 and PCNA expression in advanced colorectal cancer: response to chemotherapy and long-term prognosis. *International Journal of Cancer*, 1996. **69**(6): p. 437–441.
81. Wosikowski, K., et al., Normal p53 status and function despite the development of drug resistance in human breast cancer cells. *Cell Growth and Differentiation-Publication American Association for Cancer Research*, 1995. **6**(11): p. 1395–1404.
82. Gudas, J.M., et al., CANCER BIOLOGY: Drug-resistant breast cancer cells frequently retain expression of a functional wild-type p53 protein. *Carcinogenesis*, 1996. **17**(7): p. 1417–1427.
83. Kobayashi, S., et al., Clinical significance of bcl-2 gene expression in human breast cancer tissues. *Breast Cancer Research and Treatment*, 1997. **42**: p. 173–181.
84. Miyashita, T., et al., Identification of a p53-dependent negative response element in the bcl-2 gene. *Cancer Research*, 1994. **54**(12): p. 3131–3135.
85. Toshiyuki, M. and J.C. Reed, Tumor suppressor p53 is a direct transcriptional activator of the human bax gene. *Cell*, 1995. **80**(2): p. 293–299.
86. Oltval, Z.N., C.L. Milliman, and S.J. Korsmeyer, Bcl-2 heterodimerizes in vivo with a conserved homolog, Bax, that accelerates programed cell death. *Cell*, 1993. **74**(4): p. 609–619.
87. Suzuki, K., et al., Drug-induced apoptosis and p53, BCL-2 and BAX expression in breast cancer tissues in vivo and in fibroblast cells in vitro. *Japanese Journal of Clinical Oncology*, 1999. **29**(7): p. 323–331.

16 The Impact of Nutrition on p53 Activity

Implications for Preventing and Treating Breast Cancer

*Tabish Javeed, Nusrat Jan, and Manzoor Ahmad Mir**
Department of Bioresources, School of Biological Sciences, University of Kashmir, Srinagar, J&K, India
*drmanzoor@kashmiruniversity.ac.in

16.1 INTRODUCTION

Cancer is a major cause of death globally, with 18.1 million new cases and 9.6 million deaths reported in 2018 [1–3]. In the US, the National Institutes of Health estimated 1.8 million new cancer cases in 2020 and 606,520 deaths [3]. Traditional cancer treatments include surgery, radiotherapy, chemotherapy, endocrine therapy, and targeted therapy [4]. However, these treatments often come with significant limitations, such as severe side effects and dose-limiting toxicities [5]. Common adverse effects of cancer treatments include nausea, vomiting, peripheral neuropathy, pain, and insomnia, all of which reduce the quality of life [5, 6]. Therefore, there is an urgent need for alternative therapeutic agents that can provide better patient outcomes. Recent epidemiological studies have found a strong link between reduced cancer risk and the consumption of fruits and vegetables [7–9]. Plants produce various defensive secondary metabolites, including polyphenols, isoprenoids, alkaloids, sulforaphanes, and certain vitamins and their precursors [10, 11]. These phytochemicals generally act as antioxidants at low concentrations, scavenging free radicals such as reactive oxygen species (ROS), and protecting cells from oxidative damage to proteins, lipids, DNA, and RNA [12]. Numerous studies have indicated that regularly consuming fruits, vegetables, and products containing phytochemicals can help prevent various types of cancer [13–15]. Phytochemicals also demonstrate anticancer activity through various signaling pathways, including the death receptor or extrinsic pathway, the mitochondrial or intrinsic pathway, and the perforin/granzyme apoptotic pathway [16–19].

The p53 protein, discovered in 1979, was named based on its molecular mass of 53 kDa, as determined by SDS-PAGE analysis [20]. In humans, the p53 gene is located on the short arm of chromosome 17 [21]. Known as the "guardian of the genome," p53 is a potent tumor suppressor composed of 393 amino acid residues and three main domains: the transcriptional activation domain (TAD), the DNA-binding domain (DBD), and the tetramerization (TET) domain [22]. The TAD employs RNA polymerase and initiates the DNA-reading process. The DBD, which is rich in arginine and lysine residues and highly susceptible to mutations, binds to specific regulatory sites on DNA response elements. The TET domain facilitates the assembly of p53 monomers into oligomers [23].

The primary function of the p53 protein, encoded by the TP53 gene on human chromosome 17, is to suppress tumors. p53 achieves this by interacting with multiple signaling pathways that are crucial for cell division, genomic stability, apoptosis, autophagy, immune response, and the regulation of the tumor microenvironment (TME) [22]. When the wild-type p53 protein binds to specific DNA

DOI: 10.1201/9781003520771-16

response elements, it triggers the expression of various genes that protect against cancer development and progression [24, 25]. Under normal conditions, cells exposed to different stress signals activate the p53 signaling pathway. This activation allows cells to initiate several transcriptional programs, including cell cycle arrest, DNA repair, senescence, and apoptosis, all of which contribute to suppressing tumor growth [3].

In most human cancers, the TP53 gene is inactivated, usually through loss-of-function mutations or negative regulation of wild-type p53 proteins. This inactivation promotes invasion, proliferation, and cell survival, facilitating cancer progression and metastasis [3]. Over 75% of TP53 gene mutations lead to the loss of wild-type p53's activities. Mutated p53 proteins can act as dominant negatives over wild-type p53 or acquire new tumorigenic properties that counteract the protective function of wild-type p53 [26, 27]. Two homologs of the tumor-suppressive transcription factor p53, namely, p73 and p63, also play crucial roles in cancer development. Due to structural similarities within the p53 family, p73 and p63 can bind to most p53-responsive promoters and initiate transcription. In addition to shared functions with p53, such as activating apoptosis in response to cellular stress, p63 and p73 have unique roles due to structural differences. These family members have overlapping and distinct responsibilities in development and homeostasis. The functional connections between p53, p73, and p63 can be better understood by examining the expression of p73 and p63 isoforms in human tissues. TP63 expression is significantly correlated across various tissues, and in tissues with concurrent mRNA expression, both proteins are often co-expressed in the nuclei of the majority of cells [28].

This book chapter will explore recent advancements in understanding how mutant p53 proteins may modulate molecular signaling pathways involved in cancer progression and protection. Furthermore, the significance, regulation, and signaling pathway modulated by dietary antioxidants influencing p53 are discussed in detail.

16.2 SIGNIFICANCE OF p53

The primary function of p53 is to regulate cell cycle progression, DNA repair, and apoptosis. In vertebrates, p53 can temporarily halt the cell cycle to allow for DNA repair. Additionally, p53 can induce cellular senescence or trigger apoptosis under certain conditions, thereby preventing the accumulation of potentially cancerous or defective cells [29].

16.2.1 Apoptosis

Apoptosis is a crucial process that prevents the spread of cells with abnormal DNA. In mammals, p53 controls apoptosis by activating genes that promote cell death through two main pathways: the extrinsic pathway and the intrinsic pathway [30, 31]. The extrinsic pathway is triggered by proteins from the tumor necrosis factor receptor (TNF-R) family. Key genes involved include the Fas cell surface death receptor (Fas), death receptor 5 (DR5), and the p53 apoptosis effector related to PMP22 (PERP). Overexpression of p53 can increase Fas levels on the cell surface, making cells more sensitive to Fas-induced apoptosis, which is activated when Fas binds to its ligand FasL, expressed by T-cells. DR5 is activated by the tumor necrosis factor-related apoptosis-inducing ligand (TRAIL), which leads to cell death through the caspase-8 pathway [23, 32].

The intrinsic pathway is regulated by the B-cell lymphoma 2 (Bcl-2) family of proteins, including Bcl-2-associated X protein (Bax), p53 upregulated modulator of apoptosis (Puma), and damage protein (Noxa). These proteins form channels in the mitochondrial membrane, allowing cytochrome c (Cyt c) to escape. BID, a Bcl-2 family member, links the extrinsic and intrinsic pathways by being cleaved by caspase-8 after TNF-R exposure and then activating Bax. p53 also promotes the formation of the apoptosome by inducing Cyt c and apoptotic protease-activating factor 1 (Apaf-1), which together activate caspase-9. Caspase-9 responds to changes in the mitochondria, while caspase-8 is triggered by death receptor activation. Both initiator caspases activate effector caspases, such as caspase-3, caspase-6, and caspase-7, which then break down essential cellular components, leading to cell death [11, 33, 34].

16.2.2 Senescence

When the cell cycle is permanently halted, it leads to cellular senescence, which helps prevent the spread of mutations and thus acts as a cancer-preventive mechanism [35]. Senescence, therefore, plays a critical role in cancer prevention. However, the loss of p53 can undermine this process, particularly senescence induced by oncogenes. Although the exact molecular mechanisms remain unclear, several microRNAs and genes targeted by p53 have been implicated in both senescence and the effects of p53 depletion [36]. The p53 protein has both prooxidant and antioxidant functions, depending on the level of stress the cell is under, which contributes to its role in tumor suppression [23, 37]. When stress is mild, p53 acts as a prooxidant, allowing cells to repair damage and survive. In conditions of extreme stress, p53 functions as an antioxidant, supporting apoptosis to prevent the survival of damaged cells [38, 39].

16.2.3 Cell Cycle Arrest

Cyclins and cyclin-dependent kinases (CDKs) are essential proteins that regulate the progression of the cell cycle. When DNA damage occurs, the cell cycle is halted at the G2/M phase to prevent the spread of mutations to daughter cells. This arrest is managed by p53 through its regulation of the protein p21 [40]. The involvement of p53 in the cell cycle was first demonstrated by Kastan and colleagues in 1991, who found that the expression of the GADD45 protein depended on the presence of wild-type p53 following exposure to ionizing radiation [41]. GADD45, induced by p53, also plays a role in DNA repair. Additionally, p53 is crucial for proper mitotic cell division, as it regulates centrosome function. By blocking the mitotic spindle assembly with nocodazole, p53 activates the ataxia telangiectasia-mutated protein kinase (ATM), a key initiator of the DNA damage repair pathway [42, 43].

16.2.4 DNA Repair

The final goal of the DNA damage response (DDR) process is to repair DNA. DNA damage can be caused by internal factors such as ROS, free radicals, and certain cellular metabolites. External factors like UV light, specific drugs, and heavy metals can also damage DNA. These factors can alter the nucleotide bases of DNA, leading to breaks in the DNA strands [44, 45].

16.3 REGULATION OF p53

Excessive p53 activity is detrimental to cell survival and normal growth, so its levels are tightly regulated through a process called ubiquitination and subsequent degradation. This regulation is mainly mediated by the E3 ubiquitin ligase known as mouse double minute 2 homolog (MDM2) [46, 47]. When cells experience various stress signals, such as oxidative stress, oncogene activation, telomere shortening, and low oxygen (hypoxia), MDM2 is induced, which activates p53 [48]. MDM2 and its close relative, double minute X human homolog (MDMX), are controlled by both negative and positive regulators, creating a feedback loop.

The primary way to suppress p53 is through its negative regulator, MDM2 [49, 50]. p53 itself induces MDM2, and this leads to a self-regulating feedback loop where MDM2 inactivates p53 by tagging it for degradation. High levels of MDM2 can disable p53's functions, such as triggering apoptosis and halting the cell cycle. MDM2 and p53 together form an autoregulatory loop that maintains cellular balance. MDM2, acting as an E3 ubiquitin ligase, attaches ubiquitin molecules to p53, marking it for degradation [51–53]. Several studies have extensively reviewed the roles of the p53–MDM2 pathway in the onset, progression, and spread of human cancers [54–56]. Consequently, the regulation of p53 and MDM2 is crucial for their proper expression and function in both normal and cancer cells [49, 57] (Figure 16.1).

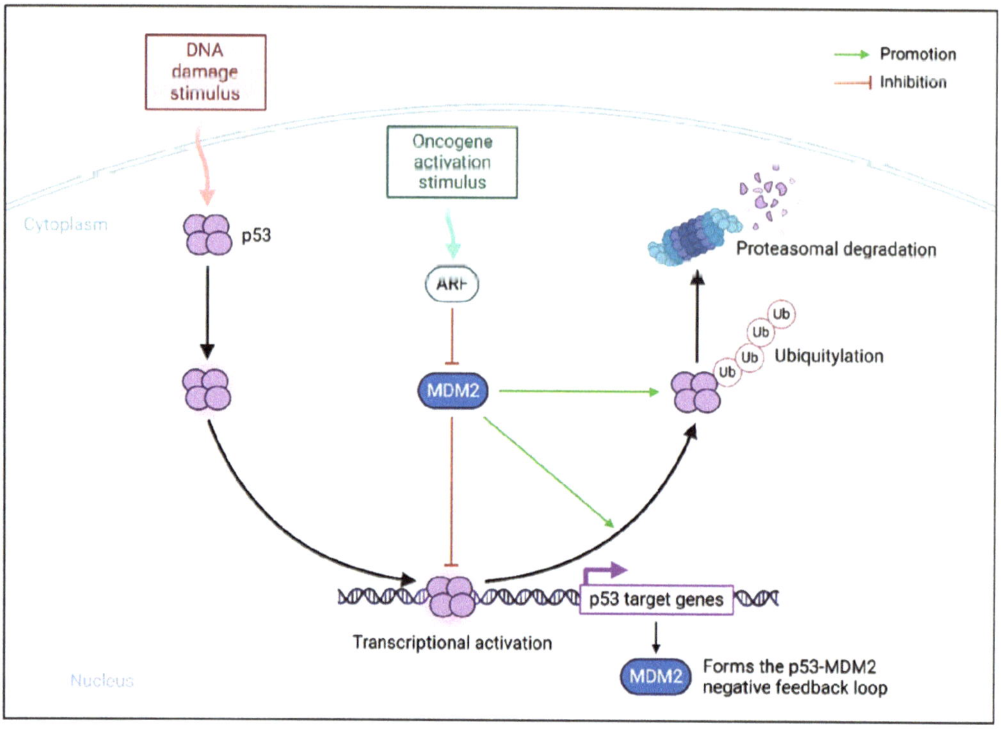

FIGURE 16.1 Mechanism of p53 regulation by MDM2.

16.3.1 Normal Cells

In normal cells, the level of p53 protein is kept very low because it is constantly tagged for degradation by MDM2 and MDMX. This regulation by MDM2 and MDMX is essential for keeping p53 in check, allowing it to be quickly activated when needed to prevent cancer. When p53 does accumulate in cells, it stimulates the production of MDM2, creating a feedback loop where MDM2 binds to p53 and inhibits its activity, ensuring p53 does not stay active for too long [58]. When DNA damage occurs, p53 is activated through a series of stress responses involving various kinases like ATM, ATR, Chk1, and Chk2, which modify MDM2 and MDMX, interrupting their suppression of p53 [59, 60]. This activation mainly occurs through post-translational modifications, increasing the stability and half-life of p53, and allowing it to accumulate in cells. p53 controls over 100 target genes involved in various critical functions [61, 62]. These include promoting apoptosis through genes like Bax, Noxa, DR5, PERP, and Puma, and causing cell cycle arrest through genes like p21, GADD45, Ypel3, and Pml [63]. These genes are involved in multiple regulatory processes, including cell signaling, extracellular matrix regulation, and maintaining cellular structure. The activity of p53 is finely tuned by several modifications, including acetylation, methylation, ubiquitination, and phosphorylation [23, 64, 65].

16.3.2 Cancer Cells

The p53 gene can exist in either a wild-type (normal) or mutant form. It is estimated that over 50% of all malignant tumors have mutations in the p53 gene [66]. Mutated p53 is more likely to promote cancer development compared to wild-type p53, which acts as a tumor suppressor by activating other genes to prevent cancer growth [67]. The loss of p53 function is closely linked to cancer development in many different organs [68]. Animals with mutant p53 have significantly reduced transcriptional activity, making them more susceptible to developing tumors [66]. Studies have found that more than half of human cancers have p53 mutations [69, 70]. About 95% of these mutations occur in the region of the gene that encodes the DNA-binding domain, and approximately 30% of mutations happen in six specific amino acids: Arg175, Gly245, Arg248, Arg249, Arg273, and Arg282 [71, 72]. These mutations disrupt the normal structure and function of p53, preventing it from activating the genes it normally regulates. Additionally, mutant p53 can interfere with wild-type p53 by forming defective complexes, further contributing to its cancer-promoting effects [73, 74]. Mutant p53 interacts with several transcription factors, including nuclear factor Y (NF-Y), E2F transcription factors (E2Fs), NF-kappa B p65 (NF-κBp65), NF-kappa B p50 (NF-κBp50), sterol regulatory element-binding protein (SREBP), Yes-associated protein (YAP), vitamin D receptor (VDR), and nuclear factor erythroid 2-related factor 2 (Nrf2). These interactions change the expression of various genes. Mutant p53 loses its ability to activate normal p53 target genes and can even suppress the function of wild-type p53 [26, 75]. In cancer cells, mutant p53 often becomes stabilized, whereas wild-type p53 has a short lifespan in both normal and cancerous tissues [76]. Like wild-type p53, mutant p53 is degraded by the proteasome, a protein complex responsible for breaking down unneeded proteins, with the help of E3 ubiquitin ligases like MDM2 [77]. However, mutant p53 can still become stabilized and active in response to cancer-related stress, similar to wild-type p53.

Studies have shown that certain cancer-derived mutant forms of p53 can activate various genes, including multiple drug resistance gene 1 (MDR1), c-myc, proliferating cell nuclear antigen (PCNA), interleukin-6 (IL-6), insulin-like growth factor 1 (IGF-1), fibroblast growth factor (FGF), epidermal growth factor receptor (EGFR), asparagine synthetase (ASNS), and telomerase reverse transcriptase (TERT) [23, 69, 78]. Therefore, mutant p53 contributes to the progression of aggressive cancers by promoting the expression of genes that support cancer growth and survival (Figure 16.2).

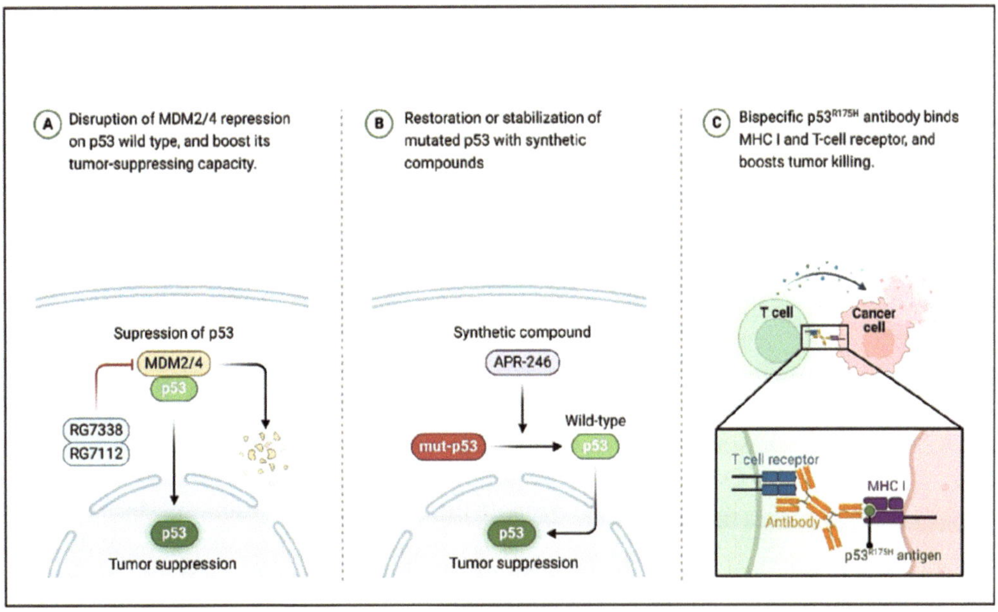

FIGURE 16.2 Cancer-targeting therapies for p53.

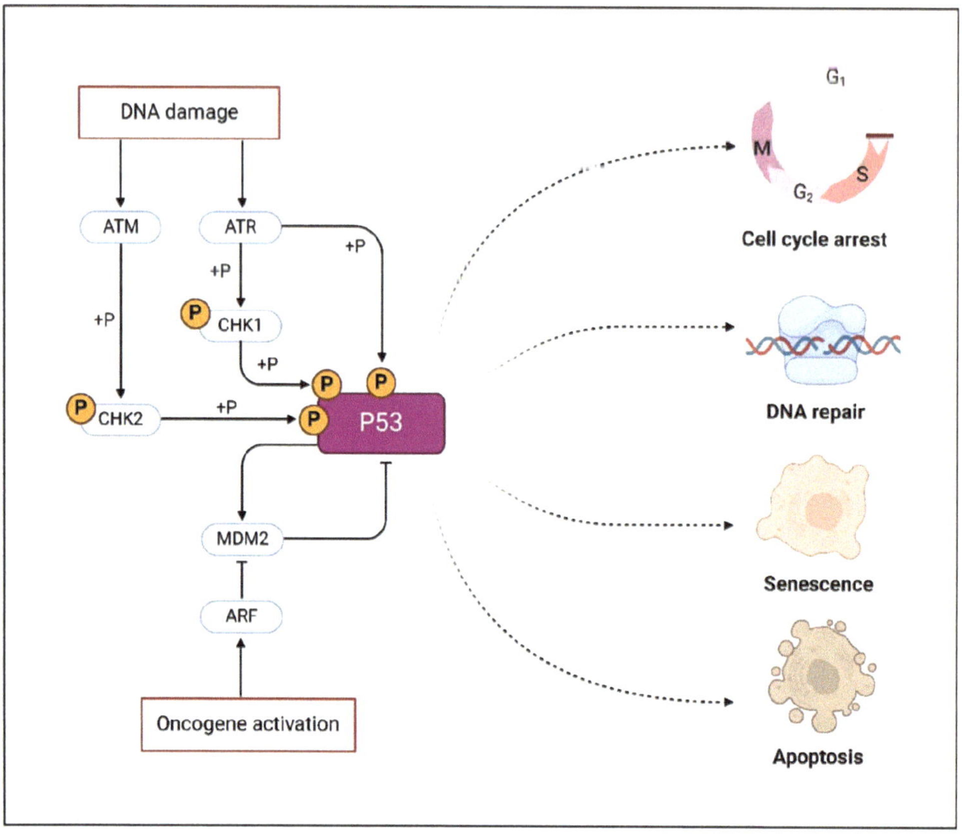

FIGURE 16.3 Signaling pathways involved in p53 regulation.

16.4 p53 SIGNALING PATHWAY MODULATED BY DIETARY ANTIOXIDANTS

Many studies have shown that bioactive compounds found in foods can strengthen the immune system and slow cancer development [79–81]. These compounds work by reducing cell growth, neutralizing cancer-causing agents, preventing the formation of new blood vessels that feed tumors, stopping the cell cycle, and triggering cell death. They also influence various cell signaling pathways. The cancer-preventing and cancer-fighting effects of dietary antioxidants have been observed in both normal and cancerous cells through the p53 signaling pathway [82–85] (Figure 16.3).

16.4.1 Vitamins

Vitamins can slow cell growth and induce cell death by increasing the levels of p53, p21, and Bax, and reducing Bcl-2 in T-cell colonies [23]. Studies have demonstrated that non-toxic doses of vitamin C boosted the expression of p53 [86, 87]. Vitamin C also enhances the effectiveness of the anticancer drug bleomycin in causing DNA double-strand breaks, making cancer cells more reliant on DNA repair mechanisms for survival [88]. Vitamin B6 activates the p53 pathway, which controls the transcription of p21 mRNA in various cancer cell lines, including HT29, Caco2, LoVo, HEK293T, and HepG2 [89]. Mice fed a diet with adequate vitamin B6 showed higher levels of p21 mRNA in their colons compared to those on a vitamin B6-deficient diet, indicating that vitamin B6's antitumor effects may be linked to the activation of p53 and increased p21 mRNA levels [23, 53].

Studies have suggested that 1,25-dihydroxyvitamin D increases oxidative stress by inhibiting the transcription of Nrf2, leading to DNA damage and activation of p16/Rb and p53/p21 signaling in a specific mouse model [90–92]. Folic acid (vitamin B9) may play a significant role in preventing gastric cancer [23]. In humans, folic acid supplementation increased p53 expression in the gastric mucosa while decreasing the expression of the oncogene protein Bcl-2. N-acetylcysteine (NAC) inhibits PDK1 expression through PPARα-mediated induction of p53 and reduction of p65 protein expression, revealing a novel mechanism by which NAC, combined with the PPARα ligand, inhibits the growth of non-small-cell lung carcinoma (NSCLC) cells [23]. Water-soluble vitamin E (Trolox) supplementation, however, promoted breast cancer growth by reducing ROS and p53 expression in mice [93]. While β-carotene, ascorbic acid, and vitamin E (α-tocopherol) protect against oxidative stress, they did not directly influence p53 expression in stressed rats [23, 94]. On the other hand, β-carotene increased DNA oxidative damage and altered p53-related pathways of cell proliferation and apoptosis in cultured RAT-1 fibroblasts exposed to tobacco smoke condensate [23, 62, 95].

16.4.2 Flavonoids

Flavonoids are thought to reduce chronic inflammation mediated by p53, which can help prevent cancer progression [96]. For example, quercetin, a type of flavonoid, can cause the phosphorylation (a type of activation) of ATM and histone H2AX, leading to the accumulation and activation of p53 even in cells without ATM, showing that quercetin can activate p53 independently of ATM [97, 98]. Quercetin also causes DNA damage and increases p53 phosphorylation, leading to apoptosis (cell death) in human leukemia cells in a dose-dependent manner. It also inhibits the growth of HeLa cells by stopping the cell cycle at the G2/M phase and inducing apoptosis through disruption of the mitochondrial membrane and activation of the intrinsic apoptotic pathway via p53 [99, 100].

Apigenin, another flavonoid, can induce the proteins p21, p53, and NAG-1 through pathways involving protein kinase C delta (PKCd) and ATM, which are crucial for stopping the growth of colorectal cancer cells [23, 101]. Kaempferol has anti-angiogenic properties, reducing the viability of human umbilical vein endothelial cells and causing DNA damage and fragmentation through activation of caspase signaling pathways mediated by ROS and p53/ATM [102]. Acacetin, an O-methylated flavone, strongly inhibits tumor growth and causes tumor shrinkage in mice by increasing p53 expression and decreasing the activity of the retinoic acid receptor gamma (RARγ) and AKT in liver cancer cells [23]. Securin and p53 are important in determining the sensitivity of human colon cancer cells to fisetin. Reducing securin levels enhances fisetin-induced apoptosis and decreases the resistance of p53-deficient cells to fisetin, making it a promising strategy for treating colon cancers [103]. Fisetin also shows an inhibitory effect against bladder cancer by activating p53 and downregulating the NF-κB pathway in a rat model, making it a safe and effective therapeutic approach [104]. Luteolin increases the expression of p53 and p21 proteins and decreases MDM4 expression in NSCLC cells and tumor tissues [105]. Theaflavins induce G2/M cell cycle arrest by modulating various proteins involved in signaling and inhibiting Bcl-2 through p53 signaling. They also interfere with phagocyte activity by modulating I-κB/NF-κB and reducing vascular endothelial growth factor (VEGF) expression and phosphorylation in LNCaP cells [106]. Epigallocatechin-3-gallate activates p53-dependent targets like p21/WAF1 and Bax and downregulates NF-κB-dependent Bcl-2, leading to growth arrest and apoptosis in LNCaP cells [106]. Apple flavonoids significantly reduce the phosphorylation of ATR, Chk1, and p53 in NNK acetate-treated BEAS-2B cells, helping protect these cells against various carcinogens by aiding DNA repair mechanisms [23]. Additionally, targeted drug delivery of encapsulated C3G chitosan nanoparticles can downregulate p53-mediated apoptosis in Kunming mice, offering a powerful cancer-preventive effect [107].

16.4.3 Phenolic Acids and Other Polyphenols

Caffeic acid increases the expression of the p53 protein in a way that depends on the concentration, and it induces cell death (apoptosis) by inhibiting the activity of Bcl-2 [108]. This inhibition leads to the release of Cyt c and the activation of caspase-3 in HeLa cells [23]. When cells were pre-treated with a specific inhibitor for p38 MAPK, it significantly reduced the phosphorylation of p53 at serine 15 [23]. However, other MAPK-related phosphorylation sites on p53 may still be activated by CAPE, which also activates extracellular signal-related kinases (ERKs) in C6 glioma cells [109]. Additionally, ellagic acid can stop cell proliferation by causing a G1 phase arrest through p21 and inducing cell death [110]. This leads to the inhibition of tumor cell growth, making ellagic acid a potential chemopreventive agent [110].

Curcumin increases p53 levels, creating a favorable environment for p53 and NAD(P)H quinone oxidoreductase (NQO1) to interact in tumor-derived cell lines like HeLa, SiHa, and CaSki [111]. This interaction reduces the binding of p53 with its negative regulator E6AP ubiquitin-protein ligase, especially when human papillomavirus E6 (HPV E6) oncoproteins are present [23]. Curcumin can also upregulate both p53 and p21 in U266 cells, leading to cell cycle arrest [23]. In contrast, curcumin reduced the expression of p53 and p21 in Wistar rats [112]. Resveratrol metabolites can induce moderate cellular aging (senescence) in breast cancer cells by inhibiting cell growth through a G2/M phase arrest via the p53/p21Cip1/WAF1 pathway [113].

16.5 CONCLUSION

Cancer remains one of the leading causes of mortality worldwide, with millions of new cases and deaths reported annually. Conventional cancer therapies, including surgery, radiotherapy, chemotherapy, and targeted therapies, are often associated with significant side effects and dose-limiting toxicities that severely impact the quality of life in patients. Therefore, there is a growing need for alternative therapeutic approaches with better patient outcomes. The p53 protein, known as the "guardian of the genome," plays a crucial role in controlling cell cycle progression, DNA repair, apoptosis, and senescence. Dietary antioxidants, including vitamins, flavonoids, phenolic acids, and other polyphenols, have shown significant potential in modulating the p53 signaling pathway, thereby exerting chemopreventive and anticancer effects. Antioxidants can modulate the mutant p53 pathway, leading to the inhibition of tumor growth and progression.

REFERENCES

1. Bray, F., et al., Global cancer statistics 2018: GLOBOCAN estimates of incidence and mortality worldwide for 36 cancers in 185 countries. *CA: A Cancer Journal for Clinicians*, 2018. **68**(6): p. 394–424.
2. Bizuayehu, H.M., et al., Global burden of 34 cancers among women in 2020 and projections to 2040: Population-based data from 185 countries/territories. *International Journal of Cancer*, 2024. **154**(8): p. 1377–1393.
3. Marei, H.E., et al., p53 signaling in cancer progression and therapy. *Cancer Cell International*, 2021. **21**(1): p. 703.
4. Debela, D.T., et al., New approaches and procedures for cancer treatment: current perspectives. *SAGE Open Medicine*, 2021. **9**: p. 20503121211034366.
5. Gadisa, D.A., S.-H. Wang, and G. Yimer, The Impact of AC and AC-T chemotherapy's toxicities on quality of life among women with breast cancer in Ethiopia: a prospective patient-reported outcomes study. *Breast Cancer: Targets and Therapy*, 2021: p. 107–132.
6. Nurgali, K., R.T. Jagoe, and R. Abalo, Adverse effects of cancer chemotherapy: anything new to improve tolerance and reduce sequelae? *Frontiers in Pharmacology*, 2018. **9**: p. 362658.
7. Key, T., Fruit and vegetables and cancer risk. *British Journal of Cancer*, 2011. **104**(1): p. 6–11.
8. Turati, F., et al., Fruit and vegetables and cancer risk: a review of southern European studies. *British Journal of Nutrition*, 2015. **113**(S2): p. S102–S110.
9. Aune, D., et al., Fruits, vegetables and breast cancer risk: a systematic review and meta-analysis of prospective studies. *Breast Cancer Research and Treatment*, 2012. **134**: p. 479–493.
10. Lobo, M., N. Hounsome, and B. Hounsome, Biochemistry of vegetables: secondary metabolites in vegetables—terpenoids, phenolics, alkaloids, and sulfur-containing compounds. *Handbook of Vegetables and Vegetable Processing*, 2018: p. 47–82. https://doi.org/10.1002/9781119098935.ch3
11. Sofi, S., et al., Clinicopathological and prognostic significance of Bcl2 in breast cancer: a comprehensive in silico and in vitro study. *Saudi Journal of Biological Sciences*, 2023. **31**(2): p. 103916.

12. Chaudhary, P., et al., Oxidative stress, free radicals and antioxidants: potential crosstalk in the pathophysiology of human diseases. *Frontiers in Chemistry*, 2023. **11**: p. 1158198.
13. Liu, R.H., Health-promoting components of fruits and vegetables in the diet. *Advances in Nutrition*, 2013. **4**(3): p. 384S–392S.
14. Rodriguez-Casado, A., The health potential of fruits and vegetables phytochemicals: notable examples. *Critical Reviews in Food Science and Nutrition*, 2016. **56**(7): p. 1097–1107.
15. Miller, P.E. and D.C. Snyder, Phytochemicals and cancer risk: a review of the epidemiological evidence. *Nutrition in Clinical Practice*, 2012. **27**(5): p. 599–612.
16. Kumar, M., et al., Phytoconstituents as apoptosis inducing agents: strategy to combat cancer. *Cytotechnology*, 2016. **68**: p. 531–563.
17. Thushara, R., et al., Differential action of phytochemicals on platelet apoptosis: a biological overview. *Current Medicinal Chemistry*, 2013. **20**(8): p. 1018–1027.
18. Adedokun, K.A., et al., Therapeutic Potentials of Medicinal Plants and Significance of Computational Tools in Anti-Cancer Drug Discovery, in *Phytochemistry, Computational Tools and Databases in Drug Discovery*. 2023, Elsevier. p. 393–455.
19. Sofi, S., et al., Elucidation of interleukin-19 as a therapeutic target for breast cancer by computational analysis and experimental validation. *Saudi Journal of Biological Sciences*, 2023. **30**(9): p. 103774–103774.
20. Patil, M.R. and A. Bihari, A comprehensive study of p53 protein. *Journal of Cellular Biochemistry*, 2022. **123**(12): p. 1891–1937.
21. Miller, C., et al., The p53 gene is located on short arm of chromosome 17 in humans. *Nature*, 1986. **319**: p. 783–784.
22. Wang, H., et al., Targeting p53 pathways: mechanisms, structures, and advances in therapy. *Signal Transduction and Targeted Therapy*, 2023. **8**(1): p. 92.
23. Merlin, J.J., et al., Role of dietary antioxidants in p53-mediated cancer chemoprevention and tumor suppression. *Oxidative Medicine and Cellular Longevity*, 2021. **2021**: p. 9924328
24. Speidel, D., The role of DNA damage responses in p53 biology. *Archives of Toxicology*, 2015. **89**(4): p. 501–517.
25. Meek, D.W., Regulation of the p53 response and its relationship to cancer. *Biochemical Journal*, 2015. **469**(3): p. 325–346.
26. Goldstein, I., et al., Understanding wild-type and mutant p53 activities in human cancer: new landmarks on the way to targeted therapies. *Cancer Gene Therapy*, 2011. **18**(1): p. 2–11.
27. Olivier, M., M. Hollstein, and P. Hainaut, TP53 mutations in human cancers: origins, consequences, and clinical use. *Cold Spring Harbor Perspectives in Biology*, 2010. **2**(1): p. a001008.
28. Marshall, C.B., et al., Tissue-specific expression of p73 and p63 isoforms in human tissues. *Cell Death & Disease*, 2021. **12**(8): p. 745.
29. Chen, J., The cell-cycle arrest and apoptotic functions of p53 in tumor initiation and progression. *Cold Spring Harbor Perspectives in Medicine*, 2016. **6**(3): p. a026104.
30. Kiraz, Y., et al., Major apoptotic mechanisms and genes involved in apoptosis. *Tumor Biology*, 2016. **37**: p. 8471–8486.
31. Kashyap, D., V.K. Garg, and N. Goel, Intrinsic and extrinsic pathways of apoptosis: role in cancer development and prognosis. *Advances in Protein Chemistry and Structural Biology*, 2021. **125**: p. 73–120.
32. Jan, N., et al., Exploring the role of trifarotene against RAR-α: an investigation of expression pattern and clinicopathological significance of RAR-α in breast cancer. *Frontiers in Pharmacology*, 2024. **15**: p. 1361679.
33. Ola, M.S., M. Nawaz, and H. Ahsan, Role of Bcl-2 family proteins and caspases in the regulation of apoptosis. *Molecular and Cellular Biochemistry*, 2011. **351**: p. 41–58.
34. Qian, S., et al., The role of BCL-2 family proteins in regulating apoptosis and cancer therapy. *Frontiers in Oncology*, 2022. **12**: p. 985363.
35. Wagh, N.S., S.R. Pai, and V.V. Sonkamble, Phytochemicals in the prevention and cure of cancers. *Plant-Derived Bioactives: Chemistry and Mode of Action*, 2020: p. 351–373.
36. Qin, S., B.A. Schulte, and G.Y. Wang, Role of senescence induction in cancer treatment. *World Journal of Clinical Oncology*, 2018. **9**(8): p. 180.
37. Jan, N., et al., Targeting breast cancer stem cells through retinoids: a new hope for treatment. *Critical Reviews in Oncology/Hematology*, 2023: p. 104156.
38. Kruiswijk, F., C.F. Labuschagne, and K.H. Vousden, p53 in survival, death and metabolic health: a lifeguard with a licence to kill. *Nature Reviews Molecular Cell Biology*, 2015. **16**(7): p. 393–405.

39. Jan, N., et al., Metronomic chemotherapy and drug repurposing: a paradigm shift in oncology. *Heliyon*, 2024. https://doi.org/10.1016/j.heliyon.2024.e24670
40. Ding, L., et al., The roles of cyclin-dependent kinases in cell cycle progression and therapeutic strategies in human breast cancer. *International Journal of Molecular Sciences*, 2020. **21**(6): p. 1960.
41. Tamura, R., et al., GADD45 proteins: central players in tumorigenesis. *Current Molecular Medicine*, 2012. **12**(5): p. 634–651.
42. Gupta, A., et al., Reactivation of p53 gene by MDM2 inhibitors: a novel therapy for cancer treatment. *Biomedicine & Pharmacotherapy*, 2019. **109**: p. 484–492.
43. Mir, M.A., M. Rashid, and N. Jan, Cytokines and Chemokines in Tumor Growth and Progression, in *Cytokine and Chemokine Networks in Cancer*. 2023, Springer. p. 33–77
44. Chatterjee, N. and G.C. Walker, Mechanisms of DNA damage, repair, and mutagenesis. *Environmental and Molecular Mutagenesis*, 2017. **58**(5): p. 235–263.
45. Mir, M.A., M. Bashir, and N. Jan, The Role of Interleukin (IL)-6/IL-6 Receptor Axis in Cancer, in *Cytokine and Chemokine Networks in Cancer*. 2023, Springer. p. 137–164.
46. Zhao, K., et al., Regulation of the Mdm2–p53 pathway by the ubiquitin E3 ligase MARCH 7. *EMBO Reports*, 2018. **19**(2): p. 305–319.
47. García-Cano, J., et al., Regulation of the MDM2-p53 pathway by the ubiquitin ligase HERC2. *Molecular Oncology*, 2020. **14**(1): p. 69–86.
48. Beyfuss, K. and D.A. Hood, A systematic review of p53 regulation of oxidative stress in skeletal muscle. *Redox Report*, 2018. **23**(1): p. 100–117.
49. Shadfan, M., V. Lopez-Pajares, and Z.-M. Yuan, MDM2 and MDMX: Alone and together in regulation of p53. *Translational Cancer Research*, 2012. **1**(2): p. 88.
50. Mir, M.A., Sumaya, N. Jan, Implications of Chemokine Heterogenicity in Cancer Metastasis, in *Cytokine and Chemokine Networks in Cancer*. 2023, Springer. p. 115–136.
51. Sparks, A., et al., The degradation of p53 and its major E3 ligase Mdm2 is differentially dependent on the proteasomal ubiquitin receptor S5a. *Oncogene*, 2014. **33**(38): p. 4685–4696.
52. Chao, C.C.-K., Mechanisms of p53 degradation. *Clinica Chimica Acta*, 2015. **438**: p. 139–147.
53. Mir, M.A., A. Manzoor, and N. Jan, CCL5/CCR5 Axis in Cancer, in *Cytokine and Chemokine Networks in Cancer*. 2023, Springer. p. 219–240.
54. Joerger, A.C. and A.R. Fersht, The p53 pathway: origins, inactivation in cancer, and emerging therapeutic approaches. *Annual Review of Biochemistry*, 2016. **85**: p. 375–404.
55. Gordon, E.M., et al., Cell cycle checkpoint control: The cyclin G1/Mdm2/p53 axis emerges as a strategic target for broadspectrum cancer gene therapy-A review of molecular mechanisms for oncologists. *Molecular and Clinical Oncology*, 2018. **9**(2): p. 115–134.
56. Lin, T., et al., Emerging roles of p53 related lncRNAs in cancer progression: a systematic review. *International Journal of Biological Sciences*, 2019. **15**(6): p. 1287.
57. Sofi, S., et al., A comprehensive analysis of notch signaling genes in breast cancer: expression pattern and prognostic significance. *Advances in Cancer Biology-Metastasis*, 2023. **7**: p. 100104.
58. Zanjirband, M. and S. Rahgozar, Targeting p53-MDM2 interaction using small molecule inhibitors and the challenges needed to be addressed. *Current Drug Targets*, 2019. **20**(11): p. 1091–1111.
59. Cheng, Q. and J. Chen, Mechanism of p53 stabilization by ATM after DNA damage. *Cell Cycle*, 2010. **9**(3): p. 472–478.
60. Mir, M.A., et al., Metronomics: toward personalized chemotherapy. *Novel Approaches in Metronomic Chemotherapy for Breast Cancer Treatment*, 2024. p. 99–119. https://doi.org/10.1201/9781032632674-8
61. Hafner, A., et al., The multiple mechanisms that regulate p53 activity and cell fate. *Nature Reviews Molecular Cell Biology*, 2019. **20**(4): p. 199–210.
62. Mir, M.A., N. Jan, and I. Noor, Therapeutic Implications of Cytokines and Chemokines Network in Cancer, in *Cytokine and Chemokine Networks in Cancer*. 2023, Springer. p. 385–414.
63. Olsson, A., et al., How important are post-translational modifications in p53 for selectivity in target-gene transcription and tumour suppression? *Cell Death & Differentiation*, 2007. **14**(9): p. 1561–1575.
64. Xu, Z., et al., Regulation of p53 stability as a therapeutic strategy for cancer. *Biochemical Pharmacology*, 2021. **185**: p. 114407.
65. Mir, M.A., N. Jan, and H. Qayoom, Conventional Chemotherapy vs. Metronomic Chemotherapy, in *Novel Approaches in Metronomic Chemotherapy for Breast Cancer Treatment*. CRC Press. p. 27–42.
66. Sabapathy, K. and D.P. Lane, Therapeutic targeting of p53: all mutants are equal, but some mutants are more equal than others. *Nature Reviews Clinical Oncology*, 2018. **15**(1): p. 13–30.
67. Cadwell, C. and G.P. Zambetti, The effects of wild-type p53 tumor suppressor activity and mutant p53 gain-of-function on cell growth. *Gene*, 2001. **277**(1–2): p. 15–30.

68. Reinhardt, H.C. and B. Schumacher, The p53 network: cellular and systemic DNA damage responses in aging and cancer. *Trends in Genetics*, 2012. **28**(3): p. 128–136.
69. Ozaki, T. and A. Nakagawara, Role of p53 in cell death and human cancers. *Cancers*, 2011. **3**(1): p. 994–1013.
70. Goh, A.M., C.R. Coffill, and D.P. Lane, The role of mutant p53 in human cancer. *The Journal of Pathology*, 2011. **223**(2): p. 116–126.
71. Balasundaram, A. and C.G.P. Doss, unraveling the structural changes in the DNA-binding region of tumor protein p53 (TP53) upon hotspot mutation p53 Arg248 by comparative computational approach. *International Journal of Molecular Sciences*, 2022. **23**(24): p. 15499.
72. Mir, M.A., N. Jan, and S. Sofi, Introduction to Metronomic Chemotherapy, in *Novel Approaches in Metronomic Chemotherapy for Breast Cancer Treatment*. 2024, CRC Press. p. 1–14.
73. Liebl, M.C. and T.G. Hofmann, The role of p53 signaling in colorectal cancer. *Cancers*, 2021. **13**(9): p. 2125.
74. Chen, X., et al., Mutant p53 in cancer: from molecular mechanism to therapeutic modulation. *Cell Death & Disease*, 2022. **13**(11): p. 974.
75. Blagosklonny, M.V., p53 from complexity to simplicity: mutant p53 stabilization, gain-of-function, and dominant-negative effect. *The FASEB Journal*, 2000. **14**(13): p. 1901–1907.
76. Alvarado-Ortiz, E., et al., Mutant p53 gain-of-function: role in cancer development, progression, and therapeutic approaches. *Frontiers in Cell and Developmental Biology*, 2021. **8**: p. 607670.
77. Li, J. and M. Kurokawa, Regulation of MDM2 stability after DNA damage. *Journal of Cellular Physiology*, 2015. **230**(10): p. 2318–2327.
78. Vaughan, C., et al., p53: its mutations and their impact on transcription, in *Mutant p53 and MDM2 in Cancer*, Subcellular Biochemistry, vol 85. 2014, Springer. p. 71–90.
79. Walia, A., A.K. Gupta, and V. Sharma, Role of bioactive compounds in human health. *Acta Scientific Medical Sciences*, 2019. **3**(9): p. 25–33.
80. Mitra, S., et al., Exploring the immune-boosting functions of vitamins and minerals as nutritional food bioactive compounds: a comprehensive review. *Molecules*, 2022. **27**(2): p. 555.
81. Afrin, S., et al., Therapeutic and preventive properties of honey and its bioactive compounds in cancer: an evidence-based review. *Nutrition Research Reviews*, 2020. **33**(1): p. 50–76.
82. Asnaashari, S., E. Amjad, and B. Sokouti, Synergistic effects of flavonoids and paclitaxel in cancer treatment: a systematic review. *Cancer Cell International*, 2023. **23**(1): p. 211.
83. Sarangi, M.K. and S. Padhi, Plants with potential anticancer activities-a Review. *International Journal of Phytomedicine*, 2014. **6**(1): p. 01.
84. Mir, M.A., et al., Imaging Techniques, Biomarkers, and Methods for Metronomic Chemotherapy, in *Novel Approaches in Metronomic Chemotherapy for Breast Cancer Treatment*. CRC Press. p. 58–71.
85. Haq, B.U., et al., Targeting p53 misfolding conundrum by stabilizing agents and their analogs in breast cancer therapy: a comprehensive computational analysis. *Frontiers in Pharmacology*, 2024. **14**: p. 1333447.
86. Böttger, F., et al., High-dose intravenous vitamin C, a promising multi-targeting agent in the treatment of cancer. *Journal of Experimental & Clinical Cancer Research*, 2021. **40**: p. 1–44.
87. Chambial, S., et al., Vitamin C in disease prevention and cure: an overview. *Indian Journal of Clinical Biochemistry*, 2013. **28**: p. 314–328.
88. Rubis, B., et al., Vitamin C increases DNA breaks and suppresses DNA damage-independent activation of ATM by bleomycin. *Free Radical Biology and Medicine*, 2019. **136**: p. 12–21.
89. Zhang, P., et al., Vitamin B6 activates p53 and elevates p21 gene expression in cancer cells and the mouse colon. *Oncology Reports*, 2014. **31**(5): p. 2371–2376.
90. Chen, L., et al., 1, 25-Dihydroxyvitamin D exerts an antiaging role by activation of Nrf2-antioxidant signaling and inactivation of p16/p53-senescence signaling. *Aging Cell*, 2019. **18**(3): p. e12951.
91. Miao, D. and D. Goltzman, Mechanisms of Action of Vitamin D in Delaying Aging and Preventing Disease by Inhibiting Oxidative Stress, in *Vitamins and Hormones*. 2023, Elsevier. p. 293–318.
92. Yang, R., et al., 1, 25-Dihydroxyvitamin D protects against age-related osteoporosis by a novel VDR-Ezh2-p16 signal axis. *Aging Cell*, 2020. **19**(2): p. e13095.
93. Diao, Q., et al., Vitamin E promotes breast cancer cell proliferation by reducing ROS production and p53 expression. *European Review for Medical and Pharmacological Sciences*, 2016. **20**(12): p. 2710–2717.
94. Khuzhakhmetova, L., et al., The role of alpha-tocopherol and cycloferon in the regulation of apoptosis in neurons of the hypothalamic suprachiasmatic nucleus and pinealocytes during stress and aging. *Journal of Evolutionary Biochemistry and Physiology*, 2019. **55**: p. 380–387.

95. Valko, M., et al., Free radicals, metals and antioxidants in oxidative stress-induced cancer. *Chemico-Biological Interactions*, 2006. **160**(1): p. 1–40.
96. Siddiqui, S.S., et al., Dietary flavonoids in p53—mediated immune dysfunctions linking to cancer prevention. *Biomedicines*, 2020. **8**(8): p. 286.
97. Majidinia, M., A. Bishayee, and B. Yousefi, Polyphenols: Major regulators of key components of DNA damage response in cancer. *DNA Repair*, 2019. **82**: p. 102679.
98. Rajendran, P., et al., Dietary phytochemicals, HDAC inhibition, and DNA damage/repair defects in cancer cells. *Clinical Epigenetics*, 2011. **3**: p. 1–23.
99. Rauf, A., et al., Anticancer potential of quercetin: A comprehensive review. *Phytotherapy Research*, 2018. **32**(11): p. 2109 2130.
100. Almatroodi, S.A., et al., Potential therapeutic targets of quercetin, a plant flavonol, and its role in the therapy of various types of cancer through the modulation of various cell signaling pathways. *Molecules*, 2021. **26**(5): p. 1315.
101. Shankar, E., et al., Plant flavone apigenin: an emerging anticancer agent. *Current Pharmacology Reports*, 2017. **3**: p. 423–446.
102. Lee, C.-F., et al., Kaempferol induces ATM/p53-mediated death receptor and mitochondrial apoptosis in human umbilical vein endothelial cells. *International Journal of Oncology*, 2016. **48**(5): p. 2007–2014.
103. Yu, S.-H., et al., Securin depletion sensitizes human colon cancer cells to fisetin-induced apoptosis. *Cancer Letters*, 2011. **300**(1): p. 96–104.
104. Rahmani, A.H., et al., The potential role of fisetin, a flavonoid in cancer prevention and treatment. *Molecules*, 2022. **27**(24): p. 9009.
105. Çetinkaya, M. and Y. Baran, Therapeutic potential of luteolin on cancer. *Vaccines*, 2023. **11**(3): p. 554.
106. Khan, H., et al., Anti-cancer effects of polyphenols via targeting p53 signaling pathway: updates and future directions. *Biotechnology Advances*, 2020. **38**: p. 107385.
107. Sachdeva, B., et al., Chitosan nanoparticles-based cancer drug delivery: application and challenges. *Marine Drugs*, 2023. **21**(4): p. 211.
108. Kleczka, A., et al., Caffeic acid phenethyl ester (CAPE) induced apoptosis in serous ovarian cancer OV7 cells by deregulation of BCL2/BAX genes. *Molecules*, 2020. **25**(15): p. 3514.
109. Wu, G.S., The functional interactions between the MAPK and p53 signaling pathways. *Cancer Biology & Therapy*, 2004. **3**(2): p. 156–161.
110. Ceci, C., et al., Experimental evidence of the antitumor, antimetastatic and antiangiogenic activity of ellagic acid. *Nutrients*, 2018. **10**(11): p. 1756.
111. Wang, Z., et al., Role of natural products in tumor therapy from basic research and clinical perspectives. *Acta Materia Medica*, 2024. **3**(2): p. 163–206.
112. Rajabi, M., T. Naji, and A. Mohamadnia, Evaluation of the efficacy of resveratrol and curcumin on the expression of Bcl-2, Bax, and P53 Genes and GAFP Protein in male wistar rats model glioblastoma multiforme. *The Journal of Applied Tissue Engineering*, 2023. **9**(1). https://doi.org/10.22034/JATE.2023.79
113. Zheng, Z., L. Zhang, and X. Hou, Potential roles and molecular mechanisms of phytochemicals against cancer. *Food & Function*, 2022. **13**(18): p. 9208–9225.

17 The Interplay between p53 and the Tumor Microenvironment in Progressing Breast Cancer

Shristi Handa[1], Mary Chatterjee[1], Nusrat Jan[2], and Manzoor Ahmad Mir[2]*

[1]Biotechnology Engineering, University Institute of Engineering and Technology, Panjab University, Chandigarh, India
[2]Department of Bioresources, School of Biological Sciences, University of Kashmir, Srinagar, J&K, India
*drmanzoor@kashmiruniversity.ac.in

17.1 INTRODUCTION TO p53 AND THE TUMOR MICROENVIRONMENT

The protein p53 serves as a critical guardian within cellular environments, diligently monitoring genomic stability and cellular equilibrium. Named for its molecular weight of approximately 53 kDa, p53 is instrumental in coordinating cellular responses to various stressors and insults. Positioned at the intersection of multiple signaling cascades, p53 acts as a master regulator of cellular fate, capable of inducing cell cycle arrest, facilitating DNA repair processes, or initiating programmed cell death (apoptosis) in response to adverse conditions (1, 2). Its functional diversity stems from a modular architecture consisting of discrete domains, including a transactivation domain facilitating gene expression, a DNA-binding domain enabling sequence-specific DNA interactions, and an oligomerization domain crucial for protein–protein interactions (3). Encoded by the TP53 gene, p53 expression is subjected to intricate regulation by a plethora of regulatory elements, ensuring precise control over its abundance and activity levels (4). Under normal physiological circumstances, usually p53 is maintained at low levels through tightly regulated degradation mediated by the E3 ubiquitin ligase MDM2. However, upon exposure to cellular stressors such as DNA damage, oncogenic activation, or hypoxia, p53 undergoes stabilization and translocates to the nucleus where it exerts its tumor-suppressive functions. This functionality is finely tuned through a series of post-translational modifications, i.e., through phosphorylation, acetylation, and ubiquitination, which allows precise modulation of downstream signaling pathways (5). Notably, p53's transcriptional targets span a broad spectrum of cellular processes, encompassing cell cycle regulation, DNA repair mechanisms, cellular senescence, and apoptosis. This versatility underscores p53's indispensable role in preserving genomic integrity and thwarting malignant transformation. Its significance in tumor suppression is underscored by frequent inactivation observed in human cancers, either through TP53 gene mutations or dysregulation of its upstream regulators and downstream effectors. As a result, elucidating the complexities of p53 biology has emerged as a focal point in cancer research, with therapeutic interventions aimed at restoring p53 function or exploiting synthetic lethal interactions with p53-deficient tumors (Figure 17.1) (6).

In essence, p53 epitomizes the molecular sentinel, serving as a stalwart defender of the genome and a guiding light in the quest for precision oncology. Furthermore, the tumor microenvironment (TME), which is known as the "dynamic ecosystem" (where cancer cells interact with surrounding

DOI: 10.1201/9781003520771-17

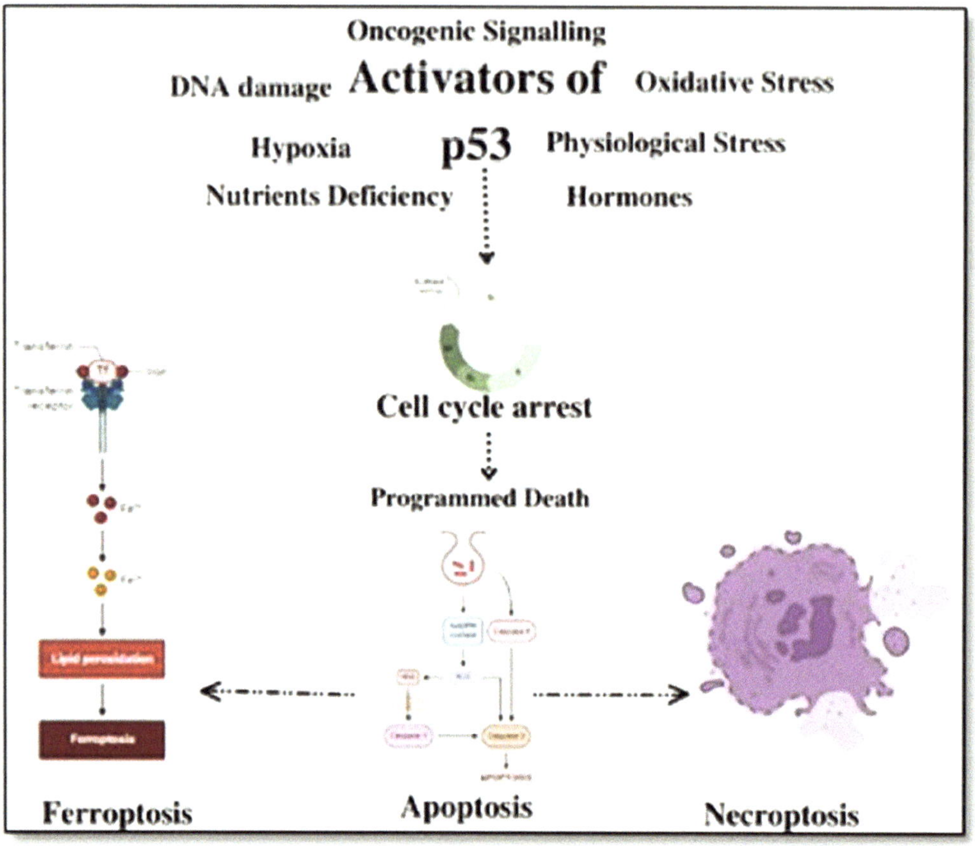

FIGURE 17.1 Schematic representation of the role of p53 as a guardian molecule.

tissues, vasculature, and immune cells), orchestrates a complex interplay that shapes disease progression and treatment outcomes (7). This intricate network of interactions governs key processes such as angiogenesis, immune evasion, and extracellular matrix remodeling, which influence the aggressiveness and therapeutic responsiveness of tumors. Emerging evidence highlights the pivotal role of p53 in modulating various aspects of the TME. One crucial function of p53 in the TME is its regulation of the immune response. p53 can influence the expression of immunomodulatory factors such as cytokines, chemokines, and immune checkpoint molecules, thereby shaping the anti-tumor immune response (8, 9). Moreover, p53 has been shown to regulate the infiltration and function of immune cells within the TME, including T cells, natural killer (NK) cells, and myeloid-derived suppressor cells (MDSCs), which can impact tumor immune evasion and immunotherapy efficacy. Additionally, p53 plays a role in regulating the tumor vasculature by modulating the expression of angiogenic factors and influencing endothelial cell function, thereby affecting tumor angiogenesis and vascular integrity (10). Furthermore, p53 can impact the metabolic landscape of the TME by regulating cellular metabolism in both cancer cells and stromal cells, which in turn affects nutrient availability, immune cell function, and tumor progression. Importantly, dysregulation of p53 in cancer cells can alter the TME, promoting immune evasion, angiogenesis, and metabolic reprogramming, thus contributing to tumor progression and therapy resistance. Understanding the role of p53 in the TME is crucial for developing effective cancer therapies that target both cancer cells and their microenvironment (11).

In breast cancer, p53 plays a critical role in tumor suppression and disease progression. While mutations in the TP53 gene are not as prevalent in breast cancer as in some other cancer types, alterations in p53 function can still significantly impact breast tumorigenesis. One of the primary roles of p53 in breast cancer is to safeguard genomic integrity by regulating cell cycle progression and DNA repair mechanisms. Functional p53 can induce cell cycle arrest in response to DNA damage, allowing time for repair or triggering apoptosis if the damage is irreparable. Moreover, p53 is involved in the regulation of cellular senescence, a state of permanent growth arrest that can prevent the proliferation of potentially malignant cells (12). Dysfunctional p53, either through mutations or dysregulation of its upstream regulators and downstream effectors leads to unchecked cell proliferation, genomic instability, and increased susceptibility to oncogenic transformation in breast epithelial cells. Additionally, p53 influences the response to breast cancer therapy, including chemotherapy, radiation therapy, and targeted therapies. Loss of functional p53 is associated with resistance to chemotherapy and poor prognosis in breast cancer patients. Furthermore, p53 status has prognostic significance in breast cancer, with tumors harboring wild-type p53 being observed to exhibit better clinical outcomes compared to those with mutated or dysfunctional p53 (13, 14).

This book chapter explores the molecular mechanisms underlying the interplay between p53 and the TME in breast cancer progression. It discusses recent advances in our understanding of how p53 influences TME components and vice versa, highlighting the implications for disease prognosis and treatment strategies. Additionally, the chapter examines emerging therapeutic approaches targeting the p53–TME axis. By elucidating the intricate interplay between p53 and the TME, the chapter aims to contribute to the growing body of knowledge in breast cancer research and paves the way for more effective therapeutic interventions.

17.2 THE TUMOR MICROENVIRONMENT IN BREAST CANCER

The TME in breast cancer is a complex milieu comprised of various cell types, extracellular matrix (ECM) components, signaling molecules, and vasculature that collectively influence tumor progression, metastasis, and response to therapy (15). At the cellular level, the TME is characterized by a heterogeneous population of cancer-associated fibroblasts (CAFs), immune cells such as tumor-associated macrophages (TAMs), lymphocytes, and endothelial cells. CAFs, the predominant stromal cells in the TME, play crucial roles in modulating the ECM, promoting angiogenesis, and secreting growth factors and cytokines that fuel tumor growth and invasion (Figure 17.2) (16).

TAMs, on the other hand, exhibit phenotypic plasticity and can adopt pro-tumorigenic (M2-like) or anti-tumorigenic (M1-like) states depending on the cues from the microenvironment. Their presence is often associated with poor prognosis in breast cancer due to their ability to promote immunosuppression, ECM remodeling, and tumor cell migration (17). Moreover, the TME harbors various immune cell subsets, including regulatory T cells (Tregs), MDSCs, and dendritic cells, which collectively contribute to immune evasion and tumor immune privilege (18). Additionally, the dysregulated ECM within the TME not only provides structural support to the tumor but also serves as a reservoir for growth factors and proteases that facilitate tumor invasion and metastasis. Furthermore, the TME is characterized by aberrant angiogenesis driven by pro-angiogenic factors secreted by tumor and stromal cells, leading to the formation of leaky and disorganized blood vessels that support tumor growth and dissemination (19). Beyond cellular components, the TME is governed by intricate signaling networks mediated by cytokines, chemokines, and growth factors, which orchestrate crosstalk between tumor and stromal cells, modulate immune responses, and promote therapy resistance. Importantly, the dynamic nature of the TME poses significant challenges for cancer therapy, as it can adapt to therapeutic interventions and promote the emergence of resistant clones. Thus, understanding the multifaceted interactions within the TME is essential for the development of effective therapeutic strategies targeting breast cancer. Emerging therapeutic approaches aimed at reprogramming the TME, such as immune checkpoint blockade, targeting of

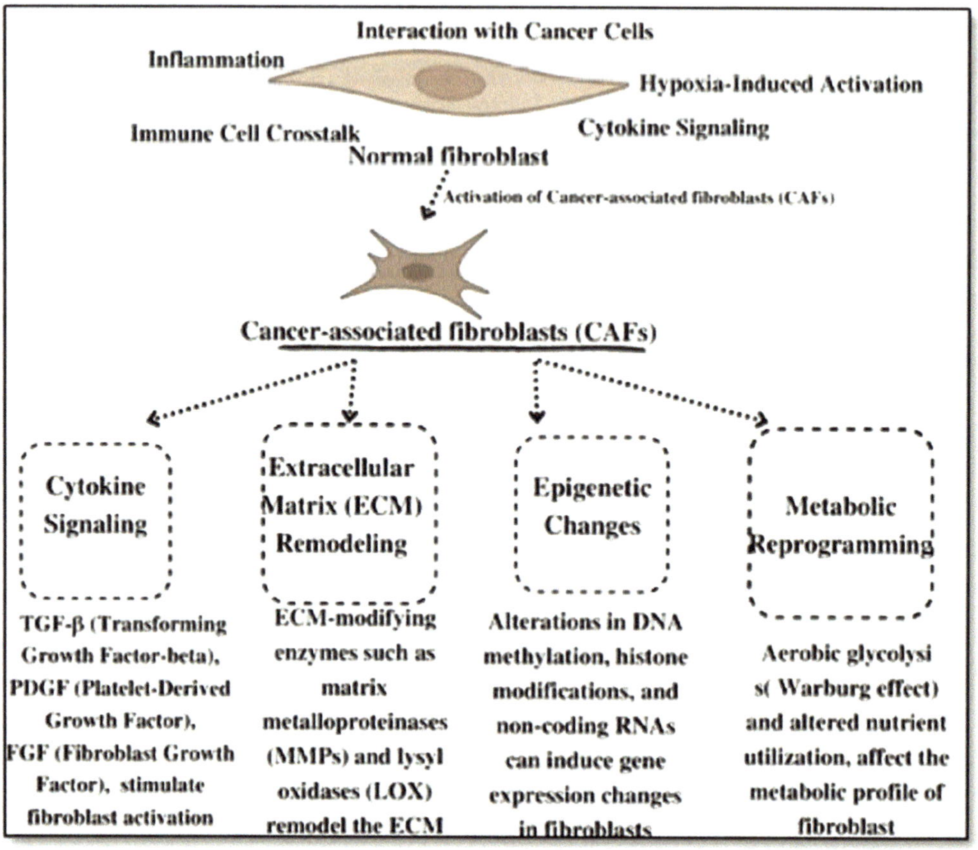

FIGURE 17.2 Schematic representation of different mechanisms that can contribute to cancer-associated fibroblast (CAF) activation.

tumor-promoting stromal components, and normalization of tumor vasculature, hold promise for improving patient outcomes by harnessing the body's own immune system and targeting the supportive niche that sustains tumor growth and metastasis (20).

17.3 REGULATION OF TUMOR MICROENVIRONMENT BY p53

Regulation of the TME by p53 represents a critical nexus in cancer biology, where the intricate interplay between a tumor suppressor protein and the surrounding milieu shapes disease progression and therapeutic responses. At its core, p53 functions as a master regulator of cellular stress responses, orchestrating a diverse array of downstream pathways that govern cell fate decisions. In the context of the TME, p53 exerts its influence through multifaceted mechanisms, modulating both the cellular and non-cellular components of the microenvironment (21). For instance, p53 has been shown to regulate the secretion of soluble factors such as cytokines and chemokines, thereby influencing the inflammatory milieu within the TME. Furthermore, p53 plays a pivotal role in modulating the activity of stromal cells, including CAFs, which contribute to tumor progression through their effects on extracellular matrix remodeling, angiogenesis, and immune modulation (22). Importantly, p53's impact on the TME extends to the immune landscape, where it influences the recruitment, activation, and function of immune cells within the tumor milieu. Notably, loss or

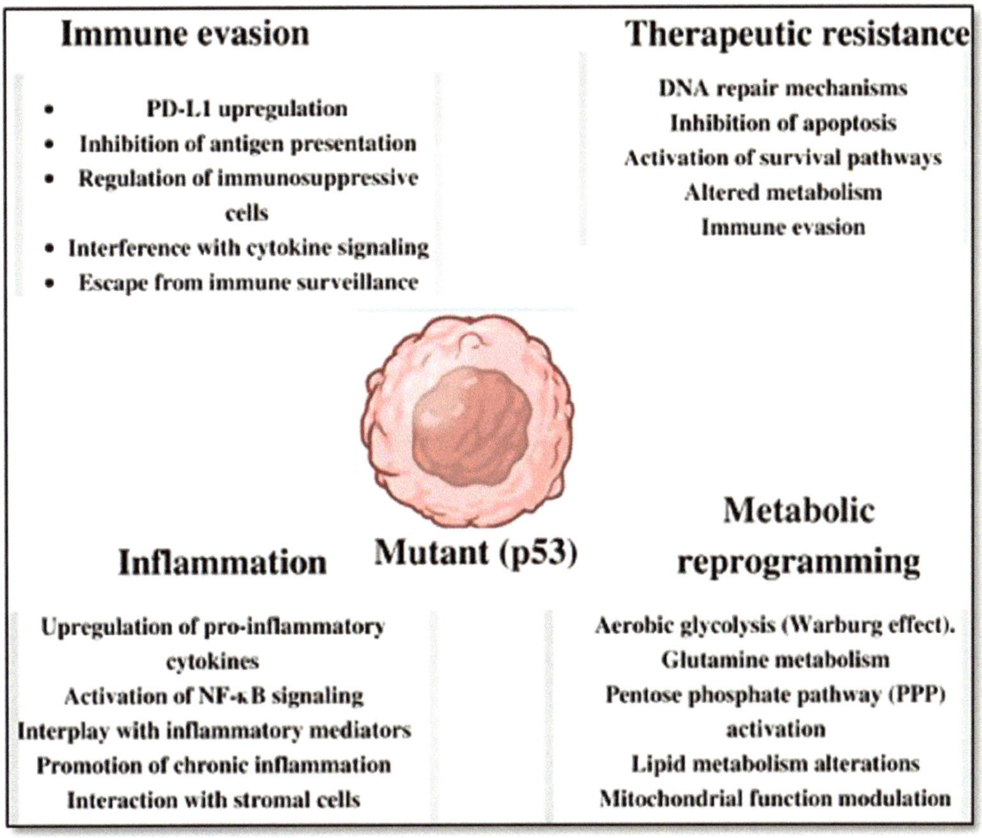

FIGURE 17.3 Schematic representation role of mutant p53 in the formation and progression of the tumor microenvironment.

mutation of p53 can disrupt these regulatory mechanisms, leading to alterations in the TME that promote tumor growth, metastasis, and therapy resistance (Figure 17.3) (23).

Conversely, restoration of p53 function or pharmacological activation of p53 pathways holds promise for reprogramming the TME toward a more hostile environment for tumor cells, thereby enhancing the efficacy of existing therapies and fostering the development of novel therapeutic strategies (24). In this way, unraveling the intricate interplay between p53 and the TME offers new insights into the complexities of cancer biology and provides a foundation for the development of targeted interventions aimed at disrupting tumor-promoting microenvironmental cues.

17.3.1 Genetic and Epigenetic Regulation of p53–Microenvironment Interactions

The genetic and epigenetic regulation of p53–microenvironment interactions constitutes a critical axis in understanding breast cancer progression and therapeutic resistance. The tumor suppressor protein p53 serves as a guardian of genomic integrity, orchestrating cellular responses to various stresses, including DNA damage, oncogenic signaling, and hypoxia (25). Genetic alterations such as mutations, deletions, and amplifications in the TP53 gene are among the most common events in breast cancer, leading to loss of p53 function or acquisition of oncogenic properties, thereby disrupting its ability to regulate cell cycle arrest, apoptosis, and DNA repair (26). Consequently, aberrant p53 signaling can fuel tumor progression by promoting genomic instability, evasion of apoptosis, and resistance to chemotherapy. Moreover, epigenetic modifications, including DNA methylation, histone modifications, and non-coding RNA-mediated regulation, exert profound effects on p53 activity and its interactions with the tumor microenvironment. Hypermethylation of the TP53 promoter region, for instance, can silence p53 expression in breast cancer cells, dampening its tumor-suppressive functions and fostering a permissive microenvironment for tumor growth and metastasis (27). Conversely, alterations in histone acetylation and methylation patterns can modulate p53 transcriptional activity and its ability to regulate the expression of genes involved in immune surveillance, angiogenesis, and ECM remodeling within the tumor microenvironment (28). Importantly, these genetic and epigenetic changes not only impact the intrinsic properties of cancer cells but also influence their interactions with stromal cells, immune cells, and the ECM, thereby shaping the dynamic TME landscape in breast cancer. For instance, loss of wild-type p53 function in tumor cells can lead to the secretion of pro-inflammatory cytokines and chemokines, promoting the recruitment of immunosuppressive cells such as MDSCs and regulatory T cells (Tregs), which in turn create an immunosuppressive niche that facilitates tumor immune evasion and therapeutic resistance (29). Moreover, dysregulated p53 signaling can perturb the balance between pro- and anti-angiogenic factors, driving aberrant angiogenesis and vascular remodeling within the TME, which sustains tumor growth and metastasis. Furthermore, alterations in p53 function can impact the secretion of extracellular vesicles by tumor cells, thereby modulating intercellular communication within the TME and promoting the dissemination of oncogenic signals to neighboring stromal and immune cells.

17.3.2 Role of p53 in Modulating Immune Response within the Tumor Microenvironment

Initially discovered for its role in preventing cancer by inducing cell cycle arrest and apoptosis in response to DNA damage, p53 has since been recognized for its multifaceted functions beyond the realm of tumor suppression. In recent years, accumulating evidence has highlighted its involvement in shaping the immune response, thus adding a new dimension to its repertoire of activities. The key mechanism through which p53 influences the immune response is by regulating the expression of genes involved in both innate and adaptive immunity (30). Upon activation, p53 can directly transactivate genes encoding various cytokines, chemokines, and immune receptors, thereby influencing immune cell recruitment, activation, and function. For instance, p53 has been shown to upregulate the expression of interleukin-6 (IL-6), a pleiotropic cytokine involved in inflammation and immune regulation. Additionally, p53 can induce the expression of chemokines such as CXCL5 and CXCL8, which play crucial roles in recruiting neutrophils and other immune cells to sites of inflammation or infection (31). Moreover, p53 activation has been linked to the upregulation of the major histocompatibility complex (MHC) class I and II molecules, facilitating antigen presentation and T cell activation.

Furthermore, p53 has been implicated in modulating the function of various immune cell types, including macrophages, dendritic cells (DCs), T cells, and NK cells. In macrophages, p53 activation can promote the production of pro-inflammatory cytokines such as tumor necrosis factor-alpha (TNF-α) and interleukin-12 (IL-12), enhancing antimicrobial and antitumor immune responses. Additionally, p53 activation in DCs has been shown to promote their maturation and antigen-presenting capacity, thereby enhancing T cell activation and adaptive immune responses. Moreover, p53 can regulate T cell function by modulating the balance between effector and regulatory T cell subsets, thereby influencing immune tolerance and autoimmune responses. Notably, p53 activation has also been reported to enhance the cytotoxic activity of NK cells, highlighting its role in orchestrating both innate and adaptive immune responses.

In addition to its direct effects on immune cells, p53 can also modulate the immune response through its crosstalk with other signaling pathways, including those involved in inflammation, oxidative stress, and metabolism. For instance, p53 has been shown to interact with nuclear factor-kappa B (NF-κB), a master regulator of inflammation, thereby influencing the expression of inflammatory cytokines and chemokines (32). Moreover, p53 can regulate the production of reactive oxygen species (ROS) and antioxidant enzymes, which play critical roles in immune cell function and redox signaling (33). Furthermore, p53 has been implicated in coordinating metabolic pathways in immune cells, such as glycolysis, oxidative phosphorylation, and fatty acid metabolism, to meet the energetic demands associated with immune activation and effector functions. Interestingly, the dysregulation of p53 signaling has been implicated in various immune-related disorders, including autoimmune diseases, chronic inflammation, and cancer. Mutations in the TP53 gene, which encodes p53, are commonly found in human cancers and can disrupt tumor-suppressive functions while also affecting its immunomodulatory activities. Moreover, alterations in the p53 pathway have been observed in autoimmune conditions such as systemic lupus erythematosus and rheumatoid arthritis, where aberrant p53 activation or inhibition may contribute to disease pathogenesis. Furthermore, chronic inflammation, a hallmark of many immune-related disorders, can perturb p53 signaling through various mechanisms, leading to immune dysfunction and tissue damage. Exhibiting, a pivotal role in modulating the immune response, p53 has emerged as a promising target for therapeutic intervention in cancer immunotherapy and immune-related diseases. Strategies aimed at restoring p53 function or targeting p53-dependent pathways could potentially enhance antitumor immunity, alleviate autoimmune responses, and mitigate chronic inflammation (34). Furthermore, the development of small molecule inhibitors or activators targeting p53 and its downstream effectors may offer new therapeutic avenues for the treatment of immune-related disorders. However, further research is needed to elucidate the complex regulatory networks governing p53-mediated immunomodulation and to effectively translate these findings into clinical applications.

17.4 CROSSTALK BETWEEN p53 AND STROMAL CELLS

The crosstalk between the tumor suppressor protein p53 and stromal cells within the tumor microenvironment is a multifaceted interplay that profoundly influences breast cancer progression and therapeutic responses (35). Stromal cells, encompassing fibroblasts, immune cells, and endothelial cells, intricately interact with cancer cells, shaping the dynamic ecosystem that supports tumor growth, invasion, and metastasis. Elucidating the intricate communication between p53 and stromal cells offers crucial insights into the underlying molecular mechanisms driving breast cancer pathogenesis and provides a foundation for the development of targeted therapeutic strategies. At the molecular level, p53 exerts regulatory control over various aspects of stromal cell function through direct and indirect mechanisms. For instance, p53 can modulate the secretion profile of stromal cells, influencing the production of cytokines, growth factors, and extracellular matrix components that regulate tumor–stromal interactions and shape the tumor microenvironment. Reciprocally, stromal cells can impact p53 activity in cancer cells through paracrine signaling pathways, highlighting the bidirectional nature of the crosstalk between p53 and stromal cells (36). A pivotal function of p53 in stromal cells is the regulation of their activation state. CAFs, a subset of activated stromal fibroblasts, play a critical role in tumor progression by fostering cancer cell proliferation, invasion, and metastasis. Dysfunctional p53 in stromal fibroblasts can drive their aberrant activation and acquisition of tumor-promoting properties, exacerbating tumor aggressiveness and therapeutic resistance. Conversely, restoration of functional p53 in CAFs has been demonstrated to suppress their tumor-promoting effects and impede tumor growth in experimental models, underscoring the therapeutic potential of targeting p53 in the stromal compartment. In addition to fibroblasts, immune cells within the tumor microenvironment engage in reciprocal crosstalk with p53-altered cancer cells. p53 orchestrates the recruitment, activation, and function of immune cells, including T cells, macrophages, and dendritic cells. Dysregulated p53 signaling in cancer cells can perturb the expression of immune checkpoint molecules, cytokines, and chemokines, fostering an immunosuppressive milieu that facilitates tumor immune evasion and progression. Conversely, activation of p53 signaling in cancer cells augments antitumor immune responses and sensitizes tumors to immunotherapy, highlighting the therapeutic implications of targeting p53 in the context of cancer-immune interactions (37).

Furthermore, the interplay between p53 and endothelial cells, crucial constituents of the tumor vasculature, is emerging as a determinant of tumor angiogenesis and vascular remodeling. p53 regulates endothelial cell function and vascular integrity, and its dysregulation can promote aberrant angiogenesis and tumor vascularization. Targeting p53 in endothelial cells represents a promising strategy to inhibit tumor angiogenesis and disrupt tumor blood supply, thereby enhancing the efficacy of anti-angiogenic therapies in breast cancer (38).

17.5 INFLAMMATORY SIGNALING PATHWAYS AND p53–MICROENVIRONMENT CROSSTALK

Inflammatory signaling pathways and their crosstalk with the tumor microenvironment (TME), particularly mediated by the tumor suppressor protein p53, represent a multifaceted axis in breast cancer progression. Chronic inflammation is a hallmark of cancer, including breast cancer, where it contributes to tumor initiation, progression, metastasis, and therapy resistance. Inflammatory cytokines, chemokines, and immune cells create a pro-tumorigenic microenvironment characterized by immune suppression, angiogenesis, and tissue remodeling (39). Importantly, p53 plays a crucial role in modulating inflammatory responses within the TME through its ability to transcriptionally regulate a myriad of target genes involved in inflammation, immune surveillance, and tissue homeostasis. Notably, wild-type p53 exerts anti-inflammatory effects by repressing the expression of pro-inflammatory cytokines such as interleukin-6 (IL-6), tumor necrosis factor-alpha (TNF-α), and interleukin-1 beta (IL-1β), while promoting the expression of anti-inflammatory mediators like interleukin-10 (IL-10) and transforming growth factor-beta (TGF-β). Moreover, p53 can modulate inflammatory signaling pathways, including NF-κB, STAT3, and JAK/STAT, by directly interacting with their components or through indirect mechanisms involving its transcriptional targets. For instance, p53 can inhibit NF-κB activation by suppressing the expression of NF-κB subunits or inducing the expression of negative regulators such as IκBα and PTEN, thereby attenuating the production of pro-inflammatory cytokines and chemokines. Additionally, p53 can inhibit STAT3 signaling by inducing the expression of suppressors of cytokine signaling (SOCS) proteins, which antagonize STAT activation and downstream target gene expression (40). Furthermore, p53 can regulate the production of reactive oxygen species and nitric oxide, which serve as signaling molecules in inflammatory pathways, by modulating the expression of antioxidant enzymes and nitric oxide synthases (41). Importantly, dysregulation of p53 function, either through genetic mutations or epigenetic alterations, can disrupt its anti-inflammatory activities and promote chronic inflammation within the TME, creating a permissive niche for tumor growth and metastasis. Conversely, inflammation can also impact p53 function by promoting its degradation, post-translational modifications, or sequestration within the cytoplasm, thereby attenuating its tumor-suppressive functions and promoting oncogenic signaling

17.5.1 Metabolic Reprogramming and p53–Microenvironment Dynamics

Metabolic reprogramming is a hallmark of cancer, including breast cancer, profoundly influencing the TME dynamics. Breast cancer cells exhibit altered metabolism characterized by increased aerobic glycolysis, enhanced glutamine dependency, and perturbed lipid metabolism to meet the bioenergetic and biosynthetic demands of rapid proliferation and survival (42). The tumor suppressor protein p53 plays a central role in regulating cellular metabolism by modulating the expression of genes involved in glycolysis, oxidative phosphorylation, and nutrient transport. In breast cancer, wild-type p53 acts as a metabolic gatekeeper, restraining glycolytic flux and promoting oxidative phosphorylation to maintain cellular energy homeostasis. Additionally, p53 regulates nutrient availability within the TME by inhibiting glucose uptake and lactate production, thereby modulating the acidic and nutrient-deprived microenvironment characteristic of tumors (43). However, mutations in the TP53 gene, which occur frequently in breast cancer, can disrupt these metabolic regulatory functions, leading to metabolic rewiring and nutrient scavenging within the TME. Mutant p53 promotes aerobic glycolysis by upregulating the expression of glycolytic enzymes such as glucose transporter 1 (GLUT1), hexokinase 2 (HK2), and lactate dehydrogenase A (LDHA) while suppressing oxidative phosphorylation through inhibition of mitochondrial respiration. Moreover, mutant p53 can enhance glutamine metabolism by promoting the expression of glutaminase (GLS) and glutamate dehydrogenase (GLUD1), fueling the tricarboxylic acid (TCA) cycle and supporting biosynthetic pathways essential for tumor growth and proliferation. Importantly, dysregulated metabolic reprogramming driven by mutant p53 contributes to the establishment of a hostile TME characterized by nutrient deprivation, hypoxia, and accumulation of metabolic byproducts, which in turn promote tumor progression, metastasis, and therapy resistance. Furthermore, mutant p53 can influence the metabolic crosstalk between cancer cells and stromal cells within the TME by promoting the secretion of metabolic intermediates and signaling molecules that facilitate tumor–stromal interactions and immune evasion (44).

17.6 ANGIOGENESIS AND VASCULAR REMODELING IN p53–MICROENVIRONMENT INTERACTIONS

Angiogenesis, the process of new blood vessel formation from preexisting vasculature, is a hallmark of tumor progression and metastasis in breast cancer, with profound implications for the TME. The tumor suppressor protein p53 emerges as a key regulator of angiogenesis and vascular remodeling within the TME, exerting both direct and indirect effects on endothelial cell behavior and angiogenic factor expression. In breast cancer, wild-type p53 functions as a potent inhibitor of angiogenesis by transcriptionally repressing the expression of pro-angiogenic factors such as vascular endothelial growth factor (VEGF), fibroblast growth factor (FGF), and angiopoietin-2 (Ang-2), while promoting the expression of anti-angiogenic factors like thrombospondin-1 (TSP-1) and endostatin. Consequently, loss or mutation of p53 disrupts this delicate balance, leading to dysregulated angiogenesis and aberrant vascular remodeling within the TME (45). Mutant p53 can enhance the expression of pro-angiogenic factors by directly binding to their promoters or by modulating the activity of transcriptional regulators such as hypoxia-inducible factor 1-alpha (HIF-1α) and nuclear factor-kappa B (NF-κB), thereby promoting endothelial cell proliferation, migration, and tube formation. Moreover, mutant p53 can impact endothelial cell behavior through non-cell-autonomous mechanisms, such as promoting the secretion of pro-angiogenic cytokines and chemokines by tumor cells or stromal cells within the TME. Importantly, dysregulated angiogenesis and vascular remodeling driven by mutant p53 contribute to tumor progression by facilitating nutrient and oxygen supply, promoting tumor cell intravasation and extravasation, and establishing a pre-metastatic niche conducive to metastatic colonization (46). Furthermore, mutant p53-mediated alterations in the TME can confer resistance to anti-angiogenic therapies by promoting alternative angiogenic pathways or enhancing the recruitment of pro-angiogenic myeloid cells. In summary, the interplay between p53 status and angiogenic processes within the TME critically influences breast cancer progression and therapeutic response, highlighting the importance of targeting mutant p53-driven angiogenesis as a promising therapeutic strategy for combating this deadly disease (47).

17.7 THERAPEUTIC IMPLICATIONS

The complex interrelationship between the tumor suppressor protein p53 and the dynamic tumor microenvironment in the progression of breast cancer presents a wide array of therapeutic opportunities grounded in fundamental molecular mechanisms. At the forefront of therapeutic exploration lies the targeting of aberrant p53 signaling pathways, offering a promising strategy to restore wild-type p53 function via gene therapy or small molecule compounds. By reinstating p53's canonical tumor-suppressive activities, these interventions aim to counteract the malignant progression driven by p53 mutations or dysregulation. Moreover, exploiting downstream effectors or synthetic lethality interactions specific to p53-deficient cells presents avenues for selective cancer cell eradication, capitalizing on vulnerabilities intrinsic to p53-mutant or p53-deficient tumors (48).

A multitude of therapeutic interventions targeting the interplay between p53 and the tumor microenvironment in breast cancer have been reported. Gene therapy approaches aim to restore wild type p53 function in mutated cells, yielding promising outcomes in preclinical studies. For instance, studies utilizing viral vectors to deliver functional p53 genes into cancer cells have shown reinstatement of p53-mediated tumor suppression and increased sensitivity to conventional therapies. Concurrently, small molecule compounds designed to reactivate mutant p53 or stabilize its conformation have demonstrated efficacy in restoring tumor-suppressive functions. These compounds, known as p53 reactivators or stabilizers, hold promise in preclinical models by inhibiting tumor growth and enhancing sensitivity to chemotherapy or radiation therapy (49). Immunotherapy, particularly immune checkpoint inhibitors, has emerged as a transformative approach to cancer treatment. Immune checkpoint inhibitors, such as pembrolizumab or atezolizumab, aim to unleash the body's immune response against cancer cells by targeting programmed cell death protein 1 (PD-1) or its ligand (PD-L1). In breast cancer, single-agent immunotherapy has shown modest responses in unselected patient populations. However, ongoing research is investigating combination approaches that integrate immune checkpoint inhibitors with agents targeting p53 or its downstream pathways. These synergistic combinations have the potential to enhance antitumor immune responses and improve treatment outcomes for breast cancer patients. Disruption of the tumor microenvironment emerges as another promising therapeutic strategy (50). Stromal components, including fibroblasts, immune cells, and the extracellular matrix, play pivotal roles in tumor progression and therapeutic resistance. Selective targeting of stromal cells or modulation of the extracellular matrix could disrupt the tumor-supportive niche, impeding cancer cell growth and metastasis. For example, inhibitors targeting components of the extracellular matrix or signaling pathways involved in stromal–cancer cell interactions, such as focal adhesion kinase (FAK) inhibitors or lysyl oxidase-like 2 (LOXL2) inhibitors, have demonstrated efficacy in preclinical models (51).

Furthermore, exploiting metabolic vulnerabilities associated with dysfunctional p53 presents a novel therapeutic avenue. Dysregulated metabolism, characterized by increased glycolysis and glutaminolysis, is a hallmark of cancer cells, partially driven by p53 alterations. Precision targeting of key metabolic enzymes or transporters could selectively impair cancer cell metabolism while preserving normal cellular function. Small molecule inhibitors targeting dysregulated metabolic pathways in cancer cells offer the potential for tailored therapeutic interventions in breast cancer treatment (52).

17.8 FUTURE OUTLOOK

The future outlook for the interplay between p53 and the tumor microenvironment in breast cancer progression holds great promise for advancing our understanding of disease dynamics and improving therapeutic strategies. As research continues to unravel the intricate molecular interactions between p53 and the TME, several key areas are poised for significant advancements and translational applications (53). With the advent of high-throughput sequencing technologies and multi-omics approaches, we anticipate a deeper characterization of the molecular landscape of breast cancer, including the genetic alterations in p53 and the TME components. Integrative analyses of genomic, transcriptomic, and epigenomic data will provide comprehensive insights into the regulatory networks governing the interplay between p53 and the TME, facilitating the identification of novel therapeutic targets and biomarkers for patient stratification (54).

Furthermore, advancements in preclinical models, such as patient-derived xenografts and organoid cultures, will enable more accurate recapitulation of the complex tumor–stromal interactions observed in breast cancer patients. These models will serve as valuable platforms for testing the efficacy of targeted therapies aimed at disrupting the p53–TME axis and evaluating their potential clinical impact. In parallel, the development of innovative therapeutic strategies targeting p53 and the TME holds great promise for improving treatment outcomes in breast cancer patients. Small molecule inhibitors targeting mutant p53 or modulating its downstream signaling pathways are under active investigation, with several compounds showing promising preclinical results (55). Combination therapies that simultaneously target p53 dysregulation and TME components, such as immune checkpoint inhibitors or stromal-targeting agents, are also being explored to overcome therapeutic resistance and enhance treatment efficacy. Moreover, the advent of precision medicine approaches, including genomic profiling and liquid biopsies, will facilitate the identification of patients who are most likely to benefit from therapies targeting the p53–TME axis (34). Personalized treatment strategies tailored to the specific molecular characteristics of individual tumors and their microenvironmental context will improve therapeutic response rates and minimize adverse effects (56). Thus, the future outlook for the interplay between p53 and the tumor microenvironment in breast cancer progression is characterized by rapid advancements in our understanding of disease biology and the development of innovative therapeutic approaches. By elucidating the molecular mechanisms underlying this intricate interplay and translating these findings into clinical practice, we aim to improve patient outcomes and ultimately transform the management of breast cancer

17.9 CONCLUSION

The intricate interplay between the tumor suppressor protein p53 and the tumor microenvironment in breast cancer progression represents a complex relationship with significant implications for disease pathogenesis and therapeutic strategies. Through its multifaceted molecular interactions, p53 exerts regulatory control over key aspects of the TME, including angiogenesis, inflammation, and immune response, while the TME reciprocally modulates p53 activity. The elucidation of these intricate interrelationships has provided invaluable insights into the underlying mechanisms driving breast cancer progression. Moreover, it has opened new avenues for therapeutic intervention, offering the potential to develop more effective and personalized treatment approaches. Moving forward, continued research efforts aimed at unraveling the molecular complexities of the p53–TME axis hold promise for improving patient outcomes and revolutionizing breast cancer management. By leveraging our understanding of the interplay between p53 and the TME, we can advance toward precision medicine approaches tailored to the specific molecular profiles of individual tumors and their microenvironmental context, ultimately enhancing therapeutic efficacy and patient care.

REFERENCES

1. Mijit M, Caracciolo V, Melillo A, Amicarelli F, Giordano A. Role of p53 in the regulation of cellular senescence. *Biomolecules.* 2020 Mar;10(3):420.
2. Friedel L, Loewer A. The guardian's choice: how p53 enables context-specific decision-making in individual cells. *The FEBS Journal.* 2022;289(1):40–52.
3. Joerger AC, Fersht AR. The p53 pathway: origins, inactivation in cancer, and emerging therapeutic approaches. *Annual Review of Biochemistry.* 2016 Jun 2;85:375–404.
4. Marcel V, Nguyen Van Long F, Diaz JJ. 40 years of research put p53 in translation. *Cancers.* 2018 May;10(5):152.
5. Chao CCK. Mechanisms of p53 degradation. *Clinica Chimica Acta.* 2015 Jan 1;438:139–147.
6. Vaddavalli PL, Schumacher B. The p53 network: cellular and systemic DNA damage responses in cancer and aging. *Trends in Genetics.* 2022 Jun 1;38(6):598–612.
7. Hainaut P. TP53: Coordinator of the processes that underlie the hallmarks of cancer. In: Hainaut P, Olivier M, Wiman KG, editors. *p53 in the Clinics* [Internet]. New York, NY: Springer; 2013 [cited 2024 Apr 29]. p. 1–23. https://doi.org/10.1007/978-1-4614-3676-8_1

8. Agupitan AD, Neeson P, Williams S, Howitt J, Haupt S, Haupt Y. P53: a guardian of immunity becomes its saboteur through mutation. *Int J Mol Sci.* 2020 Jan;21(10):3452.
9. van Weverwijk A, de Visser KE. Mechanisms driving the immunoregulatory function of cancer cells. *Nat Rev Cancer.* 2023 Apr;23(4):193–215.
10. Shi D, Jiang P. A different facet of p53 function: regulation of immunity and inflammation during tumor development. *Front Cell Dev Biol* [Internet]. 2021 Oct 18 [cited 2024 Apr 29];9. Available from: https://www.frontiersin.org/articles/10.3389/fcell.2021.762651
11. Blagih J, Buck MD, Vousden KH. p53, cancer and the immune response. Lennon-Duménil AM, editor. *J Cell Sci.* 2020 Mar 6;133(5):jcs237453.
12. Kashyap D, Garg VK, Sandberg EN, Goel N, Bishayee A. Oncogenic and tumor suppressive components of the cell cycle in breast cancer progression and prognosis. *Pharmaceutics.* 2021 Apr;13(4):569.
13. Duffy MJ, Synnott NC, O'Grady S, Crown J. Targeting p53 for the treatment of cancer. *Semin Cancer Biol.* 2022 Feb 1;79:58–67.
14. Valente JFA, Queiroz JA, Sousa F. p53 as the focus of gene therapy: past, present and future. *Curr Drug Targets.* 2018 Dec 1;19(15):1801–1817.
15. Runa F, Hamalian S, Meade K, Shisgal P, Gray PC, Kelber JA. Tumor microenvironment heterogeneity: challenges and opportunities. *Curr Mol Bio Rep.* 2017 Dec 1;3(4):218–229.
16. Bu L, Baba H, Yoshida N, Miyake K, Yasuda T, Uchihara T, et al. Biological heterogeneity and versatility of cancer-associated fibroblasts in the tumor microenvironment. *Oncogene.* 2019 Jun;38(25):4887–901.
17. Basak U, Sarkar T, Mukherjee S, Chakraborty S, Dutta A, Dutta S, et al. Tumor-associated macrophages: an effective player of the tumor microenvironment. *Front Immunol* [Internet]. 2023 Nov 16 [cited 2024 Apr 29];14. Available from: https://www.frontiersin.org/journals/immunology/articles/10.3389/fimmu.2023.1295257/full
18. de Visser KE, Joyce JA. The evolving tumor microenvironment: from cancer initiation to metastatic outgrowth. *Cancer Cell.* 2023 Mar 13;41(3):374–403.
19. Brassart-Pasco S, Brézillon S, Brassart B, Ramont L, Oudart JB, Monboisse JC. Tumor microenvironment: extracellular matrix alterations influence tumor progression. *Front Oncol.* 2020 Apr 15;10:397.
20. Nallasamy P, Nimmakayala RK, Parte S, Are AC, Batra SK, Ponnusamy MP. Tumor microenvironment enriches the stemness features: the architectural event of therapy resistance and metastasis. *Mol Cancer.* 2022 Dec 22;21:225.
21. Boutelle AM, Attardi LD. p53 and tumor suppression: it takes a network. *Trends Cell Biol.* 2021 Apr;31(4):298–310.
22. Joshi RS, Kanugula SS, Sudhir S, Pereira MP, Jain S, Aghi MK. The role of cancer-associated fibroblasts in tumor progression. *Cancers.* 2021 Jan;13(6):1399.
23. Rahnamoun H, Lu H, Duttke SH, Benner C, Glass CK, Lauberth SM. Mutant p53 shapes the enhancer landscape of cancer cells in response to chronic immune signaling. *Nat Commun.* 2017 Sep 29;8(1):754.
24. Martinez JD. Restoring p53 tumor suppressor activity as an anticancer therapeutic strategy. *Future Oncol.* 2010 Dec;6(12):1857–1862.
25. Saldaña-Meyer R, Recillas-Targa F. Transcriptional and epigenetic regulation of the p53 tumor suppressor gene. *Epigenetics.* 2011 Sep 1;6(9):1068–1077.
26. Kaur RP, Vasudeva K, Kumar R, Munshi A. Role of p53 gene in breast cancer: focus on mutation spectrum and therapeutic strategies. *Curr Pharm Des.* 2018 Aug 1;24(30):3566–3575.
27. Giancotti FG. Deregulation of cell signaling in cancer. *FEBS Lett.* 2014 Aug 19;588(16):2558–2570.
28. Wang Y, Chen Y, Chen Q, Zhang X, Wang H, Wang Z, et al. The role of acetylation sites in the regulation of p53 activity. *Mol Biol Rep.* 2020 Jan 1;47(1):381–391.
29. Li K, Shi H, Zhang B, Ou X, Ma Q, Chen Y, et al. Myeloid-derived suppressor cells as immunosuppressive regulators and therapeutic targets in cancer. *Sig Transduct Target Ther.* 2021 Oct 7;6(1):1–25.
30. Hassin O, Oren M. Drugging p53 in cancer: one protein, many targets. *Nat Rev Drug Discov.* 2023 Feb;22(2):127–44.
31. Khandia R, Munjal A. Chapter six - Interplay between inflammation and cancer. In: Donev R, editor. *Advances in Protein Chemistry and Structural Biology* [Internet]. Academic Press; 2020 [cited 2024 Apr 29]. p. 199–245. (Inflammatory Disorders, Part A; vol. 119). Available from: https://www.sciencedirect.com/science/article/pii/S1876162319300690
32. Carrà G, Lingua MF, Maffeo B, Taulli R, Morotti A. P53 vs NF-κB: the role of nuclear factor-kappa B in the regulation of p53 activity and vice versa. *Cell Mol Life Sci.* 2020 Nov 1;77(22):4449–4458.
33. Shi T, Dansen TB. Reactive oxygen species induced p53 activation: DNA damage, redox signaling, or both? *Antioxid Redox Signal.* 2020 Oct 20;33(12):839–859.

34. Hu J, Cao J, Topatana W, Juengpanich S, Li S, Zhang B, et al. Targeting mutant p53 for cancer therapy: direct and indirect strategies. *J Hematol Oncol.* 2021 Sep 28;14(1):157.
35. Akinsipe T, Mohamedelhassan R, Akinpelu A, Pondugula SR, Mistriotis P, Avila LA, et al. Cellular interactions in tumor microenvironment during breast cancer progression: new frontiers and implications for novel therapeutics. *Front Immunol* [Internet]. 2024 Mar 12 [cited 2024 Apr 29];15. Available from: https://www.frontiersin.org/journals/immunology/articles/10.3389/fimmu.2024.1302587/full
36. Baghban R, Roshangar L, Jahanban-Esfahlan R, Seidi K, Ebrahimi-Kalan A, Jaymand M, et al. Tumor microenvironment complexity and therapeutic implications at a glance. *Cell Commun Signal.* 2020 Apr 7;18(1):59.
37. Chibaya L, Snyder J, Ruscetti M. Senescence and the tumor-immune landscape: implications for cancer immunotherapy. *Semin Cancer Biol.* 2022 Nov 1;86:827–845.
38. Abou Khouzam R, Brodaczewska K, Filipiak A, Zeinelabdin NA, Buart S, Szczylik C, et al. Tumor hypoxia regulates immune escape/invasion: influence on angiogenesis and potential impact of hypoxic biomarkers on cancer therapies. *Front Immunol* [Internet]. 2021 Jan 20 [cited 2024 Apr 29];11. Available from: https://www.frontiersin.org/journals/immunology/articles/10.3389/fimmu.2020.613114/full
39. Malla RR, Kiran P. Tumor microenvironment pathways: cross regulation in breast cancer metastasis. *Genes Dis.* 2022 Mar 1;9(2):310–24.
40. Yeung YT, Aziz F, Guerrero-Castilla A, Arguelles S. Signaling pathways in inflammation and anti-inflammatory therapies. *Curr Pharm Des.* 2018 Apr 1;24(14):1449–1484.
41. Ladelfa MF, Toledo MF, Laiseca JE, Monte M. Interaction of p53 with tumor suppressive and oncogenic signaling pathways to control cellular reactive oxygen species production. *Antioxid Redox Signal.* 2011 Sep 15;15(6):1749–1761.
42. Dias AS, Almeida CR, Helguero LA, Duarte IF. Metabolic crosstalk in the breast cancer microenvironment. *Eur J Cancer.* 2019 Nov 1;121:154–171.
43. Wang YP, Lei QY. Perspectives of reprogramming breast cancer metabolism. In: Song E, Hu H, editors. *Translational Research in Breast Cancer: Biomarker Diagnosis, Targeted Therapies and Approaches to Precision Medicine* [Internet]. Singapore: Springer; 2017 [cited 2024 Apr 30]. p. 217–32. https://doi.org/10.1007/978-981-10-6020-5_10
44. Nong S, Han X, Xiang Y, Qian Y, Wei Y, Zhang T, et al. Metabolic reprogramming in cancer: mechanisms and therapeutics. *MedComm.* 2023 Mar 27;4(2):e218.
45. Madu CO, Wang S, Madu CO, Lu Y. Angiogenesis in breast cancer progression, diagnosis, and treatment. *J Cancer.* 2020 May 18;11(15):4474–4494.
46. Zhang C, Liu J, Wang J, Zhang T, Xu D, Hu W, et al. The interplay between tumor suppressor p53 and hypoxia signaling pathways in cancer. *Front Cell Dev Biol.* 2021 Feb 18;9:648808.
47. Sermeus A, Michiels C. Reciprocal influence of the p53 and the hypoxic pathways. *Cell Death Dis.* 2011 May;2(5):e164–e164.
48. Guo G, Cui Y. New perspective on targeting the tumor suppressor p53 pathway in the tumor microenvironment to enhance the efficacy of immunotherapy. *J Immunotherap Cancer.* 2015 Mar 24;3(1):9.
49. Hernández Borrero LJ, El-Deiry WS. Tumor suppressor p53: biology, signaling pathways, and therapeutic targeting. *BBA Rev Cancer.* 2021 Aug 1;1876(1):188556.
50. Muraro E, Vinante L, Fratta E, Bearz A, Höfler D, Steffan A, et al. Metronomic chemotherapy: anti-tumor pathways and combination with immune checkpoint inhibitors. *Cancers.* 2023 Jan;15(9):2471.
51. Wang DR, Wu XL, Sun YL. Therapeutic targets and biomarkers of tumor immunotherapy: response versus non-response. *Sig Transduct Target Ther.* 2022 Sep 19;7(1):1–27.
52. Stine ZE, Schug ZT, Salvino JM, Dang CV. Targeting cancer metabolism in the era of precision oncology. *Nat Rev Drug Discov.* 2022 Feb;21(2):141–162.
53. Li YR, Fang Y, Lyu Z, Zhu Y, Yang L. Exploring the dynamic interplay between cancer stem cells and the tumor microenvironment: implications for novel therapeutic strategies. *J Transl Med.* 2023 Oct 2;21:686.
54. Neagu AN, Whitham D, Bruno P, Morrissiey H, Darie CA, Darie CC. Omics-based investigations of breast cancer. *Molecules.* 2023 Jun 14;28(12):4768.
55. Guillen KP, Fujita M, Butterfield AJ, Scherer SD, Bailey MH, Chu Z, et al. A human breast cancer-derived xenograft and organoid platform for drug discovery and precision oncology. *Nat Cancer.* 2022 Feb;3(2):232–250.
56. Tang C, Fu S, Jin X, Li W, Xing F, Duan B, et al. Personalized tumor combination therapy optimization using the single-cell transcriptome. *Genome Med.* 2023 Dec 1;15(1):105.

18 Current State and Future Avenues of p53 Gene Therapy in Breast Cancer

Jahnvi Arora[1], Mary Chatterjee[1], Nusrat Jan[2], and Manzoor Ahmad Mir[2]*

[1]Biotechnology Engineering, University Institute of Engineering and Technology, Panjab University, Chandigarh, India
[2]Department of Bioresources, School of Biological Sciences, University of Kashmir, Srinagar, J&K, India
*drmanzoor@kashmiruniversity.ac.in

18.1 INTRODUCTION

18.1.1 The p53 Gene's Function in Breast Cancer

TP53 mutations frequently happen in all human cancers except that they inhibit this tumor suppressor and vital regulator transcription factor. Its broad role in maintaining the genome stability of the cells as well as the chromosomes makes p53 the "guardian of the genome." The diversity of this inhibitor of tumors can be caused by the mutations or the modifications of its expression level and the transcription factor sequence, which changes the transcription of genes. TP53 is associated with a protein that is responsible for the stability of genomic units, but it also does chromatin remodeling, repair, and recombination, other functions being included (1). Several physiological processes are regulated by TP53, which is considered the main controller of cell cycle and DNA metabolism, apoptosis, aging, energy metabolism, angiogenesis, immunological responses, and metastasis. Among all types of cancers, at least 50% of them contain mutations that modify the way TP53 functions in transcription. People with TP53 gene alterations are likely to develop various types of cancer, among them breast cancer (Figure 18.1).

There have been several genetic studies on hereditary breast cancer and basal-like cancer, which found that TP53 mutations are present in them, in addition to sporadic occurrence. We observed a positive association between p53 gene-targeted mega base-scale interactions with enhancer and promoter regions of genes related to tumor suppression such as STK11 (LKB1), CDKN1A, DLEU1, FAT1, KDM6A, TNFRSF10B, FOXO1, PTEN, WT1, and SMARCA2 (2). When there is a mutation on p53, tumors can grow either in the absence or in the presence of an external trigger, resulting in the downregulation of oncogenes that are continuously expressed in the cell and because of p53's inability to bind stress-responsive target and certain tumor suppressor genes. The TP53 gene encodes a protein with phosphate added to it and three domains of 393 amino acids (3). In the N-terminal region of the protein, are the transactivation domains 1 and 2: TAD1 is comprised of the first 40 residues of VP1 and TAD2 the next 21 residues. In the domain of transcriptional activators or corepressors, several collaborators take part in the interactions. These motifs of sequence are important for the areas of regulatory protein transcription that are involved in TAD1 and TAD2 proteins. The proline-rich region within residues 63 and 97 is one of the prominent features of the transactivation domain (4). In

 DOI: 10.1201/9781003520771-18

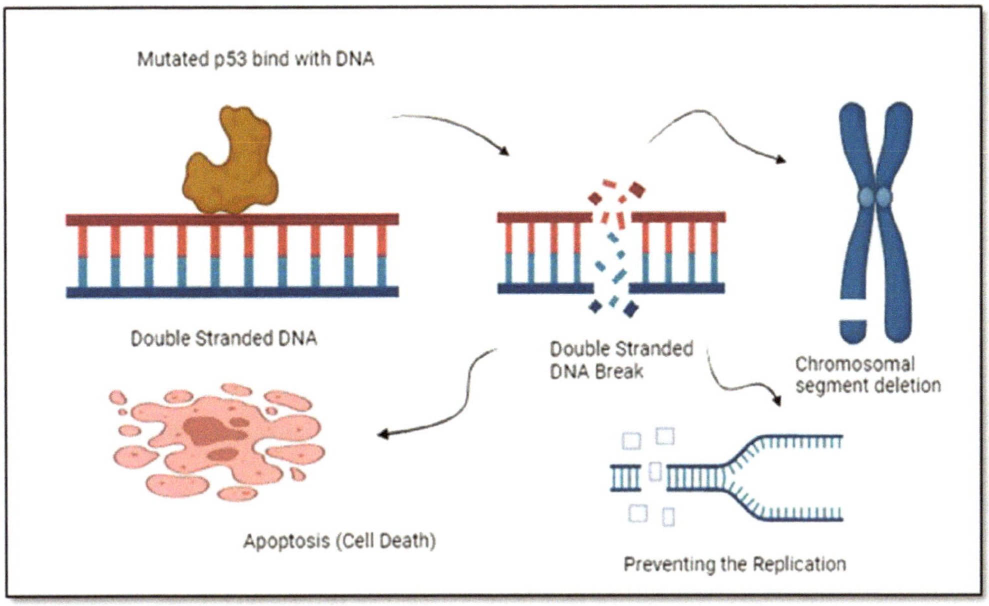

FIGURE 18.1 Binding of mutated p53 leads to various disfunctioning.

this chapter, we will be introducing the DNA binding domain, which is a highly conserved domain and is responsible for sequence-specific binding. It includes residues 102–292. Residues 301–323 form a linker region that follows the DNA binding domain and contains a signal for nuclear localization. Residues 323–356 comprise the tetramerization domain, which comes next. Finally, there is the C-terminal regulatory domain (REG), which is 363–393 residues long and mainly disorganized. The highly alkaline C-terminus contains two nuclear localization markers as well as a linker region. The C-terminus affects TP53 activity via modulating protein–protein interactions (5).

18.1.2 Importance of Gene Therapy in the Treatment of Breast Cancer

Even though there are multiple potential breast cancer gene therapy targets, no authorized gene therapy medications for breast cancer are currently available (6). It is appropriate to think that a therapeutic product will be generated soon, as cancer makes up roughly 63% of gene therapy clinical trials. As our understanding of the genetic dysregulation of the many subtypes of breast cancer develops, selecting an appropriate genetic therapy for the disease becomes increasingly difficult. The European Commission's (EC) 2003/63 regulation defines a gene therapy substance as a nucleic acid fragment administered within or outside the body for diagnosis, treatment, or prevention (Figure 18.2) (7).

The aforementioned treatments have not only reduced mortality but have also proved curative for the vast majority of patients. Metastatic lesions will reappear in a substantial proportion of tumors. Gene therapy, a potential new treatment for breast cancer, entails transferring genes that code for a variety of biological processes that may prevent tumor growth (8). However, for these strategies to be effective, several significant challenges must be solved. At the outset, our understanding of the molecular processes that lead to breast cancer remains restricted. A lack of understanding of the molecular and cellular mechanisms in action may restrict medicines aimed at halting cancer progression at the molecular level. Additionally, some vectors, such as retroviruses, cannot deliver genes into breast cancer cells due to the sluggish progression of most breast cancers. Considering that breast cancer cells grow slowly, it may be necessary to prolong gene expression beyond what is typically required to avoid immediate cell damage with gene therapy. Despite these evident

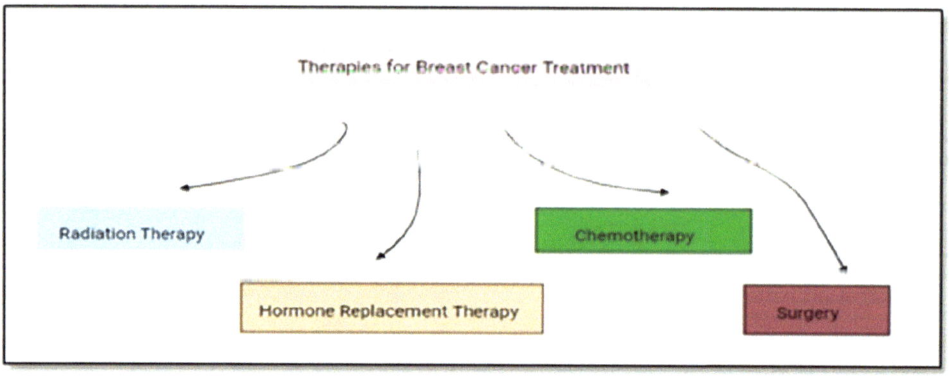

FIGURE 18.2 Treatments for breast cancer.

challenges, gene therapy techniques for breast cancer have progressed significantly. The approaches may be roughly classified into two types:

1. Those that attempt to modify the metabolic or signaling pathways of breast cancer cells.
2. Those that attempt to increase the immune response to tumor cells. Because immunologic techniques avoid many of the aforementioned issues, the second category has received the greatest attention. Breast cancer is not the only type of tumor that these treatments can be used for; in fact, they may be more effective on other tumor forms first.

18.2 BREAST CANCER: CURRENT STATUS FOR p53 GENE THERAPY

18.2.1 Existing Treatments: An Overview

Cancer is the outcome of disturbed cell development and death. Therapeutic advances need a novel medicinal chemical with an unconventional mode of action, multiple cell death pathways, and synergistic advantages with existing cancer medicines (9). These characteristics are shared by gene therapies. Cancer gene therapy includes gene-directed enzyme prodrugs, proapoptotic gene therapies, immunotherapies, anti-angiogenic gene therapies, oncolytic virotherapy, and suicide gene therapies.

18.2.2 Virotherapy with Oncolytic Properties

Cancer immunity can be increased through oncolytic virotherapy, one of the most promising approaches currently available. Oncolytic viruses (OVs) are replication-competent and preferentially infect cancer cells. Natural virus oncolytic and genetically modified virus oncolytic are two types of oncolytic. A parvovirus or Newcastle disease virus, which occurs naturally in cells, may proliferate diseases caused by viruses such as vesicular stomatitis, measles, herpes simplex virus infection, and vaccinia were made safer and more cancer-specific by modifying genes. These kinds of viruses are oncolytic; they destroy cancer cells irrespective of their genetic makeup. In addition, more established therapies like immunotherapy, which treat cancer by lysing malignant cells (10), can be used. Activating the p53 gene restores p53 production in 50% of cancers. Several recombinant OVs have been developed to produce p53, which may then be used in conjunction with the host immune system or other treatments to destroy cancer cells.

18.2.2.1 Gendicine (Recombinant Human p53 Adenovirus [Ad5RSV-p53])

Squamous cell carcinoma of the neck and head was the first gene product approved in 2003. With Gendicine, the p53 cDNA gene is inserted instead of E1 in a non-replicating adenoviral vector.

When p53 is expressed in cancer cells, it causes programmed cell death, inhibits DNA repair, and reduces cell death prevention (11). Gendicine eradicates cancer cells by restoring protein function and expression. Atypically, 90–96% of patients respond to Gendicine in a variety of therapeutic applications, with 30–40% responding completely and 50–60% responding partially. Gendicine is used by more than 30,000 patients.

18.2.2.2 Oncorine (rAd5-H101)

Non-small cell carcinoma patients who lack the p53 gene have a worse survival rate and are more resistant to medications (12). Oncorine, an ad5 virus, changes the E1B 55K gene. The wild type cannot inhibit apoptotic pathway activity without deactivating the host cell's p53 gene. The E1B 55K gene deletion restricts the virus to p53-deficient host cells by preventing healthy cells from distributing it. Oncolysis is a method of treating solid tumors that involves the development of viruses in cancer cells. After cancer cells are removed, adenoviruses enter the bloodstream and infect additional cells, triggering an Oncorine-mediated cell death cascade.

18.3 CHALLENGES AND LIMITATIONS

It is estimated that about half of all cancer cases are linked to the p53 gene, which is the most commonly altered gene in the human genome (13). Mutations in this gene can cause it to lose normal function or develop cancer-promoting characteristics. As a result of mutations in the p53 tumor suppressor, the cell cycle can be arrested, apoptosis can be induced, senescent growth can be halted, chromosomal instability can be caused, and DNA base excision repair can be inadequate. These changes promote cancer development by making it easier to evade essential cell cycle events. Cancers with gain-of-function p53 mutations, on the other hand, can enable tumors to expand faster, change target gene activation, evade programmed cell death, and become more resistant to chemotherapy (14). Researchers revealed that p53 gene mutations impact up to 96% of patients with HGSOC. These changes can induce p53 activity to increase (oncogenic) or decrease (loss of function). Most commonly, peripheral blood progenitor cells (PBPCs) have been transplanted for breast cancer patients in the United States in recent years. However, just a few randomized trials have attempted to test the effectiveness of this medication. Malignant cells inserted into a transplant following contamination of progenitor cells can cause a return of sickness, as revealed in gene tagging studies. For detecting minimal residual illness, cytochemistry, tissue culture, and polymerase chain reaction (PCR)-based methods are used. The degree of sensitivity varies across different approaches. Because the final approach can exponentially duplicate incredibly small amounts of DNA, it may be capable of achieving the highest sensitivity. For research on breast cancer, researchers often use specific markers, such as CK19, to look for epithelial cells that are usually absent in bone marrow and peripheral blood progenitor cells. Despite their high sensitivity, these approaches may produce false positives. When RT-PCR was used to identify CK19 gene transcripts in bone marrow samples, both patients with chronic myeloid leukemia and healthy individuals had false-positive findings.

18.4 SUCCESSES AND FAILURES OF CURRENT APPROACHES

Genetic engineering and molecular biology have improved dramatically in the previous two decades, enabling new gene therapy alternatives. Most of these therapies fail to cure cancer. However, a few long-term survival cases suggest this treatment may work. Many cancer types have defective p53 genes, which have been the subject of gene therapy clinical trials worldwide (15). A genetically engineered adenovirus known as ONYX-015, also known as dl1520, was used to study non-small cell lung cancer (NSCLC) patients. This modified virus lacks an E1B gene to limit its reproduction in cells with a p53 gene mutation. The virus was well tolerated and marginally reduced tumor development in early clinical studies. Gendicine, the first commercial gene therapy, created wild type-p53 with a Rous sarcoma viral promoter using a modified adenovirus. Squamous cell carcinoma of the head and neck was treated with this therapy. Sixty-four percent of 132 patients in phase III clinical trials experienced complete remission following radiation and virus injection (16). Limited information exists about this clinical study. Clinical studies of Advexin®, a similar drug, were evaluated for various cancers.

A functioning p53 detects DNA damage and stops cell development. Mutations in the p53 gene can cause cancer by removing this protective function (17). Breast cancer is complicated and caused by genetic, environmental, and lifestyle factors. Approximately 30% of breast tumors are caused by p53 gene alterations.

18.5 MECHANISM OF p53 GENE THERAPY

18.5.1 Restoring the Wild-Type Function of p53

Tumors containing mutant forms of p53 may be treated by restoring normal p53 function. It is challenging to restore p53 due to the wide variety of mutations found in cancer. As an example of a medication that restores p53 function, PRIMA-1 (APR-246) is available. It transforms into the electrophile methylene quinuclidinone when it comes in contact with Cys124 and 277 in mutant p53's core domain. MQ binding induces mutant p53 to revert to wild-type capabilities. MIRA-1, CP-31398, STIMA-1, and 3-benzoyl acrylic acid, all mutant p53-reactivating drugs, exhibited similar thiol reactivity to mutant p53. Michael's addition links them chemically to mutant p53. Inducing cell death, and inhibiting cancer growth in living beings can be achieved with small molecular weight compounds like PRIMA-1 (ARP-246) to restore the normal form of p53. When it comes to repairing p53, APR-246 is the first chemical to be examined in clinical studies, either alone or in conjunction with other therapies. Acute myeloid leukemia phase I and phase III clinical trials combining APR-246 and azacytidine are presently underway (Figure 18.3) (18).

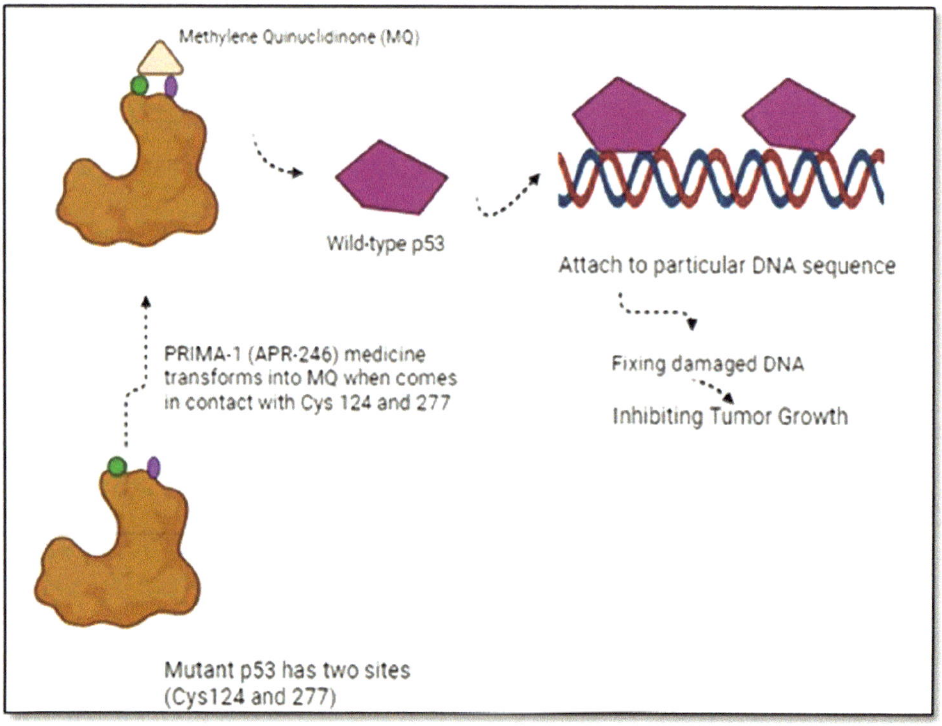

FIGURE 18.3 Wild-type p53 leads to restore p53 function.

18.5.2 Targeted Gene Delivery Systems

In recent years, gene therapy based on the adeno-associated virus (AAV) has made significant progress in treating human monogenic disorders, yielding surprising therapeutic results. Additionally, this breakthrough has enabled AAV vectors to be used in gene therapy to treat cancer. However, AAV vectors have a limited capacity to properly convey genetic information to other regions of interest since they tend to concentrate in the liver when disseminated throughout the body. Furthermore, if the vectors responsible for delivery enter the bloodstream during local delivery, the AAV capsid antigen and transgene may be dispersed throughout the body (19). Consequently, gene therapy is mainly concentrated on refining AAV vectors for better targeting of tumors.

Alexander Muick's team, on the other hand, developed chemistry that permits DARPins to be covalently bonded to the surfaces of AAV particles through PTS, which serves as a protein trans-splicing (PTS) process. Breast cancer cells carrying on epithelial cell adhesion molecule (EpCAM) were inactive with a microscopic methodology considering the combination of AAV and PTS (20). There are many doubts regarding the efficacy of DARPins-modified AAV2 vector in a gene delivery therapy that inhibits tumor cells proliferating and also distinguishes the tumor cells from other normal cells in the human cellular environment. EC1 DARPin was encoded into the AAV2 vector to give rise to AAV2MEC1, a vector skin AAV targeting EpCAM. The suicide gene HSV-TK encoded by the AAV2MEC1 construct proved efficacious in terms of invading breast cancer cells in mice and subsequent inhibition of tumors. The publication reported that AAV2MEC1 shows itself as a potential tool in breast cancer treatment because of its gene delivery method, which is groundbreaking in this field (21). We are convinced that our investigations may be the basis for the development of cancer gene therapy methods surpassing the current state of the art and more accurate gene transportation methods.

18.5.3 Immunotherapy Approaches

A tumor antigen is a small protein that contains, for example, only a few amino acids. These amino acids are called epitopes. They cause both T lymphocytes with CD8+ and CD4+ functions to recognize the antigen (22). Cellular expression of these surface epitopes happens together with those human leukocyte antigens (HLAs) in class I or class II in common. Conceptually a cancer vaccine that prevents the tumors from growing may be formulated by inducing the mutant p53 expression. Regardless of this, however, mutant p53 will not be found in the outer layer of the cell as it is found inside it (23). Scientists have come up with a mutated form of p53 protein that in conjugation with the HLA complex is now shown on the cells' surface. The development of novel immunotherapy for this p53 peptide–HLA complex might be a solution where cancer cells are showing it on their surface. This approach has those neoantigens for this purpose, which is used to enhance T-cells' ability to recognize and kill cancer cells. Vogelstein and his colleagues pioneered the development of H2-scDb, a new type of antibody that has two attached and specific arms. The p53 R175 mutant peptide–HLA complex can be seen on cancer cell surfaces with the antibody that binds partially with the T-cell receptor (24). Here, such bispecific antibody makes cancer cells have contact with T-cells and thus the latter will die. This bispecific antibody's development is the targeting of cancer cells with mutant p53 and, consequently, the tumor growth will be inhibited to a larger extent. Immunotherapy that makes use of T-cells, which gets its power from the multispecific bispecific antibody that is designed to attack p53 mutations, will be the next frontier for precision cancer medicine (Figure 18.4).

18.6 BREAST CANCER: FUTURE AVENUES FOR p53 GENE THERAPY

18.6.1 Innovations and Emerging Technologies

A chimeric protein p53-Bad contains an integrated MTS created by fusing monomeric p53 with the proapoptotic factor Bad. Mutant p53's inhibitory effects were effectively countered by chimeric

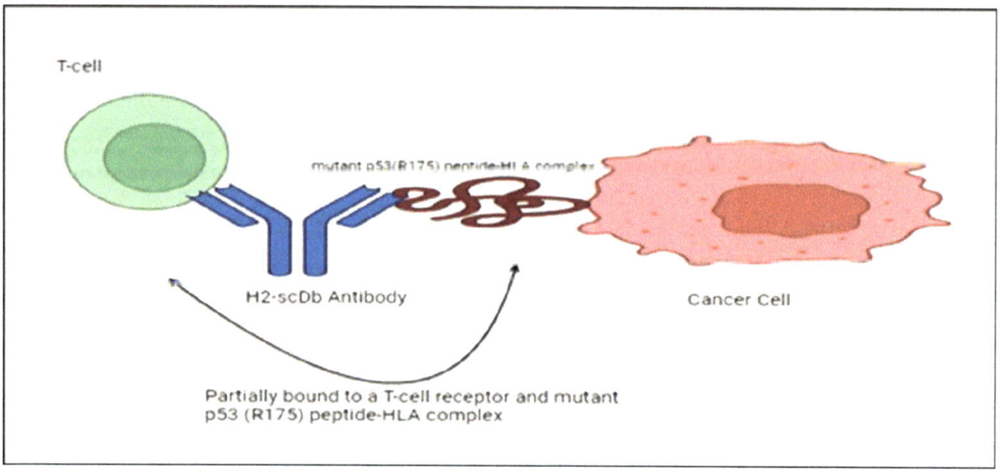

FIGURE 18.4 H2-scdb bispecific antibody leads to the ultimate destruction of cancer cells.

proteins p53-MTS and p53-Bad. Through the induction of cell death in cancer cell lines with different p53 mutations, this novel gene therapy strategy demonstrated promise as a treatment option independent of p53 status (25). Another step toward more sophisticated p53 gene therapies is the development of "super-p53," which replaces p53 with an alternate tetramerization domain (TD). For optimal transcriptional function, p53 needs its tetramerization domain. This domain not only enables dominant-negative p53 mutants and wild-type p53 to form hetero-oligomers, but it does so concurrently. To prevent this undesirable event, a modified leucine zipper with a four-stranded coiled-coil structure was used to replace the wild-type p53 protein's transactivation domain. To function properly, the engineered zipper's ability to induce tetramerization was critical because p53 molecules engineered solely for dimerization demonstrate limited efficacy as tumor suppressors (26).

Lim's study followed a similar methodology. Rather than replacing the original p53 tetramerization domain with a coiled-coil derived from B-cell receptor (BCR), the study used a coil derived from BCR, which induces apoptosis. The artificial p53-CC protein was immune to mutant p53's dominant-negative inhibition because it could not form a tetramer. Crucially, p53-CC retained its tetramer-forming and activation-triggering abilities, which are required for effective tumor suppression in living organisms.

18.6.2 Combination Therapies with p53 Gene Therapy

If a single tumor has many abnormalities in the oncogenic and signaling pathways, cancer cells may develop resistance to traditional chemotherapy. Administering two separate drugs with specific targets at the same time can improve tumor treatment efficacy compared to single-drug approaches. This approach is commonly used in clinical cancer treatment. Clinical trials have demonstrated that Adp53 gene therapy is effective when combined with radiation and chemotherapy (27). The results of studies like this provide proof for such treatment regimens. When p53 activation is added to the treatment, the likelihood of the cancer being eliminated at different stages of progression increases. The side effects are reduced and the cancer will not become resistant. Injecting chemicals of p53 restoration can cause cellular stress, which is correlated with the growth of reactive oxygen species (ROS). We can treat p53 targets with compound mixtures and then use cellular stress therapy to pursue a synergistic effect. The combination of therapies, which may include PRIMA-1, a p53-reactivating molecule that generates cellular stress, can be suggested. PRIMA-1 (APR-246) was recognized to have an activity in lowering glutathione (GSH) levels; on the other hand, it could boost ROS. SCL7A11, which is attended to xC(-) system, controls GSH levels. APR246 has been proven to be a major biomarker for the assessment of cancer patients' treatment efficiency (28). Through PRIMA plus the inhibitor of the xC(-) system, more ROS are generated that contribute to better antitumor effects. p53-reactivating compounds can be utilized more efficiently in the case when they put regulation of cellular stress-related signaling pathways in place. JNK is a signaling pathway that contributes to the positive adaptation of the organism to stress. The p53 pathway has been targeted by treatments that aim to suppress it and the result has been its activation. Cancer studies include a compound called PRIMA that restores p53 function that triggers cell death using a p53-dependent mechanism (29). One of the few other stress-related genes whose expression changed was the JNK signaling pathway in response to receiving the p53-reactivating drug RITA. These results indicate that RITA and the JNK activator operate jointly to eliminate multiple myeloma cell lines and patient samples. Because of the way small molecules trigger p53-mediated cell death via the JNK signaling pathway, combining p53-activating drugs with JNK-activating substances makes sense for treating some cancers. These findings provide new evidence for using cellular stress signaling to target mutant p53.

18.6.3 Customized Medications and Development of Biomarker

The TP53 gene, which is responsible for one of the most frequent cancer mutations, produces a p53 protein, which may be a target for future cancer treatments. Researchers are investigating several chemicals that can restore or improve normal p53 function, even though this approach is fraught with difficulties. Cancer cells with normal TP53 genes overproduce the negative regulator MDM2, effectively preventing p53 from doing its job (30). Chemicals that prevent p53 from binding to MDM2 can induce a strong p53 response, but this may result in non-cancerous cells having more p53 activity than usual. It is possible to cause significant cell death in cancer cells with a TP53 mutation by using compounds that improve the translation of nonsense mutant TP53 or reconfiguring missense mutant p53. Different types of cancer patients have been subjected to clinical trials with some of these compounds. It is still not possible to use p53-targeting medications in clinical settings. What we now understand about p53's biology may help explain why treatments to restore it have had such varying degrees of success in clinical trials. This review delves into the complex relationship between p53 and its cellular and microenvironmental context, as well as the various factors that can affect p53's function.

Using what is known about cancer suppression mechanisms, researchers created p53 biomarker profiles to predict p53 gene therapy efficacy. As a general hypothesis, we thought tumors with p53 profiles positive for gene therapy efficacy would have wild-type p53 gene configurations, where extra normal p53 would compensate for the upregulation of HDM2 and HDM4 as p53 inhibitors (31). It is hypothesized that tumors with p53 profiles unsuitable for p53 gene therapy will have higher levels of "dominant-negative" mutations, which inhibit p53 expression. These effects may render normal p53, which is introduced through gene therapy, inactive.

The Oncology Biomarker Qualification Initiative, which was launched in collaboration between the National Institutes of Health (NIH) and the Food and Drug Administration (FDA), is now live (32). The goal of this endeavor is to improve patient care and accelerate the development of new cancer medications. The ultimate goal is to discover biomarkers that can accurately identify treatment-sensitive patient populations. For terminally ill patients, identifying biomarkers that reliably indicate treatment efficacy is critical. Because there is insufficient time for trial and error, a potentially beneficial therapy may not be administered in these cases. This has led to the inclusion of predictive p53 biomarkers in clinical trials assessing the efficacy of p53 gene therapy in patients with recurrent squamous cell carcinoma of the head and neck. The trial results show that tumor p53 biomarkers can help predict which patients will benefit the most from p53 gene therapy.

18.7 CLINICAL TRIALS AND ADVANCEMENT IN RESEARCH

18.7.1 Currently Ongoing Clinical Trials

APR-246 is a small-molecular therapeutic candidate rather than a type of gene therapy. It can also be referred to as eprenetapopt or PRIMA-1^{MET}. This compound aims to rectify the unusual arrangement and function of the mutant p53, a tumor suppressor protein that is often altered and dysfunctional in cancerous tumors (33). By encouraging cell survival and proliferation, mutant p53 aids in the progression of cancer. APR-246 causes cancer cells harboring mutant p53 to undergo programmed cell death (apoptosis) by transforming the mutant p53 into a functioning version. Preclinical studies and early-phase clinical investigations using the substance have produced favorable outcomes for a wide range of cancer types. The medication designed to reactivate the mtp53 protein has progressed to the advanced phases of clinical trials. As a result, it is regarded as a superior kind of treatment. APR-246 obtained phase I and II approval for the treatment of hematological malignancies and prostate tumors about ten years after PRIMA-1 was discovered. Clinical trials in this study were designed to evaluate pharmacokinetics, maximum tolerated dose, medication safety, and dose-limiting toxicities. Participants in this research had to have at least a two-month prognosis to be considered. Around 25% of patients had the mtp53 protein, even though p53 status wasn't a determining factor. In four days of treatment with APR-246, the MTD was 60 mg/kg (34). The medicine was generally well-received due to its low risk of adverse effects when compared to other cytotoxic chemotherapy regimens. Positive pharmacokinetics were found in the study, with slight interindividual differences unaffected by delivery timing or dosage. In cancer cells, p53-targeted genes were upregulated, programmed cell death was accelerated, and the cell cycle was terminated. There were four incidences of cell cycle anomalies, including full arrest, among the six patients who had circulating cancer cells. BCL2-associated X, apoptosis regulator (Bax), p53 upregulated modulator of apoptosis (PUMA), and phorbol-12-myristate-13-acetate-induced protein 1 (NOXA) were all increased. There was also an increase in the senescence marker decoy receptor 2 (DcR2) (35).

18.8 PERSPECTIVES OF PATIENTS AND IMPLICATIONS FOR HEALTHCARE

18.8.1 Effects on Patient's Life and Its Outcomes

p53 gene therapy is a vital and integral part of the treatment paradigms in breast cancer, which has a huge effect on the treatment results and the quality of life of the patients. p53-based drugs could be very effective as they will not only help to treat the effect but also suppress the pathways connected to the molecular oncogenic processes of tumor development and progression. Further, p53 gene therapy could defy side effects usually associated with standard cancer treatments that reduce the quality of patients' lives such as fatigue, hair loss, nausea, and poor appetite. p53 gene therapy patients could experience a more priceless quality of life not only during but also after treatment without suffering severe side effects that chemotherapy inflicts such as nausea and hair loss (36). Patients with impenetrable or broad breast cancer will get new hope in the potentiality of customized p53-based treatments aligned with their genetic profile as the basis and having the objective of achieving optimal therapeutic results while minimizing the possibility of treatment resistance. Finally, the fusion of p53 gene therapy in surgical procedures is a key step toward establishing advanced and patient-oriented treatment of cancer and will be an opportunity to improve the emotional and physical aspects of cancer patients and their survivors in addition to prolonged survival.

p53 activity is regulated by several cellular stresses, such as DNA damage, hypoxia, and nucleotide shortage. Multiple types of DNA damage are the main inducers of p53. Radiation can be classified into several types, such as ionizing radiation (IR), radiomimetic medicines, ultraviolet light (UV), and compounds, e.g., methyl methane sulfonate (MMS). The short half-life of p53 is a leading factor that results in the low levels of the polypeptide. Besides the fact that p53 is usually inactive, this means that it cannot bind to DNA or initiate transcription. Improvement in p53's ability to bind to DNA and cause transcriptional activation upon DNA damage is one of the roles of p53. The very initial step of this chain reaction is the activation of multiple genes each of which can either kill the cells or help in the repairing of the damaged DNA. A recent study reported DNA damage as the main molecular mechanism that governs this phenomenon. The breakage of DNA leads to a cycle of events on the p53 peptide that includes phosphorylation, dephosphorylation, and acetylation.

18.9 GENE THERAPIES: ACCESSIBILITY AND AFFORDABILITY

Since the 1980s to 1990s of the previous centuries, new fields of human gene therapy have undergone dramatic events such as exciting discoveries and incredible outcomes, exaggerated expectations, impassable technological barriers, and poor adoption rates among the public and scientists. In the last minute, success is unavoidable because, for centuries, scientific and medical fields have advanced very rapidly in basic settings. The complicated technical device of a direct administering of useful gene-based therapies to patients at their bedside via the bedside is this great invention. As a result, a new concept of "genetic cure" for intractable diseases was created and public discussions on this topic became a common occurrence, which was unfathomable before. The phenomenon is also similar in every medical field. This way, the hypothetical principles have been removed from the initial way of success. Although it is not a panacea, this area of medicine is starting to fulfill its early expectations and the sheer possibilities are endless. Scientists have identified the genes that cause a lot of human sicknesses now. To do this, we have to come up with tools and techniques that allow us to overcome this negative influence and normalize the operation. By now, the new human disease-causing factors have become known, and some people already have their DNA (genome) and RNA machinery of cells manipulated and modified (known as genome editing) (37).

On the other hand, one of the problems in this regard is about making sure that those families and patients who are acutely in need of lifesaving discoveries get access to these marvels of medical advancements. Social and political challenges have now sprung forth as a result of the technological innovations and resolution of many scientific and technical issues; these issues will likely hinder the progress of our societies and healthcare programs as they will try to ensure that everyone has affordable and equitable access to these dynamic and therapeutic methods along with other medical innovations of the future. Scholars such as Steve Joffe and other individuals demonstrate a range of ideas for how universities can adopt approaches that will guarantee that gene-based medicines are affordable for everyone. Disappointingly, issues of cost have emerged, and they remain to be a problem for consumers, healthcare providers, and insurance companies. Only recently have new generations of therapies arrived on the market, which spotlights the problem—they are sold at sky-high prices, reaching several millions. Subsequently, a great number of patients cannot purchase them and individuals as well as public institutions are charged with a considerable cost burden. The thing that makes the situation different is that there is a different set of approval procedures from one country to another. However, others believe that the healthcare system must be restructured to make it affordable to families and hence, they conclude that the high prices are warranted and justified. The argument here is that, in the long run, the cost of treatment for patients who successfully go through treatment and the principle of preserving lives with no limits justifies the idea patients and their families should bear these costs. The bad news is that some patients know their therapies are not covered by their insurance plans, and selling their houses and liquidating their life savings is the only way left for them to afford the proper treatment.

The editors of *Gene Therapy* expressed concern about the availability and affordability of gene-based medicines (38). The United States is one example of a country whose national policies are based on complex and unjust commercial and public insurance systems, leaving healthcare insurance unavailable or too expensive for many patients and families. This is why universal healthcare is essential in these nations. Recently we held a webinar in support of gene therapy, 50 years after one of us raised particular ethical and scientific concerns. To answer the basic question of why gene therapy is so expensive, we assembled a panel of experts in gene therapy, genome editing, medical economics, and public policy. It was asked of all committee members to examine the current cost of gene-based therapies and predict how it will change with the progress of genetic medicine. This special issue of *Gene Therapy* includes five papers that provide a variety of viewpoints, analyses, and suggestions on the subject.

18.10 INDUSTRY PERSPECTIVES: INDUSTRY INVESTMENT AND MARKET TRENDS

Even though gene therapy is still a controversial issue among investors and major pharmaceutical corporations, some innovative enterprises have been able to raise more financing. A private placement of $34 million was completed by Collateral Therapeutics. With the new investment, Collateral will be able to advance its non-invasive gene therapy therapies for a variety of cardiovascular diseases. Among the well-known companies, Vical's stock price increased by more than 50% after word came that Merck intends to employ Vical's naked DNA technology in an upcoming clinical trial for an AIDS vaccine. An estimated $1 million milestone payment is owed by Merck to Vical. But if all goes as planned, Vical might earn up to $90 million in royalties by 2005 (39). Notably, following the successful completion of the phase I/II clinical trial of its GVAX prostate cancer vaccine, Cell Genesys received an additional $4.5 million. With this event, Cell Genesys has reached a significant milestone in its global relationship with Japan Tobacco, which will provide $45 million in R&D funding over the next two years. The GVAX vaccine for prostate cancer has been launched in two multicenter trials following positive results from the study.

Rhone-Poulenc Rorer has also agreed to provide Introgen Therapeutics with another $6 million as part of their collaboration agreement. Phase II clinical trials for p53 gene therapy in head and neck cancer have just been completed, and phase III trials will begin soon.

Argonex, a small biotech firm, and Rohm and Haas, a medium-sized pharmaceutical corporation, have announced a new alliance in recent months. The creators of RHeoGene set out to develop gene-flipping technologies, with an emphasis on human gene therapy. Together, Argonex and Rohm and Haas will develop immunotherapeutic products based on ecdysone-based receptor switching technology. Neurosearch, a Danish biotechnology corporation, created NsGene, a new European company that focuses on gene therapy for the central nervous system. Anders Bjoerklund from Sweden's University of Lund is engaged in this partnership. The Danish government has granted the new enterprise $6.5 million.

Companies that specialize in gene therapy have been aggressively seeking to broaden their arsenal of tumor suppressor technologies. Introgen Therapeutics, a pioneer in this medical technique, has been given an exclusive license to Corixa's mda7 cancer suppressor gene. When this gene is triggered, it suppresses the development of 24 different kinds of human cancer cells in a controlled environment, according to preliminary research. In addition, the mda7 gene inhibits cell proliferation regardless of whether the cells are mutant for p53, p16, or Rb. This opens the door to possible drug–drug interactions with Introgen's current p53-based therapies. Ingenex, a relatively unknown business, acquired the rights to a tumor-targeting technology created by Selective Genetics through a cross-license arrangement.

There are several cancer gene therapy alternatives on the market, including RB, p53, APC, and NF1 treatments, among others (40). To successfully treat various forms of cancer, these drugs target particular genes involved in cancer's origin and progression.

The use of gene therapy in the treatment of cancer and the regeneration of tissue is commercially available. Gene therapy in cancer treatment aims to eliminate cancer cells by targeting them specifically (41). Gene therapy also aids in the restoration of damaged or diseased tissues during tissue repair, hence improving patients' health and overall quality of life.

The cancer gene therapy market is expected to expand significantly in areas such as China, Europe, the United States, and Asia-Pacific. Europe and the United States are likely to dominate the market due to their sophisticated healthcare systems, favorable reimbursement policies, and increased R&D initiatives. Forecasts predict that these areas will account for more than half of the market in the near future. Rising healthcare costs and a better understanding of specialized therapy are fueling expectations of the highest growth in the Asia-Pacific region, which includes China. As a result, the gene therapy market for cancer treatment is expected to grow significantly throughout the forecast period.

A cancer patient undergoing gene therapy will have genetic material inserted into cancer cells to limit their development or cause them to die. The following gene therapy companies are driving the search for novel cancer therapies: GILEAD, REGENXBIO, Autolus, American Gene Technologies, Arcellx, Austrianova, Alphavax, Cellectis, and Chimeron. To destroy cancer cells, these businesses employ cutting-edge procedures such as CAR-T cell therapy, gene editing, and gene silencing.

18.11 CONCLUSION

Because p53 is extensively expressed in tumors and plays a crucial role in cell activity regulation, it is an appealing therapeutic target for cancer. Even though there are no medications on the market that target mutant or wild-type p53, scientists are continuously working on more complex techniques to use p53's structure and function in cancer treatment. Both wild-type and mutant variants of p53 can be targeted with drug-targeting techniques by considering MDM2. Inhibiting the interaction between MDM2 and p53 is one way to restore p53 activity. An MDM2 inhibitor was developed as a result of this. Meanwhile, stimulating MDM2-mediated ubiquitination may be a strategy to destroy mutant p53. As a result, medicines that inhibit HSP90 or HDAC, as well as NSC59984, are being investigated as potential MDM2 activators and mutant p53 destabilizers.

MDM2 inhibitors present a variety of challenges, which include resilience and toxicity, although human trials have presented significant anticancer benefits along with satisfactory toxicity profiles. The present study centers on two main areas to solve these challenges: the activation of mutant p53 and its delivery mechanisms. As for delivery systems, non-viral vectors are becoming increasingly popular as a substitute for the widely used viral vectors. This change aims to decrease immune responses and off-target consequences related to vectors of the virus while increasing the efficacy of delivery. Furthermore, although there have been few trials for p53 gene substitution therapy, CRISPR/Cas9 and other gene editing approaches are becoming increasingly popular because of their ability to correctly identify and fix p53 abnormalities. In addition, while the initial study on stimulating mutant p53 has centered on smaller molecules, a more promising path forward is toward the creation of superior activators with fewer negative consequences. Progress in this area might lead to increased safety and effectiveness of p53-targeted therapy, which could ultimately benefit breast cancer treatment and other cancer treatment options.

Cancer initiation and progression are heavily influenced by the wild-type p53 gene, which is an important tumor suppressor. Death, blood vessel creation, metabolic pathways, and epithelial–mesenchymal transition are all closely linked to the p53 gene family. Malignant solid tumors typically have p53 gene family alterations or functional issues. As a result, adenovirus-mediated gene therapy has become a popular alternative for cancer patients looking for a cure.

18.12 IMPLICATIONS FOR FUTURE RESEARCH AND CLINICAL PRACTICE

There has been great difficulty in developing drugs that target the p53 pathway. Adenovirus-based gene therapy has not gained popularity despite being clinically approved in China. This is most likely because adenovirus-based gene delivery cannot target particular cancers. The Food and Drug Administration has yet to approve targeted therapy based on the p53 pathway, the fourth major method of cancer treatment. These attempts fail for several reasons. It is important to note that TP53 mutations cause loss of function in cancer cells, making them highly druggable. Current phase III clinical studies are being conducted to demonstrate that mutant p53 can be converted back to wild-type (WT) p53 with medicines. The creation of clinical trials for targeted therapeutics is further hampered by mutant p53's gain-of-function (GOF) effects, which are dependent on certain circumstances and include several pathways. To address this issue, we need to identify biomarkers that can predict which individuals would respond well to each p53-based treatment.

Our first step must be to better understand how mutant p53 causes gain-of-function effects in each type of cancer. Our understanding of how p53 suppresses carcinogenesis is quite limited, and this is probably the most crucial aspect. In what ways does p53 suppress tumor growth by arresting cell cycle, apoptosis, or senescence? Is there any unique method that p53 can prevent tumors from developing in different cell and tissue types? Finding solutions to these fundamental issues will help us understand the p53 pathway's underlying biology and pave the way for more effective targeted therapies. Over the past four decades, researchers have barely scratched the surface of p53's vast ocean of research. The discovery of effective treatments targeting the p53 pathway might be considerably accelerated by immunotherapy techniques based on ACT (adoptive cell transfer), such as tumor-infiltrating lymphocytes, TCR-T (T-cell receptor-engineered T-cells), and CAR-T (chimeric antigen receptor T-cells). The main concept of these techniques is that cancer cells would express neoantigens produced from p53 mutations. In principle, unlike other context-dependent techniques, the efficiency of these approaches is less influenced by the complex biology associated with p53 mutations. Furthermore, TP53 mutations reduce the variety of neoantigens because they concentrate in specific hotspot regions within the DNA binding domain. By combining p53 biology with immunotherapy, future p53-based cancer treatments could be significantly improved.

18.13 A FINAL NOTE ON p53 GENE THERAPY'S CHANCES IN BREAST CANCER

There have been recent efforts to restore normal p53 suppressor activity and reduce the incidence of cancer by targeting the mutant p53 protein. Both APR-246 and COTI-2 are small-molecule drugs that are currently in clinical trials or will be soon. Gene and cell-based methods, as well as rational structure-activity drug design, are gaining popularity. Despite the latter's outstanding track record, CRISPR/Cas gene editing and adenoviral gene therapy have yet to target the mtp53 protein. Nonetheless, the investigations are set to commence. APR-246 and COTI-2, which are simple to manufacture therapeutically, are two examples of small molecules that could be used to prevent cancer growth. PRIMA-1 is efficacious in a mouse model of breast cancer prevention. Various forms of cancer are now being treated with two newer medicines, APR-246 and COTI-2, in clinical trials. Making these compounds for prophylactic purposes is a long way off, but it would be a significant advancement in science. It is critical to look for new treatments aimed at targeting mutant p53 (mtp53) since TNBC (triple-negative breast cancer) is associated with mtp53. Because there are no treatments that directly target this aggressive kind of breast cancer, this is critical for women who have it. Curcumin and luteolin, two plant-based nutraceuticals, have been demonstrated in scientific studies to have anticancer effects. Because these chemicals are frequently non-toxic, it would be immensely valuable to investigate their capacity to activate the mtp53 protein. It is expected that naturally occurring agents, such as those indicated, will provide a safe and effective treatment for persons with TNBC. There may one day be stronger forms of these molecules developed, providing non-toxic alternatives to the current pharmacological medicines.

REFERENCES

1. Gorgoulis VG, Pefani DE, Pateras IS, Trougakos IP. Integrating the DNA damage and protein stress responses during cancer development and treatment. *J Pathol* [Internet]. 2018 Sep 1 [cited 2024 Apr 30];246(1):12–40. Available from: https://pubmed.ncbi.nlm.nih.gov/29756349/

2. Pappas K, Xu J, Zairis S, Resnick-Silverman L, Abate F, Steinbach N, et al. p53 maintains baseline expression of multiple tumor suppressor genes. *Mol Cancer Res* [Internet]. 2017 Aug 1 [cited 2024 Apr 30];15(8):1051. Available from: https://pmc/articles/PMC5587155/
3. Foroutan B. A Narrative review of the TP53 and its product the p53 protein. *OBM Genet.* 2023;7(3). https://doi.org/10.21926/obm.genet.2302185
4. Pfister NT, Prives C. Transcriptional Regulation by Wild-Type and Cancer-Related Mutant Forms of p53. *Cold Spring Harb Perspect Med* [Internet]. 2017 Feb 1 [cited 2024 Apr 30];7(2). Available from: https://pubmed.ncbi.nlm.nih.gov/27836911/
5. Lei J, Qi R, Tang Y, Wang W, Wei G, Nussinov R, et al. Conformational stability and dynamics of the cancer-associated isoform Δ133p53β are modulated by p53 peptides and p53-specific DNA. *FASEB J.* 2019 Mar 1;33(3):4225–35.
6. Goswami R, Subramanian G, Silayeva L, Newkirk I, Doctor D, Chawla K, et al. Gene therapy leaves a vicious cycle. *Front Oncol.* 2019;9:297.
7. Shchaslyvyi AY, Antonenko SV., Tesliuk MG, Telegeev GD. Current State of Human Gene Therapy: Approved Products and Vectors. Vol. 16, *Pharmaceuticals.* Multidisciplinary Digital Publishing Institute (MDPI); 2023.
8. Zaimy MA, Saffarzadeh N, Mohammadi A, Pourghadamyari H, Izadi P, Sarli A, et al. New methods in the diagnosis of cancer and gene therapy of cancer based on nanoparticles. Vol. 24, *Cancer Gene Therapy.* Nature Publishing Group; 2017. p. 233–43.
9. Castañeda AM, Meléndez CM, Uribe D, Pedroza-Díaz J. Synergistic effects of natural compounds and conventional chemotherapeutic agents: recent insights for the development of cancer treatment strategies. Vol. 8, *Heliyon.* Elsevier Ltd; 2022.
10. Hamada M, Yura Y. Efficient delivery and replication of oncolytic virus for successful treatment of head and neck cancer. *Int J Mol Sci.* 2020 Oct 1;21(19):1–22.
11. Aubrey BJ, Kelly GL, Janic A, Herold MJ, Strasser A. How does p53 induce apoptosis and how does this relate to p53-mediated tumour suppression? Vol. 25, *Cell Death and Differentiation.* Nature Publishing Group; 2018. p. 104–13.
12. Canale M, Andrikou K, Priano I, Cravero P, Pasini L, Urbini M, et al. The role of TP53 mutations in EGFR-mutated non-small-cell lung cancer: clinical significance and implications for therapy. Vol. 14, *Cancers.* MDPI; 2022.
13. Levine AJ. p53: 800 million years of evolution and 40 years of discovery. *Nat Rev Cancer.* 2020 Aug 1;20(8):471–80.
14. Hientz K, Mohr A, Bhakta-Guha D, Efferth T. The role of p53 in cancer drug resistance and targeted chemotherapy [Internet]. Vol. 8, Oncotarget. 2017. Available from: www.impactjournals.com/oncotarget/
15. Hasbullah HH, Musa M. Gene therapy targeting p53 and kras for colorectal cancer treatment: a myth or the way forward? Vol. 22, *Int J Mol Sci.* MDPI; 2021.
16. Lin W, Zhao Y, Zhong L. Current strategies of virotherapy in clinical trials for cancer treatment. Vol. 93, *J Med Virol.* John Wiley and Sons Inc; 2021. p. 4668–92.
17. Ou HL, Schumacher B. DNA damage responses and p53 in the aging process. *Blood* [Internet]. 2018 Feb 1 [cited 2024 Apr 28];131(5):488–95. Available from: https://pubmed.ncbi.nlm.nih.gov/29141944/
18. Premnath N, Madanat YF. Novel investigational agents and pathways that may influence the future management of acute myeloid leukemia. Vol. 15, *Cancers.* MDPI; 2023.
19. Lugin ML, Lee RT, Kwon YJ. Synthetically engineered adeno-associated virus for efficient, safe, and versatile gene therapy applications. *ACS Nano* [Internet]. 2020 Nov 24 [cited 2024 Apr 30];14(11):14262–83. Available from: https://pubmed.ncbi.nlm.nih.gov/33073995/
20. Muik A, Reul J, Friedel T, Muth A, Hartmann KP, Schneider IC, et al. Covalent coupling of high-affinity ligands to the surface of viral vector particles by protein trans-splicing mediates cell type-specific gene transfer. *Biomaterials* [Internet]. 2017 Nov 1 [cited 2024 Apr 30];144:84–94. Available from: https://pubmed.ncbi.nlm.nih.gov/28825979/
21. Lv Y feng, Zhang H, Cui Z, Ma C jiao, Li Y ling, Lu H, et al. Gene delivery to breast cancer by incorporated EpCAM targeted DARPins into AAV2. BMC Cancer [Internet]. 2023 Dec 1 [cited 2024 Apr 30];23(1). Available from: https://pubmed.ncbi.nlm.nih.gov/38082377/
22. Raskov H, Orhan A, Christensen JP, Gögenur I. Cytotoxic CD8+ T cells in cancer and cancer immunotherapy. *Br J Cancer* [Internet]. 2021 Jan 19 [cited 2024 Apr 30];124(2):359–67. Available from: https://pubmed.ncbi.nlm.nih.gov/32929195/
23. Duffy MJ, Tang M, Rajaram S, O'Grady S, Crown J. Targeting mutant p53 for cancer treatment: moving closer to clinical use? *Cancers (Basel)* [Internet]. 2022 Sep 1 [cited 2024 Apr 30];14(18). Available from: https://pubmed.ncbi.nlm.nih.gov/36139658/

24. Mariuzza RA, Wu D, Pierce BG. Structural basis for T cell recognition of cancer neoantigens and implications for predicting neoepitope immunogenicity. *Front Immunol* [Internet]. 2023 [cited 2024 Apr 30];14. Available from: https://pubmed.ncbi.nlm.nih.gov/38045695/
25. Valente JFA, Queiroz JA, Sousa F. p53 as the Focus of gene therapy: past, present and future. *Curr Drug Targets* [Internet]. 2018 Jan 16 [cited 2024 Apr 30];19(15):1801–17. Available from: https://pubmed.ncbi.nlm.nih.gov/29336259/
26. Szewczyk-Roszczenko O, Barlev NA. The role of p53 in nanoparticle-based therapy for cancer. Vol. 12, *Cells*. Multidisciplinary Digital Publishing Institute (MDPI); 2023.
27. Xia Y, Li X, Sun W. Applications of recombinant adenovirus-p53 gene therapy for cancers in the clinic in China. *Curr Gene Ther* [Internet]. 2020 Sep 18 [cited 2024 Apr 30];20(2):127–41. Available from: https://pubmed.ncbi.nlm.nih.gov/32951572/
28. Fujihara KM, Benitez MC, Cabalag CS, Zhang BZ, Ko HS, Liu DS, et al. SLC7A11 is a superior determinant of APR-246 (eprenetapopt) response than TP53 mutation status. *Mol Cancer Ther* [Internet]. 2021 Oct 1 [cited 2024 Apr 30];20(10):1858–67. Available from: https://pubmed.ncbi.nlm.nih.gov/34315763/
29. Perdrix A, Najem A, Saussez S, Awada A, Journe F, Ghanem G, et al. PRIMA-1 and PRIMA-1Met (APR-246): From mutant/wild type p53 reactivation to unexpected mechanisms underlying their potent anti-tumor effect in combinatorial therapies. *Cancers (Basel)* [Internet]. 2017 Dec 16 [cited 2024 Apr 30];9(12). Available from: https://pubmed.ncbi.nlm.nih.gov/29258181/
30. Patil MR, Bihari A. A comprehensive study of p53 protein. *J Cell Biochem* [Internet]. 2022 Dec 1 [cited 2024 Apr 30];123(12):1891–937. Available from: https://pubmed.ncbi.nlm.nih.gov/36183376/
31. Serra F, Nieto-Aliseda A, Fanlo-Escudero L, Rovirosa L, Cabrera-Pasadas M, Lazarenkov A, et al. p53 rapidly restructures 3D chromatin organization to trigger a transcriptional response. *Nat Commun* [Internet]. 2024 Apr 1;15(1):2821. Available from: https://www.nature.com/articles/s41467-024-46666-1
32. Menetski JP, Hoffmann SC, Cush SS, Kamphaus TN, Austin CP, Herrling PL, et al. The Foundation for the National Institutes of Health Biomarkers Consortium: past accomplishments and new strategic direction. *Clin Pharmacol Ther* [Internet]. 2019 Apr 1 [cited 2024 Apr 30];105(4):829–43. Available from: https://pubmed.ncbi.nlm.nih.gov/30648736/
33. Siddiqui SS, Rahman S, Rupasinghe HPV, Vazhappilly CG. Dietary Flavonoids in p53—mediated immune dysfunctions linking to cancer prevention. *Biomedicines* [Internet]. 2020;8(8). Available from: https://www.mdpi.com/2227-9059/8/8/286
34. Juan Ribelles A, Gargallo P, Berlanga P, Segura V, Yáñez Y, Juan B, et al. Next-generation sequencing identifies potential actionable targets in paediatric sarcomas. *J Pers Med* [Internet]. 2021 [cited 2024 Apr 30];11(4):268. Available from:/pmc/articles/PMC8067272/
35. Si W, Shen J, Zheng H, Fan W. The role and mechanisms of action of microRNAs in cancer drug resistance. *Clin Epigenetics* [Internet]. 2019 Feb 11 [cited 2024 Apr 30];11(1). Available from: https://pubmed.ncbi.nlm.nih.gov/30744689/
36. Qi L, Luo Q, Zhang Y, Jia F, Zhao Y, Wang F. Advances in toxicological research of the anticancer drug cisplatin. *Chem Res Toxicol* [Internet]. 2019 Aug 19 [cited 2024 Apr 30];32(8):1469–86. Available from: https://pubmed.ncbi.nlm.nih.gov/31353895/
37. Doudna JA. The promise and challenge of therapeutic genome editing. *Nature* [Internet]. 2020 Feb 13 [cited 2024 Apr 30];578(7794):229. Available from:/pmc/articles/PMC8992613/
38. Delhove J, Osenk I, Prichard I, Donnelley M. Public acceptability of gene therapy and gene editing for human use: a systematic review. *Hum Gene Ther* [Internet]. 2020 Jan 1 [cited 2024 Apr 30];31(1–2):20–46. Available from: https://pubmed.ncbi.nlm.nih.gov/31802714/
39. Roy V. Capitalizing a cure: how finance controls the price and value of medicines. In *Capitalizing a Cure: How Finance Controls the Price and Value of Medicines*. University of California Press 2023 Jan 24;1–202. https://doi.org/10.1525/luminos.141
40. Kumar MS, Adki KM. Marine natural products for multi-targeted cancer treatment: a future insight. *Biomed Pharmacother*. 2018 Sep 1;105:233–45.
41. Belete TM. The current status of gene therapy for the treatment of cancer. *Biologics* [Internet]. 2021 [cited 2024 Apr 30];15:67. Available from:/pmc/articles/PMC7987258/

19 Insights from Genetic Studies

The Role of p53 in Hereditary Breast Cancer Syndrome

Akhil Jamwal[1], Mary Chatterjee[1], Kirti Hooda[2], Nusrat Jan[3], and Manzoor Ahmad Mir[3]*

[1]Department of Biotechnology Engineering, UIET, Panjab University, Chandigarh, India
[2]Centre for Nanoscience's and Nanotechnology, Panjab University, Chandigarh, India
[3]Department of Bioresources, School of Biological Sciences, University of Kashmir, Srinagar, J&K, India
*drmanzoor@kashmiruniversity.ac.in

19.1 INTRODUCTION

Among women in both economically developed and developing nations, breast cancer is the most common malignant illness and the primary cause of cancer-related deaths. Approximately one-third of the 1.4 million newly diagnosed cases of breast cancer worldwide each year also pass away from the illness [1, 2]. Numerous genetic and nongenetic variables predispose people to breast cancer because it is a complex illness. Numerous risk factors that predispose to breast cancer have been found based on epidemiologic research conducted on the illness. Ninety percent of instances of breast cancer are caused by nongenetic causes, with genetic factors accounting for just around 10% of occurrences [3–5]. Within the past few years, a number of genes associated with a high risk of breast cancer have been identified, including BRCA1, BRCA2, p53, and the Cowden disease gene PTEN/MMAC1. Although the mutation frequency of these genes is low in the general population, some communities have a carrier frequency of up to 1% for specific BRCA1 and BRCA2 mutations, suggesting that these genes serve as tumor suppressors. These genes' separation is probably going to shed significant light on the pathophysiology of human cancer [6–8].

A substantial inherited cancer-predisposition condition called hereditary breast and ovarian cancer condition (HBOC) is characterized by an increased chance of developing breast and ovarian cancers. Studies show that 5–10% of people with breast cancer have a hereditary predisposition to the disease; mutations in genes such as BRCA1 and BRCA2 are important in causing this syndrome. The genetic variability of HBOC has been highlighted by the discovery of non-BRCA genes linked to ovarian and breast cancers thanks to developments in next-generation sequencing (NGS). To lessen the impact of cancer on affected individuals and their families, studies highlight the significance of early detection, risk diagnosis, and the adoption of protective measures for relatives in managing HBOC. These findings highlight the need for comprehensive cancer management protocols and preventive strategies [9–12].

p53 plays a variety of roles in maintaining the integrity of the genome, including triggering apoptosis, cell cycle arrest, and DNA repair. Mdm2 and Mdmx are overexpressed in many human malignancies, which adversely affect p53 and cause genomic instability.

DOI: 10.1201/9781003520771-19

Genome instability has recently been identified as a characteristic of cancer. Chromosome or chromatid breaks, insertions, deletions, translocations, fusions, gain or loss of one or more chromosomes (aneuploidy), gain of part or an entire genome (polyploidy and tetraploidy), and centrosome amplification are examples of structural and/or numerical abnormalities in chromosomes that constitute genome instability [12–14]. The efficiency of p53 in preventing cell growth is a strong deterrent to malignant progression, but this activity must be kept tightly restrained to allow normal cell growth and development. Essential components of this regulation are the mechanisms by which the p53 protein is degraded, and efficient turnover of p53 in normal cells prevents the accumulation of the protein. It is now evident that the Mdm2 protein plays a key role in controlling p53 stability and that there are several strategies to decrease Mdm2 function [15, 16]. Cell cycle arrest and apoptosis, which are both triggered by p53, shield the organism and the cell from DNA damage that might cause genomic instability. The transcriptional u-regulation of the cell cycle inhibitor p21 (Cdkn1a) by p53 results in cell cycle arrest, which is a well-established response to many kinds of DNA damage and cellular stress. Apoptosis is induced when p53 transcriptionally activates the proapoptotic genes Bax, Noxa, and/or Puma, which block the antiapoptotic Bcl-2 proteins [2]. It is also hypothesized that p53 operates in the mitochondria, where it physically inhibits members of the Bcl-2 family that are anti-apoptotic, causing apoptosis [13, 17].

Our knowledge of hereditary breast cancer syndrome has advanced significantly as a result of genetic research on the illness. BRCA1 and BRCA2, which together account for up to 30% of hereditary breast cancers, were found to be highly penetrant susceptibility genes using linkage analysis and positional cloning in families with many affected individuals [12, 18]. More recently, over 80 loci are strongly related to sporadic breast cancer by genome-wide association studies (GWAS); nonetheless, the combined effect of these variations only accounts for 16% of the heritability of breast cancer. Due to the shortcomings of GWAS, the focus has switched to employing NGS techniques to examine the effects of uncommon genetic variants. Mutations in genes like RECQL that increase the risk of familial breast cancer have been found thanks to studies like the one by Cybulski et al. that used a staged NGS design, sequencing unrelated cases with assumed high "genetic load" first and then validating the found rare variants in larger cohorts [8, 19]. Thanks to these genetic discoveries, we can now more accurately identify people who are at a high risk of developing hereditary breast cancer syndrome. This means that affected people and their families can now receive customized cancer screening, prevention, and treatment plans.

19.2 GENETIC BASIS OF HEREDITARY BREAST CANCER SYNDROME

Most hereditary breast cancers are caused by germline mutations in the BRCA1 and BRCA2 genes. The risk of ovarian and fallopian tube cancer is also higher in women with BRCA1 or BRCA2 hereditary mutations. Furthermore, carriers of the BRCA2 mutation are more likely to develop other malignancies, including pancreatic, prostate, gastrointestinal, and male breast cancers [1, 14]. The genomic architecture of BRCA1 and BRCA2 is quite complicated, and there is no resemblance between the coding areas and any previously identified genes. The 1,863-amino-acid protein encoded by the 24 exons that make up the BRCA1 gene is much bigger than the 3,418 amino acid protein encoded by the 27 exons that make up the BRCA2 gene. Exon 11 is extremely big in both genes, while exon 1 is non-coding [1]. Tumor suppressor gene proteins are produced by the BRCA1 and BRCA2 genes. Changes or mutations in the BRCA1 gene, which is found on chr17q, can raise the chance of getting prostate, ovarian, and breast cancer. One of the acrocentric chromosomes in males, chr13q, has the BRCA2 gene. Alterations or mutations in this gene can raise the chance of developing breast, ovarian, and prostate cancer [20]. Promoter methylation, somatic mutations, and germline mutations are the causes of BRCA1 and BRCA2 malfunction. Mutations in the splice sites over the whole coding area are seen in BRCA1 and BRCA2 [21, 22].

A variety of other DNA repair genes, such as CHEK2, BRIP1 (BACH1), ATM, and PALB2, interact with BRCA1, BRCA2, and/or the BRCA pathways and cause a twofold increase in the risk of breast cancer [23, 24]. This protein is a cell cycle checkpoint regulator that is quickly phosphorylated in response to DNA damage and replication blockages in both yeast and humans. Inhibiting CDC25C phosphatase to stop mitosis and stabilizing p53 to cause cell cycle arrest in G1 are the results of activated CHEK2. BRCA1 and CHEK2 are functionally related. Through interaction and phosphorylation, CHEK2 enables BRCA1 to repair DNA damage and restore survival [25]. A protein that interacts with the BRCA1 C-terminus (BRCT) domain is encoded by BRIP1 (BACH1). Less than 1% of occurrences of breast cancer are considered to be caused by mutations in BRIP1. In women with a significant family history of breast cancer, a BRIP1 mutation is linked to a relative risk (RR) of 2.0, with an increased risk observed for early-onset breast cancer. So far, the majority of BRIP1 mutations that have been reported have involved protein truncation. Fanconi anemia type J is linked to biallelic BRIP1, although there is no appreciable rise in pediatric cancer cases. ATM is a protein kinase that controls BRCA1 and CHEK2 and is involved in the monitoring and repair of dsDNA. Ataxia–telangiectasia is an autosomal recessive illness caused by a biallelic ATM mutation. One percent is thought to be the frequency of monoallelic ATM mutations. According to a recent meta-analysis, women under 50 had a greater risk of breast cancer (RR = 2.3) when an ATM mutation was present [23]. Because of its interaction with BRCA2, PALB2 (also known as FANCN) can also generate biallelic BRCA2 mutations, which in turn can cause Fanconi anemia when biallelic mutations occur [10, 26, 27].

19.3 p53 GENE: STRUCTURE AND FUNCTION

Situated on the short arm of chromosome 17 (17p13.1), the p53 gene (TP53) spans 20 kb and comprises a first intron of 10 kb that overlaps with the Hp53int1 gene and an exon 1 that is not coding. Five areas in the p53 gene's coding sequence, mostly found in exons 2, 5, 6, 7, and 8, have a high degree of conservation in vertebrates. An N-terminal transactivation domain, a proline-rich domain, a DNA-binding domain, a tetramerization domain, and a C-terminal regulatory domain are among the several functional domains of the 393-amino-acid protein that the p53 gene encodes [28]. The most thoroughly researched region of the p53 protein is its DNA-binding domain, which includes several arginine residues that interact directly with DNA (residues 96–292). Numerous mutations in p53 that cause cancer interfere with its ability to bind DNA, which compromises its tumor suppressor properties [29, 30].

Over 50% of human malignancies have a mutation in the tumor suppressor gene p53. The reason p53 is known as the "cellular gatekeeper" or "guardian of the genome" because it keeps the body from disseminating altered DNA caused by different types of stress.

Numerous physiological reactions, such as cell cycle arrest, apoptosis, cellular senescence, and metabolic adaptability, are triggered by p53. Other cellular metabolic and energy production processes, including autophagy, antioxidation, mitochondrial quality control, fatty acid metabolism, nucleic acid metabolism, and amino acid metabolism, are also regulated by p53 [12, 31]. One tumor suppressor gene that is frequently altered in malignancies, particularly breast cancer, is TP53. Gene alterations result in changes to the expression of several genes that are either directly or indirectly controlled by p53 during transcription. Exon 4 and intron 3 of the TP53 gene are known to be often mutated in patients with breast cancer, particularly triple-negative breast cancer. Some ethnic groups have been documented to have distinct mutations in this gene [12, 32, 33]. To carry out its pro-apoptotic role, p53 is stimulated to concentrate in the cell nucleus in response to a range of cellular stressors, including DNA damage. By transactivating its target genes involved in the induction of cell cycle arrest and/or apoptosis, activated p53 promotes cell cycle arrest to allow DNA repair and/or death to stop the spread of cells with significant DNA damage. Thus, p53's ability to prevent tumor growth is closely related to its ability to bind DNA [34].

A common feature of many malignancies, including breast cancer, is the deregulation of the p53 tumor suppressor gene. Up to 30% of breast cancers have been reported to have p53 mutations, which can cause p53 function to be lost and aid in the growth and spread of tumors. Other pathways of p53 dysregulation in breast cancer have been found, including changes in p53 expression levels, post-translational modifications, and p53 isoform expression. These mechanisms extend beyond mutations. Studies have shown that in some subtypes of breast cancer, such as triple-negative breast cancer, the immunohistochemical assessment of p53 expression patterns can be a prognostic factor; higher p53 levels are associated with a worse prognosis [35, 36]. Furthermore, research has shown that p53 isoform expression may offer new pathways for cancer prognostication by contributing to the dysregulation of p53 activities. All of these results highlight how crucial it is to comprehend the intricate processes that underlie p53 dysregulation in breast cancer as doing so will help researchers create targeted treatments and enhance patient outcomes [37, 38].

19.4 MUTATIONS IN HEREDITARY BREAST CANCER SYNDROME

In hereditary breast cancer syndromes, p53 mutations are a major factor, especially in Li–Fraumeni syndrome. About 30% of all occurrences of breast cancer are caused by mutations in the TP53 gene, which codes for the p53 protein. This makes TP53 the most frequently mutated gene in breast cancer [39]. Li–Fraumeni syndrome is a hereditary cancer-predisposition disease that dramatically raises the risk of acquiring several early-onset malignancies, including breast cancer. It is caused by germline (inherited) mutations in the TP53 gene (Table 19.1) [40].

Up until recently, the dangers associated with missense variations in genes such as BRCA1, BRCA2, ATM, and CHEK2 that are linked to an elevated risk of breast cancer were not well understood. According to a study, a tiny percentage of rare missense variants for BRCA1, BRCA2, and ATM

TABLE 19.1
Types of Mutations in Hereditary Breast Cancer Syndrome

Gene	Mutation Type	Effect	Prevalence in Breast Cancer	References
TP53	Missense	Affects stability, structure, and function of p53 protein	About 30% of breast cancer	[43–45]
	Truncating	Produces truncated p53 proteins that lack key functional domains required for p53's normal tumor suppressor activities	Varies	[46–48]
	In-frame	Deleted single amino acids can disrupt the structural integrity of the p53 DNA-binding domain, leading to destabilization of the overall p53 protein structure and impairment of its normal tumor suppressor functions	Varies	[49, 50]
	Splice site	Affects stability, translation efficiency, and RNA splicing	1% of breast cancer	[51, 52]
	Frameshift	Causes loss of stability, structure, and expression patterns	Common in some subtypes of breast cancer	[53–55]
BRCA1	Missense	May affect protein–protein interactions	Varies	[56–58]
BRCA2	Missense	Harmful mutations cluster in DNA-binding domain (DBD)	Varies	[59, 60]
ATM	Missense	Risk-associated, similar to protein truncating variations (PTVs)	Varies	[61–63]
CHEK2	Missense	Risk-associated, with lower calculated risk than PTVs	Varies	[61, 62]
PALB2	Missense	Little evidence linking to breast cancer risk	Varies	[64, 65]

were linked to risks that were similar to those of protein-truncating variations (PTVs). While a larger percentage of missense variations for CHEK2 were risk-associated, the calculated risk was noticeably lower than for PTVs. On the other hand, there was little evidence linking missense variants in PALB2 to the risk of breast cancer, and very few high-risk missense variants likely exist in PALB2 [41, 42].

In contrast to the mutation spectrum seen in Western cultures, another study discovered that missense mutations in BRCA1 and BRCA2 tended to predominate over frameshift or nonsense mutations in Japanese breast cancer families. On the other hand, patients with missense and truncating mutations experienced cancer at similar ages [8, 66]. Protein stability and structure can be affected by missense mutations. A single amino acid is substituted in a protein by a missense mutation, which can cause instability and structural problems for the protein [67]. Destabilizing and harmful mutations are more likely to occur at the protein's interface or core regions, which are crucial for maintaining structural integrity [68]. For the BRCA2 gene, harmful missense mutations were discovered to cluster in the DNA-binding domain, specifically in the helical domain and OB1-fold motifs that engage the companion protein DSS1. It has been demonstrated that these pathogenic BRCA2 missense mutations reduce or eliminate DSS1's binding to BRCA2, resulting in the creation of mutant BRCA2 oligomers that are shut out of the cell nucleus [69]. Protein–protein interactions can be changed by missense mutations. The BRCA1 missense mutation study discovered that some variants, such as W1837R and S1841N, had an impact on how well BRCA1 bound to the tumor suppressor p53. The tumor suppressor properties of BRCA1 and BRCA2 may be impacted by these modifications in protein–protein interactions brought on by missense mutations [70].

In hereditary breast cancer syndrome, TP53 splice site mutations are important for the development of cancer. These mutations may significantly affect the stability, translation efficiency, and RNA splicing, which may affect the p53 protein's capacity to function. Research has demonstrated that TP53 splice mutations can affect the stability, structure, and patterns of protein production. Furthermore, these mutations may produce abnormal p53 transcripts, which could impair the protein's ability to operate normally. Along with missense, truncating, and in-frame mutations, splice mutations are one of the mutation types seen in TP53. Each of these mutant types contributes to the growth of the tumor in a different way. The existence of TP53 splice site mutations emphasizes the intricacy of the genetic changes linked to hereditary breast cancer syndrome and emphasizes the significance of comprehending the various ways in which TP53 mutations might promote the development of cancer [71, 72]. Several studies have shown differing prevalences of TP53 gene splice site mutations in patients with breast cancer. In 10 out of 13 tumors from BRCA1 mutant carriers, p53 mutations were discovered, suggesting a greater prevalence of p53 mutations in this particular population. The study focused on Ashkenazi Jewish carriers of BRCA1 mutations [73]. According to a different study, TP53 mutations account for 15–20% of all hereditary malignancies and about 1% of breast cancers, highlighting the significance of TP53 mutations in the development of breast cancer [72].

Along with missense, truncating, and in-frame mutations, frameshift mutations are among the frequently found TP53 alterations in breast cancer. The p53 protein's stability, structure, and expression patterns may be affected by these frameshift mutations, impairing the protein's typical tumor suppression function. According to research findings, TP53 frameshift mutations are more common in some subtypes of breast cancer than others. For example, in inflammatory breast cancer, up to 50% of tumors have TP53 mutations, whereas in non-inflammatory breast cancer, only 20–30% do [74]. TP53 frameshift mutations specific to breast cancer patients include a unique frameshift insertion (c.322dupG), a 2-base pair insertion, and a 1-base pair deletion [75].

Frameshift mutations in TP53 can cause the p53 protein to lose its stability, structure, and expression patterns, which will interfere with its usual function as a tumor suppressor [76]. According to research findings, frameshift mutations in TP53, namely, in exon 4 and the surrounding splice site motifs, can result in the synthesis of p53 transcripts that are abnormal, which further destabilizes the p53 protein [35].

Frameshift mutations in p53 can result in a loss of transcriptional activity, which impacts p53's ability to inhibit the proliferation of breast cancer cells. Research indicates that p53 frameshift mutants may have neomorphic characteristics, such as causing senescence and preventing cell migration in breast cancer cells, even if the gain-of-function characteristics of these mutants have not been thoroughly documented. Frameshift mutations can alter the protein levels of p53 and Mdm2 in breast cancer cells, which may result in differences between the mRNA and protein levels of important regulators such as p21, a p53 downstream target. Studying the precise effects of frameshift mutations on p53 activity in breast cancer cells can be facilitated by using isogenic cell lines that express wild-type, mutant, or no p53 from the endogenous TP53 locus [77]. About 30% of instances of breast cancer involve mutations in the most frequently altered gene, TP53. Most p53 mutations are found in the DNA-binding domain, which inhibits p53's transcriptional activity and reduces its ability to operate as a tumor suppressor. A p53 mutation in breast cancer is linked to a more aggressive course of the illness and a lower overall prognosis. Certain subtypes of breast cancer, such as those associated with BRCA1/2 and medullary breast tumors, are more likely to have p53 mutations and are typically more aggressive [78].

p53 mutations have different prognostic effects on different subtypes of breast cancer. Patients with luminal B, HER2-enriched, and normal-like breast cancers have higher mortality rates when p53 mutations are present; however, this is not the case for patients with luminal A and basal-like subtypes of the tumor [78]. In a subtype-dependent manner, the precise kind and location of the p53 mutation may also affect the prognosis for breast cancer [79].

19.5 INSIGHTS FROM GENETIC STUDIES

Studies have demonstrated how important the p53 gene is in the hereditary breast cancer syndrome. Research has demonstrated that p53 mutations are associated with an increased risk of breast cancer, especially in conditions such as Li–Fraumeni syndrome, where germline mutations of the p53 gene promote the development of cancer, including breast cancer. Furthermore, a significant proportion of non-familial breast tumors have been found to have somatic p53 mutations, highlighting the wider significance of p53 dysregulation in breast cancer. The discovery of particular p53 mutations in patients with early-onset breast cancer emphasizes how crucial it is to comprehend the functional significance of these mutations and how they may influence affected people's screening and risk assessment [80]. Additionally, studies have looked at the molecular pathways via which p53 is inhibited in breast cancer, offering insights into possible treatment approaches meant to improve outcomes for those with hereditary breast cancer syndrome and restore p53 function [78].

Research has demonstrated that p53 mutations can inhibit innate immune signals, hence fostering tumor growth. This highlights the pivotal function of p53 disruption in the advancement of cancer. Changes in genes like TP53 affect the anti-tumor immune response, and these interactions between cancer drivers and the tumor immune microenvironment are crucial in determining how cancer evolves [81]. Moreover, immune cell infiltration patterns have been associated with disruptions in pathways such as the WNT and PI3K-AKT, underscoring the intricate relationship between p53 dysregulation and the tumor microenvironment in the advancement of cancer [82]. Comprehending the molecular mechanisms underlying p53-mediated carcinogenesis is crucial for creating tailored treatments and enhancing cancer patients' results from their treatments [83]. Prospective options for furthering our comprehension of hereditary breast cancer syndrome involve researching the role of p53 in this intricate illness. Research indicates that more investigation into the functional importance of p53 mutations in susceptibility to breast cancer, especially in syndromes such as Li–Fraumeni syndrome, may yield important information on the development of cancer and risk assessment [80]. It is essential to look into the molecular pathways by which p53 dysregulation advances breast cancer and affects patient outcomes to create tailored treatment plans and targeted medications. Furthermore, investigating the relationship between immune cell responses and p53 mutations in the tumor microenvironment may reveal new treatment targets and prognostic indicators in hereditary breast cancer syndrome. Prospective investigations might concentrate on pinpointing extra genes and pathways that collaborate with p53 to regulate cancer risk and advancement, providing novel opportunities for precision medicine strategies in the treatment of patients with hereditary breast cancer syndrome [84].

The complexity of p53 mutations and their functional implications in cancer susceptibility present ongoing research problems in the investigation of p53's role in hereditary breast cancer syndrome. Although p53 mutations are linked to the development of breast cancer, it is difficult to pinpoint exactly what role these mutations have in hereditary breast cancer syndrome due to the wide range of mutations and their differing effects on p53 activity. Furthermore, given the low frequency of germline p53 mutations in this population, it is unlikely that early-onset breast cancer patients will have these mutations, suggesting that finding carriers of these variants for screening and risk assessment will remain difficult [80]. Uncovering the precise role of p53 dysregulation in breast cancer progression is further complicated by the interaction between p53 mutations and other genetic and environmental variables influencing breast cancer risk in hereditary disorders [39]. To overcome these obstacles, in-depth genetic research, functional evaluations of p53 mutations, and coordinated methods to unravel the complex mechanisms behind p53-mediated carcinogenesis in hereditary breast cancer syndrome are needed. Little molecules such as PhiKan083, PRIMA-1, and CP-31398 have been found by researchers to be able to reactivate the wild-type functions of mutant p53, therefore offering therapeutic approaches for malignancies that have p53 mutations. Targeting p53 in cancer treatment makes sense because animal research has demonstrated that reactivating wild-type p53 can effectively cause tumor regression, including the regression of liver carcinoma and lymphoma. Mechanistic research has demonstrated that mutant p53 can inhibit innate immune signals to enhance carcinogenesis, emphasizing the intricate relationship between p53 dysregulation and the tumor microenvironment in the advancement of cancer [85].

19.6 CONCLUSIONS

The complex interplay between hereditary and environmental factors that determine the risk of breast cancer highlights the significance of continued investigation into hereditary breast cancer syndrome. Given the pivotal role that p53 mutations play in both hereditary and sporadic instances, comprehending their functional consequences is imperative. Although the variety of mutations and their varying consequences make it difficult to determine the specific involvement of p53 in hereditary breast cancer, new approaches such as small-molecule therapeutics provide hope for tailored treatments. To fully understand the intricate mechanisms behind p53-mediated carcinogenesis, coordinated efforts in functional analyses and genetic studies are required. In the end, developing our knowledge of p53's function in hereditary breast cancer syndrome is essential to developing individualized treatment plans and bettering patient outcomes.

REFERENCES

1. Larsen, M.J., et al., Hereditary breast cancer: clinical, pathological and molecular characteristics. *Breast Cancer: Basic and Clinical Research*, 2014. **8**: p. BCBCR. S18715.
2. Sofi, S., et al., Clinicopathological and prognostic significance of Bcl2 in breast cancer: a comprehensive in silico and in vitro study. *Saudi Journal of Biological Sciences*, 2023. **31**(2): p. 103916.
3. De Silva, S., K.H. Tennekoon, and E.H. Karunanayake, Overview of the genetic basis toward early detection of breast cancer. *Breast Cancer: Targets and Therapy*, 2019: p. 71–80.
4. Jan, N., et al., Metronomic chemotherapy and drug repurposing: a paradigm shift in oncology. *Heliyon*, 2024. https://doi.org/10.1016/j.heliyon.2024.e24670
5. Mir, M.A., Sumaya, N. Jan, Implications of Chemokine Heterogenicity in Cancer Metastasis, in *Cytokine and Chemokine Networks in Cancer*. 2023, Springer. p. 115–136.
6. Ellisen, L.W. and D.A. Haber, Hereditary breast cancer. *Annual Review of Medicine*, 1998. **49**(1): p. 425–436.

7. Sofi, S., et al., Elucidation of interleukin-19 as a therapeutic target for breast cancer by computational analysis and experimental validation. *Saudi Journal of Biological Sciences*, 2023. **30**(9): p. 103771 103771.
8. Jan, N., et al., Exploring the role of trifarotene against RAR-α: an investigation of expression pattern and clinicopathological significance of RAR-α in breast cancer. *Frontiers in Pharmacology*, 2024. **15**: p. 1361679.
9. Yoshida, R., Hereditary breast and ovarian cancer (HBOC): review of its molecular characteristics, screening, treatment, and prognosis. *Breast Cancer*, 2021. **28**(6): p. 1167–1180.
10. Mir, M.A., N. Jan, and I. Noor, Therapeutic Implications of Cytokines and Chemokines Network in Cancer, in *Cytokine and Chemokine Networks in Cancer*. 2023, Springer. p. 385–414.
11. Mir, M.A., et al., Proteomics: Application of Next-Generation Proteomics in Cancer Research, in *Proteomics*. 2023, Elsevier. p. 55–76.
12. Mir, M.A., M. Rashid, and N. Jan, Cytokines and Chemokines in Tumor Growth and Progression, in *Cytokine and Chemokine Networks in Cancer*. 2023, Springer. p. 33–77.
13. Eischen, C.M., Genome stability requires p53. *Cold Spring Harbor Perspectives in Medicine*, 2016. **6**(6): p. a026096.
14. Mir, M.A., M. Bashir, and N. Jan, The Role of Interleukin (IL)-6/IL-6 Receptor Axis in Cancer, in *Cytokine and Chemokine Networks in Cancer*. 2023, Springer. p. 137–164.
15. Ashcroft, M. and K.H. Vousden, Regulation of p53 stability. *Oncogene*, 1999. **18**(53): p. 7637–7643.
16. Mir, M.A., A. Manzoor, and N. Jan, CCL5/CCR5 Axis in Cancer, in *Cytokine and Chemokine Networks in Cancer*. 2023, Springer. p. 219–240.
17. Jan, N., et al., Targeting breast cancer stem cells through retinoids: a new hope for treatment. *Critical Reviews in Oncology/Hematology*, 2023: p. 104156.
18. Valencia, O.M., et al., The role of genetic testing in patients with breast cancer: a review. *JAMA Surgery*, 2017. **152**(6): p. 589–594.
19. Skol, A.D., M.M. Sasaki, and K. Onel, The genetics of breast cancer risk in the post-genome era: thoughts on study design to move past BRCA and towards clinical relevance. *Breast Cancer Research*, 2016. **18**(1): p. 99.
20. Mehrgou, A. and M. Akouchekian, The importance of BRCA1 and BRCA2 genes mutations in breast cancer development. *Medical Journal of the Islamic Republic of Iran*, 2016. **30**: p. 369.
21. Mahdavi, M., et al., Hereditary breast cancer; Genetic penetrance and current status with BRCA. *Journal of Cellular Physiology*, 2019. **234**(5): p. 5741–5750.
22. Sofi, S., et al., A comprehensive analysis of notch signaling genes in breast cancer: expression pattern and prognostic significance. *Advances in Cancer Biology-Metastasis*, 2023. **7**: p. 100104.
23. Shiovitz, S. and L.A. Korde, Genetics of breast cancer: a topic in evolution. *Annals of Oncology*, 2015. **26**(7): p. 1291–1299.
24. Haq, B.U., et al., Targeting p53 misfolding conundrum by stabilizing agents and their analogs in breast cancer therapy: a comprehensive computational analysis. *Frontiers in Pharmacology*, 2024. **14**: p. 1333447.
25. Meijers-Heijboer, H., et al., Low-penetrance susceptibility to breast cancer due to CHEK2* 1100delC in noncarriers of BRCA1 or BRCA2 mutations. *Nature Genetics*, 2002. **31**(1): p. 5.
26. Rahman, N., et al., PALB2, which encodes a BRCA2-interacting protein, is a breast cancer susceptibility gene. *Nature Genetics*, 2007. **39**(2): p. 165–167.
27. Mir, M.A., M. Rashid, and N. Jan, The Interleukin-8 Pathway in Cancer, in *Cytokine and Chemokine Networks in Cancer*. 2023, Springer. p. 165–190.
28. Kamaraj, B. and A. Bogaerts, Structure and function of p53-DNA complexes with inactivation and rescue mutations: a molecular dynamics simulation study. *PLoS One*, 2015. **10**(8): p. e0134638.
29. Kato, S., et al., Understanding the function–structure and function–mutation relationships of p53 tumor suppressor protein by high-resolution missense mutation analysis. *Proceedings of the National Academy of Sciences*, 2003. **100**(14): p. 8424–8429.
30. Mir, M.A., et al., Metronomics: toward personalized chemotherapy. *Novel Approaches in Metronomic Chemotherapy for Breast Cancer Treatment*, 2024. p. 99–119. https://doi.org/10.1201/9781032632674-8
31. Hashimoto, N., H. Nagano, and T. Tanaka, The role of tumor suppressor p53 in metabolism and energy regulation, and its implication in cancer and lifestyle-related diseases. *Endocrine Journal*, 2019. **66**(6): p. 485–496.
32. Kaur, R.P., et al., Role of p53 gene in breast cancer: focus on mutation spectrum and therapeutic strategies. *Current Pharmaceutical Design*, 2018. **24**(30): p. 3566–3575.

33. Mir, M.A., N. Jan, and S. Sofi, Introduction to Metronomic Chemotherapy, in *Novel Approaches in Metronomic Chemotherapy for Breast Cancer Treatment*. 2024, CRC Press. p. 1–14.
34. Ozaki, T. and A. Nakagawara, Role of p53 in cell death and human cancers. *Cancers*, 2011. **3**(1): p. 994–1013.
35. Steffens Reinhardt, L., et al., p53 dysregulation in breast cancer: insights on mutations in the TP53 network and p53 isoform expression. *International Journal of Molecular Sciences*, 2023. **24**(12). https://doi.org/10.3390/ijms241210078
36. Shomali, N., et al., Dysregulation of P53 in breast cancer: Causative factors and treatment strategies. *Pathology – Research and Practice*, 2023. **247**: p. 154539.
37. Valente, L.J., et al., p53 deficiency triggers dysregulation of diverse cellular processes in physiological oxygen. *Journal of Cell Biology*, 2020. **219**(11): p. e201908212.
38. Zonneville, J., et al., Selective therapeutic strategy for p53-deficient cancer by targeting dysregulation in DNA repair. *Communications Biology*, 2021. **4**(1): p. 862.
39. Marvalim, C., A. Datta, and S.C. Lee, Role of p53 in breast cancer progression: An insight into p53 targeted therapy. *Theranostics*, 2023. **13**(4): p. 1421–1442.
40. Chen, X., et al., Mutant p53 in cancer: from molecular mechanism to therapeutic modulation. *Cell Death & Disease*, 2022. **13**(11): p. 974.
41. Dorling, L., et al., Breast cancer risks associated with missense variants in breast cancer susceptibility genes. *Genome Medicine*, 2022. **14**(1): p. 51.
42. Tavtigian, S.V. and G. Chenevix-Trench, Growing recognition of the role for rare missense substitutions in breast cancer susceptibility. *Biomarkers in Medicine*, 2014. **8**(4): p. 589–603.
43. Lee, H., et al., P53 immunohistochemistry is an ideal surrogate marker for TP53 mutation and a predictor of early metastasis in breast cancer: Real-world analysis in endometrial carcinoma biopsies. *The Journal of Pathology*. 2021. **31**(6): p. 907.
44. Berke, T.P., S.H. Slight, and S.M. Hyder, Role of reactivating mutant p53 protein in suppressing growth and metastasis of triple-negative breast cancer. *OncoTargets and Therapy*, 2022: p. 23–30.
45. Pollock, N.C., et al., Differences in somatic TP53 mutation type in breast tumors by race and receptor status. *Breast Cancer Research and Treatment*, 2022. **192**(3): p. 639–648.
46. Hassin, O. and M. Oren, Drugging p53 in cancer: one protein, many targets. *Nature Reviews Drug Discovery*, 2023. **22**(2): p. 127–144.
47. Gencel-Augusto, J. and G. Lozano, p53 tetramerization: at the center of the dominant-negative effect of mutant p53. *Genes & Development*, 2020. **34**(17–18): p. 1128–1146.
48. Stein, Y., R. Aloni-Grinstein, and V. Rotter, Mutant p53 oncogenicity: dominant-negative or gain-of-function? *Carcinogenesis*, 2020. **41**(12): p. 1635–1647.
49. Ellison, V., et al., Frame-shift mediated reduction of gain-of-function p53 R273H and deletion of the R273H C-terminus in breast cancer cells result in replication-stress sensitivity. *Oncotarget*, 2021. **12**(12): p. 1128.
50. Redman Rivera, L.N.R., *Evaluating Mutant p53 Gain-of-function Phenotypes and Mechanisms in Cancer* (Doctoral dissertation, Vanderbilt University). 2021.
51. Lasham, A., et al., Breast cancer patient prognosis is determined by the interplay between TP53 mutation and alternative transcript expression: insights from TP53 long amplicon digital PCR assays. *Cancers*, 2021. **13**(7): p. 1531.
52. Erson-Bensan, A.E., RNA-biology ruling cancer progression? Focus on 3′ UTRs and splicing. *Cancer and Metastasis Reviews*, 2020. **39**(3): p. 887–901.
53. Steffens Reinhardt, L., et al., p53 Dysregulation in Breast Cancer: Insights on Mutations in the TP53 Network and p53 Isoform Expression. *International Journal of Molecular Sciences*, 2023. **24**(12): p. 10078.
54. Manoharan, V., et al., Pattern of nucleotide variants of TP53 and their correlation with the expression of p53 and its downstream proteins in a Sri Lankan cohort of breast and colorectal cancer patients. *BMC Cancer*, 2020. **20**: p. 1–15.
55. Benor, G., et al., Transcriptional profiling reveals a subset of human breast tumors that retain wt TP53 but display mutant p53-associated features. *Molecular Oncology*, 2020. **14**(8): p. 1640–1652.
56. Kim, M., et al., A protein interaction landscape of breast cancer. *Science*, 2021. **374**(6563): p. eabf3066.
57. Kumar, D.T., et al., Computational structural assessment of BReast CAncer type 1 susceptibility protein (BRCA1) and BRCA1-Associated Ring Domain protein 1 (BARD1) mutations on the protein-protein interface. *Advances in Protein Chemistry and Structural Biology*, 2022. **130**: p. 375–397.
58. Cheng, F., et al., Comprehensive characterization of protein–protein interactions perturbed by disease mutations. *Nature Genetics*, 2021. **53**(3): p. 342–353.

59. Andreassen, P.R., et al., Understanding BRCA2 function as a tumor suppressor based on domain-specific activities in DNA damage responses. *Genes*, 2021. **12**(7): p. 1034.
60. Le, H.P., W. D. Heyer, and J. Liu, Guardians of the genome: BRCA2 and its partners. *Genes*, 2021. **12**(8): p. 1229.
61. Dorling, L., et al., Breast cancer risks associated with missense variants in breast cancer susceptibility genes. *Genome Medicine*, 2022. **14**(1): p. 51.
62. Wilcox, N., et al., Exome sequencing identifies breast cancer susceptibility genes and defines the contribution of coding variants to breast cancer risk. *Nature Genetics*, 2023. **55**(9): p. 1435–1439.
63. Öfverholm, A., et al., Extended genetic analysis and tumor characteristics in over 4600 women with suspected hereditary breast and ovarian cancer. *BMC Cancer*, 2023. **23**(1): p. 738.
64. Janssen, B., et al., A systematic review of predicted pathogenic PALB2 variants: an analysis of mutational overlap between epithelial cancers. *Journal of Human Genetics*, 2020. **65**(2): p. 199–205.
65. Yang, X., et al., Cancer risks associated with germline PALB2 pathogenic variants: an international study of 524 families. *Journal of Clinical Oncology*, 2020. **38**(7): p. 674–685.
66. Katagiri, T., et al., High proportion of missense mutations of the BRCA1 and BRCA2 genes in Japanese breast cancer families. *Journal of Human Genetics*, 1998. **43**(1): p. 42–48.
67. Petrosino, M., et al., Analysis and Interpretation of the Impact of Missense Variants in Cancer. *International Journal of Molecular Sciences*, 2021. **22**(11). https://doi.org/10.3390/ijms22115416
68. Kumar, R., et al., Structural and conformational changes induced by missense variants in the zinc finger domains of GATA3 involved in breast cancer. *RSC Advances*, 2020. **10**(65): p. 39640–39653.
69. Lee, M., et al., Cancer-causing BRCA2 missense mutations disrupt an intracellular protein assembly mechanism to disable genome maintenance. *Nucleic Acids Research*, 2021. **49**(10): p. 5588–5604.
70. Quaresima, B., et al., Missense mutations of BRCA1 gene affect the binding with p53 both in vitro and in vivo. *Oncology Reports*, 2006. **16**(4): p. 811–815.
71. Pinto, E.M., et al., Clinical and functional significance of TP53 Exon 4–Intron 4 splice junction variants. *Molecular Cancer Research*, 2022. **20**(2): p. 207–216.
72. Gallardo-Alvarado, L.N., et al., Prevalence of germline mutations in the TP53 gene in patients with early-onset breast cancer in the Mexican population. *BMC Cancer*, 2019. **19**(1): p. 118.
73. Phillips, K.-A., et al., Frequency of p53 mutations in breast carcinomas from Ashkenazi Jewish carriers of BRCA1 mutations. *Journal of the National Cancer Institute*, 1999. **91**(5): p. 469–473.
74. Lai, H., et al., Mutations in the p53 tumor suppressor gene and early onset breast cancer. *Cancer Biology & Therapy*, 2002. **1**(1): p. 31–36.
75. Akter, H., et al., Novel mutations in actionable breast cancer genes by targeted sequencing in an ethnically homogenous cohort. *BMC Medical Genetics*, 2019. **20**(1): p. 150.
76. Meric-Bernstam, F., et al., Survival outcomes by TP53 mutation status in metastatic breast cancer. *JCO Precision Oncology*, 2018(2): p. 1–15.
77. Tong, D.R., et al., p53 Frameshift mutations couple loss-of-function with unique neomorphic activities. *Mol Cancer Res*, 2021. **19**(9): p. 1522–1533.
78. Gasco, M., S. Shami, and T. Crook, The p53 pathway in breast cancer. *Breast Cancer Research*, 2002. **4**(2): p. 70–76.
79. Schaafsma, E., et al., Predicting clinical outcomes of cancer patients with a p53 deficiency gene signature. *Scientific Reports*, 2022. **12**(1): p. 1317.
80. Sidransky, D., et al., Inherited p53 gene mutations in breast cancer. *Cancer Research*, 1992. **52**(10): p. 2984–2986.
81. Misetic, H., et al., Mechanistic insights into the interactions between cancer drivers and the tumour immune microenvironment. *Genome Medicine*, 2023. **15**(1): p. 40.
82. Marx, C., et al., Mechanistic insights into p53-regulated cytotoxicity of combined entinostat and irinotecan against colorectal cancer cells. *Molecular Oncology*, 2021. **15**(12): p. 3404–3429.
83. Nedbal, W., et al., Mechanistic insights into p53-promoted RNA-RNA annealing. *Journal of Molecular Biology*, 1997. **266**(4): p. 677–87.
84. Lane, D. and A. Levine, p53 Research: the past thirty years and the next thirty years. *Cold Spring Harbor Perspectives in Biology*, 2010. **2**(12): p. a000893.
85. Suzuki, K. and H. Matsubara, Recent advances in p53 research and cancer treatment. *Journal of Biotechnology and Biomedicine*, 2011. **2011**: p. 978312.

20 Bridging Bench to Bedside in Breast Cancer Therapy

Translational Insights into p53

Kirti Hooda[1], Mary Chatterjee[2], Nusrat Jan[3], and Manzoor Ahmad Mir[3]*

[1]Centre for Nanosciences and Nanotechnology, Panjab University, Chandigarh, India
[2]Department of Biotechnology Engineering, UIET, Panjab University, Chandigarh, India
[3]Department of Bioresources, School of Biological Sciences, University of Kashmir, Srinagar, J&K, India
*drmanzoor@kashmiruniversity.ac.in

20.1 INTRODUCTION

One tumor suppressor gene that frequently mutates in a variety of malignancies, including breast cancer, is p53. Breast cancer can form and advance more quickly when there are mutations in the p53 gene that cause altered expression and loss of function [1, 2]. p53 is essential for the prevention of infectious illnesses and breast cancer. It also preserves genomic integrity. It is located on chromosome 17p13 and regulates cell proliferation, angiogenesis, and programmed cell death. Tumor protein 53 (TP53) mutated or not, the expression of p53 and its isoforms is a better indicator of treatment outcomes and chemotherapy responses in patients with breast cancer. Mutations in murine double minute 2 (MDM2), the negative regulator of p53, that are subtype-dependent may indicate the deactivation of p53 in breast cancer. One potential therapy approach for different kinds of breast cancer is to target both p53 mutants and wild-type cells [3]. The p53 gene codes for a transcription factor that controls the expression of genes related to cellular processes such as apoptosis, senescence, and the cell cycle when it is activated as part of the cellular stress response. Germline mutations, loss of heterozygosity (LOH) in the p53 gene, coding mutations, and p53 degradation are the pathways of p53 inactivation in breast cancer. It is possible for overexpression of MDM2 or deletion or epigenetic loss of p14ARF to unintentionally trigger p53 degradation. Additionally, the p53 protein can be inhibited and prevented from localizing to the nucleus via cytoplasmic sequestration [4]. It has been observed that the p53 gene, which shields the body from mutant cells, plays a significant role in the occurrence and progression of breast cancer. In cells with damaged DNA, mitotic activity can be sustained through mutations in the p53 gene. The non-invasive and sluggish growth of tumors, as well as their varying sizes, can be explained by the incompleteness of apoptosis [5, 6]. To introduce new paradigms in the treatment of cancer patients, translational research in breast cancer therapy entails the creation of both innovative diagnostics and treatments, which are frequently related to one another. It encompasses a wide range, from diagnosis to treatment, and fosters the creation of fresh paradigms. The following are essential elements of translational research in breast cancer therapy: The creation of innovative medicines and diagnostics are important aspects of translational research. They are frequently linked to one another and introduce fresh perspectives

DOI: 10.1201/9781003520771-20

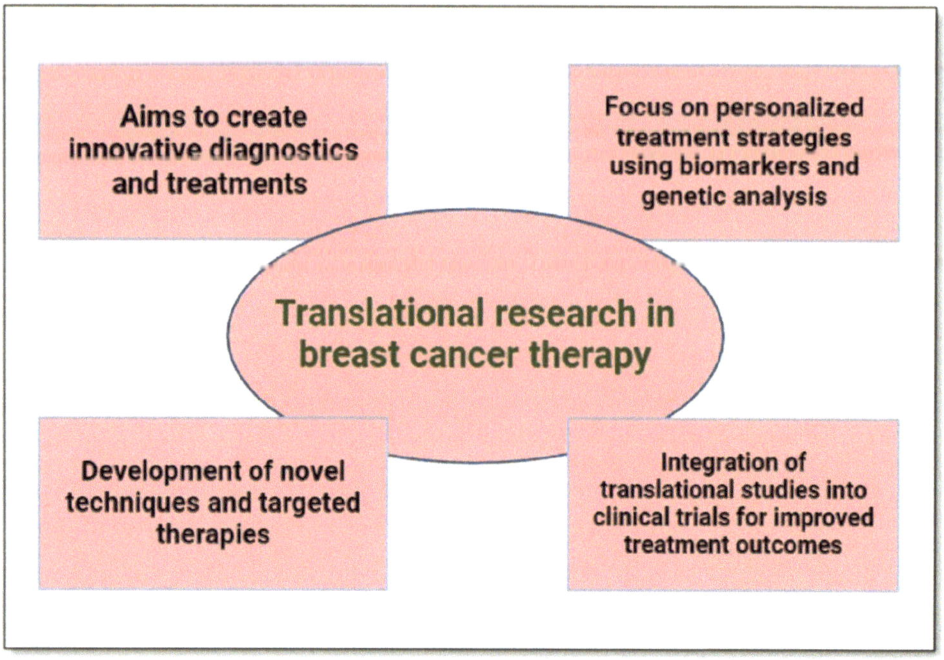

FIGURE 20.1 Elements of translational research in breast cancer therapy.

on the treatment of cancer patients. Translational research is needed to boost clinical trial efficiency and speed up the development of novel techniques, particularly in prospective clinical trials [7]. Through translational research, biomarkers for the most effective individualized treatment plans for breast cancer can be found. The incorporation of translational studies into clinical trials is crucial in the search for new and trustworthy biomarkers for a personalized treatment strategy (Figure 20.1).

A new paradigm in breast cancer treatment is signaled by genetic analysis, and translational research is essential to incorporating genomic data into clinical practice for individualized treatment plans [8]. Biomarkers, including human epidermal growth factor receptor 2, progesterone receptor, and estrogen receptor, can identify the subtype of breast cancer and provide further details on the prognosis and available treatments. Gene expression analysis provides further details on the prognosis of the disease and helps to further characterize the molecular subtype of breast cancer. While predictive biomarkers, like programmed cell death ligand 1 expression, are instruments for identifying patients who can benefit from particular therapeutic regimens to determine the optimum course of treatment, prognostic biomarkers provide information regarding recurrence risk and survival [9, 10]. Moreover, other therapeutic approaches and viable targets investigated for the treatment of metastatic triple-negative breast cancer include immunotherapy, PARP inhibition, and AKT inhibition [11–13]. While standard chemotherapy is not targeted and can impact both cancer and healthy cells, novel treatments created through translational research frequently target cancer cells directly. Because they target cancer cells directly and spare healthy cells, novel treatments created through translational research are intended to have fewer adverse effects than traditional chemotherapy. Immunotherapies, which use the patient's immune system to combat cancer, are a result of translational research on breast cancer; conventional chemotherapy does not use the patient's immune system. While traditional chemotherapy is not based on genetic information, translational research in breast cancer leads to precision medicine, where treatment is based on the exact genetic alterations present in the patient's tumor [10, 14, 15]. Promising outcomes have been observed in the enhancement of anti-PD-1 therapeutic responsiveness and induction of systemic antitumor immunity using p53 immunotherapies in breast cancer patients. Triple-negative breast cancer (TNBC) is more susceptible to anti-PD-1 immunotherapy when p53 activity is restored through intracellular protein delivery. This is achieved by causing immunogenic cell death, activating type I IFN signaling, and upregulating programmed cell death ligand 1 (PD-L1) expression. In cancers with TP53 mutations, this method has been demonstrated to be effective, safe, and possibly universal for restoring p53 activity. Furthermore, it has been proposed that patients with TNBC may benefit from immune checkpoint inhibitors in addition to p53 restoration [16, 17]. Through its ability to control DNA repair and cell proliferation, the tumor suppressor protein p53 is essential in halting the initiation and spread of breast cancer. On the other hand, poor prognosis is linked to mutations in the TP53 gene, which encodes p53 and is present in about 30–35% of instances of breast cancer. Patients with hormone receptor-negative breast cancer, especially those with basal-like and HER2-enriched subtypes, are more likely to have p53 mutations, which are linked to gain-of-function carcinogenic activity and a worse prognosis. Furthermore, p53 mutations are linked to the molecular subtype of breast cancer as opposed to a shared biologic characteristic that is characterized by triple-negative status [18–20]. Apart from TP53 mutations, many molecular processes can also affect p53 levels and functionality. These mechanisms include abnormal production of long non-coding RNAs, amplification or activation of HDM2/4, loss of function of ATM–CHEK2–p53 signaling, and TP53 isoform expression. Moreover, TP53 mutation is not as good a predictor of treatment response or outcome as p53 expression levels in breast cancer. All things considered, p53 plays a complicated role in the development and prognosis of breast cancer, involving several molecular pathways that alter p53 levels and activities. Comprehending these pathways is essential for creating new therapeutic approaches and breast cancer biomarkers [21, 22].

20.2 MOLECULAR MECHANISMS OF p53 IN BREAST CANCER

One essential component of p53's involvement in breast cancer is transcriptional regulation. One transcription factor that controls the expression of genes involved in several cellular functions, including DNA repair, cell cycle arrest, and apoptosis, is the p53 protein. When it comes to breast cancer, the tumor suppressive properties of p53 are often rendered inactive due to a mutation that affects 30–35% of instances or the overexpression of its negative regulator, MDM2. The majority of hormone receptor-positive or luminal subtypes of breast cancers maintain the wild-type p53 status, whereas hormone receptor-negative or triple-negative subtypes have a greater frequency of p53 mutations. This indicates that the incidence of p53 mutations in breast cancers is largely subtype-dependent [23, 24]. Wild-type p53 can control the expression of the estrogen receptor (ER) alpha gene in ER-positive breast cancers. With a half-life of around 20 minutes, the p53 protein is precisely regulated. It has been demonstrated that multiple ubiquitin ligases, such as MDM2, COP1, and CHIP, directly affect the stability of the p53 protein. By modifying p53 signaling, RNF187, a RING family ubiquitin ligase, promotes the growth of breast cancer and prevents apoptosis. Only in p53 wild-type groups did RNF187 expression show an increased correlation with breast cancer survival. Depletion of RNF187 promoted cell death and slowed the progression of breast cancer. According to an RNA sequencing study, RNF187 may have a significant role in regulating p53 signaling. Additional research revealed that RNF187 interacts with p53 and, independently of MDM2, facilitates its polyubiquitination, which leads to p53's degradation [12, 25]. One important part of p53's function as a tumor suppressor in breast cancer is transcriptional control. p53 is triggered in the presence of genotoxic stress to aid in apoptosis, cell cycle arrest, and DNA repair. When it comes to breast cancer, the tumor suppressive properties of p53 are often rendered inactive due to either overexpression of the negative regulator MDM2 or mutations, which affect 30–35% of cases [26]. Wild-type p53 has the ability to control the expression of the ER alpha gene in ER-positive breast cancers. With a half-life of around 20 minutes, the p53 protein is precisely regulated. It has been demonstrated that multiple ubiquitin ligases, such as MDM2, COP1, and CHIP, directly affect the stability of the p53 protein [27]. By modifying p53 signaling, RNF187, a RING family ubiquitin ligase, promotes the growth of breast cancer and prevents apoptosis. Only in the p53 wild-type groups did RNF187 expression show an increased level in breast cancer and a correlation with breast cancer survival. Depletion of RNF187 promoted cell death and slowed the progression of breast cancer. According to an RNA sequencing study, RNF187 may have a significant role in regulating p53 signaling. Additional research revealed that RNF187 interacts with p53 and, independently of MDM2, facilitates its polyubiquitination, which leads to p53's degradation [28, 29].

Another transcriptional coactivator for p53 is BRCA1, and bearers of germline mutations in BRCA1 are at risk for developing breast cancer. By maintaining the stability of the tumor suppressor p53 protein, BRCA1 controls p53 in breast cancer by causing an increase in p53 expression and consequent apoptotic cell death in epithelial cancer cells that express wild-type p53 [30]. Both in vitro and in vivo interactions between BRCA1 and p53 have been demonstrated; the interacting areas correspond to distinct BRCA1 domains and the C-terminal domain of p53. Gene expression as tumor suppressors is mostly coordinated by the connection between BRCA1 and p53, and mutations in the BRCA1 gene are frequently seen in familial breast and ovarian malignancies [13, 31]. The p53 pathway plays a pivotal role in breast cancer, and the molecular pathological examination of particular p53 pathway components holds potential for both diagnostic and prognostic purposes [4, 32].

A conserved transcription factor called HOXA5 induces apoptosis in breast cancer cell types when it is overexpressed [43]. By functioning as a positive regulator of p53 transcription and function, HOXA5 controls p53 in breast cancer. According to research, in epithelial cancer cells that express wild-type p53, HOXA5 can activate the p53 promoter, increasing p53 expression and causing apoptotic cell death (Table 20.1). Furthermore, p53 and HOXA5 mRNA and protein expression

TABLE 20.1
Transcriptional Regulators of p53 in Breast Cancer

Transcription Factor	Mechanism of Action	Relationship with p53	References
MDM2	Overexpression and negative regulation render wild-type p53 inactive	Mutations in p53 or MDM2 overexpression affect 30–35% of cases	[23, 26]
RNF187	Facilitates polyubiquitination and degradation of p53 independently of MDM2	Increased expression correlates with breast cancer survival in wild-type p53 groups	[25, 28]
BRCA1	Increases p53 expression and promotes apoptotic cell death in cells with wild-type p53	Maintains stability of p53	[30, 31]
HOXA5	Induces apoptosis by activating p53 transcription and function	Coordinated loss with p53 expression in breast cancer cells	[33, 34]
Bortezomib	Triggers apoptosis in p53 null breast cancer cells	Dependent on caspase-3 activation	[35, 36]
C-terminal peptide derived from p53	Induces apoptosis independently of p53 status	Causes cytochrome c release from mitochondria	[37, 38]
Fas, death receptor 5, BAX, Noxa, PUMA, BID	Stimulates apoptotic pathways through p53 activation	Essential for intrinsic and extrinsic pathways	[23]
HDAC inhibitors	Modify p53 transcriptional activity and affect epigenetic control	Influences p53-mediated epigenetic regulation	[39, 40]
ATM/ATR, Chk1/2 protein	Transactivate p53 to initiate senescence in response to biological stressors	Determines senescence or apoptosis based on stressor intensity	[23]
Histone modifications, DNA methylation	Epigenetic regulation of gene expression by p53	Loss of methylation at some gene promoters increased methylation at others	[41, 42]

are frequently shown to be coordinately lost in breast cancer cell lines and patient tumors, suggesting a possible regulatory link between the two [44]. Moreover, a drop in p53 expression in human breast cancers has been connected to HOXA5 expression loss, indicating that HOXA5 expression loss may be a factor in p53 loss in breast cancer. The significance of HOXA5 in controlling p53 expression and function in breast cancer cells is shown by this relationship [34]. When HOXA5 activates the p53 promoter in epithelial cancer cells that express wild-type p53, there is an increase in p53 expression and consequent apoptotic cell death [33]. A decrease in p53 expression in human breast cancers has been associated with HOXA5 expression loss, indicating that HOXA5 expression loss may be a factor in p53 loss in breast cancer [22, 33]. Moreover, reports suggest that HOXA5 may function as a transcriptional regulator of p53 expression in human breast cancer [10, 45, 46]. According to a study, p53 expression in human breast cancers can be inhibited by HOXA5 dysfunction, suggesting that HOXA5 is essential for controlling p53 expression and function in breast cancer [34, 47]. Comprehending the mechanisms underlying these transcriptional regulators is essential for devising innovative therapeutic approaches for breast cancer, as they are pivotal in the transcriptional regulation of p53 in this disease. Apoptosis in a variety of cell types, including breast cancer cells, is crucially regulated by the p53 protein. Nevertheless, p53-independent methods can also be used to cause apoptosis. For instance, a study using evidence from DNA fragmentation revealed that the proteasome inhibitor bortezomib can, in a dose-dependent way, trigger apoptosis in p53-null breast cancer cells. Additionally, the study demonstrated that bortezomib treatment dramatically activates caspase-3, suggesting that caspase-3 is responsible for inducing apoptosis in these p53-deficient cells. Furthermore, there was no change in the expression level of Mcl-1 in treated cells, and the pro-apoptotic proteins Bad, Noxa, and Puma were not important regulators of apoptosis induction in p53-null 4T1 and 4THMpc cells. However, after receiving bortezomib, these p53-deficient cells showed a highly notable increase in the anti-apoptotic protein Hsp25/27 [35]. Another study examined the mechanism of apoptosis in three human breast cancer cell lines expressing either natural wild-type or mutant p53 in response to a p53-derived C-terminal peptide. The results of the study showed that the p53-derived C-terminal peptide, independent of p53 status, caused apoptosis in all three cell lines. Additionally, the peptide adhered to the mitochondrial membrane and caused cytochrome c to be released [10, 37].

A vast network of signals that operate through either intrinsic or extrinsic apoptotic pathways are stimulated by p53. The stimulation of the expression of cell death receptors Fas, death receptor 5, and death-domain initiates the extrinsic pathway, whereas transactivation of pro-apoptotic genes belonging to the Bcl2 family, such as BAX, Noxa, PUMA, and BID, initiates the intrinsic pathway. These genes interact to encourage the multimerization and functional activation of BAX, which results in the release of cytochrome c and the activation of caspase-9 and caspase-12 [23, 48]. DNA fragmentation data demonstrated that the proteasome inhibitor bortezomib induced apoptosis in a dose-dependent manner in a study conducted on p53-null breast cancer cells. Using ubiquitin-protein conjugates, Western blot investigations demonstrated that bortezomib significantly inhibits the proteasome in 4T1 and 4THMpc cells that lack p53. The study's findings also demonstrate that bortezomib therapy dramatically activates caspase-3, suggesting that caspase-3 is responsible for inducing apoptosis in these p53-deficient cells. The further findings indicate that in p53-null 4T1 and 4THMpc cells, the pro-apoptotic proteins Bad, Noxa, and Puma are not important regulators of apoptosis induction. To induce apoptosis in breast cancer cells, p53 is essential [35].

Senescence is one of p53's other key roles. A variety of biological stressors can cause senescence, an irreversible cell cycle stop. When senescence is induced, the Rb pathway is initiated by p53 being transactivated by either ATM/ATR or Chk1/2 protein. Senescence or apoptosis, however, can be determined by the levels, kinetics, and threshold of stressor intensity [23]. Particularly in cases of breast cancer, the p53 protein is essential to the process of DNA repair. It is a transcription factor that controls several genes related to genomic stability and DNA repair. p53 is dormant in a healthy organism, but it becomes active in response to several cellular stressors, including oxidative stress, hypoxia, and damage to DNA. When p53 is activated, it controls downstream genes that prevent normal cells from transforming cancerous and, if DNA repair systems are compromised, trigger programs that cause cells to die [49]. Histone modifications and DNA methylation control gene expression as part of the molecular process of p53's epigenetic regulation of breast cancer. A deficit in p53 causes the loss of methylation at some gene promoters in breast cancer cells, including IL-6, CD44, and CD133, while increasing methylation at the ERα promoter. An autocrine loop favoring additional methylation loss at the IL-6, CD44, and CD133 promoters in addition to methylation gain at the ERα promoter is started by this loss of methylation at the IL-6 promoter. Furthermore, methylation of putative repressor sites is one of the complex alterations in genomic DNA that are induced by IL-6 treatment [50]. HDAC (histone deacetylases) drugs reduce mutant p53 transcription, cause p53 deacetylation, and modify p53 transcriptional activity through direct p53 DNA binding to influence p53-mediated epigenetic control in breast cancer. HDAC inhibitors can cause p53 to become acetylated at particular lysine sites, which increases p53 transcriptional activity and encourages the production of p21Cip1/Waf1. HDAC inhibitors also can control the production of long noncoding RNAs and noncoding microRNAs, which are critical for alternative splicing and transcription elongation [39, 51].

20.3 TARGETED THERAPIES AGAINST TUMORS WITH MUTANT p53

Translational research has revealed multiple approaches to target p53 in breast cancer, both mutant and wild type. These tactics include genetic-based methods employing vectors and designed antibodies, TP53 gene therapy, p53 vaccinations, and the recovery of mutant p53 activity. They also include novel small-molecule pharmacologic inhibitors, stapled peptides, and PROTACs. Targeted therapies against tumors with mutant p53 are being developed to reactivate or restore mutant p53 to wild type, promote degradation, induce synthetic lethality, inhibit gain-of-function-associated interactors or pathways, and incorporate wild-type p53 gene into tumor cells. The tryptamine derivative JNJ26854165 has shown promising results in a phase I trial for advanced breast cancer [23]. Some of the few instances of p53-targeted breast cancer treatments that have been created via translational research are to combat p53-mutated malignancies; TP53 gene therapy, p53 vaccinations, and mutant p53 function rescue have all been suggested. JNJ26854165, a derivative of tryptamine, prevents the MDM2–p53 complex from attaching to the proteasome, causing p53-associated death in cells expressing wild-type p53 (Figure 20.2) [52].

Immunotherapies, gene therapies use vectors to introduce the wild-type p53 gene into tumor cells, and targeted therapies against tumors containing mutant p53 that concentrate on reactivating or restoring mutant p53 to wild type [23], encouraging degradation, causing synthetic lethality, and blocking its interactors or pathways associated with gain-of-function using synthetic fatal interactions with mutant p53 to target genes or pathways that compensate for the lack of functional p53 and increase the therapeutic advantages [53]. For breast cancer, numerous ongoing clinical trials are investigating p53-targeted treatments. One such is the anti-p53 medication PK11007, which has demonstrated encouraging outcomes in preclinical studies when used to treat TNBC [54]. However, the complexity of p53 mutations in cancer cells and the absence of a known method for restoring p53 function has presented major obstacles to the development of p53-targeted therapeutics. Despite these obstacles, there is still optimism for the creation of tailored medications that specifically target particular p53 mutations and for the resurgence of gene therapy and cancer immunotherapy techniques [55]. Additionally, p53-associated pathways are interesting therapeutic targets for breast cancer via translational research. For instance, p53 signaling targeting has been shown to inhibit the development and metastasis of breast cancer cells, according to a study published in Cancer Cell International. According to this study, patients with breast cancer may benefit from a therapeutic approach that targets p53-associated pathways [56].

Research on the efficacy of p53-targeted treatments for breast cancer is ongoing, with encouraging findings and obstacles to be addressed. There is still promise for p53-targeted treatments to treat breast cancer despite these obstacles. The TP53 tumor suppressor gene mutation is quite common

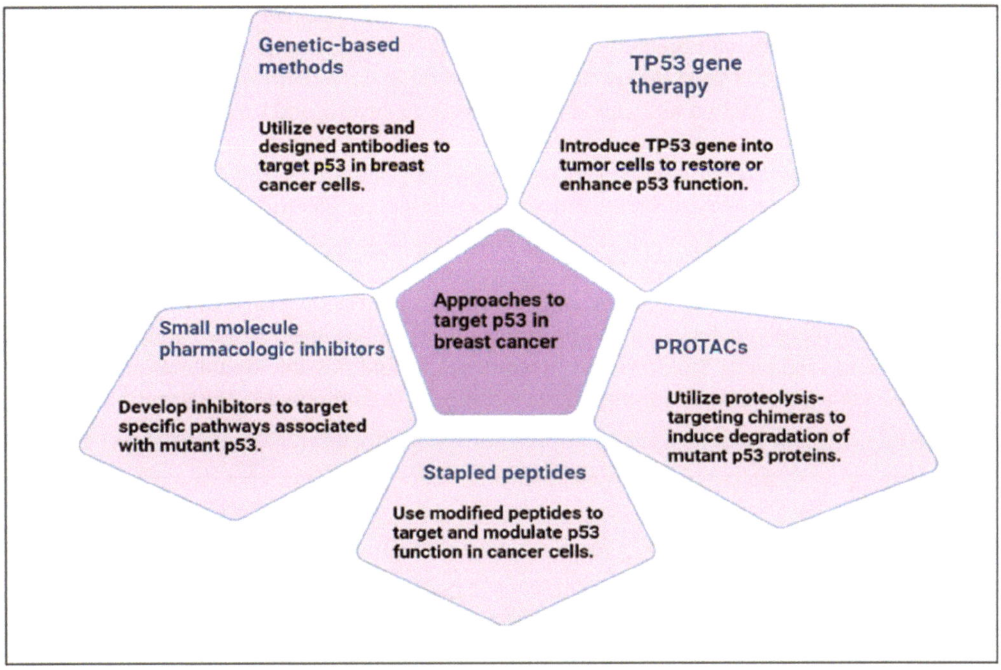

FIGURE 20.2 Different approaches to target p53 in breast cancer.

in cancer, and the p53 protein functions as a significant barrier against the genesis and progression of cancer. Though few drug research programs have advanced to late-stage clinical trials and no p53-based treatments have been authorized in the USA or Europe thus far, attempts to restore the functionality of p53 in tumors as a therapeutic strategy have encountered difficulties. The authors identify several interesting strategies for p53-based therapy, such as medications designed to target particular types of p53 mutants and small compounds that can either shield p53 from its negative regulators or restore the activity of mutant p53 proteins [57]. A fresh interest in gene therapy approaches has also resulted from recent discoveries that make the p53 pathway practically "druggable" and from advances in our understanding of the molecular regulation of the p53 protein. The majority of these tactics are indirect; they entail working with endogenous p53 modulators, including inducers of the nucleolar stress response, Sirt1/2 inhibitors, Mdm2 and Mdmx inhibitors, and inhibitors of the deubiquitinase USP7. The frequent p53 gene mutation in malignancies, the incidence of undesirable side effects, and the target selectivity of the currently available compounds are some of the obstacles that still need to be overcome to generate clinically useful p53-targeting medications. Consequently, more pre-clinical research is needed to find potential lead chemicals for p53 pathway drugging [58].

20.4 CHALLENGES AND LIMITATIONS IN HARNESSING p53 FOR BREAST CANCER THERAPY

One advantage of p53 targeting in breast cancer treatment may be the restoration of p53's regular activity in cancer cells, which may prevent tumor development and metastasis. Restoring p53 can stop tumor formation since it is a significant transcription factor involved in the regulation of multiple cellular activities, including the reduction of cell proliferation in response to different stimuli. In p53-null cells, targeting p53 can also result in MDM2-dependent activity, indicating that these drugs may have use outside of malignancies that express wild-type p53. Additionally, strategies for targeting p53 in breast cancer therapy include immunotherapies, gene therapies using vectors to incorporate wild-type p53 gene into tumor cells, promoting degradation, inducing synthetic lethality, inhibiting gain-of-function-associated interactors or pathways, and reactivation or restoration of mutant p53 to wild type [23, 59].

Because different breast cancer subtypes may respond differently to different treatment approaches, the heterogeneity of breast cancer makes targeting p53 for therapy extremely difficult. The development of universal therapeutic approaches is complicated by the diversity of subtypes of breast cancer [60]. Targeting p53 in TNBC is difficult because this subtype does not have particular targeted medicines. The lack of hormone receptors restricts the range of available treatments, emphasizing the necessity for creative approaches to close this therapeutic gap. Gene expression data can be analyzed using bioinformatics techniques to find possible treatment targets for breast cancer. Researchers employed bioinformatics techniques to find possible therapeutic targets in the

TABLE 20.2
Challenges Faced in Targeting p53 for Breast Cancer Therapy

Challenge	Details	References
Heterogeneity of breast cancer subtypes	Different breast cancer subtypes respond differently to treatment approaches, making targeting p53 for therapy extremely difficult. The development of universal therapeutic approaches is complicated by the diversity of subtypes.	[62–64]
Targeting p53 in triple-negative breast cancer (TNBC)	TNBC lacks particular targeted medicines due to the absence of hormone receptors, limiting treatment options. Creative approaches are needed to address this therapeutic gap.	[60, 65–67]
Misfolding and accumulation of altered p53 protein	The altered p53 protein in breast cancer is prone to misfolding and accumulation, making it difficult to restore normal p53 function. Stabilizing agents and analogs are required to address this challenge.	[2, 68, 69]
Complexity of p53 mutations and inactivation mechanisms	p53 mutations and mechanisms underlying p53 inactivation are complex, posing challenges in restoring or reversing normal p53 activity in breast cancer cells. Novel therapeutic strategies are needed to effectively alter p53 function.	[70–72]
Identification of Mutp53 protein structure	Difficulty in identifying the structure of mutp53 protein presents challenges in developing effective p53-based therapeutics.	[71, 73, 74]
Challenges in developing combination therapies	Combination regimens of MDM2 inhibitors with other treatments and nanomedicine-based therapy show potential for anticancer therapy, but identifying the mutp53 protein structure and using multiple medicines targeting mutp53 present difficulties.	[68, 75]
Difficulty in targeted therapy for specific breast cancer subtypes	Targeted therapy is challenging in some breast cancer subtypes, such as TNBC, due to the lack of hormone receptors.	[65, 66, 76]
Obstacles in analyzing and utilizing large datasets for target identification	Analyzing large quantities of proteomic and genomic data using machine learning algorithms to find possible targets for breast cancer treatments presents challenges.	[77–79]
Challenges in translational research and clinical trials	Developing p53-targeted treatments for breast cancer requires overcoming various challenges encountered in translational research and clinical trials.	[73, 80]
Resistance of mutant p53 cells to certain treatments	Mutant p53 cells exhibit resistance to certain treatments, impacting the efficacy of p53-targeted therapies.	[68]

PI3K/Akt signaling system, which is frequently dysregulated in breast cancer, in a work published in the journal *Biomolecules* [61].

Amyloid aggregates are created when the p53 protein, which is changed in breast cancer, misfolds and accumulates. The misfolding dilemma makes it more difficult to target p53 in breast cancer therapy, which calls for the creation of stabilizing agents and analogs to solve the problem. A computer technique called molecular docking is used to forecast how tiny compounds will bind to a protein target. The p53 protein is prone to misfolding and accumulation in breast cancer cells; possible stabilizing drugs for this protein can be found using this technique. Researchers employed molecular docking in a study published in *Frontiers in Pharmacology* to find substances that might attach to the p53 protein and stop its misfolding and buildup [2]. Because p53 mutations and the mechanisms underlying p53 inactivation are so complex, restoring or reversing the normal activity of p53 in breast cancer cells is a substantial problem. To overcome this obstacle, novel therapeutic strategies that can efficiently alter p53 function in breast cancer are needed [23].

Large quantities of proteomic and genomic data can be analyzed using machine learning algorithms to find possible targets for breast cancer treatments. Researchers employed machine learning techniques to find synthetic lethal interactions with mutant p53 in breast cancer cells in a study published in the *Journal of Hematology & Oncology* (Table 20.2) [53]. One of the drawbacks of p53-based breast cancer treatments is that targeted therapy is challenging in some breast cancer subtypes, such as TNBC because these subtypes lack hormone receptors. It is also difficult to restore normal p53 function because the altered p53 protein in breast cancer is prone to misfolding and accumulation.

The development of effective p53-based therapeutics is hampered by the intricacy of p53 mutations and their implications on the survival and proliferation of cancer cells. Moreover, combination regimens of MDM2 inhibitors with other treatments and nanomedicine-based therapy may be potential approaches for anticancer therapy; however, the identification of the mutp53 protein structure and the usage of numerous medicines targeting mutp53 present difficulties [61, 81].

20.5 CONCLUSION

In conclusion, the tumor suppressor gene p53's complex role in breast cancer highlights the importance of this gene as a therapeutic target. A significant number of instances of breast cancer, especially those with hormone receptor-negative subtypes, have mutations in the TP53 gene, which codes for p53. These mutations may result in altered p53 expression or loss of function, which would accelerate the disease's course and worsen its prognosis. Translational research has shed light on several approaches, including genetic-based techniques and small-molecule pharmacologic inhibitors, to target p53 in breast cancer therapy. There are still obstacles in the way of effectively using p53 to treat breast cancer, despite encouraging advancements.

One major challenge is the multiplicity of breast cancer subtypes, which calls for creative solutions to deal with them. Furthermore, the tendency of the mutant p53 protein to misfold and aggregate makes therapeutic targeting more difficult, necessitating the creation of stabilizing agents. Interdisciplinary approaches in breast cancer research are crucial because machine learning algorithms and bioinformatics techniques provide useful tools for discovering possible targets and synthetic lethal interactions with mutant p53. Reaching these obstacles will be essential to maximizing the benefits of p53-targeted treatments and enhancing patient outcomes for breast cancer.

REFERENCES

1. Kaur, R.P., et al., Role of p53 gene in breast cancer: focus on mutation spectrum and therapeutic strategies. *Current Pharmaceutical Design*, 2018. **24**(30): p. 3566–3575.

2. Haq, B.U., et al., Targeting p53 misfolding conundrum by stabilizing agents and their analogs in breast cancer therapy: a comprehensive computational analysis. *Frontiers in Pharmacology*, 2024. **14**: p. 1333447.
3. Moftah Abuhagr, A., et al., Targeting P53 Gene in Breast Cancer. *Journal of Advanced Zoology*, 2023.
4. Gasco, M., S. Shami, and T. Crook, The p53 pathway in breast cancer. *Breast Cancer Research*, 2002. **4**(2): p. 70.
5. Abdullaevna, K.D., The role of P53 and BCL-2 GENE expression in breast cancer therapy. *Frontline Medical Sciences and Pharmaceutical Journal*, 2023. https://doi.org/10.37547/medical-fmspj-03-01-01
6. Jan, N., et al., Metronomic chemotherapy and drug repurposing: a paradigm shift in oncology. *Heliyon*, 2024. https://doi.org/10.1016/j.heliyon.2024.e24670
7. Mir, M.A., et al., *Proteomics: A Groundbreaking Development in Cancer Biology, in Proteomics*. 2023, Elsevier. p. 31–53.
8. Starzer, A., A. Berghoff, and R. Bartsch, Biomarkers and translational research approaches in breast cancer—an update. *memo - Magazine of European Medical Oncology*, 2022. **16**. https://doi.org/10.1007/s12254-022-00855-0
9. Bernier, J., Translational breast cancer research: Recent advances through the lens of experimental radiotherapy. *The Breast*, 2010. **19**(1): p. 23–27.
10. Mir, M.A., M. Rashid, and N. Jan, *Cytokines and Chemokines in Tumor Growth and Progression, in Cytokine and Chemokine Networks in Cancer.* 2023, Springer. p. 33–77.
11. Nagayama, A., N. Vidula, and A. Bardia, Novel therapies for metastatic triple-negative breast cancer: spotlight on immunotherapy and antibody-drug conjugates. *Oncology (08909091)*, 2021. **35**(5). https://doi.org/10.46883/onc.2021.3505.0249
12. Sofi, S., et al., A comprehensive analysis of notch signaling genes in breast cancer: expression pattern and prognostic significance. *Advances in Cancer Biology-Metastasis*, 2023. **7**: p. 100104.
13. Jan, N., et al., Exploring the role of trifarotene against RAR-α: an investigation of expression pattern and clinicopathological significance of RAR-α in breast cancer. *Frontiers in Pharmacology*, 2024. **15**: p. 1361679.
14. Toi, M., Y. Takebayashi, and L.W. Chow, Translational research in breast cancer. *Breast Cancer*, 2005. **12**(2): p. 86–90.
15. Toi, M., Y. Takebayashi, and L. Chow, Translational research in breast cancer. *Breast cancer (Tokyo, Japan)*, 2005. **12**: p. 86–90.
16. Yang, Z., et al., Restoration of p53 activity via intracellular protein delivery sensitizes triple negative breast cancer to anti-PD-1 immunotherapy. *Journal of Immunotherapy Cancer*, 2022. **10**(9). https://doi.org/10.1136/jitc-2022-005068
17. Sofi, S., et al., Elucidation of interleukin-19 as a therapeutic target for breast cancer by computational analysis and experimental validation. *Saudi Journal of Biological Sciences*, 2023. **30**(9): p. 103774–103774.
18. Steffens Reinhardt, L., et al., p53 Dysregulation in Breast Cancer: Insights on Mutations in the TP53 Network and p53 Isoform Expression. *International Journal of Molecular Sciences*, 2023. **24**(12): p. 10078.
19. Jan, N., et al., Targeting breast cancer stem cells through retinoids: a new hope for treatment. *Critical Reviews in Oncology/Hematology*, 2023: p. 104156.
20. Mir, M.A., Sumaya, N. Jan, Implications of Chemokine Heterogenicity in Cancer Metastasis, in *Cytokine and Chemokine Networks in Cancer.* 2023, Springer. p. 115–136.
21. Powell, E., D. Piwnica-Worms, and H. Piwnica-Worms, Contribution of p53 to metastasis. *Cancer Discovery*, 2014. **4**(4): p. 405–414.
22. Mir, M.A., M. Rashid, and N. Jan, The Interleukin-8 Pathway in Cancer, in *Cytokine and Chemokine Networks in Cancer.* 2023, Springer. p. 165–190.
23. Marvalim, C., A. Datta, and S.C. Lee, Role of p53 in breast cancer progression: An insight into p53 targeted therapy. *Theranostics*, 2023. **13**(4): p. 1421–1442.
24. Mir, M.A., M. Bashir, and N. Jan, The Role of Interleukin (IL)-6/IL-6 Receptor Axis in Cancer, in *Cytokine and Chemokine Networks in Cancer.* 2023, Springer. p. 137–164.
25. Li, X., et al., Regulation of P53 signaling in breast cancer by the E3 ubiquitin ligase RNF187. *Cell Death & Disease*, 2022. **13**(2): p. 149.
26. Sullivan, K.D., et al., Mechanisms of transcriptional regulation by p53. *Cell Death & Differentiation*, 2018. **25**(1): p. 133–143.
27. Shirley, S.H., et al., Transcriptional regulation of estrogen receptor-alpha by p53 in human breast cancer cells. *Cancer Res*, 2009. **69**(8): p. 3405–3414.

28. Li, X., et al., Regulation of P53 signaling in breast cancer by the E3 ubiquitin ligase RNF187. *Cell Death & Disease - Nature*, 2022. **13**(2): p. 149.
29. Mir, M.A., N. Jan, and I. Noor, Therapeutic Implications of Cytokines and Chemokines Network in Cancer, in *Cytokine and Chemokine Networks in Cancer.* 2023, Springer. p. 385–414.
30. Scata, K.A. and W.S. El-Deiry, *BRCA1 Regulation of p53 Stability and Target Expression in Cancer Research*, 2006. American Association for Cancer Research.
31. Zhang, H., et al., BRCA1 physically associates with p53 and stimulates its transcriptional activity. *Oncogene*, 1998. **16**(13): p. 1713–1721.
32. Mir, M.A., N. Jan, and S. Sofi, Introduction to Metronomic Chemotherapy, in *Novel Approaches in Metronomic Chemotherapy for Breast Cancer Treatment.* 2024, CRC Press. p. 1–14.
33. StasinopoulosI.A., et al., HOXA5-twist interaction alters p53 homeostasis in breast cancer cells. *Journal of Biological Chemistry*, 2005. **280**(3): p. 2294–2299.
34. Raman, V., et al., Compromised HOXA5 function can limit p53 expression in human breast tumours. *Nature*, 2000. **405**(6789): p. 974–978.
35. Yerlikaya, A., E. Okur, and E. Ulukaya, The p53-independent induction of apoptosis in breast cancer cells in response to proteasome inhibitor bortezomib. *Tumor Biology*, 2012. **33**(5): p. 1385–1392.
36. Alwahsh, M., et al., Bortezomib advanced mechanisms of action in multiple myeloma, solid and liquid tumors along with its novel therapeutic applications. *EXCLI Journal*, 2023. **22**: p. 146–168.
37. Kim, A.L., et al., Conformational and molecular basis for induction of apoptosis by a p53 C-terminal peptide in human cancer cells. *Journal of Biological Chemistry*, 1999. **274**(49): p. 34924–34931.
38. Guo, X., et al., The influence of a modified p53 C-terminal peptide by using a tumor-targeting sequence on cellular apoptosis and tumor treatment. *Apoptosis*, 2023. https://doi.org/10.1007/s10495-023-01926-1
39. Delcuve, G.P., D.H. Khan, and J.R. Davie, Roles of histone deacetylases in epigenetic regulation: emerging paradigms from studies with inhibitors. *Clinical Epigenetics*, 2012. **4**(1): p. 5.
40. Brancolini, C., T. Gagliano, and M. Minisini, HDACs and the epigenetic plasticity of cancer cells: Target the complexity. *Pharmacology & Therapeutics*, 2022. **238**: p. 108190.
41. Vrba, L., et al., p53 induces distinct epigenetic states at its direct target promoters. *BMC Genomics*, 2008. **9**(1): p. 486.
42. Mrakovcic, M., et al., Epigenetic targeting of autophagy via HDAC inhibition in tumor cells: role of p53. *International Journal of Molecular Sciences*, 2018. **19**(12). https://doi.org/10.3390/ijms19123952
43. Saldaña-Meyer, R. and F. Recillas-Targa, Transcriptional and epigenetic regulation of the p53 tumor suppressor gene. *Epigenetics*, 2011. **6**(9): p. 1068–1077.
44. Raman, V., et al., Compromised HOXA5 function can limit p53 expression in human breast tumours. *Nature*, 2000. **405**(6789): p. 974–978.
45. Gendronneau, G., et al., Influence of Hoxa5 on p53 tumorigenic outcome in mice. *Am J Pathol*, 2010. **176**(2): p. 995–1005.
46. Mir, M.A., et al., Metronomics: toward personalized chemotherapy. *Novel Approaches in Metronomic Chemotherapy for Breast Cancer Treatment*, 2024. p. 99–119. https://doi.org/10.1201/9781032632674-8
47. Mir, M.A., A. Manzoor, and N. Jan, *CCL5/CCR5 Axis in Cancer, in Cytokine and Chemokine Networks in Cancer.* 2023, Springer. p. 219–240.
48. Sofi, S., et al., Clinicopathological and prognostic significance of Bcl2 in breast cancer: a comprehensive in silico and in vitro study. *Saudi Journal of Biological Sciences*, 2023. **31**(2): p. 103916.
49. Yasuko, K., K. Mayumi, and M. Satoru, DNA Repair Molecules and Cancer Therapeutical Responses, in *Oncogene and Cancer*, S. Yahwardiah, Editor. 2013, IntechOpen. Ch. 5.
50. D'Anello, L., et al., Epigenetic control of the basal-like gene expression profile via Interleukin-6 in breast cancer cells. *Molecular Cancer*, 2010. **9**(1): p. 300.
51. Li, G., Y. Tian, and W.-G. Zhu, The roles of histone deacetylases and their inhibitors in cancer therapy. *Frontiers in cell and developmental biology*, 2020. **8**: p. 576946.
52. Berke, T.P., S.H. Slight, and S.M. Hyder, Role of reactivating mutant p53 protein in suppressing growth and metastasis of triple-negative breast cancer. *OncoTargets and Therapy*, 2022: p. 23–30.
53. Hu, J., et al., Targeting mutant p53 for cancer therapy: direct and indirect strategies. *Journal of Hematology & Oncology*, 2021. **14**(1): p. 157.
54. Duffy, M.J., et al., Targeting p53 for the treatment of cancer. *Seminars in Cancer Biology*, 2022. **79**: p. 58–67.
55. Wang, H., et al., Targeting p53 pathways: mechanisms, structures, and advances in therapy. *Signal Transduction and Targeted Therapy*, 2023. **8**(1): p. 92.
56. Marei, H.E., et al., p53 signaling in cancer progression and therapy. *Cancer Cell International*, 2021. **21**(1): p. 703.

57. Hassin, O. and M. Oren, Drugging p53 in cancer: one protein, many targets. *Nature Reviews Drug Discovery*, 2023. **22**(2): p. 127–144.
58. Jiang, F., C. G. Li, and S. W. Seto, Editorial: Drugging p53 for non-cancer diseases. *Frontiers in Pharmacology*, 2022. **13**. https://doi.org/10.3389/fphar.2022.1101742
59. Duffy, M.J., N.C. Synnott, and J. Crown, Mutant p53 in breast cancer: potential as a therapeutic target and biomarker. *Breast Cancer Research and Treatment*, 2018. **170**(2): p. 213–219.
60. Chapdelaine, A.G. and G. Sun, Challenges and opportunities in developing targeted therapies for triple negative breast cancer. *Biomolecules*, 2023. **13**(8): p. 1207.
61. Wallis, B., et al., The challenges and prospects of p53-based therapies in ovarian cancer. *Biomolecules*, 2023. **13**(1). https://doi.org/10.3390/biom13010159
62. Sulaiman, A., et al., CSCs in breast cancer—one size does not fit all: Therapeutic advances in targeting heterogeneous epithelial and mesenchymal CSCs. *Cancers*, 2019. **11**(8): p. 1128.
63. Jacquemin, V., et al., Dynamic cancer cell heterogeneity: diagnostic and therapeutic implications. *Cancers*, 2022. **14**(2): p. 280.
64. Khan, M.M., et al., Recent strategies to overcome breast cancer resistance. *Critical Reviews in Oncology/Hematology*, 2024: p. 104351.
65. Gupta, G.K., et al., Perspectives on triple-negative breast cancer: current treatment strategies, unmet needs, and potential targets for future therapies. *Cancers*, 2020. **12**(9): p. 2392.
66. Obidiro, O., G. Battogtokh, and E.O. Akala, Triple negative breast cancer treatment options and limitations: future outlook. *Pharmaceutics*, 2023. **15**(7): p. 1796.
67. Webb, M.J. and C. Kukard, A review of natural therapies potentially relevant in triple negative breast cancer aimed at targeting cancer cell vulnerabilities. *Integrative Cancer Therapies*, 2020. **19**: p. 1534735420975861.
68. Hu, J., et al., Targeting mutant p53 for cancer therapy: direct and indirect strategies. *Journal of Hematology & Oncology*, 2021. **14**(1): p. 157.
69. Duffy, M.J., et al. *Targeting p53 for the Treatment of Cancer in Seminars in Cancer Biology*. 2022. Elsevier.
70. Kwok, M., et al., Targeting the p53 pathway in CLL: State of the art and future perspectives. *Cancers*, 2021. **13**(18): p. 4681.
71. Gomes, A.S., et al., Structural and drug targeting insights on mutant p53. *Cancers*, 2021. **13**(13): p. 3344.
72. Rahman, M.A., et al., p53 modulation of autophagy signaling in cancer therapies: perspectives mechanism and therapeutic targets. *Frontiers in Cell and Developmental Biology*, 2022. **10**: p. 761080.
73. Hassin, O. and M. Oren, Drugging p53 in cancer: one protein, many targets. *Nature Reviews Drug Discovery*, 2023. **22**(2): p. 127–144.
74. Foroutan, B., A Narrative Review of the TP53 and Its Product the p53 Protein. *OBM Genetics*, 2023. **7**(3): p. 1–71.
75. Bansal, M.P., *Perspectives in ROS/Redox Regulation Cancer Therapy in Redox Regulation and Therapeutic Approaches in Cancer*. 2023, Springer. p. 411–431.
76. Yang, R., et al., Therapeutic progress and challenges for triple negative breast cancer: Targeted therapy and immunotherapy. *Molecular Biomedicine*, 2022. **3**(1): p. 8.
77. Shaikh, N., et al., A review on computational analysis of big data in breast cancer for predicting potential biomarkers. *Current Topics in Medicinal Chemistry*, 2022. **22**(21): p. 1793–1810.
78. Kaur, P., A. Singh, and I. Chana, Computational techniques and tools for omics data analysis: state-of-the-art, challenges, and future directions. *Archives of Computational Methods in Engineering*, 2021. **28**(7): p. 4595–4631.
79. Wen, B., et al., Deep learning in proteomics. *Proteomics*, 2020. **20**(21–22): p. 1900335.
80. Lu, Y., et al., The development of p53-targeted therapies for human cancers. *Cancers*, 2023. **15**(14): p. 3560.
81. Szewczyk-Roszczenko, O. and N.A. Barlev, The role of p53 in nanoparticle-based therapy for cancer. *Cells*, 2023. **12**(24): p. 2803.

Index